A Practical Guide to Contemporary Pharmacy Practice
Second Edition

A PRACTICAL GUIDE TO CONTEMPORARY PHARMACY PRACTICE

SECOND EDITION

Judith E. Thompson, R.Ph., M.S.

Clinical Associate Professor
School of Pharmacy
University of Wisconsin-Madison
Madison, Wisconsin

With CD/audiovisuals by

Lawrence W. Davidow, Ph.D., R.Ph.

Director, Integrated Laboratories
Department of Pharmacy Practice
The University of Kansas
Lawrence, Kansas

LIPPINCOTT WILLIAMS & WILKINS
A **Wolters Kluwer** Company
Philadelphia · Baltimore · New York · London
Buenos Aires · Hong Kong · Sydney · Tokyo

Editor: David Troy
Managing Editor: Matt Hauber
Marketing Manager: Chris Kushner
Production Editor: Christina Remsberg
Compositor: Maryland Composition
Printer: Quebecor World—Dubuque

Printed in the United States of America

First Edition, 1998

Library of Congress Cataloging-in-Publication Data

Thompson, Judith E.
 A practical guide to contemporary pharmacy practice / Judith E. Thompson; with
CD/audiovisuals by Lawrence W. Davidow.—2nd ed.
  p. ; cm.
 Includes bibliographical references and index.
 ISBN 0-7817-4177-7
  1. Pharmacy—Outlines, syllabi, etc. 2. Pharmacy—Handbooks, manuals, etc. I.
Davidow, Lawrence W. II. Title.
 [DNLM: 1. Drug Compounding—Handbooks. 2. Pharmaceutical
Preparations—administration & dosage—Handbooks. 3. Pharmacy—methods—Handbooks.
QV 735 T473p 2004]
RS98.T47 2004
615'.1—dc21

                                                      2003054532

The publishers have made every effort to trace the copyright holders for borrowed material. If they have inadvertently overlooked any, they will be pleased to make the necessary arrangements at the first opportunity.

To purchase additional copies of this book, call our customer service department at **(800) 638-3030** or fax orders to **(301) 824-7390**. International customers should call **(301) 714-2324**.

Visit Lippincott Williams & Wilkins on the Internet: http://www.LWW.com. Lippincott Williams & Wilkins customer service representatives are available from 8:30 am to 6:00 pm, EST.

                                        03 04 05 06 07
                                        1 2 3 4 5 6 7 8 9 10

To Wayne, with deep appreciation for the love, support, encouragement, and patience.

PREFACE

The aim of this second edition of *A Practical Guide to Contemporary Pharmacy Practice* remains the same as that for the original text: to provide a functional handbook for practicing pharmacists and pharmacy students. This essential purpose has served as the focal point amidst an amazing array of changes that have occurred in the practice of pharmacy and health care in the last 5 years. Some of the changes are the result of the continuing evolution and publication of improved practice standards, which have become so important to modern pharmacy. Many changes have been made possible by progress in computer technology and the widespread access to information via the internet. Some advances in compounding practice have been the result of the general availability of new pharmaceutical ingredients and equipment. All of these are reflected in this second edition.

The most obvious change and improvement in this new text is the inclusion of a compact disk and text photographs, which have enabled us to illustrate, both verbally and visually, compounding equipment, techniques, calculations, and even patient consultations. I am deeply indebted to Dr. Larry Davidow for his collaboration in providing both the CD and the majority of the text photographs for this edition. Dr. Davidow paired his experience with teaching pharmacy students at the University of Kansas School of Pharmacy together with his extensive computer technology experience and savvy to create a CD companion for this text that really brings the printed material to life. To enable readers to closely integrate their reading of the text with the instructional materials on the CD, a special CD icon ▦ has been placed alongside in-text discussions that have corresponding material on the CD.

As I researched information to update the printed text, I was truly astounded by the rich resources that are now available to anyone who has access to the internet. I was also surprised at the rapid pace with which documents and practice guidelines are now revised and updated. As a result, for documents available on the internet, I included internet site addresses rather than print versions of the presently current documents. In doing this, I realize that the addresses will continue to change (most of those listed in the text were accessed in fall of 2002), but if an address is no longer active, the URL will give the reader a starting point for an organization or government agency that may provide the newest and most up-to-date information. Prime examples of this are the ASHP technical assistance bulletins and practice guidelines; ASHP updates these regularly and has generously made them available on their internet site for anyone to access and use. As a result, printed copies are no longer available in the appendix section of this text. I want to express my appreciation to ASHP, NABP, and USP for generously allowing the reproduction of definitions, drug and chemical specifications, practice guidelines, and model rules and practice acts that are included or referenced in this text or the companion CD.

I have continued to include with this book as many useful hints and practical facts and figures as possible. The companion CD has greatly expanded our ability to include some lengthy reference items, such as pK_a tables and NABP model acts, without having to include them in the printed text (as I observe my students with their heavy loads of books, I am sure that they appreciate this feature).

As was true with the first edition, the material for this book is organized in outline form, since this seems to offer the fastest and easiest format for finding information. This recognizes that pharmacists and pharmacy students are busy professionals who need to read and access information as expeditiously as possible. You will notice that the chapters on calculations show several different methods for solving a given problem, since I recognize that pharmacists and students have different styles of problem solving. I have also attempted to show the practical application of these calculations in the sample prescriptions and have referred the reader to these additional examples whenever this would seem helpful. As an added feature, many calculations are also presented and explained on the CD.

A major emphasis of this book is on modern techniques and materials for compounding; the reference sections on pharmaceutical ingredients have been greatly expanded to include more helpful information on the properties, uses, and methods of preparation for these materials. The sample prescriptions all have added sections on compatibility, stability, and beyond-use date considerations with examples of useful resources and references for determining this information. Each sample prescription also contains a brief section on quality control considerations for that product. These sections should serve as useful guides for students and pharmacists who compound extemporaneously. Sample standard operating procedures are illustrated for the most commonly encountered procedures, but these are not a main focus of this text since these are currently available from other sources.

I wish to thank the following chapter contributors, who revised two of the chapters for this edition:

Chapter 33
Gordon S. Sacks, Pharm.D., BCNSP
Clinical Associate Professor
University of Wisconsin—Madison

Chapter 5
Kathleen A. Skibinski, RPh, MS
Clinical Assistant Professor
School of Pharmacy
University of Wisconsin—Madison

I also wish to express my appreciation to my students and colleagues who have generously offered their time and invaluable advice and assistance with both editions of *A Practical Guide*. I wish to especially acknowledge:

My colleagues in the AACP Laboratory Instructors Special Interest Group and the USP Pharmacy Compounding Expert Committee for their continued support and for freely sharing their expertise.

University of Kansas Clinical Assistant Professor Lawrence Davidow, not only for the major contribution of the companion CD, but also for offering helpful advice and insight with the text material. Larry has been a truly wonderful collaborator.

Senior Managing Editor Matt Hauber of Lippincott, Williams and Wilkins for his constant guidance and support with this project.

Assistant Dean Mary Ann Kirkpatrick of Shenandoah University for her encouragement and suggestions and for supplying the written materials on the Hazard Communication Standard, which are contained in chapter 12.

University of Wisconsin Emeritus Professors Kenneth Connors and George Zografi continue as my pharmaceutical mentors and have generously given their time in editing some of the compounding sections of this book, offering advice and helpful suggestions both on content and format.

Robert Schwartz, a model pharmacist, teacher, and friend helped write many of the original sample prescriptions and patient consultations.

Several of my former students researched and tested formulations described in this book and offered helpful suggestions; I wish to particularly acknowledge Michael Brown, Susan

Stein, John Dopp, Susan Kreul, Kimberly Buchfinck, Tony Bridgeman, Jenna Bakkum, Eileen Cobb, Tait Waege, Ronald Popp, Tom Heckenkamp, and Matthew Chambers.

Program Assistants Mary Capener, Audrey Fish, and Joni Mitchell used their creative talents and word processing skills in helping to formulate the tables and equations for this book.

My good friend and laboratory co-worker Bonnie Fingerhut continues to assist and encourage me in so many ways. She works with our students on a daily basis and provides me with the feedback needed to improve the content and experiences presented in *A Practical Guide*.

Dean Melvin Weinswig has, as always, been an enthusiastic supporter, offering encouragement and advice when I have needed it.

Finally, I wish to thank my families, both my academic family, students and faculty colleagues at the University of Wisconsin and elsewhere, and my nuclear family, my husband, children, grandchildren, siblings, and mother—they have encouraged and supported me and shown great patience with me as I have been writing and rewriting "the book."

Judith E. Thompson
Madison, Wisconsin

PREFACE TO COMPANION CD-ROM

We began using Judy Thompson's book, *A Practical Guide to Contemporary Pharmacy Practice*, in 1998 for teaching laboratory courses at the University of Kansas. We chose the textbook because it is well written and organized with many prescription examples. Over the years I have asked students their opinion of the *Practical Guide*. Collectively students have praised the textbook. Some students commented that they felt overwhelmed by the depth of subject matter and struggled with trying to visualize compounding procedures from only a written description. Because of limited class time, I needed some way outside of class to address these student needs. To accomplish this Robert Emerson, the lab coordinator, and myself began to develop a multimedia CD-ROM that would be used as a companion to the *Practical Guide*. The CD-ROM companion was developed to: 1) enhance reading comprehension by providing study guides for key chapters of the text, 2) encourage student self-assessment by quizzing on basic concepts, and 3) help students visualize compounding procedures using a narrated slide show. We chose a slide show format because it has a step-by-step feel and the high-resolution images taken at close range better illustrate the compounding process. In addition to developing these slide shows we also reviewed calculations, pharmacist documentation, product labeling, and included audio of a pharmacist's counseling a patient on the product.

Use of the CD-ROM in lab has been a positive experience. It allows us to make better use of class time because students are better prepared, ask intelligent clarifying questions before beginning procedures, and feel more confident about what they are doing.

Robert Emerson and I owe much thanks to Judy Thompson for her help in determining what should be included on the CD-ROM as well as her assistance in revising and reviewing the content. We are also thankful for the support of our families and colleagues while completing this project. Special thanks should be given to Mr. Harold Godwin and Dr. Jack Fincham for encouraging, granting us the time, and helping fund the necessary equipment and software. A debt of gratitude is owed to Ms. Trudy Bowen for her exceptional administrative assistance. Lastly, we thank all of our former students who supported and encouraged our efforts despite suffering through failed auto-starts, incompatible web browsers, and no sound. They have reminded us of the value of patience and perseverance.

Lawrence W. Davidow
Lawrence, Kansas

CONTENTS

CD-ROM CONTENTS

PART 1

PROCESSING THE PRESCRIPTION

CHAPTER 1

Prescription and Medication Orders

I. OUTPATIENT PRESCRIPTION DRUG ORDERS

A. Definitions
1. A "Prescription Drug Order" is defined in the National Association of Boards of Pharmacy (NABP) Model State Pharmacy Act as "a lawful order from a Practitioner for a Drug or Device for a specific patient, including orders derived from Collaborative Pharmacy Practice, that is communicated directly to a Pharmacist in a licensed Pharmacy" (1). The terms prescription drug order, prescription order, and prescription are used interchangeably by health care workers and the public and are most commonly used to describe drug orders for ambulatory patients (also referred to as "outpatients") who get their prescribed medications from retail or clinic pharmacies.
2. The term "medication order" is usually used when referring to drug orders for persons who are patients in hospitals, nursing homes, or other institutional settings. These patients are often referred to as "inpatients."
3. The NABP Model Act defines "Medical Order" as "a lawful order of a Practitioner that may or may not include a Prescription Drug Order" (2).
4. The term "Collaborative Pharmacy Practice Agreement" refers to a written and signed agreement between a pharmacist and licensed prescriber that allows the pharmacist to initiate or modify a patient's drug regimen within the guidelines of an agreed protocol for the purpose of drug therapy management (3,4). Collaborative Pharmacy Practice Agreements are often used by pharmacists to help physicians manage patients with specific disease states such as diabetes or asthma or intense drug therapy such as anticoagulation.

B. Prescribing authority
1. State statutes regulate which licensed health care providers may prescribe drug products for outpatients in that state.
2. Although medical and osteopathic doctors, podiatrists, dentists, and veterinarians have traditionally been the practitioners given this authority, some states now give prescribing authority to optometrists, nurse practitioners, physician assistants, psychologists, and/or pharmacists. In the later cases, certain restrictions may apply. For example, such practitioners may be required to possess advanced degrees or to pass special certification exams, or they may be restricted to prescribing only under the su-

pervision of a licensed physician, or under a limited, established protocol. It is the duty of the pharmacist to keep informed about state laws regulating current prescribing authority.

3. In all cases, practitioners are restricted to prescribing within the scope of their practice and for a legitimate medical purpose (5). For example, veterinarians can only prescribe for animals; dentists are limited to prescribing medications required by their dental patients for their dental problems, and so on.

C. Information required on prescription drug orders

1. In addition to regulating who may prescribe, state statutes also spell out what information is required on prescription drug orders and what must be kept in records of dispensing.

2. The information given in the next section concerning recommended legal requirements for prescription drug orders comes from the NABP "Model Rules for Pharmaceutical Care." NABP has written a Model State Pharmacy Act and model rules for various areas of practice. States are encouraged to use these in formulating individual state laws for the practice of pharmacy. (A copy of the 2001-2002 NABP "Model Rules for Pharmaceutical Care" and several other NABP model rules are available in the Appendices section of the CD that accompanies this book.) The *Model State Pharmacy Act and Model Rules of the National Association of Boards of Pharmacy* are revised and updated frequently; a current copy can be obtained from: National Association of Boards of Pharmacy, 700 Busse Highway, Park Ridge, IL 60068 (phone 708/698-6227); or through the NABP Internet site at www.nabp.org.

3. The NABP-recommended legal requirements for a prescription drug order are outlined below and are illustrated in Figures 1.1 and 1.2 (5). To learn the specific legal requirements for the state where you are practicing, consult the applicable state statutes. For the samples in Figures 1.1 and 1.2, the elements that are printed in simulated handwriting type denote those items which are normally entered on the prescription order by the prescriber. Those elements on the samples that are printed in italics are added by the pharmacist at the time of dispensing and are described in section D., Records of dispensing.

■ **Figure 1.1** Prescription order for a generic drug product.

Contemporary Physicians Group Practice
20 S. Park Street, Triturate, WI 53706
Tel: (608) 555-1333 Fax: (608) 555-1335

R # *123456*

Name *John Doe*   Date *00/00/00*

Address *123 N. Main Street*   Age   Wt/Ht

℞

Rugby Labs   *J. Thompson 00/00/00*
Amoxicillin Capsules 250 mg
 # 30
Sig: i cap tid for 10 days.

Refills *0*   *Linus Ashman*   M.D.

DEA No. _____

■ **Figure 1.2** Prescription order for a branded, controlled substance drug product.

```
┌─────────────────────────────────────────────────────────┐
│              Contemporary Physicians Group Practice        │
│              20 S. Park Street, Triturate, WI  53706       │
│              Tel: (608) 555-1333  Fax: (608) 555-1335     │
│                                    ℞    123457            │
├─────────────────────────────────────────────────────────┤
│ Name  Jane Doe                    Date   00/00/00         │
├─────────────────────────────────────────────────────────┤
│ Address  123 N. Main Street       Age         Wt/Ht       │
├─────────────────────────────────────────────────────────┤
│  ℞                        J. Thompson 00/00/00            │
│                                                           │
│     Tylenol w/Codeine  No. 3 Tablets    #30              │
│                                                           │
│     Sig:  i tab q 4-6 hr prn severe pain                 │
│                                                           │
│  Refills  1x                    Lysander Coupe      MD    │
│  Note: No red "C" – Record   DEA No.  AC 3936199          │
│  kept electronically                                      │
└─────────────────────────────────────────────────────────┘
```

a. Full name and address of the patient
b. Date of issue
c. Name and address of the prescriber
d. Name, strength, dosage form, and quantity of the drug product prescribed
e. Directions for use
f. Refills authorized, if any
Note: Accepted interpretation of refill, or lack of refill, information, may be specified in state law or state pharmacy licensing board rules. Common interpretations include:
(1) For drug products available only on prescription, the absence of refill information usually means zero refills are authorized.
(2) The number of allowed refills for controlled substances is specified in both state and federal law. Information on this topic can be found in Chapter 3, Controlled Substances.
(3) The designation "prn" refills for prescription medications that are not controlled substances is limited to authorizing refills for 1 year, or other specified time period, from the date of issue.
g. Prescriber's signature (written orders)
h. For controlled substances, the following additional requirements apply:
(1) DEA registration number of the prescriber
(2) The **prescriber's signature is required** on all prescription orders for **Schedule II** drugs; however, most states allow oral or electronic transmission, including voice telephoned prescription orders, for Schedule II medications in emergency situations, provided the quantity prescribed is limited to the amount needed for the emergency period and a written, signed document is received within a specified time period. In 1997 the federal law set this time period as 7 days, but because the most stringent law (i.e., federal or state) always applies, check your current state statutes for the standard at your practice site (6).

4. Often the prescriber neglects to include on the written order a required element, such as the patient address. The pharmacist must then ascertain this missing information from pharmacy records, or by asking the patient, the prescriber, or the agent of the patient or prescriber. The omission of some items of information by the prescriber, such as the date of issue on an order for a controlled substance, may render the order invalid.

5. Except for Schedule II prescription orders in non-emergency situations, telephone and verbal prescriptions orders are allowed. Because verbal orders may be misunderstood, they can be the source of medication errors. Eliminating miscommunications of this sort is one of the National Patient Safety Goals for 2003 as set by the Joint Commission on Accreditation of Healthcare Organizations (JCAHO). One of their recommendations is to require verification of the complete order by the person taking a verbal or telephone order (7). It is good practice to repeat back to the prescriber any verbal or telephone order and to clarify any part of a prescription order that may be confusing.

D. Records of dispensing

1. At the time of dispensing a prescription, the pharmacist must make a record of the dispensing.

2. The NABP model rules recommend that this information be kept by pharmacies for five years (8), and some other authorities suggest that it be kept for at least the time of state and federal statute of limitations. This time period varies with the type of offense alleged, but for felony offenses, it would be 5 or 6 years from the date when the crime was alleged to have occurred (9).

3. It is recommended that, because the prescription order is a legal document, information on it should be written in ink or indelible pencil or be typed. Although the ink requirement may actually be specified in the law only for legal requirements on prescription orders for controlled substances in Schedule II, use of ink is prudent practice for information recorded on all prescription orders.

4. The elements listed below and printed in italics on the samples are the items recommended or required for inclusion in the dispensing record (8). Some of these items are now kept by pharmacies in their computer system, and if recorded in this way, it is not required that they be entered directly on the hard copy of the prescription document.

   a. Quantity dispensed, original and all refills, if different from that prescribed

   b. Dispensing pharmacist's identification

   c. Date of dispensing

   d. Retrieval designation (e.g., serial number of the prescription order)

   e. Brand name or manufacturer of manufactured drug products prescribed generically

   Note: In Figure 1.1, the prescriber ordered amoxicillin. At the time of dispensing, the pharmacist specified the manufacturer of the brand dispensed, Rugby Labs in this example.

   f. Record of all refills

   g. For controlled substances, additional dispensing records are required to permit the identification and retrieval of prescription orders for controlled substances. These requirements are part of Title 2 of the federal Controlled Substances Act of 1970, which is described in more detail in Chapter 3, Controlled Substances. Below are given documentation methods commonly employed for identification and retrieval of prescription orders for controlled substances. To learn the specific legal requirements for the state where you are practicing, consult the applicable state statutes.

      (1) Schedule II prescriptions are filed separately.

      (2) A red "C" no less than 1 inch in height is applied to the lower right-hand corner of prescription orders in Schedules III–V unless these are filed separately in a three-file system (as described in Chapter 3, Controlled Substances). Since 1997, DEA regulations allow waiver of the red "C" requirement for

pharmacies that use electronic record-keeping systems which permit identification by prescription number and which allow retrieval of original documents by prescriber's name, patient's name, drug dispensed, and date filled (10). Check your current state statutes to determine if the state in which you practice has adopted this standard.

E. Recommended records for compounded prescription drug orders

1. The compounding record is intended to make it easier for the pharmacist who is preparing a refill of the prescribed drug preparation to make an identical preparation. It is also a quality control device and facilitates tracking if there are problems with a compounded preparation, and it enables the pharmacist to make appropriate alterations in the formulation based on feedback from the patient about the acceptability of the preparation.

2. The following informational items are recommended for inclusion on completed prescription drug orders or formula records and control logs for compounded drug preparations. When compounding is done infrequently, pharmacists often record this information on the front and back of the prescription order. A better method is to use a separate control and/or formula sheet, which is cross-referenced on the prescription document. Since some states may have specific record-keeping requirements for compounded prescriptions, consult the applicable state laws or regulations for the state in which you practice. The recommendations given here are a composite of information given in 1) NABP Good Compounding Practices Applicable to State Licensed Pharmacies (see CD accompanying this book), 2) ASHP Technical Assistance Bulletin on Compounding Nonsterile Products in Pharmacies (available on the ASHP Internet site, www.ashp.org, Accessed November 2002, and 3) USP/NF General Chapter ⟨795⟩, Pharmaceutical Compounding: Nonsterile Preparations. Multiple examples of prescription orders with compounding records that comply with these recommendations are given in later chapters of this book.

   a. Name and quantity of all ingredients, including both active ingredients and compounding aids (vehicles, solvents, levigating agents, flavors, colors, buffers, preservatives)

   b. Source of all ingredients: manufacturer or distributor, lot number and expiration date of each ingredient; brand name or manufacturer and strength or concentration of manufactured drug products used as ingredients; capsule size and color for capsules

   c. Calculations, quantities of ingredients weighed or measured for intermediate steps when making aliquots or dilutions

   d. Amount of preparation made, including number of extra doses made to allow for loss on compounding

   e. Order of mixing, compounding procedures, and equipment used

   f. Accurate account of the amount of a controlled drug weighed, dispensed, and discarded when preparing excess dosage units and/or aliquots

   g. Quality control methods used to ensure the identity, strength, quality, and purity of the preparation

   h. Containers used, and storage and beyond-use date recommendations

   i. Name(s) of person or persons who prepared and who are responsible for the preparation. In some cases a pharmacy technician compounds the preparation under the supervision of a pharmacist. Both individuals should be identified on the record.

II. INPATIENT MEDICATION ORDERS

A. Inpatient medication orders are used to order medications for persons who are patients in hospitals, nursing homes, or other institutional settings. Sample orders are given in Figure 1.3.

MEDICAL CENTER HOSPITAL
Triturate, Wisconsin 53706

PATIENT ORDERS

Patient Name: David John
History Number: 120579   Room Number: 430
Weight: 125 lb   Height: 5'9"
Age: 62 y.o.
Attending Physician: R. Farrell

Date	Time	Orders
00/00/00	1300	10,000 units Heparin Sodium in 250 mL NS.
		Infuse IV over 4 hr. R. Farrell, MD
		J. Thompson, 00/00/00
00/0/00	1600	Penicillin G K IM Inj. Give 200,000 units stat
		then 100,000 units q 4 hr. R. Farrell, MD
		J. Thompson, 00/00/00
00/00/00	1400	Morphine sulfate 10 mg and Atropine sulfate
		0.4 mg Injection Give IM
		On call for surgery at 0800 on 00/00/00.
		R. Farrell, MD
		J. Thompson, 00/00/00

■ **Figure 1.3** Inpatient medication orders.

B. Although there are no legal requirements for information to be included on medication orders for inpatients, there are recommendations for good practice. Some institutions have written requirements in their policy and procedure manuals.

C. Items commonly included on completed inpatient medication orders are:
1. Patient identification
   a. Name
   b. History number (this is a patient-specific number used to verify the identity of a patient)
2. Patient location (that is, room/bed number)
3. Date and time of order
4. Name, quantity, and dosage form of medications ordered

5. Route of administration
6. Dosage schedule
7. Prescriber identification (that is, signature of prescriber or, for verbal or telephone orders, the prescriber's name and the name or initials of the nurse or pharmacist taking the order)
8. Name or initials of person(s) who transcribed the order (often this includes both a nurse and a pharmacist)
9. Date of transcription

III. MEDICAL ABBREVIATIONS AND SYMBOLS

A. As can be seen in Figures 1.1 through 1.3, many abbreviations and symbols are used in writing prescription and medication orders. The use of this sort of shorthand, while perhaps time-saving for the writer, has been criticized because of the possibility of confusion or misinterpretation.

B. Appendix A gives a brief list of some commonly used abbreviations. (For a more complete list, access that section on the CD that accompanies this book, or consult one of the published books of medical abbreviations, such as *Medical Abbreviations: 15,000 Conveniences at the Expense of Communications and Safety* by Dr. Neil M. Davis.)

C. Because of the confusion caused by abbreviations, the JCAHO requires hospitals to formulate and publish a list of abbreviations that are approved for use in that institution, as well as abbreviations, acronyms, and symbols not to use (7).

D. Some abbreviations or notations have become notorious because they are commonly misinterpreted or because their misinterpretation may have serious consequences. They should be avoided.

1. The symbol *u* for unit, when hand-written, can be read as an *0*, with a possible resulting ten-fold overdose. Always write out the word *unit*.
2. *Mcg* is the acceptable abbreviation for microgram because μg can easily be read as *mg*.
3. When writing whole numbers for medication strengths or dosages, never add a decimal point with a trailing zero: that is, write 25 mg, not 25.0 mg. If the decimal point is not seen, 250 mg may be read rather than the desired 25 mg.
4. When writing a decimal fraction for a number less than one, always precede the decimal point with a zero: that is, write 0.25 mg, not .25 mg. In this case, if the decimal point is not seen, 25 mg would be administered rather than the desired 0.25 mg.
5. The abbreviation *q.o.d.*, used to indicate *every other day*, has been read both as *q.d.* for *daily* or *q.i.d.* for *four times daily*. To avoid confusion, write out *every other day*.
6. The period after the *q* in the abbreviation *q.d.*, meaning every day, can be mistaken for an *i*, causing the medication to be given four times a day.
7. The abbreviations *SC* and *SQ*, with the intended meaning of subcutaneous, could be misinterpreted as *SL*, meaning sublingual or sublingually.
8. The abbreviation *T.I.W.*, meaning *three times a week*, has been misread as *three times a day* or misinterpreted as *two times a week*.
9. When the same abbreviations have more than one meaning, misinterpretation may result. Common examples include *D/C*, which can mean either *discontinue* or *discharge; HS*, which can mean either *at bedtime* or *half-strength;* and *IVP*, which can mean *IV push* or *intravenous pyelogram*.
10. The Latin abbreviations *au, as,* and *ad,* which mean, respectively, *both ears, left ear,* and *right ear,* have been misread or misinterpreted as *ou, os,* or *od,* meaning *both eyes, left eye,* and *right eye.* Obviously, the opposite misinterpretation may also occur.
11. When writing or typing the names, strengths, and units of drugs, do not omit the spaces between the words, unit abbreviations, or set of numbers. For example, write

Propranolol 40 mg, not Propranolol 40mg or Propranolol40mg.

12. Avoid the symbols "/" and "&." The "/" symbol can be taken for a number 1, and the "&" symbol, when handwritten, can look like the number 4 (11,12).

IV. RECOMMENDED PRESCRIPTION WRITING PRACTICES TO PREVENT MEDICATION ERRORS

A. The National Coordinating Council for Medication Error Reporting and Prevention (NCC MERP) is a public/private group of national organizations formed in 1995 with the purpose of reducing medication errors in health care delivery (13,14). In July 1996 the Council met and identified a set of recommendations that, if followed, could reduce the potential for medication errors in prescription and medication orders. Their recommendations were reported in the Sept./Oct. 1996 edition of *The Standard, News from the United States Pharmacopeia.*

B. The Council recommendations, which are summarized below, are intended to foster safer prescription writing, which would be a first step in ensuring the five basic rights of patients in receiving drug therapy: the right drug in the right dose by the right route of administration to the right patient at the right time (12).

1. **All written prescription or medication orders must be legible.** In reviewed reports of the USP Medication Errors Reporting Program, the Council found that illegible handwriting on prescription and medication orders is the most widely recognized cause of medication error. Because of the inherent difficulty in reading individual handwriting, the Council encourages progress toward direct, computerized, medication order entry systems for prescribers.

2. **Prescribers should avoid the use of abbreviations,** both for drug names and Latin directions for use. The abbreviations the Council found to be particularly dangerous are included in the list of dangerous abbreviations given previously.

3. **All prescriptions and medications orders should be written using the metric system.** Excepted are those therapies that use standard units, such as insulin and some vitamins and antibiotics. The apothecary and avoirdupois systems were singled out as archaic systems whose symbols may easily be misinterpreted. Furthermore, these older systems often require conversions and calculations that provide an additional and unnecessary potential for error.

4. **Prescribers should provide the age and, when appropriate, weight of the patient on the prescription order.** This information, especially for pediatric and geriatric patients, can aid the pharmacist, nurse, or other health care provider in double-checking appropriateness of drug and dose.

5. **The prescription or medication order should include the drug name, metric weight or concentration, and dosage form.** The pharmacist should check with the prescriber if any information is missing or questionable.

6. **A leading zero should always precede a decimal point in quantities less than one, and a trailing zero should never be used after a decimal point.**

7. **Prescription and medication orders should include, when possible, a notation of purpose of the medication.** This gives the provider of the medication a useful double-check for the appropriateness of the drug and dose. The Council recognized that there may be instances in which confidentiality issues warrant the omission of this information. However, if this information is not written on the order, the pharmacist should always discreetly ask the patient about the intended use of the medication. This is an important double-check safeguard.

8. **Prescribers should not use imprecise instructions such as "Take as directed" or "Take as needed."** Even if the patient has been given more exact verbal instructions, these may be forgotten or misinterpreted. When written orders are vague, the pharmacist should check with the prescriber (12).

C. To track, monitor, and analyze the incidence of medication errors from a systems viewpoint, health care professionals are encouraged to report medication errors or potential errors to one of the organizations that are collaborating to develop and maintain a national database on medication errors. There are several ways that the reporting can be done easily.

   1. The USP operates three medication error reporting programs: the Medication Errors Reporting (MER) Program, the Veterinary Practitioners' Reporting (VPR) Program, and MedMARx. Each program can be accessed on the Internet through the USP's web site at www.usp.org.

     a. The MER Program, operated in cooperation with the Institute for Safe Medication Practices (ISMP), is a spontaneous, voluntary reporting program that health care professionals can use to report medication errors to USP. This can be done directly online through USP's web site or by printing a report form from the web site and mailing or faxing the report to USP. Practitioners can also report by calling toll-free anytime 1-800-23-ERROR. Practitioners who report medication errors through this program are assured of confidentiality and may, if preferred, make their report anonymously. USP staff review these reports for any possible general patient safety concerns. Information from the reports is sent to FDA and to the manufacturers of the drug product involved. The information is then added to the MER database for analysis of error type and cause.

     b. With the VPR Program, USP works in cooperation with the American Veterinary Medical Association. This program collects data on veterinary product problems and adverse reactions in addition to medication errors or misadventures. As with the MER Program, reports can be filed online using USP's web site, or a printed report form may be faxed or mailed. Practitioners may also telephone USP at 1-800-4-USP-PRN.

     c. MedMARx is an Internet-accessible program that enables participating hospitals to anonymously report and track medication errors for the purpose of internal quality improvement. The information is also entered into USP's national database for analysis. Summary reports of information submitted through the MedMARx system have been available through USP's web site.

   2. Practitioners can use the web site of the Institute for Safe Medication Practices (www.ismp.org) to file a confidential report to ISMP, USP, or FDA (for adverse drug reactions). There is even an international option for participating countries. Reports may also be e-mailed to ismpinfo@ismp.org.

D. Drug products that have names that look and/or sound alike have been recognized as potential sources of medication errors.

   1. Although the FDA and pharmaceutical manufacturers make a concerted effort to avoid and eliminate this problem through the careful selection of both brand and generic names for drugs, problems still exist. In an effort to provide more visual differentiation of the established names of particularly problematic drug pairs with look-alike names, the FDA Office of Generic Drugs asked manufacturers of these drugs to use "Tall Man" letters on their labels. An example would be ChlorproMAZINE and ChlorproPAMIDE. Sixteen additional pairs can be seen at FDA's Name Differentiation Project web site at www.fda.gov/cder/drug/MedErrors.

   2. Confusion over medications with similar names, written or spoken, was reported to account for approximately 15% of all reports to the MER Program between Jan. 1, 1996, and Dec. 31, 2000 (15).

   3. Lists of drugs with similar names, look-alike/sound-alike drug pairs, are available. It is helpful for pharmacists and pharmacy technicians to be familiar with drug names that have caused confusion so that special caution is used when dealing with these medications.

     a. The USP regularly publishes in *USP Quality Review*, a current list of drug names that have caused confusion as reported to the MER Program. A copy of the most current list can be printed from the USP web site by accessing issues of *USP*

Quality Review, which are archived under the practitioner reporting section. USP has also made its list available in an Adobe Acrobat (pdf) version through its web site at www.usp.org/reporting/review.

b. Similar lists are published occasionally in various pharmacy journals or publications. The journal *Hospital Pharmacy* has published these lists in chart form, which can be posted in the pharmacy for easy reference (16).

c. The National Association of Chain Drug Stores maintains on its web site (www.nacds.org) a more modest list of look-alike/sound-alike drug pairs commonly encountered in ambulatory pharmacy practice.

4. Confusion with look-alike/sound-alike drug names has been found to be aggravated by the following factors (15):

a. Illegible handwriting on prescription or medication orders

b. Lack of information or incomplete knowledge of drug names or products, especially newly available products with which pharmacists, nurses, or technicians are not yet familiar

c. Similar packaging, labeling, or product strengths

d. Dispensing software systems that employ computerized drug product lists, which make incorrect selection of a product with a similar name more likely. This is exacerbated by the fact that most dispensing software systems use mnemonics, several-letter abbreviations for long drug names (e.g., CPZ for Chlorpromazine), which can easily be confused or used incorrectly for another drug name.

References

1. Model State Pharmacy Act and Model Rules of the National Association of Boards of Pharmacy. National Association of Boards of Pharmacy, Park Ridge, IL, 2001; 9.

2. Model State Pharmacy Act and Model Rules of the National Association of Boards of Pharmacy. National Association of Boards of Pharmacy, Park Ridge, IL, 2001; 7.

3. Model State Pharmacy Act and Model Rules of the National Association of Boards of Pharmacy. National Association of Boards of Pharmacy, Park Ridge, IL, 2001; 3.

4. Pharmacist Scope of Practice. American College of Physicians–American Society of Internal Medicine. Ann Intern Med. 2002; 136: 84.

5. Model State Pharmacy Act and Model Rules of the National Association of Boards of Pharmacy. National Association of Boards of Pharmacy, Park Ridge, IL, 2001; 75.

6. 21 CFR § 1306.11.

7. National Patient Safety Goals for 2003, JCAHO, Oakbrook Terrace, IL, July 24, 2002.

8. National Association of Boards of Pharmacy Model Rules for Pharmaceutical Care. National Association of Boards of Pharmacy, Park Ridge, IL, 2001; 88.

9. Fink JL, III, Vivian JC, Reid KK, eds. Pharmacy law digest, 36th ed. St. Louis: Facts and Comparisons, Inc., 2002; 36.

10. 21 CFR § 1304.04[h].

11. Cohen MR, Davis NM. Expressing strengths, doses, and drug names properly. Am Pharm 1992; NS32: 32–33.

12. The Standard. Rockville, MD: The United States Pharmacopeial Convention, Inc., Sept./Oct. 1996; 1, 4-5.

13. National council focuses on coordinating error reduction efforts. USP Quality Review. No. 57. Rockville, MD: The United States Pharmacopeial Convention, Inc., Jan.1997.

14. Dispensing strategies devised. USP Quality Review. No. 67. Rockville, MD: The United States Pharmacopeial Convention, Inc., June 1999.

15. USP Quality Review No. 76. Rockville, MD: The United States Pharmacopeial Convention, Inc., March 2001.

16. Baker DE. Sound-alike and look-alike drug errors. Hosp Pharm 2002; 37(3): 225.

CHAPTER 2

Labeling Prescriptions and Medications

I. LABELS FOR OUTPATIENT PRESCRIPTION DRUG ORDERS

A. Definitions

1. The terms "label" and "labeling" are defined differently for manufactured drug products and for products dispensed by the pharmacist to a patient on prescription order.

2. For manufactured drug products, the USP defines the terms "labeling" and "label" as follows: "The term 'labeling' designates all labels and other written, printed, or graphic matter upon an immediate container of an article or upon, or in, any package or wrapper in which it is enclosed, except any outer shipping container. The term 'label' designates that part of the labeling upon the immediate container" (1). Labels and labeling of manufactured drug products are strictly controlled by the FDA.

3. NABP Model Rules for Pharmaceutical Care defines the term "labeling" for the purposes of pharmacists dispensing drug products to patients as "the process of preparing and affixing a label to any Drug container exclusive, however, of the Labeling by a Manufacturer, packer, or Distributor of a Non-Prescription Drug or commercially packaged Legend Drug or Device" (2).

B. Labeling of outpatient prescriptions is regulated by federal law and state statutes.

1. Section 503(b)(2) of the Federal Food, Drug, and Cosmetic Act requires that drug products dispensed on prescription orders be labeled with "the name and the address of the dispenser, the serial number and the date of the prescription or of its filling, the name of the prescriber, and, if stated in the prescription, the name of the patient, and directions for use and cautionary statements, if any, contained in such prescription."

2. State laws often have additional labeling requirements. The pharmacist must label the drug product with those items specified in the federal law plus any additional state requirements.

C. Required and recommended elements on labels for outpatient prescriptions

1. As with prescription drug orders, the NABP Model Rules for Pharmaceutical Care (see CD that accompanies this book) contain recommendations for state statutes on required items of information for the prescription product label (3). These are listed below and are illustrated in the label examples shown in Figures 2.1 and 2.2. The labels correspond to the prescription orders given in Figures 1.1 and 1.2 of Chapter 1.

   a. Name and address of pharmacy that dispensed the drug

■ Figure 2.1   Prescription label for a generic drug product.

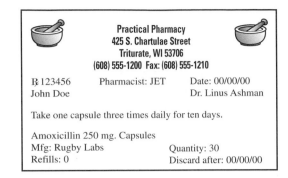

Practical Pharmacy
425 S. Chartulae Street
Triturate, WI 53706
(608) 555-1200 Fax: (608) 555-1210

℞ 123456   Pharmacist: JET   Date: 00/00/00
John Doe   Dr. Linus Ashman

Take one capsule three times daily for ten days.

Amoxicillin 250 mg. Capsules
Mfg: Rugby Labs   Quantity: 30
Refills: 0   Discard after: 00/00/00

   b. Name of patient; if the patient is an animal, label with the species of animal and the owner's name
   c. Name of prescriber
   d. Directions for use as stated on the prescription order
   e. Date dispensed
   f. Cautionary statements, if any
   g. Serial number of prescription
   h. Name or initial of the dispensing pharmacist
   i. Name (proprietary or generic) and strength of drug product dispensed; special requirements with regard to the name of the product may apply if an equivalent drug product is dispensed
   j. Name of the manufacturer or distributor of the product dispensed
   k. Beyond-use date of the product

Note: For controlled substances in Schedules II–IV, the following auxiliary label is required: "Caution: Federal law prohibits the transfer of this drug to any person other than the patient for whom it was prescribed."

  2. Some states have additional requirements for the label. Examples are given below. It is the duty of each pharmacist to be informed about the specific legal requirements for labeling for the state in which he or she is practicing.
   a. Quantity dispensed
   b. Number of refills

D. Computerized dispensing software, created for a national market, is now used extensively for generating prescription labels. Although most labeling software includes additional non-required information, it is important that pharmacists ensure that, at a minimum, all labeling elements required by their state law are included in the dispensing software package purchased for their practice.

■ Figure 2.2   Prescription label for a branded, controlled substance drug product.

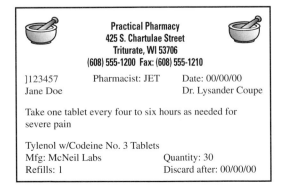

Practical Pharmacy
425 S. Chartulae Street
Triturate, WI 53706
(608) 555-1200 Fax: (608) 555-1210

]123457   Pharmacist: JET   Date: 00/00/00
Jane Doe   Dr. Lysander Coupe

Take one tablet every four to six hours as needed for severe pain

Tylenol w/Codeine No. 3 Tablets
Mfg: McNeil Labs   Quantity: 30
Refills: 1   Discard after: 00/00/00

Auxiliary Labels: May Cause Drowsiness; Alcohol and Operating Car or
Machine Warning; Federal "Do Not Transfer" label

E. Two of the labeling requirements merit additional discussion: 1) directions for use, and 2) name and strength of product/active ingredients.

1. Directions for Use

a. The directions for use should be written in clear, concise English using terminology that the general public (including patients with minimal education) can understand. Avoid abbreviations such as GI and SOB and medical terms that the patient may not understand. For patients who do not speak English, be certain that they understand how to use their medication. Some dispensing software programs have labeling in Spanish as an option. Remember that verbal instruction to the patient in techniques of administration is an excellent opportunity for the pharmacist to provide professional service to the patient. For difficult-to-use dosage forms, such as inhalers, written labels and product instructions are rarely sufficient: demonstrate the appropriate technique to the patient, and then have the patient show you how he or she will use it.

b. Directions for use should be in complete sentences including a verb: "Take one tablet three times daily" as opposed to "One tablet three times daily." Use easily understood verbs such as take, give, apply, insert, place, use, and put. Avoid outdated terms such as "instill" unless you are certain the patient understands. For topical administration, the adverbs "topically" or "locally" are sometimes used, but are optional.

c. The route of administration should be specified in most cases, including eye, ear, nose, rectum, vagina, and urethra. For medications given by mouth, the route is usually understood from the directions and is not required unless the prescriber has specifically written this in the directions for use, or if there is a possibility of confusion. Some states require the route of administration to be specified in all cases, including oral products. In some cases this additional requirement is mandated only for prescription products dispensed to patients in long-term care facilities.

d. Numbers, when part of the directions for use, should be spelled out whenever possible. This is a safety feature. Because the numbers are next to each other on the keyboard, it would be easy to type a 2 when a 3 is desired. A typing error made in spelling the number, such as "tjree" for three, would be detected easily, and the patient would not confuse the misspelling with another number.

e. Volume doses such as teaspoons should be written with the suffix "-ful" (e.g., teaspoonful). Teaspoonfuls is the preferred plural of teaspoonful, but according to "Webster's New Collegiate Dictionary," teaspoonsful is also acceptable. If the prescription is for a bulk powder, specify "level" (e.g., level teaspoonful).

f. While the directions for use should be as close as possible to those on the prescription order, the pharmacist may clarify the instructions as long as the intent of the prescriber is not changed.

g. Vague labeling instructions, such as "Take as directed" or "Take as needed," are not sufficient directions for use. They assume that the patient was given adequate additional oral instructions, and that he or she had a correct interpretation and understanding of these instructions. Furthermore, they rely on the memory of the patient, which is always risky. If vague instructions are indicated on the prescription order, the prescriber should be consulted for more specific instructions (4).

2. Name and quantity of active ingredients

a. If permitted by the applicable state law, prescriptions may be labeled either with the generic name or the brand name of the product dispensed, as long as the legal standard for trademarks is followed. Trademark law holds that a drug product may be labeled with a company's brand name only when that brand is the one dispensed. Some states require that drug products be labeled with both the brand and the generic name of the drug product; others specify that prescription products that are labeled generically must have the name of the manufacturer or distributor of the product. NABP Model Rules for Pharmaceutical Care recommend that when a equivalent drug product is dispensed, the word "Interchange" or the letters "IC" should be included with the generic name and manufacturer of the product (3).

    b. For branded combination products or official USP or NF formulations, the brand name or the official name of the product is sufficient because the ingredients are specified in the official or brand formula. If a generic version of a fixed combination is dispensed, NABP model rules allow the pharmacist to use professional judgment in labeling the active ingredients (3).

    c. For topical products, the concentration usually is expressed as a percent using the conventions for percentage measurement as set down in the General Notices of the USP and described in Chapter 7 of this book, Quantity and Concentration Expressions and Calculations. Topical antibiotics are sometimes labeled in units or milligrams of active ingredient per gram of solid or semisolid or per milliliter of liquid product. Some drug products that are used in very dilute concentrations have traditionally been labeled in ratio strength. This is acceptable.

    d. For individual dosage forms (e.g., capsules, divided powders, lozenges, suppositories), the strength is expressed as a metric weight of each active ingredient per dosage unit (1). The dosage system is understood and need not be identified. For example, when dispensing a bottle of capsules with each capsule containing 15 mg Codeine, the active ingredient may be labeled merely as Codeine 15 mg.

    e. For prescription labeling, when the salt form is identified, chemical symbols for the common inorganic salts are permitted: HCl for hydrochloride, HBr for hydrobromide, Na for sodium, and K for potassium. However, by USP convention, when Sodium or Potassium appears at the beginning of a drug name, as for example Sodium Nitroprusside, the word rather than the chemical symbol is used (1).

    f. For oral liquids and oral bulk powders, label either: 1) the quantity of active ingredient per standard volume (e.g., Amoxicillin 250 mg/5 mL or Digoxin 50 mcg/mL); or 2) the quantity of active ingredient(s) per dosage volume specified in the directions for use on the label. For example, with directions for use of "Take one tablespoonful one hour after each meal," the label may specify the quantity of active ingredient as, for example, Calcium Carbonate 20 mg/mL, Calcium Carbonate 100 mg/5 mL, or Calcium Carbonate 300 mg/tablespoonful.

    g. The content of electrolytes for replacement therapy should be stated in milliequivalents (mEq) of the electrolyte(s). The weight of the ingredient(s) providing the electrolyte should also be given (1). For example, Potassium Chloride packets or capsules could be labeled as Potassium Chloride 8 mEq (600 mg).

    h. It is recommended as a safety feature that labels for phosphorus supplements include the number of millimoles of phosphorus **and** the number of milliequivalents of potassium and/or sodium. For example, K-Phos Neutral® Tablets would be labeled K Phos Neutral (phosphorus 8 mmol, potassium 1.1 mEq, and sodium 13 mEq) (5).

    i. The content of alcohol in a liquid dosage form should be stated as a percentage v/v of C_2H_5OH (1).

II. LABELS FOR INPATIENT DRUG ORDERS

A. Although many states have no legal requirements for labeling inpatient drug products, the NABP Model Rules for Pharmaceutical Care do address this issue (3).

    1. The following are recommendations for drug products used by inpatients in health care facilities where the product is administered by a health care professional and therefore is not in the possession of the ultimate user until time of administration. The recommendations are divided into products available in single-unit packages and those in multiple-dose containers.

        a. The label for single-unit or unit-dose packages should include:

            (1) Name (proprietary or generic) of the drug product

            (2) Route of administration, unless oral

            (3) Strength and, if applicable, volume of the product, expressed when possible in the metric system

    (4) Control number and expiration date

    (5) If repackaged, identification of the repackager

    (6) Special storage conditions, if needed

  b. If a multiple-dose distribution system is used, the container should be labeled with:

    (1) Identification of the dispensing pharmacy

    (2) Patient's name

    (3) Date of dispensing

    (4) Name (proprietary or generic) of the drug product

    (5) Strength, expressed when possible in the metric system

2. If a drug product for an inpatient is to be self-administered, the label should conform to the standards of outpatient prescriptions.

3. Labeling standards for parenteral products are addressed both by the NABP Model Rules for Pharmaceutical Care (3) and by a technical assistance bulletin (TAB) published by the American Society of Health-System Pharmacists (6). (A copy of the 2001-2002 NABP Model Rules for Pharmaceutical Care is available on the CD that accompanies this book.) The ASHP TAB on Quality Assurance for Pharmacy-prepared Sterile Products is available on the ASHP Internet site, www.ashp.org, Accessed November 2002. The following list is a combination of the labeling recommendations from both documents. These recommendations are illustrated in Figures 2.3 through 2.5, which correspond to the inpatient medication orders given in Figure 1.3 of Chapter 1. Some information listed below is optional on the label if it is easily retrieved from a product control log.

  a. For patient-specific products: the patient's name and any other appropriate patient identification (e.g., location, identification number)

  b. For batch-prepared products: control or lot number

  c. Bottle sequence number or other system control number

  d. All solution and ingredient names, amounts, strengths, and concentrations (when applicable)

  e. Date of preparation (and time, when applicable)

  f. Beyond-use date (and time, when applicable)

  g. Prescribed administration regimen, when appropriate (including infusion rate and route of administration)

  h. Appropriate auxiliary labeling (including precautions)

  i. Storage requirements

  j. Identification (e.g., initials) of the responsible pharmacist and, if applicable, the technician making the product

  k. Device-specific instructions (when appropriate)

  l. Any additional information, in accordance with state and federal requirements

4. The following are additional guidelines for labeling parenteral products:

  a. Labels for parenteral products should be affixed on the container such that the contents can be inspected, the volume can be identified, and the capacity markings can easily be read. For large-volume parenterals, the name, type of solution, and lot number on the manufacturer's label should be visible. The label should be positioned so that it can be read as the product is being administered. For example, for large-volume parenterals and piggyback bags, the label should be upright when the IV is hanging.

■ **Figure 2.3**   Patient-specific syringe label.

```
David John  H.N. 120579  Rm 430     ℞ 105124
Morphine SO₄ 10 mg, Atropine SO₄ 0.4 mg/2 mL
This syringe contains 0.1 mL excess for priming
On call for surgery at 0800 00/00/00   Give IM
Do not use after 0900   00/00/00   Control #000000-1
```

■ **Figure 2.4**   Batch-prepared syringe label.

```
Control #000000-2   Prep'd: 00/00/00  1700 JET
Penicilin G K 200,000 units/mL   For IM use
Do not use after 00/02/00   1700
This syringe contains 0.1 mL excess for priming
Refrigerate, Do not freeze
```

   b. Abbreviations, such as KCl for Potassium Chloride, are permissible on labels for parenteral products because they are intended to be read by health professionals.

   c. **For injections, the concentration**, not just the quantity, of the drug **must be specified** on the label. For example, "Atropine SO$_4$ 0.4 mg" is not sufficient labeling for a syringe. The label must give a concentration such as "Atropine SO$_4$ 0.4 mg/mL." This is necessary because the person giving the dose to the patient must verify the dose and volume at the time of administration. It is recommended that the concentration be given as the amount of active ingredient in metric units (or units for some antibiotics and insulin) per specified volume in milliliters of one dose. This makes verification easier for the person administering the dose.

   d. When excess volume is added to a syringe to allow for priming a needle prior to administration, the label should state this fact; for example, "This syringe contains 0.1 mL excess to prime needle." Because desired priming volume may vary by institution, by nursing unit within an institution, by drug solution to be administered, and by route of administration (e.g., IM versus IV), the pharmacist should always verify the desired priming volume when preparing syringes. Some drug solutions require larger priming volumes to allow for priming of IV tubing used to administer the drug solution; this information must be stated clearly and boldly on the label because not including the needed priming volume for this procedure would result in a significant dosage error.

   e. For IV additives, the strength of the additive is not given as a concentration. The product is labeled with both the name and quantity of active ingredient added and the name, concentration, and volume of the large-volume parenteral.

■ **Figure 2.5**   Patient-specific IV admixture label.

```
                    MEDICAL CENTER HOSPITAL
                    Triturate, Wisconsin 53706

David John Rm 430                    Bottle #1
History Number:. 120579              Control #000000-3


              Heparin Na 10,000 units

IN: 0.9% Sodium Chloride   250 mL

Infuse     over 4 hours
           at 62 mL/hr
           10 drop/min using 10 drop/mL IV set

Date/Time prepared:  00/00/00  1400  By: JET
Do not use after:      00/2/00  1400  Chk'd; BJF
Refrigerate, Do not Freeze
```

III. AUXILIARY LABELS

A.   Auxiliary labels are placed on drug product containers to give the patient, caregiver, or health care provider important information needed for storing or using the product. Auxiliary labels may be used to clarify directions, provide additional instructions, or reinforce directions given on the regular label. They are not intended to be used in place of patient consultation.

B.   Common auxiliary labels and some recommended uses are given below. Although some labels are required (e.g., "Shake Well" labels for disperse systems), in most cases the pharmacist must exercise professional judgment in deciding what, if any, auxiliary labels to use.

1. **Shake Well** Required on all liquid disperse systems, such as suspensions and emulsions, unless specific product labeling instructs otherwise.

2. **Keep in the Refrigerator, Do Not Freeze** Required on products that are chemically unstable at room temperature (e.g., many reconstituted antibiotics) and on products that are physically unstable at room temperature (e.g., cocoa butter suppositories). It is recommended for parenteral products that have been manipulated and that are not being used immediately, especially those that do not contain a preservative.

3. **Do Not Use After** Required on all manipulated parenteral products, reconstituted antibiotics and liquids, compounded preparations, and other products known to have limited stability. Recommended on all other dispensed products.

4. **Refrigerate, Shake Well, Discard After** Used to avoid multiple auxiliary labels when all three messages, 1, 2, and 3 above, are required, such as on most oral reconstituted antibiotic suspensions.

5. **External Use Only** Recommended on external use products, especially those that would potentially be dangerous if ingested.

6. **May Cause Drowsiness; Alcohol and Operating Car or Machine Warning** Used for adult ambulatory patients. Required for all Schedule II narcotics and other medications, such as some muscle relaxants, that cause significant drowsiness. Recommended on other narcotics, antianxiety agents, tranquilizers, long-acting barbiturates, sedating antiseizure agents, antihistamines and antidepressants, and any other medication that may cause drowsiness. The use of this label on products prescribed as sleeping aids is a matter of professional judgment.

7. **May Cause Drowsiness** Used for pediatric patients and non-ambulatory adults. Same requirements and recommendations as for #6 above.

8. **Do Not Drink Alcohol** Required for medications that give a disulfiram reaction, such as disulfiram, metronidazole, and chlorpropamide. Recommended with hypnotic drugs or others in which the additive CNS effect may be hazardous. Oral explanation should also be given.

9. **Avoid Sun Exposure** Required on drugs that cause photosensitivity reactions, such as tetracyclines, sulfonamides, griseofulvin, nalidixic acid, thiazides, and phenothiazines.

10. **Take with Food** Recommended for drugs that cause stomach upset when this effect may be decreased by taking the medication with food. Examples of medications in this group include nitrofurantoin, valproic acid, erythromycin, NSAIDs, and aspirin.

11. **Take on an Empty Stomach** Recommended for drugs that have decreased absorption or increased destruction in the stomach when taken with food, such as tetracycline and ampicillin.

12. **Take with Plenty of Water** Recommended for sulfonamides to decrease the likelihood of crystalluria, for expectorants to enhance viscosity reduction of bronchial secretions, for bulk laxatives to increase stool bulk and decrease the likelihood of compaction, and for irritating drugs, such as potassium supplements, chloral hydrate, certain antibiotics, and theophylline products.

13. **Finish all this Medication** Recommended as a compliance aid for antibiotics and anti-infectives when a specific time course is not given in the directions for use.

14. **Do not Take with Dairy Products, Antacids . . . .** Required for tetracycline products to prevent inactivation of the drug by polyvalent ions. Recommended for enteric-coated products because milk products and antacids create a basic pH in the stomach that could cause premature dissolution of the enteric coating.

15. **May Cause Discoloration of Urine or Feces** Recommended for drugs that discolor urine or feces, such as methylene blue, nitrofurantoin, and phenazopyridine.

16. **Do not Take Aspirin** Required on warfarin-type anticoagulants.

17. **Caution: Federal Law Prohibits Transfer of this Drug to Another Person** Required by law on all outpatient drug containers for controlled substances in Schedules II–IV.

18. **This Prescription May be Refilled _____ Times** An optional label informing the patient of the number of refills. This information is now often printed directly on the prescription label by dispensing software.

19. **Keep out of the Reach of Children** May be used for any drug product container, but required for drug containers without safety closures.

20. **Protect from Light** Required for parenteral products that are photosensitive, such as sodium nitroprusside, furosemide, and phenothiazines. This label is especially important when the immediate container for these products is not amber or opaque. It is appropriate labeling for all photosensitive drugs.

21. **Cancer Chemotherapy, Dispose of Properly** Required for containers of cytotoxic drug products.)

References

1. The 2002 United States Pharmacopeia 25/National Formulary 20. Rockville, MD: The United States Pharmacopeial Convention, Inc., 2001;10.
2. National Association of Boards of Pharmacy Model Rules for Pharmaceutical Care. National Association of Boards of Pharmacy: Park Ridge, IL, 2002; 69.
3. National Association of Boards of Pharmacy Model Rules for Pharmaceutical Care. National Association of Boards of Pharmacy: Park Ridge, IL, 2002; 80–81.
4. Sitowitz J, Roberts SB. Danger of "as directed" instructions. Am J Health-Syst Pharm 2001; 58: 1657.
5. Cohen MR. ISMP medication error report analysis. Hosp Pharm 2002; 37: 593.
6. ASHP technical assistance bulletin on quality assurance for pharmacy-prepared sterile products. Am J Hosp Pharm 2000; 57: 1156.

CHAPTER 3

Controlled Substances

I. LEGAL JURISDICTION FOR CONTROLLED SUBSTANCES

Controlled substances are regulated by both federal and state laws.

A. The federal law known as the Controlled Substances Act of 1970 is Title 2 of the Comprehensive Drug Abuse Prevention and Control Act (Public Law 91-513). The applicable portions of the law can be found in Title 21 of the U.S. Code (U.S.C.).

B. The Controlled Substances Act (CSA) is enforced by the Drug Enforcement Administration (DEA), which is a section of the Federal Bureau of Investigation (FBI) under the Department of Justice. The DEA regulations that spell out the provisions and applications of 21 U.S.C. are found in Title 21 of the Code of Federal Regulations (CFR).

C. All states have similar regulations, but states may have provisions that are stricter than the federal act. The pharmacist must follow the most stringent regulations that apply for the state in which he or she is practicing.

D. The information given in this chapter is a brief synopsis of the federal regulations of controlled substances that affect general dispensing activities of pharmacists. For more complete information on this subject, consult the applicable sections of the Code of Federal Regulations (21 CFR §1300 and following), the U.S. Code (21 U.S.C. §801 and following), current state pharmacy practice acts, and/or reference books and Internet sites on the subject.

1. The latest revision of the text of the U.S. Code and the Code of Federal Regulations can be accessed on the Internet through the U.S. Government Printing Office site: www.access.gpo.gov. This site has a section "Access to Government Information Products" that provides a link to various important public documents such as the U.S.C., the CFR, and the Federal Register. You can purchase printed copies of the documents through this site, but the site also provides selected documents online in text and pdf formats. These documents are subject to revision, and the information and subsections given in this chapter are from the April 1, 2001 revision of 21 CFR §1300 and following. For the most up-to-date revision, consult the U.S. Government Printing Office Internet site.

2. The DEA Diversion Control Program maintains an excellent resource for pharmacists and pharmacy students to assist them in understanding and complying with the provisions of the CSA. Called the *Pharmacist's Manual*, it is available in print or on the Internet at: www.deadiversion.usdoj.gov/pubs/manuals/pharm2/index.htm, Accessed June 2002

The Pharmacist's Manual explains the applicable regulations in very understandable language and includes tables that give easy comparisons for requirements for the various classes.

II. DEA REGISTRATION

A. The CSA regulates all aspects of narcotic and nonnarcotic stimulants, depressants, and hallucinogenic drugs through the medium of registration (1). To aid government officials in administering and enforcing the controlled substance regulations, all importers and exporters, manufacturers, distributors, researchers, prescribers, and dispensers of controlled substances must register with the DEA. In fact, 21 CFR § 1301.13 lists nine different classes of registrants.

B. Upon registration, these parties are issued DEA registration numbers. Registrants must record their DEA numbers on all documents that they use for the transfer or distribution of controlled substances up to the ultimate consumer.

C. The class "Dispensing and Instructing" includes practitioners, hospitals, clinics, retail pharmacies, and teaching institutions. This class uses DEA application form 224 for initial registration and 224a for renewal, which is required every 36 months (2).

D. Prescribers of Controlled Substances
1. Traditionally, practitioners who were registered with the DEA to prescribe controlled substances included physicians, dentists, and veterinarians.
2. In 1993, the DEA established a new category of registrant called "mid-level practitioner" (MLP). A MLP is anyone other than a physician, veterinarian, dentist, or podiatrist who is licensed or registered and authorized by the state in which he or she practices to dispense controlled substances (3). Depending on the state, this category includes health care professionals such as advanced-practice nurses and physician assistants, provided they have been given prescribing authority by the state in which they practice. Specific privileges and restrictions on prescribers of controlled substances are defined by each state.
3. The DEA registration number of the prescriber must appear on any outpatient prescription order for a controlled substance.

E. Dispensers of Controlled Substances
1. Although prescribers register as individuals, dispensers, such as pharmacists, do not. A pharmacist who is dispensing controlled substances is considered an agent of a registered pharmacy.
2. Pharmacies that order, receive, handle, and dispense controlled substances must be registered with the DEA and must have a DEA registration number.
3. The pharmacy's DEA number is required when the pharmacy orders controlled substances from manufacturers or distributors. It is imprinted on DEA Form 222, which is the form required for ordering controlled substances in Schedule I or II.

F. DEA numbers are unique, nine-character numbers that are computer-generated to contain check digits that help pharmacists identify invalid registration numbers and fraudulent prescription orders for controlled substances. Many dispensing software packages automatically check for invalid numbers when new prescription orders for controlled substances are entered into the computer. DEA numbers can be manually checked by following these steps:

➤ **EXAMPLE:** DEA # AD5426817
1. The first digit should be a letter: A or B for prescribers and dispensers, M for mid-level practitioners, and P for distributors.

2. The second digit is usually a letter, specifically the first letter of the registrant's last name. In the above case, if the prescriber's last name is Jones, the second letter of a valid DEA number would be J, so the above example DEA number would be invalid. If the registrant is a business with a name that starts with a number, such as "5th Avenue Pharmacy," the second digit should be the number "9."

3. The third through the eighth positions of the DEA number should contain numbers that are used to calculate the number in the ninth position, the check digit.
    a. Add the 1st, 3rd, and 5th digits: $5 + 2 + 8 = 15$
    b. Add the 2nd, 4th, and 6th digits and multiply the sum by 2:
        $$4 + 6 + 1 = 11 \times 2 = 22$$
    c. Add the two results: $15 + 22 = 37$
    d. The far right-hand digit of this check number should be the same as the ninth digit of the DEA number. In this example, both numbers are 7, so the DEA number is a valid number.

III. SCHEDULES FOR CONTROLLED SUBSTANCES

A. Controlled substances are divided into five classes, Schedules I–V, based on their potential for abuse. Drugs in Schedule I have the highest abuse potential and no accepted medical use; Schedule V drug products have the lowest abuse potential. The CSA also allows class exemptions for certain nonnarcotic scheduled substances when in combination with other therapeutic agents if it can be shown that the drug product has a very low potential for abuse. Manufacturers of these products must apply for this exemption (4).

B. A brief but representative list of drugs and drug products in the various schedules is given below. For an official list of all drugs and drug products in Schedules I–V, see 21 CFR § 1308.11-1308.15. In professional practice, the easiest way to determine the schedule of a drug product is to look at the drug package; the CSA requires that the schedule symbol (e.g., C-II, C-III, etc.) be imprinted on the label of the manufactured product container (5).

1. Schedule I
    a. High potential for abuse, no accepted medical use, and lack of accepted safety even under medical supervision
    b. Examples of drugs in this schedule include (6):
        (1) Heroin
        (2) Lysergic acid diethylamide (LSD), Mescaline, Peyote, Psilocybin
        (3) Marihuana (Marihuana has been used investigationally for treatment of nausea and vomiting associated with chemotherapy used to treat cancer patients.)
        (4) Methaqualone
2. Schedule II
    a. High potential for abuse; therefore, drugs in Schedule II are treated more stringently than those in Schedules III through V.
    b. Examples of drugs in this schedule include (7):
        (1) All narcotic agonists such as Codeine, Morphine, Meperidine, Hydromorphone, Methadone, Oxycodone, and Fentanyl when not combined with another therapeutic agent
        (2) Certain potent narcotic agonists even when in combination products such as Oxycodone with Acetaminophen and Powdered Opium with Belladonna Suppositories
        (3) Codeine, Morphine, and several other narcotic combination products may be in Schedules II, III, or V, depending on the amount of the narcotic in the product. These levels are listed under Schedules III and V below.
        (4) Cocaine
        (5) Stimulants, such as Amphetamine, Methamphetamine, and Methylphenidate

(6) Short-acting barbiturates, such as Amobarbital, Pentobarbital, and Secobarbital, except when in combinations or in suppository form (they are then in Schedule III) and certain other depressants such as Glutethimide

3. Schedule III

    a. Less potential for abuse than drugs in Schedule II

    b. Examples of drugs in this schedule include (8):

        (1) Specified narcotics combined with other therapeutically active nonnarcotic drugs where the amount of narcotic is restricted to a given level. Several common examples are given below. When the quantity of narcotic exceeds the given amount, the product is in Schedule II.

            (a) Codeine or Dihydrocodeine in combination with one or more nonnarcotic drugs where the maximum amount of Codeine or Dihydrocodeine is 90 mg/unit or 18 mg/mL

            (b) Hydrocodone or ethylmorphine in combination with one or more nonnarcotic drugs where the maximum amount of Hydrocodone or ethylmorphine is 15 mg/unit or 3 mg/mL

            (c) Morphine in combination with one or more nonnarcotic drugs where the maximum amount of Morphine is 0.50 mg/mL or g

        (2) All barbiturates alone or in combination not listed in another schedule. Examples include injectable Thiopental, which is used for anesthesia; short-acting barbiturates such as Amobarbital, Pentobarbital, and Secobarbital when in combinations or in suppository form; and some intermediate-acting barbiturates such as Butabarbital.

        (3) Certain specified stimulants, such as Benzphetamine and Phendimetrazine

        (4) Anabolic steroids, such as Testosterone, unless excepted or listed in another schedule

4. Schedule IV

    a. Lower potential for abuse than Schedule III, but usually treated the same as products in Schedule III

    b. Examples of drugs in this schedule include (9):

        (1) Specified sedative/hypnotics, such as Phenobarbital, Chloral Hydrate, and Meprobamate

        (2) Benzodiazepines, such as Alprazolam, Diazepam, Lorazepam, and Triazolam

        (3) Dextropropoxyphene when formulated into a drug product, alone or in combination

        (4) Certain stimulants, such as Pemoline and Phentermine

        (5) Miscellaneous substances such as Fenfluramine and Pentazocine

5. Schedule V

    a. Lowest potential for abuse among the controlled substance drugs

    b. Examples of drugs in this schedule include (10):

        (1) Narcotic drugs in combination with other therapeutic agents when the amount of the narcotic does not exceed the specified level. Most commonly, the examples given here are used therapeutically as cough suppressants.

            (a) Codeine not more than 2 mg/mL or g

            (b) Dihydrocodeine or ethylmorphine not more than 1 mg/mL

        (2) The following combination medications, usually used as antidiarrheals, when the amount of the narcotic does not exceed the specified level:

            (a) Opium not more than 1 mg/mL or g

            (b) Not more than 2.5 mg of Diphenoxylate HCl with not less than 25 mcg of Atropine Sulfate per dosage unit

IV. REQUIREMENTS FOR PRESCRIPTION DRUG ORDERS FOR CONTROLLED SUBSTANCES

A. The federal requirements for prescription orders for controlled substances are given below. These are the requirements as of the April 1, 2001, revision of 21 CFR § 1300. Because these regulations change from time to time, it is best to access the most up-to-date revision. As described at the beginning of this chapter, this can be done on the Internet through the U.S. Government Printing Office site. State controlled substance laws may add additional requirements. Furthermore, federal and state laws concerning required elements for all prescription orders also apply. For information on these laws, see Chapter 1, Prescription and Medication Orders.

B. All schedules
Prescription drug orders for all controlled substances have the following requirements (11):
  1. Date of issue
  2. Full name and address of the patient
  3. The drug name, strength, dosage form, quantity prescribed
  4. Directions for use
     (Note: For states that limit prescription orders for controlled substances to a 34-day supply, the directions for use must be specific enough to ascertain that amount.)
  5. Full name, address, and DEA number of the prescriber
  6. For written prescription orders, the signature of the prescriber
  7. When an oral order is not permitted (e.g., Schedule II), the prescription must be written in ink, indelible pencil, or typewriter and must be manually signed.

C. Schedule II
Because of the high potential for abuse, drugs in Schedule II have additional requirements.
  1. The dispenser must have a **written or typed prescription order, signed by the prescriber,** at the time of dispensing. As stated in Chapter 1, most states allow oral or electronic transmission, including voice telephoned prescription orders, for Schedule II medications in emergency situations, provided (12):
     a. The quantity prescribed is limited to the amount needed for the emergency period.
     b. The prescription order, containing all required information except the signature, is immediately put in written form.
     c. The pharmacist makes a good faith effort to verify that the order came from a registered practitioner if the prescriber is not known to the pharmacist.
     d. A written, signed document is received within a specified time period. In 1997 the federal law set this time period as 7 days, but because the most stringent law (i.e., federal or state) always applies, check your current state statutes for the standard at your practice site.
  2. Faxed prescriptions are permitted in non-emergency situations provided the pharmacist is given the original signed prescription order for review prior to the actual dispensing of the controlled drug. Facsimile orders without original signed prescriptions are permitted in certain practices such as IV infusion services, long-term care, and hospice (12).
  3. Refills are prohibited (13).
  4. Partial filling of a prescription is permissible, but the remaining portion must be filled within a 72-hour time period (14).
  5. Although there is no federal limitation, some states have quantity limitations such as a 34-day supply or 120 doses, although exceptions may be permitted in special circumstances (15).

D.   Schedules III and IV

Drugs and drug products in Schedules III and IV have less potential for abuse than drugs in Schedule II. Although Schedule III substances have greater abuse potential than those in Schedule IV, drugs in these two schedules are treated essentially the same, with the same requirements and restrictions.

1. Prescription orders may be transmitted by phone or fax (16).
2. Refills are permitted with a maximum of five refills or 6 months from date of the original order, whichever is first. Records of refills must be kept and may be either in writing on the prescription order or recorded electronically. The specifics of refill records can be found in 21 CFR §1306.22 (17).
3. In a two-file system (described in the next section), a red "C" no less than 1 inch in height must be applied to the lower right-hand corner of prescription orders in Schedule III, IV, and V. As stated in Chapter 1, since 1997, DEA regulations allow waiver of the red "C" requirement for pharmacies that use electronic record-keeping systems that permit identification by prescription number and that allow retrieval of original documents by prescriber's name, patient's name, drug dispensed, and date filled (18). Check your current state statutes to determine if the state in which you practice has adopted this standard.
4. Although there is no federal limitation, some states have quantity limitations such as a 34-day supply or 120 doses (15), but some states allow exceptions such as a 90-day supply for anticonvulsant drug products that are in Schedule IV.

D.   Schedule V

1. Drug products in Schedule V have the lowest potential for abuse among the controlled substance drug products.
2. There are some drug products in this schedule which the FDA has determined may be sold without a prescription drug order.
3. For drug products dispensed on a prescription order, most of the prescription order requirements are the same as for Schedule III and IV. One exception is the treatment of refills. These are handled like non-scheduled prescriptions; that is, a specific number of refills must be indicated, but there is no time or number limit.
4. For drug products in this class that the FDA has determined may be sold without a prescription, the following CSA restrictions apply (19):
   a. May be dispensed only by a pharmacist (although the cash or credit transaction may be done by a nonpharmacist)
   b. The purchaser must be at least 18 years old, and any person, if not known by the pharmacist, must provide identification and when appropriate proof of age.
   c. Limitations of quantity and frequency of purchase:
      (1) 240 mL (8 ounces) or 48 dosage units of an opium product per 48-hour period (Most of these products are antidiarrheal products.)
      (2) 120 mL (4 ounces) or 24 units of any other controlled substance per 48-hour period (Most of these products are Codeine-containing cough suppressants.)
   d. Special record-keeping requirements include a bound log with date of purchase, name and quantity of product, name and address of purchaser, and name or initials of the pharmacist. Some states also require the signature of the purchaser and the pharmacist.

V. RECORD-KEEPING FOR CONTROLLED SUBSTANCES

A.   Although different restrictions apply to drug products based on their schedule, the receipt and delivery of all controlled substances must be accounted for by registered pharmacies. The specifics of the inventory requirements can be found in 21 CFR § 1304.11.

B.   Controlled substances must be inventoried every 2 years (20).

C. Because they have the greatest abuse potential of drugs with legitimate medical use, Schedule II drugs are singled out. They must be ordered on special narcotic ordering forms, DEA Form 222.

D. For drug products in the other schedules, invoices must be kept to document their receipt in the pharmacy.

E. Pharmacies must also follow specified record-keeping requirements for the dispensing of controlled drug products and substances.

   1. The CSA requires the following on records of dispensing (21):
      a. Name and address of the patient
      b. Date of dispensing
      c. The name, dosage form, and quantity dispensed of the product
      d. The name or initials of the dispenser

   2. Pharmacists may choose to file prescription orders for controlled substances in either a two- or three-file system as described below (18). These systems are designed so that scheduled prescriptions can be easily identified and retrieved. Because of the higher abuse potential for drugs in Schedule II, these prescriptions must either be kept separately or, if filed with other scheduled prescriptions, they must be easily identified.

      a. Three-file system:
         (1) Schedule II prescription orders are in one file.
         (2) Schedules III–V orders are in a second file.
         (3) All non-controlled prescription orders are in a third file.

      b. Two-file system, Option A
         (1) Schedule II orders are in a separate file.
         (2) Schedule III–V orders are filed with non-controlled prescription orders. The Schedule III–V prescription orders must be distinguished from the non-Scheduled prescription orders by having a 1-inch, red "C" in the bottom right-hand corner of the prescription document. This marking enables law enforcement officials, when they are inspecting the pharmacy's records, to easily distinguish the orders for the controlled prescriptions. As stated previously, since 1997, DEA regulations allow waiver of the red "C" requirement for pharmacies that use electronic record-keeping systems that permit identification by prescription number and that allow retrieval of original documents by prescriber's name, patient's name, drug dispensed, and date filled (18). Check your current state statutes to determine if the state in which you practice has adopted this standard.

      c. Two-file system, Option B
         (1) Schedule II–V orders are filed together, but separately from prescription orders for non-controlled products. Again, the Schedule III–V prescription orders must have a 1-inch, red "C" in the bottom right-hand corner of the prescription document. This is to allow easy separation of the Schedule III–V orders from those in Schedule II. The same waiver of the red "C" is allowed for pharmacies that use electronic record-keeping as stated above.
         (2) Prescription orders for non-controlled products are in a separate file.

VI. LABELING OF OUTPATIENT PRESCRIPTIONS FOR CONTROLLED SUBSTANCES

A. The federal requirements for labeling controlled substances are given in the following sections of 21 CFR § 1306: Schedules II, 21 CFR § 1306.14, Schedules III–V, 21 CFR § 1306.24, and Schedule V when dispensed without a prescription, 21 CFR § 1306.31. These requirements are summarized below. State laws may add additional requirements.

   1. Date of dispensing (date of initial dispensing for Schedules III, IV, and V)

2. Pharmacy name and address
3. Prescription identification or serial number
4. Name of patient
5. Name of prescriber
6. Directions for use and cautionary statements, if any
7. A federal transfer label is required on prescriptions in Schedules II, III, and IV but not Schedule V. This label states:

   Caution: Federal law prohibits the transfer of this drug to any person other than the patient for whom it was prescribed. (21)

B. Notice that while the federal labeling requirements for controlled substances do not require the name and strength of the drug product dispensed, these are requirements for general prescription labels in most states. See Chapter 2, Labeling Prescriptions and Medications, for general information on labeling prescriptions.

VII. OTHER REQUIREMENTS

As stated at the beginning of this chapter, the above provides an overview of the requirements for handling controlled substances in the pharmacy. The specifics of registration, storage and security, inventory records, order forms, transferring of prescriptions, detoxification programs, required institutional records, and complete schedules for drug products are beyond the scope of this text. For more information refer to the current revisions of appropriate sections of the CFR, the U.S.C., state pharmacy practice acts, and/or reference books on pharmacy law.

References

1. Fink JL III, Vivian JC, Reid KK, eds. Pharmacy Law Digest, 36th ed. St. Louis: Facts and Comparisons, Inc., 2001; 135.
2. 21 CFR § 1301.13.
3. 21 CFR § 1300.01.
4. 21 CFR § 1308.31.
5. 21 CFR § 1302.03.
6. 21 CFR § 1308.11.
7. 21 CFR § 1308.12.
8. 21 CFR § 1308.13.
9. 21 CFR § 1308.14.
10. 21 CFR § 1308.15.
11. 21 CFR § 1306.05.
12. 21 CFR § 1306.11.
13. 21 CFR § 1306.12.
14. 21 CFR § 1306.13.
15. Fink JL III, Vivian JC, Reid KK, eds. Pharmacy Law Digest, 36th ed. St. Louis: Facts and Comparisons, Inc., 2001; 156.
16. 21 CFR § 1306.21.
17. 21 CFR § 1306.22.
18. 21 CFR § 1304.04.
19. 21 CFR § 1306.26.
20. 21 CFR § 1304.11.
21. 21 U.S.C. § 825(c).

CHAPTER 4

Expiration and Beyond-Use Dating

I. DEFINITIONS

A. **Expiration Date:** This is the date put on the label of a drug product by the manufacturer or distributor of the product. The *United States Pharmacopeia (USP)* defines expiration date in the following way:

> "The expiration date identifies the time during which the article may be expected to meet the requirements of the Pharmacopeial monograph, provided it is kept under the prescribed storage conditions. The expiration date limits the time during which the article may be dispensed or used. Where an expiration date is stated only in terms of the month and the year, it is a representation that the intended expiration date is the last day of the stated month" (1).

B. **Beyond-Use Date:** This is the date put on the dispensing container by the pharmacist. According to the *USP:*
    1. "The dispenser shall place on the label of the prescription container a suitable beyond-use date to limit the patient's use of the article based on any information supplied by the manufacturer and the *General Notices and Requirements* of this Pharmacopeia. The beyond-use date placed on the label shall not be later than the expiration date on the manufacturer's container" (1).
    2. "The beyond-use date is the date after which an article must not be used" (1).

C. It should be noted that these definitions use the term "article," which is defined in the *USP* as "an item for which a monograph is provided whether an official substance or an official preparation" (2). Therefore, technically these definitions apply only to official *USP* articles. In practice these definitions are generalized to include other non-official drug entities, nutrients and dietary supplements, pharmaceutical ingredients, and preparations.

II. REGULATION OF EXPIRATION AND BEYOND-USE DATING

A. Manufactured drug products in their original containers
    1. Manufactured products are covered by federal regulations because they are shipped in interstate commerce.
    2. Prior to the late 1960s, except for insulin and antibiotics, most commercial packages of drug products carried no expiration date. It was common to find drug products in

prescription departments of pharmacies that were 20 to 30 years old. This gradually changed during the 1970s so that by Sept. 28, 1978, Good Manufacturing Practice regulations required expiration dates on almost all drug products manufactured and distributed to pharmacies.

3. The General Notices of the *USP* contains the following statement about the requirement for expiration dates on *USP* products:

> "The label of an official drug product, nutritional or dietary supplement product shall bear an expiration date. All articles shall display the expiration date so that it can be read by an ordinary individual under customary conditions of purchase and use" (1).

4. Currently, the only exceptions for the requirement of expiration dating on manufactured drug products are for: drug products or nutritional supplements packaged in containers for sale at retail without a prescription drug order, and labeling which allows no limitation of dosage, and the product must be shown to be stable for at least 3 years under the recommended conditions of storage (1).

B.   Drug products labeled, packaged, and dispensed by the pharmacist on prescription orders
1. Because dispensing drug products to patients is regulated by state law, the requirements for beyond-use dates on most prescription containers are regulated by state statutes. The NABP Model Rules for Pharmaceutical Care, which is used as a model for state pharmacy laws, recommends that a beyond-use date be included on the prescription label (3). As a result, many states have adopted this standard. Check the regulations for the state in which you are practicing for information about requirements for labeling prescription containers with beyond-use dates.
2. As quoted above in the definitions section, the General Notices of the *USP* states that the dispenser (this includes both pharmacists and dispensing physicians) shall label a prescription container with a beyond-use date (1).
3. One area in which federal law has jurisdiction in regulating the labeling of prescriptions is for drug products dispensed for nursing home patients; the Code of Federal Regulations specifies that FDA and USP requirements be followed for prescriptions dispensed to nursing home patients in intermediate-care and skilled nursing facilities. Therefore, prescriptions for these patients must be labeled with beyond-use dates.
4. Even when it is not required by law, most pharmacists feel that the labels of all prescription containers should include beyond-use dates; they feel it is their professional responsibility to provide their patients with a date after which a medication may no longer have its labeled potency. It is well known that many patients keep any unused portion of their prescriptions in case they need it in the future, so many households have partially used prescription drug products that could unknowingly be used well past their expiration date if the container was not labeled with a beyond-use date.
5. Many dispensing software programs automatically place beyond-use dates on all labels for prescriptions.

III. DIFFICULTIES IN ASSIGNING BEYOND-USE DATES

A.   A major stumbling block to assigning and labeling dispensed drug products with beyond-use dates has been the lack of adequate stability information available to the pharmacist. The questions is, how should the pharmacist determine a valid beyond-use date without the benefit of stability studies conducted with the drug product in the dispensing container stored in the uncontrolled home environment?

B.   This problem was recognized in Resolution No. 11 at the 1990 United States Pharmacopeial Convention:

> "The United States Pharmacopeial Convention is encouraged to explore with the Food and Drug Administration the development of mechanisms by which reliable data and

information can be generated to establish scientifically sound beyond-use dates for repackaged products" (4).

C. Over the next 10 years, USP took the initiative to address this concern. Studies were conducted by USP and pharmaceutical manufacturers, conferences were held, and the *Pharmacopeial Forum* of the USP was used as a medium for exchanging ideas and soliciting information from pharmacists, regulatory bodies, pharmacy professional organizations, and the pharmaceutical industry. The results of these deliberations can be seen in the current General Notices of the *USP* and are summarized here.

1. Manufacturers are given responsibility for providing the pharmacist with needed information to use in assigning beyond-use dates, and, as indicated above, the dispenser is to use any information provided by the manufacturer in assigning a beyond-use date (1).

2. Pharmacists are directed to dispense only in or from containers labeled with an expiration date, and the product dispensed must be within the labeled expiry time period (1). This has implications for pharmacies that serve institutional or long-term care facilities in that unused drug products that are returned to stock should not be co-mingled with products that have a different (especially longer) expiration date.

3. Pharmacists are reminded to use professional judgment when using the available information for determining beyond-use dates.

   a. For products requiring reconstitution before use, the manufacturer's recommendations on the product labeling should be followed.

   b. For all other products, pharmacists are instructed to take into account the following factors:

   (1) The nature of the drug

   (2) The characteristics of the container used by the manufacturer and the expiration date on the product label

   (3) The properties of the dispensing container

   (4) The expected storage conditions for the product during the time of use, including any unusual conditions to which it may be exposed

   (5) The expected length of time that the product will be used (1).

4. For manufactured drug products, pharmacists are given default guidelines to use in assigning beyond-use dates that are based on the type of dispensing packaging used: multi-dose containers, unit-dose containers, and customized patient medication packages. These are described in the next section.

5. Pharmacists are also given guidelines for determining beyond-use dates for compounded preparations. These are described in a later section.

IV. ASSIGNING BEYOND-USE DATES TO MANUFACTURED DRUG PRODUCTS DISPENSED BY THE PHARMACIST

A. Multi-dose containers

1. For prescription drug products dispensed in multi-dose containers, the *USP* allows use of the manufacturer's expiration date or 1 year from the date the drug product is dispensed, whichever is earlier (1).

   a. Remember that this is the **maximum** length allowed, and that the factors given above must be considered, including the drug, the container, and the storage conditions.

   b. The pharmacist should be conscious of the recommended storage conditions for a drug product. Many products require storage at controlled room temperature. Therefore, it is prudent to be conservative with beyond-use dates when a product is dispensed in hot weather, especially when it cannot be assured that the product will be stored under controlled conditions. Furthermore, many tablets and capsules are sensitive to moisture, and dispensing them in a prescription vial, even though it is classified as a tight container, may decrease their shelf-life; the patient will be opening and closing the dispensing container often as doses are taken, thus exposing the drug product to the atmosphere.

    c. Although it is usually satisfactory to use the maximum allowable time when the drug product is dispensed in its original container, and the patient will be storing the product as directed, an exception to this would be a volatile drug like nitroglycerin. Even though this drug is dispensed in its original glass container, it will lose potency over time as the patient opens and closes the bottle to remove doses.

    d. Dispensing software packages that automatically label prescriptions with expiration dates of 1 year from the date dispensed should be used with discretion; the manufacturer's expiration date should always be consulted and a shorter dating should be printed on the prescription label when this is warranted.

2. The *USP* specifies that the facility in which drug products are packaged and stored has a temperature that is maintained so as not to exceed a mean kinetic temperature of 25°C. Temperature records are to be kept by the pharmacy (1). A discussion and a sample calculation of mean kinetic temperature are given in Chapter 12, Compounding Equipment and Ingredients.

3. To protect the product from humidity or moisture permeation, any plastic packaging material must provide protection better than that given by polyvinyl chloride (1). For multi-dose containers, this specification can easily be met by using tight containers.

B. Single-unit and unit-dose containers for nonsterile dosage forms

    1. For nonsterile solid and liquid dosage forms dispensed in single-unit or unit-dose containers, the *USP* allows use of the manufacturer's expiration date or 1 year from the date the drug product is packaged in the unit container, whichever is earlier (1).

        a. Longer beyond-use dates are allowed if the product labeling allows this, or if independent stability studies have been done that justify a longer dating (1).

        b. Notice that this recommendation uses the date **packaged**, while that for multi-dose containers uses the date **dispensed**. These recommendations assume that drugs repackaged in multi-dose containers are dispensed at that time, while unit-dose packaging is often carried out in advance of the dispensing act.

    2. All of the other considerations stated above for multi-dose packaging also apply to single-unit or unit-dose packaging. Of special concern for this type of packaging is the requirement that plastic packaging materials give better moisture permeation protection than polyvinyl chloride; the dispenser must confirm that materials used for this type of packaging meet this specification.

    3. There are some additional requirements.

        a. In addition to a temperature requirement, there is a maximum relative humidity requirement for nonsterile solid and liquid dosage forms repackaged in unit containers. These products are to be repackaged and stored under conditions specified in the product monograph; if the monograph does not specify the conditions, then the conditions should be controlled room temperature and relative humidity should not exceed 75% at 23°C (5).

        b. *USP* Chapter ⟨661⟩ also prohibits reprocessing of repackaged unit-dose containers. In other words, the dispenser may not remove dosage units from one unit-dose container and dispense it in another unit-dose container (5).

C. Customized patient medication packages (5)

    1. A customized patient medication package, or patient med-pak, is a package prepared by a pharmacist for a specific patient. It comprises a series of packets or containers that contain two or more prescribed solid oral dosage forms. It is intended as a compliance aid for the patient so that each packet or container is labeled with the day and time that the contents of that container are to be taken.

    2. The *USP* has separate recommendations for labeling of patient med-paks. These can be found in their entirety in *USP* Chapter ⟨661⟩ Containers, Customized Patient Medication Packages.

3. With regard to assigning a beyond-use date to a patient med-pak, Chapter ⟨661⟩ directs that it be no longer than the shortest recommended beyond-use date for any dosage form in the med-pak or not longer than 60 days from the date of preparation, and that it not exceed the shortest expiration date on the original manufacturer's bulk container for any of the dosage forms in the med-pak.

4. Chapter ⟨661⟩ also contains requirements for packaging materials for patient med-paks: unless there are more strict packaging requirements for any units contained in the med-pak, the materials for these med-paks must meet the specifications for Class B single-unit or unit-dose containers as described in *USP* Chapter ⟨671⟩ Containers—Permeation. Pharmacists who repackage in single-unit, unit-dose, or patient med-paks should consult the applicable chapters of the *USP* for complete information on packaging materials and storage and packaging requirements.

V. ASSIGNING BEYOND-USE DATES TO COMPOUNDED DRUG PREPARATIONS

A. The *General Notices* of the USP state that compounded drug preparations shall be labeled with a beyond-use date. Guidance for assigning beyond-use dates to extemporaneously compounded nonsterile drug preparations is given in *USP* Chapter ⟨795⟩, Pharmacy Compounding. Guidelines on beyond-use dates for sterile products is discussed in *USP* Chapter ⟨1206⟩ and in the American Society of Health-System Pharmacists *Technical Assistance Bulletin on Quality Assurance for Pharmacy-prepared Sterile Products*; these are discussed in Chapter 32 of this textbook.

B. In applying these standards, it is important to keep in mind the general rules for assigning beyond-use dates, which state that you must take into account the nature of the drug or drugs involved, the characteristics of the preparation container, and the expected storage conditions.

C. Before compounding any drug product, consult the available literature for stability information.

1. Numerous references are available that give helpful information on drug product stability. A partial list of these references appears in Chapter 34. If you are unable to find needed information, or if you do not have access to a particular reference, you may be able to obtain the needed information by consulting with a College of Pharmacy faculty member or colleague, or by calling the library at a School or College of Pharmacy or a Drug Information Service at a teaching hospital. Some companies that specialize in selling compounding supplies also maintain customer service departments that can help you with your questions. One very helpful reference that gives specific compatibility and stability information on a large number of drugs is *Trissel's Compatibility of Compounded Formulations*, published by the American Pharmaceutical Association.

2. If information specific to the situation cannot be found, judgment of stability can be based on several factors, including the structural formula of the drug, the availability of similar manufactured dosage forms of the drug, and published stability information on drugs with similar chemistry. When extrapolating information from the literature, be conscious of significant differences between the study conditions and those of your preparation: containers, storage conditions, vehicles, and excipients, to name a few. Details on compatibility and stability considerations are discussed in Chapter 34.

D. When assigning a beyond-use date to a compounded preparation, you must take into consideration the expiration dates of all the ingredients used in formulating the preparation. In addition, because you are manipulating these ingredients and are usually mixing them with other drugs, excipients, and pharmaceutic ingredients, the new preparation should have a shorter expiration date than that assigned to any of the single original ingredients. How much should you reduce the beyond-use date? There are six key factors to consider:

1. The nature of each ingredient. For example, we know that some drugs, such as potassium chloride and calamine, are intrinsically very stable chemically, whereas others, like penicillin and aspirin, are subject to chemical decomposition.

2. The combination of ingredients. For example, an isoniazid suspension formulated with 50% sorbitol solution is stable for approximately 3 weeks, whereas an isoniazid suspension made with sugar-base syrups is not nearly that stable (6).

3. The final pharmaceutical dosage form. Most drugs formulated as dry powders, such as bulk powders, chartulae, or capsules, are much more stable than when these same drugs are dispensed in systems that contain water, such as aqueous solutions, suspensions, and emulsions. Keep in mind, however, that while hard capsule shells look "dry," the material for gelatin capsule shells contains 10% to 15% water (7), and a very vulnerable drug in close contact with the capsule shell may be subject to some instability.

4. Compounding procedures. Variation in compounding procedures and equipment used for making a formulation can affect the stability of the final preparation. For example, the physical properties of product uniformity and rate of sedimentation for suspensions can be altered by passing the preparation through a hand homogenizer. Use of heat during compounding can have a negative effect on the chemical properties of some ingredients in the final preparation.

5. Packaging used for the preparation. Many drugs are sensitive to moisture and are more stable when packaged in a tight container than in a well-closed container. Other preparations need protection from light.

6. Possible storage conditions. Most drugs with limited stability degrade more rapidly as temperatures increase. Many preparations are sensitive to high humidity. Although the pharmacist tries to control storage conditions through proper labeling and consultation with the patient, this is one variable over which control is relinquished once the preparation leaves the pharmacy.

E. As indicated above, *USP* Chapter ⟨795⟩ on pharmacy compounding has established some basic guidelines that are useful in assigning beyond-use dates for nonsterile compounded preparations.

1. To avoid any misinterpretations of this information, the guidelines are quoted directly here.

"In the absence of stability information that is applicable to a specific drug and preparation, the following maximum beyond-use dates are recommended for nonsterile compounded drug preparations that are packaged in tight, light-resistant containers and stored at controlled room temperature unless otherwise indicated.

For Nonaqueous Liquids and Solid Formulations *(Where the manufactured drug product is the source of active ingredient)*—The beyond-use date is not later than 25% of the time remaining until the product's expiration date or 6 months, whichever is earlier.

(Where a USP or NF substance is the source of active ingredient)—The beyond-use date is not later than 6 months.

For Water-Containing Formulations (prepared from ingredients in solid form)—The beyond-date is not later than 14 days when stored at cold temperatures.

For All Other Formulations—The beyond-use date is not later than the intended duration of therapy or 30 days, whichever is earlier. These beyond-use date limits may be exceeded when there is supporting valid scientific stability information that is directly applicable to the specific preparation (i.e., the same drug concentration range, pH, excipients, vehicle, water content, etc.)" (8).

2. To illustrate the application of the above maximum default beyond-use dates, consider the following examples:

a. The pharmacist is crushing Diazepam tablets for incorporation into compounded capsules. If the bulk package of tablets has a labeled expiration date of 1 year from the date of compounding, the **maximum** possible beyond-use date for this compounded nonaqueous solid preparation would be 3 months (25% of 1 year). This assumes that the capsules will be dispensed in a tight, light-resistant container and stored at controlled room temperature.

b. If the same situation were to occur but the capsules were made using pure Diazepam USP powder, the maximum beyond-use date would be 6 months. This assumes that the expiration date on the Diazepam powder is longer than 6 months; if it is less than 6 months, the beyond-use date on the capsules would have to be shortened appropriately. For example, if the powder had an expiration date of 4 months, the assigned beyond-use date for the capsules might be 1 or 2 months.

c. If either crushed manufactured tablets or pure powder were used to make a Diazepam aqueous oral suspension, the maximum default beyond-use date would be 14 days. This assumes that the suspension will be stored in a cold place such as a refrigerator. In the case of Diazepam, there have been numerous stability studies for compounded suspensions, and some formulations have acceptable stability for up to 60 days. If one of these specific formulations is used, the beyond-use date could be lengthened to that given in the study. A good review of these studies is given in *Trissel's Stability of Compounded Formulations* (9).

d. If either crushed manufactured tablets or pure powder were used to make Diazepam suppositories, the pharmacist would have the option to select 3 months (if using the crushed tablets described above) or 6 months (if using pure drug powder) because this is a nonaqueous formulation, or the 30 days or intended length of therapy guideline as recommended for "other formulations." In this case the pharmacist would have to use professional judgment in selecting an appropriate date. Because heat is used in the compounding procedure for making suppositories, a conservative beyond-use date would be recommended. A stability study for a Diazepam suppository formulation has also been reported (9).

F. As indicated at the beginning of this section, guidelines on beyond-use dates for sterile products is discussed in *USP* Chapter ⟨1206⟩ and in the American Society of Health-System Pharmacists *Technical Assistance Bulletin on Quality Assurance for Pharmacy-prepared Sterile Products.* Because of the added requirement for sterility, assigning beyond-use dates for these preparations is more complex; this is discussed in Chapter 32 of this textbook.

VI. SUMMARY

A. Because the subject of assigning scientifically based beyond-use dates is one that continues to be debated, it is important to be knowledgeable about the latest published standards.

1. For all dispensing and for repackaging of drug products in unit-dose or single-unit packages, check the *General Notices* of the most current *USP*.
2. For compounded nonsterile preparations, check *USP* Chapter ⟨795⟩.
3. For sterile products, check the current USP Chapter ⟨1206⟩ and ASHP's most current technical assistance bulletin on sterile products prepared by the pharmacy.

B. As professionals charged with protecting the health of their patients, pharmacists want to be sufficiently conservative in assigning beyond-use dates so that the label adequately reflects the actual potency of the product or preparation. At the same time, the dates should not be so conservative that patients are unnecessarily inconvenienced with frequent visits to the pharmacy, and drug products or preparations are not wasted by discarding items that are still within labeled limits.

C. Although it has been pointed out that there is only one reported case in which a degraded drug (tetracycline) has caused human toxicity (10), it must be remembered that therapeutic failure, especially in the case of a critical drug, a critical disease, or a critical patient, caused by a subpotent drug product or preparation may be just as serious as a case of toxicity caused by a degraded drug. This should always be kept in mind when assigning beyond-use dates, and the patient should be instructed to monitor the results of the therapy.

References

1. The 2003 United States Pharmacopeia 26/National Formulary 21. Rockville, MD: The United States Pharmacopeial Convention, Inc., 2002; 10–11.
2. The 2003 United States Pharmacopeia 26/National Formulary 21. Rockville, MD: The United States Pharmacopeial Convention, Inc., 2002; 3.
3. National Association of Boards of Pharmacy Model Rules for Pharmaceutical Care. National Association of Boards of Pharmacy: Park Ridge, IL, 2002; 80–81.
4. Pharmacopeial Forum. Rockville, MD: The United States Pharmacopeial Convention, Inc., 1998;24: 43–56.
5. The 2003 United States Pharmacopeia 26/National Formulary 21. Rockville, MD: The United States Pharmacopeial Convention, Inc., 2002; 2148–2149.
6. ASHP Handbook on Extemporaneous Formulations. American Society of Hospital Pharmacists. Bethesda, MD, 1987; 27.
7. The 2003 United States Pharmacopeia 26/National Formulary 21. Rockville, MD: The United States Pharmacopeial Convention, Inc., 2002; 2399.
8. The 2003 United States Pharmacopeia 26/National Formulary 21. Rockville, MD: The United States Pharmacopeial Convention, Inc., 2002; 2198.
9. Trissel LA. Trissel's Stability of Compounded Formulations, 2nd ed., Washington, DC: American Pharmaceutical Association, 2000; 121–124.
10. Drug past their expiration date. The Medical Letter. New Rochelle, NY: The Medical Letter, Inc., 2002; 44: 93–94.

CHAPTER 5

Drug Utilization Review/ Medication Use Evaluation

I. DEFINITIONS

A. **"Drug Utilization Review (Drug Use Review, DUR, and Drug Use Evaluation)** — process used to assess the appropriateness of drug therapy by engaging in the evaluation of data on drug use in a given health care environment against predetermined criteria and standards" (1).

    a. This definition was published as part of a report called *Principles of a Sound Drug Formulary System*. The report was prepared and endorsed by a coalition of national organizations with a primary interest in promoting rational, clinically appropriate, safe, and cost-effective drug therapy (1).

    b. The coalition working group was broad-based and included representatives from the Academy of Managed Care Pharmacy, the American Medical Association, the American Society of Health-System Pharmacists, the Department of Veterans Affairs, the National Business Coalition on Health, and the United States Pharmacopeia.

B. **Drug Use Evaluation** or **Drug Use Review (DUE/DUR)**

    1. The terms **Drug Use Evaluation** and **Drug Use Review** have been used interchangeably but should **not** be **interchanged** with **Drug Utilization Review** (DUR), described below.

    2. The DUE/DUR process involves the development, use, monitoring, refinement, and adjustment of objective, measurable criteria that describe the appropriate use of a drug (2). The underlying concepts of DUE/DUR are now contained as just one part of the more current and broader concept of Medication Use Evaluation (MUE), which is described below.

    3. DUR can be used prospectively and retrospectively by any health care entity (hospital, community pharmacy, ambulatory practice setting, third-party payers, etc.) in an effort to provide appropriate medication management.

C. **M24edication Use Evaluation (MUE)**

    1. MUE is a process of prospective assessment that focuses on the outcome of the patient's medication therapy according to predetermined criteria. The goal of the evaluation is to *optimize medication management and improve the patient's quality of life throughout all phases of the medication use process* (3).

2. The medication use process includes the responsibilities of *prescribing, preparation and dispensing, administration, and monitoring of medications*. The evaluation is concerned with the inter-relatedness of these functions and the continuum of care.

3. MUE is a "performance improvement method that focuses on evaluating and improving medication-use processes with the goal of optimal patient outcomes" (3). It is a prospective method of evaluation that can be applied in any health care setting. MUE augments DUE/DUR beyond utilization of drug products and appropriateness of prescribing and dispensing. MUE assesses the individualization of the medication management throughout the medication-use process in relation to standards of care, and evidence-based medicine.

4. MUEs can be initiated for a variety of reasons and are not restricted to the prescribing and dispensing functions of a pharmacist. MUEs can evaluate specific medications, classes of medications, pharmacologic treatment of disease states, and actual or potential medication-use process problems. Categories of reasons prompting MUE include:
   a. Problem-prone drugs
   b. High-volume and high-cost drugs
   c. High-risk medications
   d. High-risk patient populations
   e. New drug entities
   f. New therapeutic plans

5. The development of the evaluation criteria is the collaborative responsibility of interdisciplinary practitioners and administrators throughout the medication-use process. The criteria should be based on standards of practice and evidence-based medicine found in the primary literature. Other resources applicable to MUE criteria can be computer software programs and external standard-setting organizations.

6. MUE can be conducted in any health care setting provided the process is interdisciplinary, collaborative, and prospective and has access to comprehensive patient information.

7. MUE is compatible with the performance improvement model. The performance improvement steps of Plan, Do, Check, and Act are paramount to the MUE process. The evaluation process not only provides guidance for optimal therapeutic management of patients, prevention of medication-related problems, cost control, and patient safety, but also provides insight into the appropriateness of the criteria and optimal functioning of the medication-use process.

D.   Drug Utilization Review (DUR)

1. There are two distinct types of DUR: prospective DUR (ProDUR) and retrospective DUR (RDUR).
   a. ProDUR is the review that a pharmacist conducts before dispensing a new prescription order. The new prescription order is reviewed with the intent of maximizing therapy and detecting problems caused by incorrect dosage, route of administration, duration of therapy, therapeutic duplication, drug-allergy or drug-disease contraindications, undesirable drug-drug interactions, inappropriate therapeutic use, or over- or underutilization of medication. To perform ProDUR well, the pharmacist should have access to information about the patient's lifestyle, medical history, current diagnosis, past and present medication use, and laboratory values. Some of this information can be found on the patient's medication profile record, which is available in the pharmacy. Needed information not on the profile record may sometimes be obtained from the patient or the prescriber.
   b. RDUR is a review (often involving comparative statistics) of a large number of prescription orders that have already been dispensed. This large database is examined for potential problems, such as fraud, abuse, gross overuse, or inappropriate or medically unnecessary care among physicians, pharmacists, and patients. The goal of RDUR is to maximize cost-effective, rational therapy. In most cases,

identified problems are handled by educating those involved with the intent of avoiding the problems in the future. In cases of fraud or abuse by practitioners or patients, legal action may be taken.

E. Standards

1. Although in DUE/DUR the term "standards" is sometimes used interchangeably with the term "criteria," standards are technically defined as "deviations from the criteria screens which we are willing to accept" (4).

2. In RDUR, standards may be set using statistics. For example, the standard for prescribing patterns may be set at two standard deviations from the mean for prescribers in a given peer group. This means that those setting the standard are willing to accept prescribing patterns that are within two standard deviations of the mean; those that fall outside two standard deviations are questioned. In this example, if statistical analysis of a set of nursing home patients shows that $15\% \pm 3\%$ of these patients are taking sleeping medications, then if more than 21% ($15\% + 2 \times 3\% = 21\%$) of the nursing home patients for a given practitioner are taking sleeping meds, the prescribing patterns of that particular practitioner exceed the set standard. The prescriber is said to "except out." He or she is contacted to determine if there are extenuating circumstances to justify this exceptional pattern. If not, the practitioner is given educational materials about currently accepted practices in the prescribing of sleeping medications for the elderly. Notice that the practice patterns are compared within the peer group of nursing home patients, not the population as a whole. This procedure is called **exception processing**. It often uses claims data for the statistical analysis and for the identification of practitioners who are outliers.

3. A standard may be tied to a DUE or MUE criterion. For example, a DUE criterion for a drug may be a dosage range of 50 to 100 mg daily. A standard for ProDUR based on this criterion may say that any medication orders outside this range must be checked by a pharmacist. The DUE criteria may also be used to set a standard for RDUR. In setting RDUR standards using DUE criteria, it is understood that a certain number of situations exist in which a dose outside the given range is medically necessary. Therefore, a possible RDUR standard might be: 75% of all prescription orders should be within the DUE dosage range criteria. The hospital or insurer monitors prescription or medication orders. If more than 25% of orders for this drug fall outside the 50 to 100 mg per day range, the situation is investigated and reviewed.

4. Pharmacists should realize that criteria and standards are used in the DUR computer packages available as part of dispensing systems. For example, software packages that screen for drug-drug interactions are based on set standards. The level at which a flag for a drug-drug interaction appears when a new prescription order is entered may be set anywhere from "serious interactions of major clinical significance" to "minor or moderate interactions." Pharmacists should be knowledgeable about their software system and should know the level of significance for these flags. With some software, the standard or level of significance can be selected by the pharmacist. Pharmacists should never rely solely on these computer aids. An interaction of minor significance in the general population may be important to an individual patient under certain circumstances.

II. HISTORY

A. Drug Utilization Review (DUR)

1. DUR is a DUE/DUR process of evaluation that has been mandated by our federal and state governments for several decades and is required by organizations that seek government funding for medical services provided to the elderly (patients 65 years of age and older, Medicare recipients) and indigent (Medicaid recipients) patient populations.

2. The funding of health care began in the 1930s with the creation of the Social Security Act. Medicare and Medicaid came into existence in the 1960s to address

the financial needs of patients in nursing facilities. In 1967 Congress authorized the first set of standards (Federal Indicators) for nursing facilities. Since that time, several regulations have been adopted and amended. Although Long-Term Care (LTC) facilities and hospitals have been under these regulations for the longest period of time, outpatient providers of care, including Managed Care Organizations (MCO), Home Health Care agencies, mail order pharmacies, and so forth, are also included under these regulations. Outpatient prescribing practices were brought into the review process in the 1990s with the passage of the Omnibus Budget Reconciliation Act of 1990 (OBRA 90).

3. OBRA 90 mandated the formation of state DUR boards for use in state Medicaid programs providing outpatient prescription services. The intent of OBRA 90 was to increase patient education and to promote the appropriate use of medication through prescribing practices and therefore to control health care costs funded by the government (5).

4. The United States Pharmacopoeia (USP) developed and published standards of care to be incorporated by these DUR boards. Standards are set by regulation and enforced by the Health Care Finance Administration (HCFA). The focus of these standards was to prevent:
   a. Over/underutilization of drug
   b. Duplication of therapy
   c. Drug-drug, drug-food, drug-disease, and drug allergy interactions
   d. Incorrect dosage or duration
   e. Clinical abuse or misuse

5. In addition to these standards, in 2001 the USP adopted Principles Supporting Appropriate Drug Use (6) to guide prescribers and health care systems in decisions affecting pharmacotherapy in regards to patient care, formulary management, and reimbursement issues. These principles address:
   a. Drug selection
   b. Individualization of patient care
   c. Monitoring of medication therapy
   d. Education of patients
   e. Utilization

6. OBRA was revised by the HCFA in 1999 to incorporate quality indicators into the review of nursing facilities. The indicators are intended to evaluate the quality of the process and the outcomes of care. There are 24 indicators grouped into 11 domains of care. Medications are a focus of evaluation in these specific domains (clinical management, infection control, psychotropic drug use, and quality of life indicators) but should not be excluded from the evaluations set forth in the other domains of care.

7. LTC facilities are evaluated according to the OBRA regulations as well as the Beers Criteria (7), which were published in 1997 and were included in the revision of OBRA in 1999. These criteria were also incorporated to assist in the evaluation of potential inappropriateness of medication use by elderly patients in LTC facilities. The criteria are categorized according to high and low severity levels and identify specific medications as well as disease and medication combinations that could be inappropriate.

B. Medication Use Evaluation (MUE)

1. MUE is a more recent concept than DUE or DUR. "ASHP Guidelines on Medication-Use Evaluation" was approved in 1996 (3) and was adopted to replace the "ASHP Guidelines on the Pharmacist's Role in Drug-Use Evaluation," dated Nov. 19, 1987 (2).

2. Unlike DUR, MUEs are not mandated by government regulations. Health care practices seeking accreditation status will be subjected to an evaluation of the MUE processes by the appropriate agency/organization.

3. MUE satisfies JCAHO's Medication Use Standards TX.3: address the medication use processes of an organization (8). Medication-use evaluation is addressed in several of the standards and addresses the availability of patient medication information, the review of

the medication order prior to dispensing, the evaluation of the medication use in terms of prescribing, preparation and dispensing, administration and monitoring, the presence of a collaborative approach to medication management, and the incorporation of the evaluation results into the organization's performance improvement process.

III. PROFESSIONAL ASSOCIATION PRACTICE STANDARDS COVERING DUR

The codes of ethics and practice standards for professional associations of pharmacists address the issue of the responsibility of the pharmacist for conducting DUR and DUE.

A. The American Pharmaceutical Association Code of Ethics for Pharmacists addresses this issue in a general sense with these statements:

   1. "Pharmacists are health professionals who assist individuals in making the best use of medications."

   2. "[A] pharmacist promises to help individuals achieve optimum benefit from their medications, to be committed to their welfare, and to maintain their trust" (9).

B. The American Society of Health-System Pharmacists (ASHP) has adopted and published a series of documents that speak to the responsibility of the pharmacist in this area of practice.
   1. The most current guidelines for DUE are contained in "ASHP Guidelines on Medication-Use Evaluation."
   2. A second document, "ASHP Statement on Pharmaceutical Care," states the ASHP philosophy that pharmaceutical care "merits the highest priority in all practice settings" (10). In providing this type of service, ASHP sees as major functions of the pharmacist the identification, resolution, and prevention of medication-related problems caused by untreated indications, improper drug selection, subtherapeutic dosage, failure to receive medication, overdosage, adverse drug reactions, drug interactions, and medication use without indication (10).
   3. A third document, also approved in April 1996, is "ASHP Guidelines on a Standardized Method for Pharmaceutical Care." All three documents can be accessed through the ASHP web site at www.ashp.org.

IV. GOVERNMENT REGULATIONS CONCERNING DUR

A. Federal Law
   DUR is addressed in OBRA 90. It requires that the states establish DUR regulations for Medicaid patients. Refer to the discussion in the History section above for a more detailed description of OBRA 90. Specifically, in 42 U.S.C. §1396r-8:

   (i) "The state plan shall provide for a review of drug therapy before each prescription is filled or delivered to an individual receiving benefits under this subchapter, typically at the point-of-sale or point of distribution. The review shall include screening for potential drug therapy problems due to therapeutic duplication, drug-disease contraindication, drug-drug interactions (including serious interaction with nonprescription or over-the-counter drugs), incorrect drug dosage or duration of drug treatment, drug-allergy interactions and clinical abuse/misuse."

   (ii) "As part of the State's prospective drug use review program—applicable state law shall establish standards for counseling of individuals receiving benefits— by pharmacists which includes . . . (5)"

B. State Laws
   1. DUR is required in all states, as described in OBRA 90 federal regulations. Pharmacists should be knowledgeable about the applicable statutes requiring DUR activities for the states in which they are practicing.

2. The NABP "Model Rules for Pharmaceutical Care" states that:

> "A Pharmacist shall review the patient record and each Prescription Drug Order presented for Dispensing for purposes of promoting therapeutic appropriateness by identifying:
>
> **(1)** Over-utilization or under-utilization;
>
> **(2)** Therapeutic duplication;
>
> **(3)** Drug-disease contraindications;
>
> **(4)** Drug-Drug interactions;
>
> **(5)** Incorrect Drug dosage or duration of drug treatment;
>
> **(6)** Drug-allergy interactions; and
>
> **(7)** Clinical abuse/misuse" (11).

V. PATIENT MEDICATION PROFILE RECORDS

A. Comprehensive and accurate patient medication profile records are necessary tools in performing any form of medication evaluation.

B. The "National Association of Boards of Pharmacy Model Rules for Pharmaceutical Care" addresses the issue of recommended patient records systems for pharmacies. (This document can be accessed on the CD that accompanies this book.) Note that these Model Rules recommend that these patient records be kept for not less than 5 years from the date of the last profile entry (11).

C. Reviewing the prescription order
The following list identifies information that should be available and reviewed. Some of the items in the list are in the NABP Model Act, and some of the information is required by law in some states for inclusion on patient medication profile records that are to be maintained by pharmacies. Be sure to check the applicable laws for the state in which you practice.
1. Patient identification information: name, address, telephone number, date of birth, gender
2. Patient medical history: allergies, adverse drug reactions, idiosyncrasies, history of chronic conditions and medical and surgical events, use of drug products or devices (either prescription or over-the-counter) that are not in the dispensing record, and pharmacists' comments or interventions. If there are none, this should be indicated.
3. Other useful patient information: height, weight, occupation, any additional helpful information such as inability to use safety closures or swallow tablets or capsules
4. If applicable, information on third-party payers (insurance, medical assistance)
5. Information for each prescription order dispensed
    a. Drug product information—name (generic and/or brand), strength, and dosage form
    b. Quantity dispensed
    c. Directions for use—should identify dose, frequency and route of administration, and, if not treating a chronic lifetime condition, duration of use
    d. Therapeutic indication or when known the diagnosis related to the prescription order
    e. Supplemental information and warnings (i.e., administration instructions)
    f. Prescriber identification and contact information

    g. Retrieval designation assigned to the prescription order

    h. Date of dispensing, initial and all renewals

    i. Identification of dispensing pharmacist

VI.   PROSPECTIVE DUR ELEMENTS

When a new or renewal prescription order is presented to the pharmacist, the following elements should be considered when evaluating the medication management:

A. Accuracy and completeness of the prescription order

B. Appropriateness of dose, route of administration, dosage schedule and dosage form in relation to disease, patient- and medication-specific characteristics

C. Previous allergic reaction or adverse events with the prescribed drug or with a drug that is similar structurally or therapeutically. Be sure to ask the patient or caregiver about both allergies and adverse events.

D. Unexpected changes in dose and/or schedule when presented with a new prescription order for a currently used medication

E. Quantitative misuse of current medications by the patient, which could indicate adherence problems or therapeutic failures of the medication management
    1. Overutilization
    2. Underutilization

F. Undesired medication management due to:
    1. Contraindications
    2. Drug-drug interactions
    3. Drug-disease interactions
    4. Drug-laboratory interactions
    5. Therapeutic duplication, including specific ingredients, therapeutic class, or possible additive effects of dissimilar drug entities (e.g., sedating antihistamines and narcotic analgesics)

G. Check prescription and nonprescription product usage as well as self-management with alternative therapies.

H. Drugs that have a high risk profile due to interaction potential, narrow therapeutic window, unknown reactions due to new drug entity, interaction with specific patient populations (chronic illness, life-threatening illness, multiple medication regimen, greater than or equal to 9 doses per day, 65 years of age or older, etc.)

I. Specific medications as well as disease and medication combinations that could be inappropriate

VII.   WHAT TO DO WHEN A PROBLEM IS IDENTIFIED

A. General rules for dealing with patients and other health professionals concerning a problem with drug therapy:
    1. Always be tactful.
    2. No matter what the problem (including overutilization, failure to adhere to prescribed therapy, illogical prescribing, etc.), approach patients, caregivers, and health care providers with the assumption that there is a good reason or a logical explanation for the prescribed therapy or the present course of action.

B. Considerations

1. Severity of the problem. This must be considered because it affects your course of action.

2. A potential problem with a new prescription or medication order

    a. The problem is manageable.

        (1) Dispense the order as written. For example:

            (a) There may be an interaction, but no special precautions are necessary.

            (b) There may be an interaction, but it can be accommodated with appropriate patient consultation on use of the medication and/or therapy monitoring.

        (2) A change in therapy is possibly needed.

            (a) Contact the prescriber first:

                i. Briefly describe the problem.

                ii. If possible, give a reference source for your information.

                iii. Have suggestions ready for alternatives.

    b. The problem is non-manageable.

        (1) If the problem cannot be resolved to your satisfaction, you may decide not to dispense the medication.

        (2) You should fully inform the patient of your concerns and actions on his or her behalf.

        (3) Document your intervention.

3. A potential problem with current existing therapy

    a. There is a problem with overuse or adherence in the use of a current medication.

        (1) Talk with the patient. Remember to be tactful and assume there is a logical reason for the suspected overuse or nonadherence.

        (2) If a problem exists, alert the patient's physician so that together you can work with the patient to solve the problem.

        (3) Document the intervention.

    b. There is a new adverse event as a result of current therapy.

        (1) Get detailed information from the patient about the adverse reaction: for example, what happens, when, specific circumstances, and medications being used concurrently.

        (2) Discuss the problem with the patient's physician:

            (a) Briefly describe the problem.

            (b) Have suggestions ready for alternatives.

        (3) Document the intervention.

        (4) If this is a serious adverse event, report it to the FDA. Report forms, including both on-line and printed forms that can be mailed or faxed, are available on the FDA web site at www.fda.gov under the MedWatch system.

References

1. Principles of a Sound Drug Formulary System. www.usp.org/information/principle.htm. Accessed December 2002.
2. ASHP guidelines on the pharmacist's role in drug use evaluation. Am J Hosp Pharm 1988; 45: 385–386.
3. ASHP guidelines on medication-use evaluation. Am J Health-Syst Pharm. 1996; 53: 1953–1955.
4. Palumbo FB. Drug use review under OBRA 90. US Pharmacist 1993; 18: 84–92.
5. Omnibus Budget Reconciliation Act of 1990, 42 U.S.C. §1396r-8.
6. Guiding principles supporting appropriate drug use at the patient and population level. Statement of scientific policy, Council of Experts Information Executive Committee, United States Pharmacopeia Convention, Inc., March 12, 2001. www.usp.org/information/index.htm Accessed December 2002.
7. Explicit criteria for determining potentially inappropriate medication use by the elderly: An update. Arch Int Med 1997; 157: 1531–1536.

8. Comprehensive accreditation manual for hospitals, The official handbook. Joint Commission on Accreditation of Healthcare Organizations. Oakbrook Terrace, IL, 2000.

9. Code of Ethics for Pharmacists' adopted by the membership of the American Pharmaceutical Association. Washington, DC, October 27, 1994.

10. ASHP statement on pharmaceutical care. Am J Hosp Pharm 1993;50: 1720–1723.

11. National Association of Boards of Pharmacy Model Rules for Pharmaceutical Care. National Association of Boards of Pharmacy. Park Ridge, IL, 2001; 83.

CHAPTER 6

Patient Consultation

I. PROFESSIONAL STANDARDS OF PRACTICE

A. Although it may seem to you that talking with patients about their medications is a normal function of pharmacists, this has not always been true. From the 1940s until the late 1960s, ethical codes for pharmacists advised them *against* discussing medications with their patients. There was concern that pharmacists could disrupt the patient–physician relationship if they discussed with patients topics like therapeutic indications, side effects, precautions, and so on. To give you a sense of the evolution of standards of practice concerning sharing information with patients during this era, consider the following excepts from the codes of ethics of the American Pharmaceutical Association (APhA) in 1952 versus 1969 (1):

1952 "The pharmacist does not discuss the therapeutic effects or composition of a prescription with a patient. When such questions are asked, he suggests that the qualified practitioner (physician or dentist) is the proper person with whom such matters should be discussed."

1969 "A pharmacist should hold the health and safety of patients to be of first consideration; he should render to each patient the full measure of his ability as an essential health practitioner."

B. The current codes of ethics and standards of practice promulgated by APhA, the American Society of Health-System Pharmacists (ASHP), the American Association of Colleges of Pharmacy (AACP), and other pharmacy associations promote patient education as a primary professional responsibility of pharmacists.

   1. The APhA Code of Ethics is given in Appendix I. Statements from this Code that address the issue of patient consultation and pharmacist-patient communication include:

      a. "Pharmacists are health professionals who assist individuals in making the best use of medications."

      b. "A Pharmacist promotes the right of self-determination and recognizes individual self-worth by encouraging patients to participate in decisions about their health. A pharmacist communicates with patients in terms that are understandable. In all cases, a pharmacist respects personal and cultural differences among patients."

      c. "[A] pharmacist promises to help individuals achieve optimum benefit from their medications, to be committed to their welfare, and to maintain their trust" (2).

   2. The "ASHP Guidelines on Pharmacist-Conducted Patient Education and Counseling" is a three-page document that, as its name implies, provides more complete guidelines to the pharmacist on this area of practice. These guidelines are very well written and useful and are recommended reading for pharmacy students and pharmacists in all practice settings. The full document can be accessed on the ASHP web site at www.ashp.org. The first paragraph in the introductory "Purpose" section states the following:

> "Providing pharmaceutical care entails accepting responsibility for patients' pharmacotherapeutic outcomes. Pharmacists can contribute to positive outcomes by educating and counseling patients to prepare and motivate them to follow their pharmacotherapeutic regimens and monitoring plans. The purpose of this document is to help pharmacists provide effective patient education and counseling" (3).

II.   STATE LAW

A. Because professions like pharmacy, medicine, and law are regulated by state laws, the legal responsibilities of these professionals vary from state to state. As part of their pharmacy practice acts, some states have had requirements for pharmacist consultation of their patients for some years. Other states have codified this requirement more recently.

B. To provide more uniformity of regulation from state to state, the National Association of Boards of Pharmacy (NABP) published in 1990 its version of a model patient counseling requirement. A copy of this resolution is shown in Figure 6.1. It includes a definition of patient counseling and lists the specific areas of counseling.

C. The NABP "Model Rules for Pharmaceutical Care" (see the CD that accompanies this book) states that

> "Upon receipt of a prescription drug order and following a review of the patient's record, a Pharmacist shall personally initiate discussion of matters which will enhance or optimize drug therapy with each patient or caregiver of such patient (4)."

The pharmacist is encouraged to consult with the patient or caregiver in person but may use the telephone, if necessary. The "Model Rules" further state that alternative means of communication, such as information leaflets, pictogram labels, or videotapes, shall be used to **supplement** the discussion when this is appropriate (4).

D. The elements recommended in the "Model Rules" for discussion with patients include:
   1. Name and description of the drug
   2. Dosage form, dose, route of administration, and duration of drug therapy
   3. Intended use of the drug and expected action
   4. Special directions and precautions for preparation, administration, and use by the patient
   5. Common severe side effects or adverse effects or interactions and therapeutic contraindications that may be encountered, including their avoidance, and the action required if they occur
   6. Techniques for self-monitoring drug therapy
   7. Proper storage
   8. Prescription refill information
   9. Action to be taken in the event of a missed dose
   10. Pharmacist comments relevant to the individual's drug therapy, including any other information peculiar to the specific patient or drug (4).

E. To further emphasize the importance of patient consultation, Section 5 (the section of the "Model Rules" that addresses unprofessional conduct) lists the following as an act of unprofessional conduct on the part of a pharmacist or pharmacy: "Attempting to circumvent the Patient Counseling requirements, or discouraging patients from receiving Patient Counseling concerning their Prescription Drug Orders" (5).

F. Although NABP may recommend model pharmacy practice legislation, it is up to individual state governments to introduce and pass recommended legislation. States may and

■ **Figure 6.1** NABP Model Regulations for Patient Counseling.

NATIONAL ASSOCIATION OF BOARDS OF PHARMACY

Resolution No.: 86-5-90

Title: Model Regulation for Patient Counseling

Source: Committee on Law Enforcement/ Legislation & Committee on Pharmacy Practice

COMMITTEE RECOMMENDATIONS:

DO PASS

WHEREAS, the membership of NABP at its 84th Annual Meeting overwhelmingly supported mandatory patient counseling and endorsed the development of model regulations,

THEREFORE BE IT RESOLVED, that the committees on law Enforcement/Legislation and Pharmacy Practice recommend the inclusion of the following Model Regulation for Patient Counseling in the Model State Pharmacy Act and Model Regulations:

SECTION 1. DEFINITION OF PATIENT COUNSELING

"Patient Counseling" shall mean the effective communication by the pharmacist of information, as defined in this act, to the patient or caregiver, in order to improve therapeutic outcomes by maximizing proper use of prescription medications and devices. Specific areas of counseling shall include:

a) Name and description of the medication;
b) Route dosage, administration, and continuity of therapy;
c) Special directions for use by the patient as deemed necessary by the pharmacist;
d) Side effects or interactions that may be encountered, which may interfere with the proper use of the medication or device as was intended by the prescriber, and the action required if they occur;

SECTION 2. PATIENT INFORMATION

In order to effectively counsel patients, the pharmacist shall make a reasonable effort to obtain, record, and maintain the following patient information:

a) Name, address, telephone number;
b) Date of birth (age), gender;
c) Medical History
   1. Disease state(s)
   2. Allergies/drug reactions
   3. Current list of medications and devices;
d) Pharmacist comments

SECTION 3. COMMUNICATION TO THE PATIENT

a) A pharmacist shall counsel the patient or caregiver "face to face" when possible or appropriate. If this is not possible, a pharmacist shall make a reasonable effort to counsel the patient or caregiver;
b) Alternative forms of patient information may be used to supplement patient counseling;
c) Patient counseling as described above and defined in the "Practice of Pharmacy," Section 104 of this Model Act, shall also be required for outpatient and discharge patients of hospitals and institutions;
d) Patient counseling as described above and defined in the "Practice of Pharmacy," Section 104 of this Model Act, shall not required for inpatients of a hospital or institution where a nurse or other licensed health care professional is authorized to administer the medication(s); and
e) The pharmacist shall maintain appropriate patient-oriented reference materials for use by the patient upon request.

do customize such rules for their own purposes. Because all states have now codified requirements for patient counseling by pharmacists, consult the pharmacy practice act for the state in which you are practicing to determine the specific requirements of your state law on patient counseling.

III. FEDERAL LAW

A. If regulation of professional practice is left to the states, just how does the federal government get involved? You are surely aware of the concern the federal government has for bringing and keeping medical costs under control. The government is particularly concerned about medical costs when it has to pay the bill. With this in mind, Congress included in the Omnibus Budget Reconciliation Act (OBRA) of 1990 provisions aimed at controlling escalating medical costs for entitlement programs. Under OBRA 90, pharmacists are held responsible for patient counseling and are required to perform drug utilization review (DUR). This was the result of a series of studies issued by the Office of the Inspector General (OIG) for the Department of Health and Human Services. Essentially, the studies found that clinical functions performed by pharmacists that monitor drug therapy and that help patients to use their medications appropriately are valuable medical services and ultimately reduce the costs of providing medical care (6–8). Although OBRA technically covers just Medicaid patients, most pharmacists feel they are ethically bound to provide these services to all their patients.

B. Excerpts from OBRA 90 (42 U.S.C.§ 1396r—8) that are relevant to patient consultation requirements for pharmacists are given in Figure 6.2.

C. For an excellent review article on this subject, see "OBRA 90: Patient Counseling—Enhancing Patient Outcomes" in *U.S. Pharmacist,* January 1993 (9).

IV. GENERAL GUIDELINES FOR PATIENT COUNSELING

There are many excellent journal articles, books, and programs available to pharmacy students and pharmacists on the subject of educating and counseling patients concerning their medications and pharmacotherapy. A good list of references can be found at the end of the ASHP "Guidelines on Pharmacist-Conducted Patient Education and Counseling." The sections that follow provide a basic introduction to this subject. Although this information is written primarily from the point of view of a patient receiving counseling in an ambulatory setting, the principles can be easily applied to any practice setting.

A. Appropriate physical environment
   1. Discussion with patients or caregivers about health, pharmacotherapy, and other medical issues is a very private activity. This aspect of patient counseling is critical and should be respected no matter what the practice site is: hospital room, clinic, busy community pharmacy, or drive-up window. Some means of conducting this activity in a confidential area is essential. If the environment precludes privacy (e.g., a drive-up window), the pharmacist should make arrangements with the patient to discuss the relevant issues by telephone.
   2. To perform this service well, the pharmacy should also provide an environment that feels comfortable and unrushed. Although this may be difficult in some pharmacy practice sites, the option is always available to make a telephone call to the patient at a later, mutually convenient time. Patients and caregivers should understand that optimal medication use is achieved as a cooperative effort, and the communication between the pharmacist and patient is a vital link in this process.

B. Before you prepare the prescription:
   The consultation process begins not when you transfer the prescription to the patient, but as you receive the prescription order from the patient or the agent of the patient.
   1. Input from the patient
      a. Ask the patient or caregiver if there is any information you should have before preparing the prescription. For example, has the doctor given the patient any special instructions? Can the patient open child-resistant safety closures? What about language issues; can the patient read labeling in English?

■ **Figure 6.2** Excerpts from the Omnibus Budget Reconciliation Act of 1990.

101st Congress   House of Representatives   Report
2nd Session   101-934

Omnibus Budget Reconcilation Act of 1990

Excerpts from OBRA 90(42 U.S.C. § 1396r-8)

(ii) As part of the State's prospective drug use review program—applicable state law shall establish standards for counseling individuals receiving benefits—by pharmacists which includes at least the following:

(I) The pharmacist must offer to discuss with each individual—or caregiver of such individual (in person, whenever practicable, or through access to a telephone service which is toll-free for long-distance calls)—who present a prescription, matters which in the exercise of the pharmacist's professional judgement (consistent with State law respecting the provision of such information), the pharmacist deems significant including the following:

    (aa) The name and description of the medication.
    (bb) The route, dosage form, dosage, route of administration and duration of drug therapy.

    (cc) Special directions and precautions for preparation, administration and use by the patient
    (dd) Common severe side effects or adverse effects or interactions and therapeutic contraindications that may be encountered, including their avoidance and the action required if they occur.
    (ee) Techniques for self-monitoring drug therapy.
    (ff) Proper storage.
    (gg) Prescription refill information.

(II) A reasonable effort must be made by the pharmacist to obtain, record and maintain at least the following information regarding individuals receiving benefits under this subchapter:

    (aa) Name, address, telephone number, date of birth (or age) and gender.
    (bb) Individual history where significant including disease state or states, known allergies and drug reactions and a comprehensive list of medications and relevant devices.
    (cc) Pharmacist comments relevant to the individual's drug therapy. Nothing in this clause shall be construed as requiring a pharmacist to provide consultation when an invidual receiving benefits under this subchapter or carefiver of such individual refused such consultation.

October 27 (Legislative Day October 26, 1990).—Ordered to be printed

---

    b. An issue of increasing relevance is that of third-party coverage for prescription medications. Some plans have formulary restrictions concerning what medications will be covered. Patients may need help in understanding that a formulary restriction does not mean that they cannot obtain a prescribed medication, but it may mean that the patient has to pay for that medication or the pharmacy may need prior authorization for payment. These can be complex issues, especially for patients, but they are important in patient care, and explanations and discussions should take place in an atmosphere of patience and mutual respect.

    c. If the prescription order is for a branded product, check if a generic equivalent can legally be dispensed. If so, does the patient want a generic product? What are the implications with respect to both therapy and cost to the patient and third-party coverage and co-payments?

  2. Review of the patient's medication record

    a. Perform the normal prospective DUR assessments as described in Chapter 5. Are there any contraindications to the new therapy, any drug-drug interactions, etc.?

    b. Look for problems with the new prescription, and also review the patient's total drug therapy.

    (i)   Do there appear to be problems with adherence to or overutilization of existing therapy? (See the final section of Chapter 5 on "What to Do When a Problem is Identified.")

    (ii)   Does this patient need a "pep talk" or advice on strategies concerning adherence issues?

    (iii)   Are there possible helpful hints you may give the patient? For example, if the patient is taking other medications, he or she would probably like to know about taking more than one drug product at the same time.

    (iv)   Would a dosing aid, such as a pill reminder box, a tablet crusher, or a pocket pill box, be helpful?

C. When delivering the prescription to the patient:

Imagine yourself as the patient, and then practice "the golden rule."

1. It is helpful to give the patient an estimate of the length of time the consultation requires. Recognize the patient's right to refuse counseling. Most patients are appreciative of your professional advice and counsel; however, circumstances may exist that interfere with a complete counseling encounter. For example, a patient may be very ill and just want or need to get home to bed. Perhaps the patient is a sick child, and the parent or caregiver is not, at this moment, in a position to be attentive to your counseling. Be sensitive of these types of needs. In cases like this, you may want to give only the essential information and offer to call the patient or caregiver later, or ask the patient or caregiver to call you at a mutually convenient time for a more complete consultation. Patients who are in pain or other distress probably are not able to concentrate on what you are saying. When they have returned to the familiar surroundings of their home and have experienced some relief, they probably are better able to understand you and remember what you have told them. Questions about the use of their medication may also have come to mind.

2. Maintain a professional, sincere attitude. Use a professional but friendly, relaxed, and sincere demeanor. This attitude should help put the patient at ease and foster an atmosphere that encourages the patient to ask questions.

3. Use language appropriate to the needs and level of understanding of the patient. Avoid technical medical terms and jargon unless you are talking with a fellow medical practitioner, such as a nurse or physician. At the same time, do not "talk down" to the patient. Many patients are very knowledgeable; assessing their level of understanding is essential to a good counseling experience. Listening to the patient and discussing the medication with the patient rather than lecturing about it helps you to assess the patient's level of knowledge and understanding.

4. The pharmacist's role in promoting the right of self-determination for patients is explicitly stated in the APhA Code of Ethics, so it is essential that pharmacists inform patients about both positive and negative aspects of their therapy. By the same token, necessary precautions should be disclosed in a tactful way. Think about how you would feel about taking a medication if you were warned by your pharmacist that you may cough up blood, stop breathing, or go into convulsions. Would you want to take such a medication?

5. Notice the patient's body language. Watch the patient's face for feedback. Do the eyes indicate that you are being understood? Does the patient appear to be interested in what you are saying, or have you obviously lost contact?

6. Be aware of cultural differences among patients. If you deal with patients who have different cultural backgrounds from your own, make it a point to learn about cultural issues that will help you in communicating most effectively with these patients.

V. TOPICS FOR PATIENT COUNSELING

Guidelines that give recommended patient counseling topics have been published by professional pharmacy associations and government agencies. Below are some suggestions concerning consultation topics using the consultation template shown in Figure 6.3.

■ **Figure 6.3** Patient consultation template

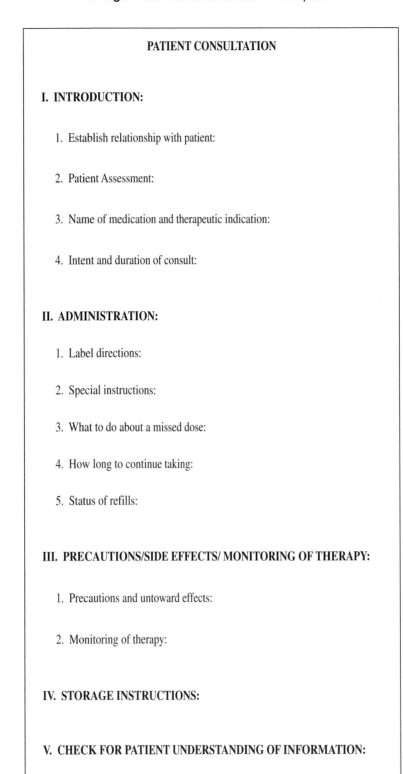

PATIENT CONSULTATION

I. INTRODUCTION:

    1. Establish relationship with patient:

    2. Patient Assessment:

    3. Name of medication and therapeutic indication:

    4. Intent and duration of consult:

II. ADMINISTRATION:

    1. Label directions:

    2. Special instructions:

    3. What to do about a missed dose:

    4. How long to continue taking:

    5. Status of refills:

III. PRECAUTIONS/SIDE EFFECTS/ MONITORING OF THERAPY:

    1. Precautions and untoward effects:

    2. Monitoring of therapy:

IV. STORAGE INSTRUCTIONS:

V. CHECK FOR PATIENT UNDERSTANDING OF INFORMATION:

I. Introduction

   1. Establish relationship with patient.

   Introduce yourself to the patient if he or she is not known to you. Find out whether you are talking directly with the patient, a family member, or some other agent of the patient. You may want to find out how the patient prefers to be addressed. Some patients liked to be called by their first names, whereas others may be offended by such familiarity. This is also your opportunity to get an initial sense of the level of understanding of the patient.

   2. Patient assessment

   a. Find out the patient's understanding of the prescribed medication and the medical condition it is intended to treat. What did the prescriber tell the patient? Does he or she know what the medication is called, its usual therapeutic intent, and why it was prescribed for this patient? Did the prescriber tell the patient how to take or use the medication and for how long? What is the patient to expect from this therapy?

   b. Ask the patient if he or she has ever taken medication like this before. If so, what was the result? Has the patient ever had either an unusual or allergic reaction to a medication of this type?

   c. Is the patient taking any other medications that might not be listed on the medication profile, including nonprescription drugs like aspirin or cough-and-cold medications? What about alternative therapies such a nutritional or dietary supplements, herbals, etc.?

   d. If the prescription is a refill, ask questions to determine the effectiveness of the therapy. Rather than just asking if the patient has any questions, find out if he or she thinks that the medication is "working." Is he or she experiencing any side effects? What times of day are the doses being taken? Are there problems with scheduling doses or adherence to the prescribed schedule? How is the patient feeling? What kind of medication or health-related problems, if any, is he or she experiencing?

   3. Name of medication and therapeutic indication

   a. From the patient assessment, you know the patient's current understanding of the medication. Therefore, you need not repeat any information that the patient already knows.

   b. It is **essential** to establish with the patient the name and therapeutic indication of the medication being dispensed. This is an important safeguard in preventing dispensing errors. Many drug names look or sound alike. You can provide some protection against dispensing errors if you cover this quick and easy point of information. Be sure to do this in a confidential and private manner. Nothing can destroy the rapport that you are building with the patient so rapidly as breaching confidentiality concerning his or her health and medical status.

   4. Intent and duration of consult

   a. Offer to spend a few minutes with the patient to give advice on the effective use of the prescribed medication and to answer any questions.

   b. If the use and monitoring of the medication is complicated and needs an extended consult, be honest with the patient about this. He or she may want to be told the essentials with an agreed time for a more complete conversation.

   c. Be sensitive to patients who are obviously ill. They may need a brief consult with a follow-up phone call.

II. Administration

   1. Label directions

   a. Repeat the directions for use on the label, including information on auxiliary labels.

   b. This is a convenient time to open the container and show the patient the physical appearance of the product. It is also a good last check that the correct medication is in the container.

   c. Check the label one last time as you do this.

   2. Special instructions

   a. Give any special instructions, such as take on an empty stomach or swallow tablets whole.

b. If you have a special dosage form, such as an inhaler, ophthalmic drops, or suppositories, make sure that the patient knows how to use the product. In some cases you may need to demonstrate the use of the product. Helpful leaflets or visual aids may be given to the patient; these are especially helpful because the multiple steps involved in using these dosage forms are difficult to remember until they have been reinforced by the patient's use of the product.

   3. What to do about a missed dose

    a. Help the patient to establish clear, **specific** guidelines for deciding when, and if, to skip or double forgotten doses. Just what does the phrase "almost time for your next dose" mean in their particular case?

    b. Offer strategies to aid adherence with therapy.

   4. How long to continue taking

   Patients need to know if medications should be taken only when needed, on schedule until the prescription is all gone, for the rest of their life, or until told to discontinue by their doctor.

   5. Status of refills

    a. Are refills authorized? If so, how many? How does the patient order needed refills?

    b. Are there any special circumstances? For example, if the patient is seriously ill and is taking Schedule II pain medication, be sure you give information on how he or she can get more needed medication. Do not just say that there are no refills with this medication.

III.   Precautions/side effects/monitoring therapy

   1. Precautions and untoward effects

   Communicating about precautions and untoward effects is probably the area of greatest difficulty for pharmacists: How much should I say? What are the most important issues? Will I scare the patient if I talk about possible serious side effects? As discussed above, current philosophy concerning drug therapy holds that patients have the right to self-determination and that they should be given full information about proposed therapy so that they can make informed decisions about their own health care. (See the excerpts of the APhA Code of Ethics for Pharmacists at the beginning of this chapter.)

    a. Some drugs have many potential side effects; emphasize those side effects or precautions that are of major or moderate clinical significance.

    b. Distinguish between those side effects that may be annoying but of no clinical harm, and those that require a physician's attention.

    c. If a side effect can be minimized by timing of administration, such as by taking the medication with food or by taking on an empty stomach, communicate this information to the patient.

   2. Monitoring of therapy

   Monitoring of therapy can be anything from encouraging the patient to see the physician for follow-up checks or lab work, to giving instructions on how to watch for signs of improvement or sharing warning signals of potential drug toxicity.

➤ *EXAMPLE*

    To give you some sense for what and how to cover information in this section, read the information below that one veteran clinical pharmacist typically relates to her patients about side effects, precautions, and therapy monitoring for the use of controlled-release theophylline products with initial prescription orders for these products. Although theophylline is now used less frequently because of issues with safety and drug interactions, as well as the introduction and use of effective long-acting beta-agonists, this example illustrates very well how to give information on a medication with a complex profile.

      1. This is a potent medication that should be used with caution. Take it as directed; do not switch brands without first checking with your doctor; let your doctor know if you start any new medications or if you stop taking any medications that you are currently taking.

2. The most common side effects are those usually associated with drinking too much coffee or caffeinated soda—jittery, can't sleep, headaches. These usually go away as your body adjusts to the medicine and are minimized if you avoid or limit extra stimulants, such as caffeinated beverages.

3. Some people experience stomach upset (nausea, vomiting, heartburn). This is minimized by taking your medication with food.

4. If any side effect continues or if you notice anything more serious, such as diarrhea or pounding heart, consult your doctor immediately.

5. Be sure to keep any follow-up appointments with your physician and report any problems with control of your asthma or adverse effects of this medication to your physician or to me so appropriate action can be taken.

IV. Storage instructions

1. These instructions are given in the *USP/DI* and product package inserts. The usual instructions are to keep out of the reach of children, in a place with moderate temperature, and away from high humidity.

2. You may have to balance proper storage recommendations against adherence issues. If the patient explains that he or she can only remember to take medication by keeping it in a place that is routinely accessed like the kitchen cupboard, your professional judgment may say that adherence is more important than providing perfect protection from the relatively high humidity found in many kitchens.

V. Check for patient understanding of information.

Ask questions to be sure that the patient understands all necessary information, but do this in a pleasant way– you obviously do not want to sound like a teacher giving a quiz. Perhaps you can determine patient understanding in a way that puts the responsibility for any missed or inadequate communication on yourself rather than on the patient. You may want to say, "I know I covered a lot of information. So that I am sure I didn't forget any important points, why don't you tell me about your understanding of what I've said?"

VI. ASSESSMENT OF CONSULTATION SKILLS

To aid you in evaluating your consultation skills and to help you monitor your progress, an assessment tool is shown in Figure 6.4. This is a sample form used by pharmacy preceptors and clinical faculty to evaluate the patient consultations of pharmacy students in their clerkships and internships. You might want to ask a friend or family member to use this tool in evaluating your skills as you practice this aspect of professional practice.

References

1. Higby GJ. Pharmacy in the American century. Pharmacy Times 1997; 63:16–24.
2. Code of Ethics for Pharmacists adopted by the membership of the American Pharmaceutical Association, October 27, 1994.
3. American Society of Health-System Pharmacists. ASHP Guidelines on Pharmacist-Conducted Patient Education and Counseling. Am J Health-Syst Pharm 1997; 54: 431–434.
4. National Association of Boards of Pharmacy Model Rules for Pharmaceutical Care. National Association of Boards of Pharmacy, Park Ridge, IL, 2001; 84.
5. National Association of Boards of Pharmacy Model Rules for Pharmaceutical Care. National Association of Boards of Pharmacy, Park Ridge, IL, 2001; 95.
6. Office of Inspector General-Office of Analysis and Inspections. The clinical role of the community pharmacist. Department of Health and Human Services. Publication OAI-01-89-89020. January 1990.
7. Office of Inspector General-Office of Analysis and Inspections. State discipline of pharmacists. Department of Health and Human Services. Publication OAI-01-89-89160. January 1990.
8. Office of Inspector General-Office of Analysis and Inspections. Medication regimens: causes of noncompliance. Department of Health and Human Services. Publication OAI-04-89-89121. March 1990.
9. Hatoum HT, Hutchinson RA, Lambert BL. OBRA 90: Patient counseling—enhancing patient outcomes. US Pharmacist 1993; 18:76–84.

■ **Figure 6.4** Evaluation form for student/pharmacist-conducted patient consulting.

Student Name: _____

Date: _____

Instructor/Preceptor: _____

The evaluation of each patient consultation is based on both the process and content of the patient counseling session using this EVALUATION OF PATIENT CONSULTING document.

EVALUATION OF PATIENT CONSULTING

I. PROCESS

    A. Introduction / Establishment of Rapport

                Prescription Number:_____

                Score:_____

      1. No introduction by student to the patient including name, explanation of role, purpose of medication counseling session and estimated time of the session.
      2. Needs improvement in introduction, explanation of the purpose of the session; however, some of this information provided.
      3. Good. Introduces self, attempts to establish rapport with patient and describes purpose of session and duration to patient.
      4. Very good. Establishes rapport with patient via introduction of self, with a patient specific focus to reasons for the counseling session.
      5. Outstanding. Patient specific rapport established which is an asset to the counseling session and discussion of intent, session duration.

    B. Verbal: Audible, Articulate, Appropriate Rate, Variable Tone

                Prescription Number:_____

                Score:_____

      1. Poor, hard to hear or understand. Mumbles and/or delivery shows lack of interest. Rate too fast or too slow. Many pronunciation errors or inappropriate use of medical terms.
      2. Needs improvement in loudness. Sometimes monotone without interest in material. Some pronunciation errors or inappropriate use of medical terms.
      3. Good. Adequate loudness but some words lost to mumbling. Tone and rate reflect interest in material. Some errors in pronunciation or inappropriate use of medical terms.
      4. Very good. Audible with good enunciation. Tone and rate reflect interest in material. No error in pronunciation or inappropriate use of medical terms.
      5. Outstanding. Audible, good enunciation. Appropriate rate and tone to reflect interest. Easy to listen to. Proper pronunciation and use of medical terms

    C. Nonverbal: Distracting Mannerisms, Eye Contact

                Prescription Number:_____

                Score:_____

      1. Poor. Mannerisms so distracting, presentation content was lost. No eye contact.
      2. Needs improvement. Mannerisms very distracting. Little eye contact. Reads all of medication handouts.
      3. Good. Few distracting mannerisms. Good eye contact. Relies on reading notes and prescription labels.
      4. Very good. No distracting mannerisms; appropriate gestures. Very good eye contact. Notes and labels used only as a reference.
      5. Outstanding. No distractions. Shows polish, poise as speaker. Outstanding eye contact, rarely relies on notes.

    D. Confidence

                Prescription Number:_____

                Score:_____

      1. Fails to display confidence in self.
      2. Seldom displays confidence in self during the session.
      3. Occasionally displays confidence in self.
      4. Frequently displays confidence in self.
      5. Consistently and appropriately to the situation displays a high degree of confidence in self.

■ **Figure 6.4** *(continued)*

E. Summary/Feedback and Checking for Understanding

Prescription Number:_____

Score:_____

1. No summary or checking with the patient to verify understanding of information provided.
3. Attempts to summarize or check for patient understanding.
5. Provides a comprehensive and appropriate summary of information. Verifies patient understanding and expands upon questions/issues raised.

PRESCRIPTION NUMBER:_____

TOTAL SCORE:_____

II. CONTENT

Please use the scale below to evaluate each of the criteria concerning the content of the medication counseling session.

1 Deficits Exit	2 Marginal	3 Good	4 Very Good	5 Truly Exceptional	6 N/A
Needs extensive intervention; Sometimes the preceptor must complete the task.	Needs consistent intervention; Preceptor must provide directed questioning in a problem-solving manner.	Requires only occasional intervention consisting of a single limited prompt.	Requires no intervention; Performs within expections.	Requires no intervention; Performs above exceptions; The student teaches faculty something new.	Not applicable.

CRITERIA	Prescription Number:
Data Gathering (Allergies, ADRs, Current Medications, Insurance, Disability)	
Medication Name and Indication (Brand and/or Generic Name. Indication Patient Specific with time to benefit).	
Administration- When, How, Duration (Information is patient specific. First dose information provided. Duration and administration issues (food, empty stomach, etc addressed).	
Untoward Effects (Major adverse effects which are patient specific are addressed).	
Self-Monitoring/Cautions (Patient specific therapeutic endpoints, management for adverse effects and cautions addressed).	
Storage, Refill (Patient specific refill, storage information provided).	

Prescription Number
_____

Section I (Process):
Total Points   _____

Section II (Content);
Total Points   _____

TOTAL   _____

PART 2

CALCULATIONS

CHAPTER 7

Quantity and Concentration Expressions and Calculations

I. INTRODUCTION

An essential function of pharmacy service is to ensure that patients get the intended drug in the correct amount. These are two important components of the five recognized "rights" of patients in receiving medication: the right drug in the right dose by the right route of administration to the right patient at the right time. Although providing the correct drug in the correct amount is considered a basic right of medical care, the difficulty of ensuring that it occurs for all patients 100% of the time is evident in the various studies of medical errors, including the famous 1999 Institute of Medicine report, "To Err is Human." That the health professions continue to struggle with this issue is evident in that incorrect doses and administration of the wrong drug product continue to be in the top tier of causes of medication errors as reported by hospitals that are part of USP's MedMARx error reporting network (1). Although medication safety is a joint responsibility of all members of the health care team, it is clearly an area in which pharmacists can and do play a major role.

Basic to providing the correct amounts of drug products to patients is a firm understanding of the dimensions or units of measurement for drugs and the expressions of quantity and concentration for drug products. Further, the pharmacist must know how to use this information to perform the calculations needed in providing correct and intended drug therapy. The purposes of this chapter address this subject:

1. To review the dimensions of quantity that are used pharmaceutically
2. To explain and illustrate accepted methods of expressing drug concentration in pharmaceutical products and preparations
3. To present sample calculations that illustrate different methods for determining quantities of ingredients and concentration of drugs when preparing or dispensing drug products
4. To discuss and illustrate special cases of expressing quantities and concentrations.

This information forms the basis for understanding the important topic of evaluating doses and dosage regimens, which is presented in Chapter 8. It will also be used in Part 5 of this book, Dosage Forms and Their Preparation. Most importantly, this information is vital to providing safe and effective therapy to patients.

▮ II. ▮ EXPRESSIONS OF QUANTITY OF DRUG

A. The following factors determine the accepted method for representing the quantity of a drug.

1. Accurate representation of the amount of the active principle, a drug molecule, acting at a receptor

2. Convenience of measurement

3. Route of administration

4. Tradition

B. Pharmaceutically useful dimensions of quantity

Note: Appendix C contains the units for the International (SI), Metric, and Common Systems of measurement.

1. Weight of drug (microgram [mcg], milligram [mg], gram [g], grain [gr]); for example, Diazepam 5 mg

CAUTION:

- The abbreviation "gr" is for the Apothecary grain, not the Metric gram. If there is any uncertainty, check with the prescriber.

- The SI symbol for micro is "μ," so the abbreviation for microgram would be "μg"; because when handwritten this symbol can be misread as mg, in health care the recommended abbreviation for microgram is mcg.

2. Volume of drug (milliliter [mL], liter [L], drop [gtt]); for example, Glacial Acetic Acid 2 drops

3. Units (used for insulin, some antibiotics, some vitamins, and certain other natural products); for example, NPH Insulin 25 units

CAUTION: A unit is an expression of potency that differs for each biological substance measured in units. Therefore, the unit markings on a U-100 Insulin syringe can be used to measure only Insulin, and only U-100 Insulin (that is, Insulin that has a concentration of 100 units per mL).

4. Molecules, moles, millimoles, and molecular weights

a. One **molecule** of a substance is too small a quantity to be pharmaceutically useful because we always deal with fairly large numbers of molecules. Instead of counting molecules, it is therefore convenient to measure in terms of a larger unit. Usually the unit used for this purpose is the **mole** (abbreviated mol), which is Avogadro's number (6.023×10^{23}) of molecules.

b. The **molecular weight** (MW) of a compound is the weight in grams of one mole of the compound; that is, it is the weight in grams of 6.023×10^{23} molecules. For example, the MW of water is 18.0, meaning that 18.0 g of water contains 6.023×10^{23} molecules of water. Similarly, the MW of phenobarbital is 232.2, meaning that 232.2 g of phenobarbital contains 6.023×10^{23} molecules of phenobarbital. Because elements, ions, and molecules react in integral ratios (1:1, 1:2, and so on), the mole is a more fundamentally useful unit than is the gram, but the gram offers convenience of measurement.

c. **Millimoles** (mmol) often are used in pharmacy and medicine rather than moles because the required quantities and concentrations of drugs are relatively small. There are 1,000 mmol per mole of a compound. The number of grams per mole (the molecular weight) is also equal to the number of mg per mmol; for example, 1 mmol of phenobarbital weighs 232.2 mg.

One example of a drug that traditionally has had its dose expressed in millimoles is phosphate when administered for electrolyte replacement. In this case we are interested in the amount of phosphorus, the P part of the phosphate, and we need a way to get at this. One millimole of phosphate, whether in the form $H_2PO_4^{-1}$, HPO_4^{-2}, or PO_4^{-3}, contains the same amount of phosphorus, P, but all three forms have different weights (and different numbers of milliequivalents).

➤ *EXAMPLE CALCULATION 7.1:*

Calculate the weight in grams from moles:

You have a formula that calls for 0.5 moles of Sodium Hydroxide (NaOH). Sodium Hydroxide is available as a solid. How many grams of NaOH should you weigh? The MW of NaOH = 40.

$$\left(\frac{40\,g\,NaOH}{mole\,NaOH}\right)\left(\frac{0.5\,moles\,NaOH}{}\right) = 20\,g\,NaOH$$

➤ *EXAMPLE CALCULATION 7.2:*

Calculate millimoles from weight in milligrams:

You have a liquid formulation that has 600 mg of Potassium Chloride (KCl) in each teaspoonful of syrup. You want to know how many millimoles of KCl this would be. The MW of KCl is 74.5.

$$\left(\frac{mmol\,KCl}{74.5\,mg\,KCl}\right)\left(\frac{600\,mg\,KCl}{}\right) = 8\,mmol\,KCl$$

5. Equivalents, milliequivalents, and equivalent weights

   a. When dealing with electrolytes in solution, we are at times interested in only one of the ion pair. For example, with mineral acids, we may be interested only in the number of H^+ ions in solution. We do not care about the counter ion, the Cl^-, the $SO_4^=$, the NO_3^-, and so on. Therefore, we do not care about the weight of the acid present, or the number of moles of compound present; we want to know how many moles of H^+ are present. The concept of equivalents evolved from this special need.

   b. **Equivalents,** sometimes referred to as combining power, is the number of univalent counter ions needed to react with each molecule of the substance. Hydrochloric acid (HCl) has one equivalent per mole because one mole of the univalent ion OH^- reacts exactly with one mole of H^+ in HCl. (Also note that one mole of Na^+ reacts exactly with one mole of Cl^- in HCl.) Sulfuric acid (H_2SO_4) contains two equivalents per mole because two moles of OH^- are required to react with one mole of sulfuric acid. The compound $Al_2(SO_4)_3$ has six equivalents per mole because in aqueous solution two Al^{+3} ions are obtained for each $Al_2(SO_4)_3$ and they would react with six univalent anions, such as six Cl^-s. The sulfate ($3\,SO_4^{-2}$) also reacts with six univalent counter ions, such as six H^+s.

   c. The definition of equivalent depends upon the particular type of reaction undergone, so it is subject to some ambiguity. The number of equivalents per mole for electrolytes with variable valence like phosphate and carbonate depends on the pH of solution (Na_2HPO_4 with two equivalents/mol is predominant at high pH, whereas NaH_2PO_4 with one equivalent/mol predominates at lower pH). For this reason, phosphate concentration for replacement therapy is always expressed in terms of mmol rather as mEq.

   d. The **equivalent weight** of an element or compound is that weight which combines chemically with one equivalent of another element or compound. The equivalent weight of HCl is its molecular weight because this compound has one equivalent per mole and reacts with one equivalent of another compound. The equivalent weight of sulfuric acid is its molecular weight divided by 2 because sulfuric acid has two equivalents per mole. The equivalent weight of aluminum sulfate is its molecular weight divided by 6 because there are six equivalents per mole. This can be expressed by the general equation:

$$Equivalent\,Weight = \frac{Atomic\,or\,Molecular\,Weight\,of\,the\,Substance}{Number\,of\,Equivalents\,per\,Atomic\,or\,Molecular\,Weight}$$

   e. **Milliequivalents** (mEq), rather than equivalents, are used often in pharmacy and medicine because, when dosing electrolytes, we are usually dealing with small quantities. There are 1,000 mEq per equivalent. The number of equivalents/mol for a given compound equals the number of mEq/mmol for that substance.

f. Electrolytes such as potassium, sodium, calcium, and chloride often are dosed in terms of milliequivalents because, from a therapeutic point of view, it is the individual ion that is of interest. Often the method of expressing the dose of an electrolyte may be a matter of tradition. For example, oral doses of calcium usually are given in terms of milligrams or grams of the compound (e.g., calcium carbonate 500 mg), whereas parenteral electrolyte replacement doses usually are expressed in terms of milliequivalents of calcium (e.g., Ca^{++} 4.6 mEq).

g. There is a trend toward expressing electrolyte doses in terms of milligrams of the pertinent ion rather than as milliequivalents of the ion or milligrams of the salt.

   (1) This method has the advantage of being unambiguous, and it is the system now used internationally. For example, the intravenous dose of Calcium Chloride is given in the *2002 USP/DI* as "500 mg to 1 gram (136 to 272 mg of calcium ion)" rather than as milliequivalents of calcium.

   (2) As is often the case when there is a change in systems, errors of misinterpretation can occur; there have been reports of doses written in terms of milligrams of the salt (e.g., 500 mg Calcium Chloride) and interpreted and administered as milligrams of the ion (e.g., 500 mg calcium ion, which is 1,836 mg of the Calcium Chloride, nearly a four-fold overdose). Pharmacists must be **very careful** when interpreting these orders.

➤ *EXAMPLE CALCULATION 7.3:*

Calculate weight in milligrams of the **salt** from milliequivalents:

A potassium supplement tablet contains 10 mEq of KCl. How many milligrams of KCl are in each tablet? The MW of KCl = 74.5.

$$\left(\frac{74.5\ mg\ KCl}{mmol\ KCl}\right)\left(\frac{mmol\ KCl}{1\ mEq\ KCl}\right)\left(\frac{10\ mEq\ KCl}{}\right) = 745\ mg\ KCl$$

➤ *EXAMPLE CALCULATION 7.4:*

Calculate weight in milligrams of **salt** from milligrams of the **ion**:

A dose of Calcium Chloride is given as 136 mg of calcium ion. How many milligrams of Calcium Chloride are needed? Calcium Chloride is available as the monohydrate ($CaCl_2 \cdot H_2O$), which has a MW = 147; calcium ion has an atomic weight of 40.

$$\left(\frac{147\ mg\ CaCl_2 \cdot H_2O}{40\ mg\ Ca}\right)\left(\frac{136\ mg\ Ca}{}\right) = 500\ mg\ CaCl_2 \cdot H_2O$$

➤ *EXAMPLE CALCULATION 7.5:*

Calculate milliequivalents from weight in milligrams of salt:

The powder for oral solution for a bowel cleansing product contains 568 mg of anhydrous Sodium Sulfate (Na_2SO_4). How many milliequivalents of Na are in this product? The MW of Na_2SO_4 = 142.

$$\left(\frac{2\ mEq\ Na}{1\ mmol\ Na_2SO_4}\right)\left(\frac{mmol\ Na_2SO_4}{142\ mg\ Na_2SO_4}\right)\left(\frac{568\ mg\ Na_2SO_4}{}\right) = 8\ mEq\ Na$$

6. Osmols and milliosmols

a. Osmotic pressure is discussed in some detail in Chapter 10. Basically, pharmaceutical solutions that come in contact with cell membranes should have the same osmotic pressure as the cell contents to prevent tissue damage and discomfort. Because osmotic pressure is a colligative property, it depends on the number of individual solute particles (ions or molecules) per given volume of solution.

    b. An **osmol** is the number of moles of solute present multiplied by the number of particles per molecule obtained when the solute is dissolved in water. Nonelectrolytes, such as dextrose, do not dissociate in solution, so one mole of dextrose yields one osmol. Sodium chloride dissociates into two ions in aqueous solution, so one mole of sodium chloride gives two osmols. Sodium sulfate (Na_2SO_4) gives three ions per molecule, so there are three osmols per mole of sodium sulfate.

    c. **Milliosmols** (mOsmol), rather than osmols, are used often in pharmacy and medicine. There are 1,000 mOsmol per osmol. The number of osmol/mol for a given compound equals the number of mOsmol/mmol for that substance.

    d. If a drug or chemical is present in solid form as a hydrate (e.g., $MgSO_4 \bullet H_2O$), the water molecules do not count as particles because they merely become part of the solvent in aqueous solution.

➤ *EXAMPLE CALCULATION 7.6:*
    Calculate osmols from weight in grams:
    Isotonic Sodium Chloride Solution has 9 g of NaCl in each liter of solution. How many osmols are there in each liter of solution? The MW of NaCl = 58.5.

$$\left(\frac{2\ osmol}{mol\ NaCl} \right)\left(\frac{mol\ NaCl}{58.5\ g\ NaCl} \right)\left(\frac{9\ g\ NaCl}{L} \right) = 0.308\ osmol/L$$

➤ *EXAMPLE CALCULATION 7.7:*
    Calculate milligrams from milliosmols:
    You want to add solute to a liter of water so that there are 300 mOsmol in this solution. Your source of solute is Magnesium Sulfate Heptahydrate ($MgSO_4 \bullet 7H_2O$), which has MW = 246.5. How many milligrams of this solute should you add?

$$\left(\frac{246.5\ mg\ MgSO_4}{mmol\ MgSO_4} \right)\left(\frac{mmol\ MgSO_4}{2\ mOsmol} \right)\left(\frac{300\ mOsmol}{} \right) = 36,975\ mg\ MgSO_4$$

III. EXPRESSIONS OF CONCENTRATION

    A. Concentration gives **quantity of drug** or active ingredient **per** amount (volume or weight) of product or preparation.

    B. Concentrations are always used for expressing doses for topical preparations. In this case, concentration has conceptual importance because concentration gradient is the driving force for transfer of the drug across the membrane or barrier, such as the skin.

    C. Concentration also is used to express the strength of liquid systemic products; for example, Amoxicillin 250 mg/5 mL, or Dextrose 5% in Water.

    D. For individual dosage units such as capsules, tablets, and suppositories, the dose is expressed as a quantity of drug rather than as a concentration (e.g., Diazepam 5 mg). However, because pure drug is almost never dispensed, these quantities are technically concentrations. For example, when the label on a bottle of Aspirin states Aspirin 325 mg, what is really meant is Aspirin 325 mg **per** tablet. Because the tablet contains other ingredients (excipients such as binders, disintegrants, lubricants) besides the Aspirin, the tablet weighs more than 325 mg and the content could be given as a concentration; for example, Aspirin 325 mg per 450 mg of tablet material.

    E. Pharmaceutically useful expressions of concentration
      1. Weight of active ingredient per weight of product; for example, Gentamicin Ophthalmic Ointment 3 mg/g is 3 mg of gentamicin in each 1 g of ointment

2. Weight of active ingredient per volume of product; for example, Tobramycin Ophthalmic Solution 3 mg/mL is 3 mg of Tobramycin in each 1 mL of solution; Amoxicillin Suspension 250 mg/5 mL is 250 mg of Amoxicillin per 5 mL of suspension

3. Molarity, molality, mmol/L
   a. **Molarity** (M) is the number of moles of solute per **liter of solution**. For example, a 1 M solution of sodium hydroxide contains one mole of sodium hydroxide per liter of solution. Because the molecular weight of sodium hydroxide is 40.0, a 1 M solution of sodium hydroxide contains 40.0 grams of sodium hydroxide per liter of solution (40 g/L) or 40 mg/mL.
   b. **Molality** (m) is the number of moles of solute per **1,000 grams of solvent.**
   c. For dilute aqueous solutions, the numeric values of molarity and molality are nearly equal. This is because water has a density of approximately 1.0 g/mL, and because the small amount of solute takes up very little volume in the solution, and the density of the solution is also very close to 1.0 g/mL. This does not hold true for solutions with a large amount of solute, and when the densities of the solvent and solution are not equal to 1.0. The example given below for Syrup NF is a good illustration of the large difference in molarity and molality for a concentrated solution.
   d. Other concentration terms used in pharmacy include mmol/mL or mmol/L.

➤ **EXAMPLE CALCULATION 7.8:**

Calculate molarity from grams of solute per milliliter of solution:

Diluted Hydrochloric Acid NF contains 10 g of HCl in 100 mL of solution. Calculate its molarity. The MW of HCl = 36.5.

$$\left(\frac{mol\ HCl}{36.5\ g\ HCl}\right)\left(\frac{10\ g\ HCl}{100\ mL}\right)\left(\frac{1000\ mL}{L}\right) = 2.74\ mol/L = 2.74\ M$$

➤ **EXAMPLE CALCULATION 7.9:**

Calculate the grams of solute per liter from molarity:

You want to make 500 mL of a 1 M solution of Sulfuric Acid (H_2SO_4). How many grams of H_2SO_4 do you need? The MW of H_2SO_4 = 98.1.

$$\left(\frac{98.1\ g\ H_2SO_4}{mol\ H_2SO_4}\right)\left(\frac{1\ mol\ H_2SO_4}{L}\right)\left(\frac{0.5\ L}{}\right) = 49.1\ g\ H_2SO_4$$

➤ **EXAMPLE CALCULATION 7.10:**

Calculate the molarity and the molality of a solution from its weight/volume concentration and the density of the solution:

Syrup NF contains 850 g of Sucrose in 1000 mL of solution. The solution has a density of 1.3. The MW of Sucrose = 342.

Molarity (*M*) of the solution:

$$\left(\frac{mol\ Sucrose}{342\ g\ Sucrose}\right)\left(\frac{850\ g\ Sucrose}{1000\ mL\ solution}\right)\left(\frac{1000\ mL\ solution}{L}\right) = 2.49\ mol/L = 2.49\ M$$

Molality (*m*) of the solution:

To calculate the molality of the solution, we first must calculate the weight of the solution using its density, and then calculate the weight of the solvent, water.

Grams of solution per L:

$$\left(\frac{1.3\ g\ solution}{mL\ solution}\right)\left(\frac{1000\ mL\ solution}{L}\right) = 1300\ g\ solution/L\ solution$$

Remembering that weights are additive,

Grams of solute + Grams of solvent = Grams of solution

850 g Sucrose + x g of water = 1,300 g of solution/L

x g of water = 1,300 g solution—850 g Sucrose = 450 g water/L solution

Calculation of molality of the solution:

$$\left(\frac{mol\ Sucrose}{342\ g\ Sucrose}\right)\left(\frac{850\ g\ Sucrose}{L\ solution}\right)\left(\frac{L\ solution}{450\ g\ water}\right)\left(\frac{1000\ g\ water}{kg\ water}\right) = 5.5\ mol/kg = 5.5\ m$$

➤ **EXAMPLE CALCULATION 7.11:**

Calculate mmol/L from milligrams per milliliter:

To conform with the international system of units, reporting of cholesterol blood plasma levels has changed from milligram per deciliter (1 dL = 100 mL) to millimoles per liter. A patient's medical record from a former hospitalization shows a cholesterol level of 230 mg/dL. What is the equivalent of this level in mmol/L? The MW of cholesterol = 387.

$$\left(\frac{mmol\ Choles.}{387\ mg\ Choles.}\right)\left(\frac{230\ mg\ Choles.}{100\ mL}\right)\left(\frac{1000\ mL}{L}\right) = 5.94\ mmol\ Cholesterol/L$$

4. Normality and mEq/L
   a. **Normality** (N) is the number of equivalents per liter of solution.
      (1) A 1 N solution of HCl has one equivalent/liter. Because the molecular weight of HCl is 36.5 g and because there is one equivalent per mole, a 1 N solution has 36.5 g of HCl per liter of solution, and a 1 N solution of HCl equals a 1 M solution of HCl.
      (2) A 1 N solution of sulfuric acid also has one equivalent/liter. However, because sulfuric acid has two equivalents per mole, a 1 N solution of sulfuric acid has 49.0 g (half the molecular weight) of sulfuric acid per liter of solution. In this case, a 1 N solution of H_2SO_4 equals a 0.5 M solution of H_2SO_4.
      (3) Both solutions, 1 N HCl and 1 N H_2SO_4, provide the same number of H^+ ions in each liter of solution.
   b. Other concentration terms used in pharmacy include mEq/L and mEq/mL.

➤ **EXAMPLE CALCULATION 7.12:**

Calculate grams per liter from normality:

You want to make 500 mL of a 1 N solution of Sulfuric Acid (H_2SO_4). How many grams of H_2SO_4 do you need? The MW of H_2SO_4 = 98.1.

Note: This problem is similar to that given in the molarity section except that it asks for a 1 N solution rather than a 1 M solution.

$$\left(\frac{98.1\ g\ H_2SO_4}{mol\ H_2SO_4}\right)\left(\frac{mol\ H_2SO_4}{2\ Equiv.}\right)\left(\frac{1\ Equiv.}{L}\right)\left(\frac{0.5\ L}{}\right) = 24.5\ g\ H_2SO_4$$

➤ **EXAMPLE CALCULATION 7.13:**

Calculate mEq/mL from grams per milliliter:

You have a pint of Potassium Chloride Syrup that is labeled 10% (10 g KCl per 100 mL of solution). You want to know the concentration in mEq per 15 mL (one tablespoonful). The MW of KCl is 74.5.

$$\left(\frac{1\ mEq\ K^+}{mmol\ KCl}\right)\left(\frac{mmol\ KCl}{74.5\ mg\ KCl}\right)\left(\frac{1000\ mg}{g}\right)\left(\frac{10\ g\ KCl}{100\ mL}\right)\left(\frac{15\ mL}{}\right) = 20.1\ mEq\ K^+$$

5. Osmolality and osmolarity
   a. The concepts of osmolality and osmolarity apply to aqueous solutions in contact with biological membranes.

b. For aqueous solutions, **osmolality** is the number of osmols per kilogram of water. For a nonelectrolyte that behaves ideally (no dissociation or association), a 1 molal (m) solution (one mole of the compound per kilogram of water) is also a 1 osmolal solution. For example, if the 85% sucrose solution in Example Calculation 7.10 behaved ideally, the 5.5 m solution would also be a 5.5 osmolal solution. For an aqueous solution of a univalent-univalent electrolyte such as NaCl, if behaving ideally and giving two ions per molecule, a 1 m solution would have an osmolality of 2 osmol/kg of water.

c. **Osmolarity** is the number of osmols per liter of solution. For a compound that does not ionize in water, a 1 molar (M) solution, which contains one mole of the compound per liter of solution, is also a 1 osmolar solution. For the 85% sucrose solution in Example Calculation 7.10, the 2.49 M solution would also be a 2.49 osmolar solution. For an aqueous solution of the univalent-univalent electrolyte NaCl, if behaving ideally and giving two ions per molecule, a 1 M solution would have an osmolarity of 2 osm/L of solution.

d. The concept of osmolarity/osmolality is an important one when dealing with solutions that come in contact with sensitive body tissues.

(1) The osmolarity of a solution that is isotonic with body fluids is approximately 0.307 osmol/L or 307 mOsmol/L.

(2) We try to match this osmolarity as closely as possible when we prepare pharmaceutical solutions that are administered parenterally or applied topically to sensitive membranes, such as the eye.

(3) For most adults, the lining of the gastrointestinal tract can tolerate highly hypertonic solutions (those of high osmolarity). In contrast, the gastrointestinal lining of neonates is sensitive to hypertonic solutions. Oral solutions for these infants should be close to 300 mOsmol/L.

e. As with molarity and molality, the numeric values for osmolality and osmolarity are very close in dilute solutions but can vary substantially with concentrated solutions. This is clearly illustrated with the 85% Sucrose Solution, which has calculated osmolality and osmolarity values of 5.5 osmol/kg and 2.49 osmol/L, respectively. It is very important to keep this difference in mind when you are given values in either osmolarity or osmolality.

(1) In clinical practice, osmolarity is used most frequently because we usually make pharmaceutical solutions to a volume, and we can calculate an estimate of osmolarity from the weights of the solutes, their molecular weights, and the expected number of particles per mole for each specie. The values obtained from such calculations are only estimates, because these calculations assume that the particles behave ideally: electrolytes completely dissociate and do not interact with each other, and none of the particles self-associate or interact with the water molecules. In reality, solutions, especially concentrated solutions, do not behave ideally. In the example above for the 85% Sucrose Solution (2.49 M or 5.5 m), the osmotic coefficient for this solution has been measured and it is approximately 1.45; that is, the effective osmotic pressure is approximately 1.45 times greater than the calculated value (2). The osmotic coefficient varies both with the solute and with concentration. Therefore, when true effective osmolarity is needed, it should be measured with an osmometer.

(2) Unfortunately, osmolarity cannot be measured directly. Osmometers, which are used in hospitals and laboratories, measure osmolality rather than osmolarity. For example, the specifications for the manufactured syrup vehicle Ora-Sweet® give the osmolality as 3,240 mOsm/kg. It is possible to calculate osmolarity from osmolality if the density of the solution is also known and if the concentration(s) of the solute(s) in the solution are known. In this case, the following equation can be used.

$$\text{Osmolarity} = \text{osmolality} \times (\text{solution density in g/mL} - \text{anhydrous solute concentration in g/mL})$$

➤ *EXAMPLE CALCULATION 7.14:*

Calculate milliosmols per liter from grams per milliliter:

Sodium Chloride Injection is 0.9% NaCl (0.9 g per 100 mL). Calculate its concentration in mOsmol/L. The MW of NaCl = 58.5.

$$\left(\frac{2\,mOsmol}{mmol\,NaCl}\right)\left(\frac{mmol\,NaCl}{58.5\,mg\,NaCl}\right)\left(\frac{900\,mg\,NaCl}{100\,mL}\right)\left(\frac{1000\,mL}{L}\right)=307.7\,mOsmol\,/\,L$$

➤ *EXAMPLE CALCULATION 7.15:*

Calculate milligrams per liter from mOsmol/L:

You need to make an oral calcium supplement for a neonate. You will use Calcium Gluconate as the source of calcium and you want the concentration of the solution to be 300 mOsmol/L. How many milligrams of Calcium Gluconate will you need to make a liter of solution? The MW of Calcium Gluconate = 430.4, and the formula is Ca(Gluconate)$_2$, which means that each molecule of Calcium Gluconate give 3 ions.

$$\left(\frac{430.4\,mg\,Ca\,Gluc.}{mmol\,Ca\,Gluc.}\right)\left(\frac{mmol\,Ca\,Gluc.}{3\,mOsmol}\right)\left(\frac{300\,mOsmol}{L}\right)=4304\,mg\,Ca\,Gluc.$$

6. Percent

a. Definitions

The General Notices of the *USP* state:

"The term *percent* used without qualification means, for mixtures of solids and semisolids, percent weight in weight; for solutions or suspensions of solids in liquids, percent weight in volume; for solutions of liquids in liquids, percent volume in volume; and for solutions of gases in liquids, percent weight in volume" (3).

These conventions are uniformly accepted in the scientific and medical communities.

b. In pharmacy and medicine, percentages are used for expressing concentrations of:

(1) Active ingredients in topical products

(2) Alcohol in both internal and external products

(3) Some ingredients in large-volume parenteral products

(4) Active ingredients in dosage forms for internal use (this is less common)

c. The various types of percent concentrations are illustrated by the examples given here. Numerous example calculations are given in section IV, Calculations of Concentration.

(1) Percent weight in weight (% w/w) for solids in solids: Hydrocortisone 1% Ointment is 1 gram Hydrocortisone powder in 100 grams of ointment mixture.

(2) Percent weight in volume (% w/v) for solids in liquids: Dextrose 5% in Water is 5 grams of Dextrose powder in 100 mL of solution.

(3) Percent volume in volume (% v/v) for liquids in liquids: Isopropyl Alcohol 70% is 70 mL of Isopropyl Alcohol in 100 mL of solution.

d. Exceptions to the General Notices rules on percent

(1) There are several major exceptions to the General Notices rules on percent. These include:

(a) Ethyl Alcohol

(b) Concentrated acids

(c) Formaldehyde

(2) In each of these cases, the active ingredient generally is not available to the pharmacist in pure form. It is available as a concentrated solution, which contains something less than 100% of the active ingredient.

(a) With Ethyl Alcohol we have a compound that requires special procedures to be made in pure form, so the commonly used form is a 95% v/v aqueous solution, Alcohol USP. In this case, although the pure compound, Dehydrated Alcohol USP, is available, it is much more expensive and it is not in general use.

   (b) In several instances, such as Hydrochloric Acid and Formaldehyde, the active ingredient is a gas. The only form generally available to the pharmacist is a concentrated aqueous solution.

   (3) When the above compounds are prescribed by percent, the pharmacist must determine whether the prescriber wants a v/v percent of the official liquid in the prescribed liquid vehicle (as described above for mixtures of liquids in liquids), or a percent (either by weight or volume) of the **pure compound** in the prescribed liquid vehicle.

   (4) For Alcohol, the situation is simplified by official notices in the *USP* that specify how the interpretation is to be made. These specifications can be found in the General Notices of the *USP*. They also are quoted in the section of this chapter devoted to special calculations involving Alcohol. To aid you in understanding how to apply these specifications when preparing compounded drug products, numerous examples are given in that section.

   (5) For concentrated acids and Formaldehyde, there are no official rules. Some examples and guidelines concerning percent mixtures of these compounds are discussed in section VI of this chapter, Special Calculations Involving Concentrated Acids.

7. Ratio Strength

   a. Concentrations of **very dilute** solutions or solid mixtures are sometimes expressed as ratio strengths rather than as percents. This notation has been used for many years, possibly because some pharmacists and physicians may think it is easier to visualize a dilute concentration written as 1:10,000 rather than as the percent 0.01%.

   b. The use of ratio strength notation is to be discouraged because the 1:x symbolism may be interpreted in two ways: the colon may be interpreted either as q.s. ad or as plus. By standard pharmaceutical definition, the colon stands for q.s. ad (4). That is, when a ratio strength of 1:1,000 is indicated, this is interpreted as follows:

   (1) *For solids in liquids*: 1 gram of solute or solid in 1,000 milliliters of solution or liquid preparation

   (2) *For liquids in liquids*: 1 milliliter of liquid constituent in 1,000 milliliters of solution or liquid preparation

   (3) *For solids in solids*: 1 gram of solid constituent in 1,000 grams of solid mixture

   c. An example of a preparation with concentration expressed as a ratio strength is the solid in liquid preparation Potassium Permanganate Solution 1:5,000, which is 1 gram of Potassium Permanganate crystals in 5,000 mL of solution.

   d. Not all prescribers are knowledgeable about the above conventions. You may get prescription orders that use ratio strength notation, and the prescriber intends the colon to be interpreted as a plus rather than the conventional q.s. ad.

   (1) Example:

   ℞

   Gentamicin ointment
   White Petrolatum   Mix 1:2
                          Dispense 30 g

   Two interpretations are possible:

   (a) If interpreted by official convention, this would be made by weighing one part of Gentamicin Ointment, then q.s. ad to two parts with White Petrolatum. In other words, there would be one part of Gentamicin Ointment and one part of White Petrolatum for a total of two parts.

   (b) The alternative *plus* interpretation would mean to mix one part of Gentamicin Ointment with two parts of White Petrolatum for a total of three parts.

(2) This ambiguity of interpretation causes no great inaccuracy if the solution or mixture is very dilute. If, however, as in the above example, the preparation is concentrated, a rather large error in product concentration would result from using the unintended interpretation. In cases like these, consult the prescriber for clarification.

(3) At times, internal evidence may give you a hint as to the intention of the prescriber. For example, if 8 ounces is prescribed and the ratio strength designation is 1:7, the desired interpretation of the colon is probably a plus; that is, 1 ounce of component A plus 7 ounces of component B to give a total of 8 ounces. In contrast, if 8 ounces is prescribed and the ratio strength designation is 1:8, the desired interpretation of the colon is probably a q.s. ad; that is, 1 ounce of component A plus 7 ounces of component B to give a total of 8 ounces. In the Gentamicin prescription given above, the internal evidence, 30 grams of product and three parts total product, would favor the plus interpretation. However, the prescriber should be consulted concerning the actual intent.

IV. CALCULATIONS OF CONCENTRATIONS

Below are examples illustrating several different methods of calculating amounts of ingredients and concentrations of finished products when making pharmaceutical preparations. In most cases four methods are illustrated for each problem: alligation, percent, proportion, and dimensional analysis. (The alligation method is also illustrated on the CD that accompanies this book.) When performing calculations like this, use the method that makes the most sense to you for the type of problem presented. Often a combination of methods is the most convenient. Although the examples below use liquids and solutions, the same general principles apply to calculations for solids.

Note: Although the alligation method is shown in the examples below, a mathematical description of this method is beyond the scope of this text. The relationships can be derived algebraically. For an explanation of this method, see a book on pharmaceutical calculations.

A. Calculate the amounts of two solutions of different strengths that must be combined to get a third solution of a specified strength.
General steps:
  1. Calculate the **quantity** of drug or chemical needed in the third solution.
  2. Calculate the volume(s) of each of the two given solutions that will give you this amount.

➤ **EXAMPLE 7.16:**

   You want to make 120 mL of a 50% solution of Isopropyl Alcohol (IPA). You have available pure 100% IPA and water. How many milliliters of each will you need?

• **By alligation:**

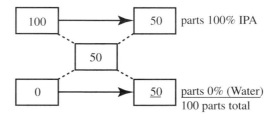

   In this case, in which you need to mix the solution in equal parts (50 parts of each), inspection shows that for 120 mL of final solution, you need 60 mL of each initial solution:
   ■ Pour 60 mL of 100% IPA into a graduated cylinder and add sufficient Purified Water to give 120 mL of solution.

- **By percent:**

  Rate (Percent) × Whole = Part

  50% × 120 *mL solution* = 60 *mL IPA*

  ■ Pour 60 mL of 100% Isopropyl Alcohol and add sufficient Purified Water to give 120 mL of solution.

- **By proportion:**

  By definition a 50% v/v solution of IPA means 50 mL of IPA/100 mL solution. Therefore,

$$\frac{50\ mL\ IPA}{100\ mL\ solution} = \frac{x\ mL\ IPA}{120\ mL\ solution};\ x = 60\ mL\ IPA$$

  ■ Pour 60 mL of 100% IPA and add sufficient Purified Water to give 120 mL of solution.

- **By dimensional analysis:**

  Again, by definition a 50% v/v solution of IPA means 50 mL of IPA/100 mL solution. Therefore,

$$\left(\frac{50\ mL\ IPA}{100\ mL\ solution}\right)\left(\frac{120\ mL\ solution}{}\right) = 60\ mL\ IPA\ needed$$

  ■ Pour 60 mL of 100% IPA and add sufficient Purified Water to give 120 mL of solution.

➤ *EXAMPLE 7.17:*

  You want to make the same solution (50% v/v IPA), but you only have available 70% IPA and water. How many milliliters of each do you need?

- **By alligation:**

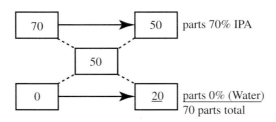

In this case, the numbers are less obvious, so you need to use extra math to calculate the volumes of the initial solutions to give the respective required parts. For example, by proportion:

$$\frac{50\ parts\ 70\%\ IPA}{70\ parts\ total} = \frac{x\ mL\ 70\%\ IPA}{120\ mL\ solution};\ x = 86\ mL\ 70\%\ IPA$$

  ■ Pour 86 mL of 70% IPA and add sufficient Purified Water to give 120 mL of solution.

- **By percent:**

  Rate (Percent) × Whole = Part

As in Example 7.16, we first need to calculate the amount (the *Part*) of IPA needed:

  50% × 120 mL solution = 60 mL IPA needed

Next, we need to find out how many milliliters of the 70% solution (the only one of the initial solutions to contain IPA) contain this needed 60 mL of IPA. We use the same general equation, but instead solve for the *Whole* term:

$$x = \frac{60\ mL\ IPA}{0.7} = 86\ mL\ of\ 70\%\ IPA\ solution$$

  70% × x mL of 70% IPA soln = 60 mL IPA

  ■ Pour 86 mL of 70% Isopropyl Alcohol and add sufficient Purified Water to give 120 mL of solution.

- **By proportion:**

Again, first determine the number of mL of IPA needed:

$$\frac{50 \; mL \; IPA}{100 \; mL \; solution} = \frac{x \; mL \; IPA}{120 \; mL \; solution}; x = 60 \; mL \; IPA$$

Then calculate the number of mL of 70% IPA that contains this amount:

$$\frac{70 \; mL \; IPA}{100 \; mL \; 70\% \; solution} = \frac{60 \; mL \; IPA}{x \; mL \; 70\% \; solution}; x = 86 \; mL \; 70\% \; IPA \; solution$$

- ■ Pour 86 mL of 70% Isopropyl Alcohol and add sufficient Purified Water to give 120 mL of solution.

- **By dimensional analysis:**

Again, first determine the number of mL of IPA needed:

$$\left(\frac{50 \; mL \; IPA}{100 \; mL \; solution} \right) = \left(\frac{120 \; mL \; solution}{} \right) = 60 \; mL \; IPA \; needed$$

Then calculate the number of mL of 70% IPA that contains this amount:

$$\left(\frac{100 \; mL \; 70\% \; IPA \; solution}{70 \; mL \; IPA} \right) \left(\frac{60 \; mL \; IPA}{} \right) = 86 \; mL \; 70\% \; IPA \; solution$$

- ■ Pour 86 mL of 70% Isopropyl Alcohol and add sufficient Purified Water to give 120 mL of solution.

➤ *EXAMPLE 7.18:*

You want to make the above solution (50% v/v IPA) and you want to use a 70% IPA solution and a 30% IPA solution (no pure water). How many milliliters of each will you need?

This example is a little more difficult. It can be solved using either algebra or alligation (a method derived from algebra).

- **By alligation:**

$$\frac{20 \; parts \; 70\% \; IPA}{40 \; parts \; total} = \frac{x \; mL \; 70\% \; IPA}{120 \; mL \; solution}; x = 60 \; mL \; 70\% \; IPA$$

$$\frac{20 \; parts \; 30\% \; IPA}{40 \; parts \; total} = \frac{x \; mL \; 30\% \; IPA}{120 \; mL \; solution}; x = 60 \; mL \; 30\% \; IPA$$

- ■ Pour 60 mL of 70% Isopropyl Alcohol and add 60 mL of 30% Isopropyl Alcohol to give 120 mL of solution.

- **By algebra:**

Let: x = the number of mL of 30% solution needed

y = the number of mL of 70% solution needed

Then: $x + y = 120 \; mL$

$x = 120 - y$

Also: $30\% \; x + 70\% \; y = 50\% \; (120 \; mL)$

Substituting for x and solving:

$$0.3\,(120 - y) + 0.7\,y = 0.5\,(120)$$
$$36 - 0.3\,y + 0.7\,y = 60$$
$$0.4\,y = 24$$
$$y = 60$$
$$x = 120 - y = 120 - 60 = 60$$

- Pour 60 mL of 70% Isopropyl Alcohol and add 60 mL of 30% Isopropyl Alcohol to give 120 mL of solution.

B. Calculate the final strength of a diluted or mixed solution when given the original strength(s) and volume(s).

General steps:
1. Calculate the **amount** of drug in the original solution(s).
2. Calculate the final volume of the new solution.
3. Calculate the concentration of the new solution by dividing the **amount** calculated in part 1 by the new volume calculated in part 2.
4. Express the final answer in the desired format (g/mL, mg/mL, percent).

➤ *EXAMPLE 7.19:*

You have 4 mL of Tobramycin Ophthalmic Solution 0.3%. You dilute it with 2 mL of Sterile Saline Solution. What is the percent strength of Tobramycin in the final solution?

1. Calculate the amount of drug Tobramycin in the original solution. By definition, 0.3% Tobramycin (Tob.) is 0.3 g per 100 mL. Multiply the concentration times the volume to get the amount of tobramycin in the given volume:

$$\left(\frac{0.3\ g\ Tob.}{100\ mL\ solution} \right)\left(\frac{4\ mL\ solution}{} \right) = 0.012\ g\ Tob.$$

Or, by proportion:

$$\frac{0.3\ g\ Tob.}{100\ mL\ solution} = \frac{x\ g\ Tob.}{4\ mL\ solution};\ x = 0.012\ g\ Tob.$$

2. Calculate the final volume of the new solution:

$$4\ mL + 2\ mL = 6\ mL$$

3. Calculate the concentration of the new solution by dividing the **amount,** 0.012 g, by the final volume, 6 mL.

$$\frac{0.012\ g\ Tob.}{6\ mL\ final\ solution} = 0.002\ g/mL$$

4. For a percent concentration, calculate the amount of drug per 100 mL.

$$0.002\ g/mL \times 100\ mL = 0.2\ g\ in\ 100\ mL\ or\ 0.2\%$$

You may want to use the information in this problem to check your understanding of the previous section. An example is given below.

➤ *EXAMPLE 7.20:*

Say that you want 6 mL of a 0.2% solution of Tobramycin. You have available a 0.3% solution and Sterile Saline. How much of each do you need? As shown above, there are several ways to approach solving this problem; one example is given below.

1. Calculate the amount of drug needed in the final solution.

$$0.2\% \times 6\ mL = 0.012\ g$$

2. Calculate the volume(s) of the given solutions that give you this amount.

$$\frac{0.3 \; g \; Tob.}{100 \; mL \; solution} = \frac{0.012 \; g \; Tob.}{x \; mL \; solution}; \; x = 4 \; ml \; solution$$

Measure 4 mL of the 0.3% solution and q.s. ad 6 mL with the Sterile Saline Solution.

➤ **EXAMPLE 7.21:**

You again have 4 mL of Tobramycin Ophthalmic Solution 0.3%. This time you fortify it with Tobramycin Injection 80 mg/2 mL. What is the concentration of Tobramycin in the final solution?

1. Calculate the amount of drug Tobramycin in the original solutions.

$$\left(\frac{0.3 \; g \; Tob.}{100 \; mL \; solution}\right) = \left(\frac{4 \; mL \; solution}{}\right) = 0.012 \; g \; Tob.$$

$$\left(\frac{80 \; mg \; Tob.}{2 \; mL \; solution}\right)\left(\frac{2 \; mL \; solution}{}\right) = 80 \; mg \; Tob. \; or \; 0.08 \; g \; Tob.$$

Total Tobramycin in both solutions $= 0.012 \; g \; + 0.08 \; g \; = 0.092 \; g \; \; Tob.$

2. Calculate the final volume of the new solution:

$$4 \; mL \; + 2 \; mL \; = 6 \; mL$$

3. Calculate the concentration of the new solution by dividing the **amount,** 0.092 g, by the final volume, 6 mL.

$$\frac{0.092 \; g \; Tob.}{6 \; mL \; final \; solution} = 0.0153 \; g \, / \, mL$$

4. For a percent concentration, calculate the amount of drug per 100 mL.

$$0.0153 \; g/mL \; \times \; 100 \; mL \; = 1.53 \; g \; in \; 100 \; mL \; or \; 1.53\%$$

Again, you may want to use the information in this problem to check your understanding of the previous section. An example is given below.

➤ **EXAMPLE 7.22:**

You receive a medication order for 6 mL of a fortified 1.5% ophthalmic solution of Tobramycin. You have available the 0.3% ophthalmic solution and the 80 mg/2 mL sterile injection. How many milliliters of each do you need?

This is a more difficult question, but it is similar to the third example in section A in which either alligation or algebra may be used. This problem occurs in practice situations, so it is important that you know how to solve a problem of this sort. One possible method is given below. No matter what method is used, consistent dimensional units must be used. In the sample calculation given below, all of the concentrations are expressed as percents by converting 80 mg/2 mL to a percent, 4%.

Let: $x =$ the number of mL of 0.3% solution needed
      $y =$ the number of mL of 4% (the 80 mg/2 mL injection) solution needed

Then: $x + y = 6 \; mL$
      $x = 6 - y$

Also: $0.3\% \; x + 4\% \; y = 1.5\% \; (6 \; mL)$

Substituting for x and solving:

$$0.003 \; (6 - y) + 0.04 \; y = 0.015 \; (6)$$
$$0.018 \; - 0.003 \; y + 0.04 \; y = 0.09$$
$$0.037 \; y = 0.072$$
$$y = 1.95 \; mL \; or \; 2 \; mL$$
$$x = 6 - y = 6 - 2 = 4$$

Note that the slight difference in the answer (1.95 mL versus 2 mL) is due to rounding the 1.53% of the previous problem to 1.5% in this problem.

➤ **EXAMPLE 7.23:**

You have an IM injectable solution of Edetate Solution 200 mg/mL. You put 10 mL of it in an empty sterile vial and dilute it with 3.3 mL of Procaine HCl 2% injection. What is the final concentration of the Edetate in mg/mL? What is the final concentration of the Procaine HCl in percent?

Edetate:

1. 200 mg/mL × 10 mL = 2,000 mg

2. 10 mL + 3.3 mL = 13.3 mL

3. 2,000 mg/13.3 mL = 150 mg/mL

Procaine HCl:

1. 2% = 2 g/100 mL   2 g/100 mL × 3.3 mL = 0.066 g

2. 10 mL + 3.3 mL = 13.3 mL

3. 0.066 g/13.3 mL = 0.005 g/mL

4. 0.005 g/mL × 100 = 0.5%

V.   SPECIAL CALCULATIONS INVOLVING ALCOHOL USP

In the General Notices section of the *USP,* it states:

"**Alcohol**–All statements of percentages of alcohol, such as under the heading *Alcohol content,* refer to percentage, by volume of C_2H_5OH at 15.56°. Where reference is made to "C_2H_5OH," the chemical entity possessing absolute (100 percent) strength is intended.

Alcohol–Where "alcohol" is called for in formulas, tests, and assays, the monograph article *Alcohol* is to be used" (5).

The General Notices in the *USP* also state that for labeling alcohol content:

"The content of alcohol in a liquid preparation shall be stated on the label as a percentage (v/v) of C_2H_5OH" (6).

The examples that follow are intended to aid you in understanding how to apply these specifications when preparing compounded drug preparations.

➤ **EXAMPLE 7.24:**

Contemporary Physicians Group Practice
20 S. Park Street, Triturate, WI 53706
Tel: (608) 555-1333 Fax: (608) 555-1335

℞ #

Name *Dalia Duck*   Date *00/00/00*

Address *521 Mill Pond Circle*   Age   Wt/Ht

℞

Clindamycin	*1%*
Alcohol	*15%*
Propylene Glycol	*5%*
Distilled Water *q s ad*	*100 mL*

Sig: Apply to areas of acne bid

Refills   0   *Linus Ashman*   M.D.

DEA No. _____

---

1. Calculate the amount of Alcohol needed:

In this prescription order, the Alcohol 15% means 15% v/v of C_2H_5OH, or 15 mL of C_2H_5OH for each 100 mL of solution in the final product. Because the normal source of C_2H_5OH is Alcohol USP, you are required to calculate the number of milliliters of Alcohol USP needed to give 15 mL of C_2H_5OH:

$$\frac{95 \ mL \ C_2H_5OH}{100 \ mL \ Alcohol \ USP} = \frac{15 \ mL \ C_2H_5OH}{x \ mL \ Alcohol \ USP}; \ x = 15.8 \ mL \ Alcohol \ USP$$

Therefore, we need 15.8 mL of Alcohol USP for this product.

2. Labeling of the alcohol content:

Because all labeling of alcohol is percentage v/v of C_2H_5OH, the alcohol content of this product would be labeled: Alcohol 15%.

➤ **EXAMPLE 7.25:**

Contemporary Physicians Group Practice
20 S. Park Street, Triturate, WI 53706
Tel: (608) 555-1333 Fax: (608) 555-1335

R #

Name *Willard Coyote*   Date *00/00/00*

Address *459 Grand Canyon Drive*   Age   Wt/Ht

℞

Castor Oil	*40 mL*
Acacia	*qs*
Alcohol	*15 mL*
Cherry Syrup	*20 mL*
Distilled Water *q s ad*	*100 mL*

M et ft Emulsion

Sig: *Take two tablespoonfuls at bedtime prn for constipation*

Refills   0   *Linus Ashman*   M.D.

DEA No. _____

---

1. Determine the amount of Alcohol needed:

Because the monograph article Alcohol USP is to be used when "alcohol" is called for in formulas, simply measure 15 mL of Alcohol USP. As an esteemed colleague says, when alcohol is written in milliliters, "Pour and go."

2. Labeling of the alcohol content:

Because alcohol is to be labeled by percentage v/v of C_2H_5OH, the percent concentration of C_2H_5OH in this product must be calculated:

$$95\% \times 15 \ mL \ Alcohol \ USP = 14.25 \ mL \ of \ C_2H_5OH$$

Percent content of C_2H_5OH in this ℞:

$$\frac{14.25 \ mL \ C_2H_5OH}{100 \ mL \ preparation} = 14.25\%$$

➤ *EXAMPLE 7.26:*

Contemporary Physicians Group Practice
20 S. Park Street, Triturate, WI 53706
Tel: (608) 555-1333 Fax: (608) 555-1335

R #

Name *Roddy Runner*	Date *00/00/00*
Address *429 Desert Blvd.*	Age Wt/Ht

℞

Guaifenesin		*2.4 g*
Tussend		*90 mL*
Cherry Syrup	*q s ad*	*120 mL*

Sig: One teaspoonful q 4-6 hr prn cough

Refills   0   *Linus Ashman*   M.D.

DEA No. _____

---

1. Determine the amount of Alcohol needed:

   Guaifenesin has limited solubility in water but is freely soluble in alcohol (1 g/1–10 mL). The pharmacist determined that 12 mL of Alcohol USP is required to dissolve the 2.4 g of Guaifenesin.

2. Labeling of the alcohol content:

   Determine the total C_2H_5OH content of the formulation:

   a. The content in the 12 mL of Alcohol USP added to dissolve the Guaifenesin:

   $$95\% \times 12 \text{ mL Alcohol USP} = 11.4 \text{ mL}$$

   b. The labeled alcohol content of Tussend Liquid® is 5%.

   $$5\% \times 90 \text{ mL Tussend®} = 4.5 \text{ mL}$$

   c. Cherry syrup (soda fountain type) was used as the flavored vehicle. It contained no alcohol.

   d. The total amount of C_2H_5OH in the prescription is calculated:

   $$11.4 \text{ mL} + 4.5 \text{ mL} = 15.9 \text{ mL}$$

   Calculate the percent by volume content of C_2H_5OH in the final formulation:

   $$\frac{15.9 \text{ mL } C_2H_5OH}{120 \text{ mL preparation}} = \frac{x \text{ mL } C_2H_5OH}{100 \text{ mL preparation}}; x = 13.25 \text{ mL} = 13.25\%$$

➤ **EXAMPLE 7.27:**

Contemporary Physicians Group Practice
20 S. Park Street, Triturate, WI 53706
Tel: (608) 555-1333 Fax: (608) 555-1335

R #

Name *B. J. Bunny*	Date *00/00/00*
Address *756 Carrot Patch Lane*	Age Wt/Ht

℞

	Phenobarbital		*15 mg/5 mL*
	Flavored Elixir	*q s ad*	*100 mL*

Sig: Take one teaspoonful at 8 AM and 2 PM and two teaspoonfuls hs

Refills   0   *Linus Ashman*   M.D.

DEA No. _____

---

1. Calculate the amount of Alcohol in the formulation:

    a. This is an example of a formula in which the drug, Phenobarbital, is not very wa-
        ter-soluble and needs a certain concentration of alcohol to remain in solution.
        Tables 7.1 and 7.2 give the solubility of Phenobarbital in various water-alcohol
        concentrations and in water–glycerin–alcohol concentrations (7,8). Note that the
        concentrations of Phenobarbital in these tables are given in w/v%, so the first step
        is to calculate the w/v percent of Phenobarbital in this prescription.

$$\frac{0.015 \text{ g Phenobarb.}}{5 \text{ mL preparation}} = \frac{x \text{ g Phenobarb.}}{100 \text{ mL preparation}} ; x = 0.3\%$$

    b. From the table of solubility of phenobarbital in alcohol–aqueous systems (Table
        7.1), it is determined that approximately 20% alcohol is needed to maintain the
        solubility of 0.3% phenobarbital at pH 2–6. (Specifically, the chart shows that at
        pH = 2–6, a 0.27% Phenobarbital solution requires 20% alcohol to maintain a
        solution.)

    c. The vehicles available are: Orange Syrup, which has a pH of 3 and contains no
        alcohol and Alcohol USP.

        Amount of C_2H_5OH needed: *20% × 100 mL = 20 mL*
        Number of mL of Alcohol USP to give 20 mL of C_2H_5OH:

$$\frac{95 \text{ mL } C_2H_5OH}{100 \text{ mL Alcohol USP}} = \frac{20 \text{ mL } C_2H_5OH}{x \text{ mL Alcohol USP}} ; x = 21 \text{ mL Alcohol USP}$$

    d. Dissolve the phenobarbital in 21 mL of Alcohol USP and q.s. to 100 mL with
        Orange Syrup.

2. Labeling of alcohol content: Alcohol 20%

Table 7.1. Solubility[a] of Phenobarbital in Alcohol-aqueous Systems at Various pH Values (7)

Alcohol, % (v/v)	PH				
	2–6	7	8	9	10
0	0.11[b]	0.17	0.41	1.40	2.90
5	0.12	0.18	0.41	1.19	2.71
10	0.16	0.22	0.41	1.01	2.53
15	0.20	0.26	0.41	0.94	2.34
20	0.27	0.33	0.49	0.94	2.15
25	0.40	0.47	0.63	1.01	1.99
30	0.61	0.70	0.85	1.15	1.98
35	0.94	1.03	1.16	1.40	2.07
40	1.46	1.45	1.60	1.80	2.28
45	1.94	2.10	2.20	2.36	2.64
50	2.68	2.84	3.02	3.20	3.49

a. The solubility was determined at $25 \pm 0.02°$.
b. Denotes % phenobarbital *(w/v)*.

Reprinted with permission from Urdang A, Leuallen EE. The effect of pH upon the solubility of phenobarbital in alcohol-aqueous solutions. JAPhA Sci Ed 1956;40:526.

Table 7.2. Solubility of Phenobarbital in Alcohol–glycerin–water Systems at $25°C \times 0.1°$ (8)

Alcohol	Glycerin										
	0%	10%	20%	30%	40%	50%	60%	70%	80%	90%	100%
0%	0.12	0.19	0.20	0.21	0.23	0.28	0.37	0.48	0.66	0.82	1.16
10%	0.19	0.22	0.30	0.37	0.50	0.64	0.84	1.14	1.59	2.25	
20%	0.30	0.42	0.57	0.83	1.13	1.54	2.11	2.77	4.13		
30%	0.64	0.93	1.35	1.89	2.67	3.45	4.45	6.79			
40%	1.46	2.16	2.87	4.09	5.37	6.83	9.40				
50%	3.21	4.26	5.57	7.18	9.29	12.01					
60%	5.33	7.47	9.19	11.23	14.25						
70%	8.53	10.73	12.75	15.74							
80%	11.56	13.58	16.27								
90%	13.38	15.30									
100%	12.30										

Note: Where the sum of the percentages of alcohol and glycerin mixtures does not equal 100, the difference is water. Where the sum equals 100, no water is present in such mixtures.

Reprinted with permission from Krause GM, Cross JM. Solubility of phenobarbital in alcohol-glycerin-water systems. JAPhA Sci Ed 1951;40:139.

➤ *EXAMPLE 7.28:*

Contemporary Physicians Group Practice
20 S. Park Street, Triturate, WI 53706
Tel: (608) 555-1333 Fax: (608) 555-1335

R #

Name *Elmo Phudd*	Date *00/00/00*
Address *762 Shotgun Circle*	Age Wt/Ht

℞

Phenobarbital		*15 mg/5 mL*
Tylenol w/Codeine Elixir		*60 mL*
Flavored Elixir	*q s ad*	*100 mL*

Sig: Take one -two teaspoonfuls q 4-6 hr prn tension headache

Refills   0   *Linus Ashman*   M.D.

DEA No. _____

---

1. Determine the amount of alcohol and other ingredients:

   a. Note that the concentration of Phenobarbital in this prescription is the same as for Example 7.27; therefore, 20% C_2H_5OH is needed.

   b. The vehicles and other ingredients are:

      Cherry syrup (soda fountain type), which contains no alcohol,

      Tylenol w/Codeine Elixir®, which contains 7% alcohol, and Alcohol USP.

      Amount of C_2H_5OH needed: *20% × 100 mL = 20 mL*

      Amount of C_2H_5OH in the Tylenol Elixir: *7% × 60 mL = 4.2 mL*

      Amount of C_2H_5OH still needed: *20 mL − 4.2 mL = 15.8 mL*

      Number of mL of Alcohol USP to give 15.8 mL of C_2H_5OH:

$$\frac{95\ mL\ C_2H_5OH}{100\ mL\ Alcohol\ USP} = \frac{15.8\ mL\ C_2H_5OH}{x\ mL\ Alcohol\ USP}; x = 16.6\ mL\ Alcohol\ USP$$

   c. Dissolve the phenobarbital in 16.6 mL of Alcohol USP, add 60 mL of Tylenol w/Codeine Elixir®, and q.s. to 100 mL with Cherry syrup.

2. Labeling of alcohol content: Alcohol 20%

VI. SPECIAL CALCULATIONS INVOLVING CONCENTRATED ACIDS

A. Irrespective of the physical state of the pure chemical, the concentrations of concentrated acid solutions have traditionally been expressed as percent w/w (Hydrochloric Acid NF is 36.5% to 38.0% by weight of HCl; Phosphoric Acid NF is 85.0% to 88.0% by weight of H_3PO_4; Sulfuric Acid NF is 95.0% to 98.0% by weight of H_2SO_4; Glacial Acetic Acid USP is 99.9% to 100.5% by weight of $C_2H_4O_2$).

B. Although diluted solutions of concentrated acid are solutions of liquids in liquids, their concentrations, as given in official monographs, are not expressed as percent v/v of the concentrated acid solution in water, but rather as percent w/v of the pure acid in water. For example, Diluted Hydrochloric Acid NF is 10% w/v of HCl in water, and Diluted Phosphoric Acid NF is 10% w/v of H_3PO_4.

C.   To get a better idea of the complexity of the situation, consider the following acetic acid preparations. Keep in mind that the situation with most concentrated acids is made more difficult by the fact that the same name applies to both the pure chemical and an official solution, which usually contains less than 100% of the pure chemical.

1. Glacial Acetic Acid USP is acetic acid ($C_2H_4O_2$) in pure form. Its monograph follows the convention for concentrated acids by expressing its concentration as 99.5% to 100.5% w/w.

2. Acetic Acid NF is a diluted acid. Its monograph gives its concentration as 36.0% to 37.0%, by weight (that is, percent w/w), of $C_2H_4O_2$. This follows **neither** the General Notices rule for expressing the concentration of a mixture of a liquid in a liquid as percent v/v, **nor** the convention for expressing concentrations of diluted solutions of concentrated acids as percent w/v. Perhaps, although diluted, this acid is still fairly concentrated and is therefore considered a concentrated acid. The line between concentrated and dilute solutions is hazy.

3. Diluted Acetic Acid NF has its concentration expressed as 5.7 to 6.3 grams of $C_2H_4O_2$ per 100 mL of solution, or 6% w/v. This follows the traditional mode for expressing the concentration of diluted acids as percent w/v.

4. Acetic Acid Irrigation USP has its concentration specified in mg $C_2H_4O_2$/100 mL of solution.

5. Acetic Acid Otic Solution USP contains Glacial Acetic Acid in a nonaqueous solvent. Here the monograph states, "It contains not less than 85.0 percent and not more than 130.0 percent of the labeled amount of $C_2H_4O_2$" (9), but there is no indication whether this percent is w/w or w/v. Consider the situation if glycerin is chosen as the nonaqueous solvent. Does the stated percent give the amount of Glacial Acetic Acid per 100 mL of Glycerin solution or per 100 grams of Glycerin solution? (The latter would be approximately 125 mL of Glycerin because Glycerin has a specific gravity of 1.25.)

6. Acetic Acid (6%) BP (*British Pharmacopeia*) follows the same convention as Diluted Acetic Acid NF. Several other pharmacopeias have similar products, but the percent strengths vary.

7. Acetic Acid (33%) BP follows the pattern of Acetic Acid NF with the exception that its concentration is 33.0% by weight rather than the 37% by weight in the Acetic Acid NF product. Again, several other pharmacopeias have similar products, but the percent strengths vary.

8. Acetic Acid 2% in Spirit Drops. The 29th edition of *Martindale The Extra Pharmacopoeia* listed this product from The Royal National Throat, Nose, and Ear Hospital, London, England. From the above examples one might expect this product to contain 2% w/w or 2% w/v of $C_2H_4O_2$. Neither was true. This product was formulated following the *USP* General Notices convention for a mixture of a liquid in a liquid. Its formula is given as: Acetic Acid (33%) 2 mL, industrial methylated spirit 50 mL, water to 100 mL (10). This product is 2% v/v with respect to Acetic Acid (33%) BP. It is only 0.66% w/v with respect to the chemical, acetic acid ($C_2H_4O_2$). Fortunately, the 30th and later editions of *Martindale* have recognized and addressed this problem. It states, "The nomenclature of acetic acid often leads to confusion as to whether concentrations are expressed as percentages of glacial acetic acid ($C_2H_4O_2$) or of this diluted form. In *Martindale*, the percentage figures given against acetic acid represent the amount of $C_2H_4O_2$" (11).

D.   With all these conflicting examples in mind, consider the following simple prescription order.

℞

Hydrochloric Acid	10%
Purified Water q.s. ad	100 mL

How should this prescription be compounded?

1. **Possibility #1**

   Make this solution 10% v/v of Hydrochloric Acid NF in water. This follows the convention in the General Notices for a mixture of a liquid in a liquid.

   $$10\% \times 100\ mL = 10\ mL\ of\ Hydrochloric\ Acid\ NF$$

   Procedure: Measure **10 mL** of Hydrochloric Acid NF and q.s. to 100 mL with water. (Remember, of course, that we add acid to water, so add the concentrated acid to some of the water first before final q.s.'ing with water.)

2. **Possibility #2**

   Make this solution 10% w/v with respect to pure HCl in water. This follows the convention for dilute solutions of concentrated acids (see Diluted Hydrochloric Acid NF).

   $$10\% \times 100\ mL = 10\ g\ of\ HCl$$

   How would you measure this? Hydrochloric Acid NF is 37.3% w/w or 37.3 g HCl/100 g of Hydrochloric Acid NF. How many grams of Hydrochloric Acid NF solution will you need for 10 g of pure HCl?

   $$\frac{37.3\ g\ HCl}{100\ g\ HCl\ NF\ soln} = \frac{10\ g\ HCl}{x\ g\ HCl\ NF\ soln}; x = 26.8\ g\ HCl\ NF\ soln$$

   We could weigh the 26.8 g of Hydrochloric Acid NF solution by taring a graduated cylinder and then weighing 26.8 g of the solution. An easier method is to convert this weight to a volume. Conversions like this are done using the density or specific gravity of the liquid. Hydrochloric Acid NF has a specific gravity of 1.18.

   $$\frac{1.18\ g\ HCl\ NF\ soln}{1\ mL\ HCl\ NF\ soln} = \frac{26.8\ g\ HCl\ NF\ soln}{x\ mL\ HCl\ NF\ soln}; x = 22.7\ mL\ HCl\ NF\ soln$$

   These last two calculations also can be done in one process using dimensional analysis:

   $$\left(\frac{1\ mL\ HCl\ NF}{1.18\ g\ HCl\ NF}\right)\left(\frac{100\ g\ HCl\ NF}{37.3\ g\ HCl}\right)\left(\frac{10\ g\ HCl}{}\right) = 22.7\ mL\ HCl\ NF$$

   Procedure: Measure **22.7 mL** of Hydrochloric Acid NF and q.s. to 100 mL with water.

E. As you can see, there can be considerable differences in the potencies of these products, each made following accepted conventions. Which is the correct interpretation? One obvious approach is to ask the prescriber. Often this is not helpful because the prescriber got the formula from a colleague, a reference book, or a journal article, and the nameless percent is all that was given.

F. You easily can think of even more complex scenarios. For example, what happens when you have a mixture of a concentrated acid in a semisolid? Consider the common example of a prescription order that calls for Lactic Acid 5% in an ointment base. What does this mean? Bear in mind that Lactic Acid USP is 87% by weight and has a specific gravity of 1.2. For 100 grams of product, would you use: 5 grams of the liquid Lactic Acid USP (%w/w with respect to Lactic Acid USP)? 5 grams of lactic acid, the chemical (%w/w with respect to pure lactic acid, $C_3H_6O_3$)? 5 mL of the liquid Lactic Acid USP (%v/w [is there such a thing?] with respect to Lactic Acid USP)? When you read the label of a manufactured ointment containing 5% lactic acid, how is this to be interpreted?

VII. SPECIAL CALCULATIONS INVOLVING FORMALDEHYDE SOLUTIONS

A. Another exception to the General Notices rules is Formaldehyde Solution USP. It is a solution of a gas in a liquid and, by the general convention as stated in the General Notices, it should have its concentration expressed as percent w/v; instead, its monograph gives its concentration as a percent w/w.

B. Formaldehyde Solution USP, also known by the common name as formalin, is 37% by weight of formaldehyde (CH₂O), with 10% to 15% methanol present to prevent polymerization. *The Merck Index* states, "This soln is the full strength and also known as Formalin 100% or Formalin 40 which signifies that it contains 40 grams of formaldehyde within 100 mL of the soln" (12).

C. If one should get a prescription order requesting a given percent of formaldehyde, how is this to be interpreted?

   1. If the order calls for Formaldehyde Solution 37% or Formalin 40%, it would seem logical, because of the coincidental numbers, to conclude that the prescriber really wants the full-strength Formaldehyde Solution. Obviously, it is always best to check.

   2. What if the order calls for Formaldehyde 10% Solution, Dispense one liter?

   a. One convention is the use of the word **formalin** or **formaldehyde solution** to indicate the USP solution and the term **formaldehyde** to indicate the compound CH₂O (13). With this in mind, this prescription order asking for formaldehyde 10% would require 100 grams of formaldehyde (CH₂O), or 250 mL of Formaldehyde Solution (containing 40% w/v of formaldehyde), to make one liter of product.

   b. *Martindale The Extra Pharmacopoeia* gives a different interpretation and is very clear in its explanation of the accepted interpretation for the United Kingdom. It states:

   Formaldehyde solution is sometimes known as formalin or just formaldehyde and this has led to confusion in interpreting the strength and the form in which formaldehyde is being used. In practice formaldehyde is available as formaldehyde solution which is diluted before use, the percentage strength being expressed in terms of formaldehyde solution rather than formaldehyde (CH₂O). For example in the UK formaldehyde solution 3% consists of 3 volumes of Formaldehyde Solution (B.P.) diluted to 100 volumes with water and thus contains 1.02 to 1.14% w/w of formaldehyde (CH₂O); it is not prepared by diluting Formaldehyde Solution (B.P.) to arrive at a solution containing 3% w/w of formaldehyde (CH₂O) (14).

   Unfortunately, no similar statement of official interpretation for the United States is given in the *USP–NF*.

   3. Although this discussion creates many questions but no satisfactory answers, it should serve to alert you to the problem and gives some possible interpretations.

VIII. CALCULATIONS INVOLVING SALTS AND COMPOUNDS CONTAINING WATER OF HYDRATION

A. Drugs and Chemicals That May Contain Water of Hydration

   1. When a solid drug or chemical is available in both the anhydrous form and as one or more hydrates, there may be ambiguity when calculating quantities or concentrations. An example is given below for one such case, Magnesium Sulfate, but the same difficulties exist for any drug or chemical that is available in both anhydrous and hydrated form.

  a. The USP monograph for Magnesium Sulfate Injection states that it "contains magnesium sulfate equivalent to not less than 93.0 percent and not more than 107.0 percent of the labeled amount of $MgSO_4 \cdot 7H_2O$" (15). In other words, when you have Magnesium Sulfate Injection labeled 50%, it is not 50% with respect to the pure magnesium sulfate, but rather 50% with respect to the heptahydrate.

  b. At one time this made logical sense because this was how magnesium sulfate was available, and the solid magnesium sulfate that was official in the USP was the heptahydrate. This is no longer true; magnesium sulfate is available in both anhydrous and hydrated forms, and the official monograph for magnesium sulfate now lists the anhydrous, the monohydrate, and the heptahydrate forms. Yet to make changes now in how the concentration of Magnesium Sulfate Injection is expressed could cause confusion and could lead to wrong doses being given.

  c. Consider another example, this one for a non-parenteral dosage form. A pharmacist receives the following prescription order: Magnesium Sulfate 25% in Purified Water, Dispense 100 mL. How should this be made? What did the prescriber intend?

    (1) If the pharmacy has both the anhydrous and heptahydrate forms, which form should be used? Because of the large differences in the molecular weights of the anhydrous (120 g) versus the heptahydrate (246 g), there would be a great difference in the final concentration of magnesium sulfate in the preparation, depending on the form used.

    (2) If the pharmacy stocks only one form, is this the form intended? If not, the amount weighed must be altered to compensate for the presence of the water of hydration or the lack of it. This is not a difficult calculation, but it must be considered. For example, if the pharmacist determines that the intent of the order is for 25 g of Magnesium Sulfate heptahydrate ($MgSO_4$ hh) and has only the anhydrous form, the amount of the anhydrous powder that will give the correct amount of magnesium sulfate can be calculated:

$$\left(\frac{120 \text{ g } MgSO_4 \text{ anhy.}}{246 \text{ g } MgSO_4 \text{ hh}} \right) \left(\frac{25 \text{ g } MgSO_4 \text{ hh}}{} \right) = 12.195 \text{ g } MgSO_4 \text{ anhy.}$$

B. Salt and Complex Forms of Drugs

  1. Many drugs are also available in both the free form of the drug and as a salt or complex. The salt or complex forms are made primarily to confer water solubility on poorly soluble organic drug molecules. If the counter ion contributes significantly to the weight of the molecule, the same problems can occur as with anhydrous and hydrate forms of a drug.

  2. In some cases the situation is even more complex because the drug, the salt, or the complex may also contain various amounts of water of hydration. Two examples illustrate this problem:

    a. Theophylline is available as:

Theophylline, anhydrous:	MW 180
Theophylline monohydrate:	MW 198
Theophylline ethylenediamine 2:1(Aminophylline):	MW 420
Theophylline ethylenediamine 2:1 dihydrate:	MW 456

Obviously, problems could occur with dosing and measuring this drug. In this case, the drug also has a narrow therapeutic window, so that incorrectly determined amounts of this drug could have severe consequences. Fortunately, drug information references and package labeling carefully specify which dose belongs to which form of the drug, but the pharmacist must be careful in dealing with this drug.

    b. Morphine is another classic example. Morphine Sulfate (anhydrous and pentahydrate) is the official USP form of morphine. The Morphine Sulfate monograph states that it is calculated on the anhydrous basis. One of the official morphine dosage forms, Morphine Sulfate Injection USP, has its labeled amount based in the pentahydrate. Morphine is also available as the free base, the base monohydrate, the hydrochloride salt, and several other forms (see *The Merck Index*). In this case, drug information references are not specific with respect to dose-form of the drug (see Morphine dosing information in the *USP/DI*).

C. Dealing With These Issues

1. If all practitioners were knowledgeable about these issues, and if drug information references were always specific in expressing doses, this issue would be handled more easily. Unfortunately, many prescribers, and even some pharmacists, do not realize that this problem exists or are unaware of its complexity or possible ramifications. Fortunately, in some cases, drug information references and product labeling are now addressing the problem. There is still room for improvement.

   For example, take the case of Magnesium Sulfate Injection. The *USP/DI* gives the usual adult intramuscular dose for electrolyte replenishment as "1 to 2 grams of a 50% solution (8.1 to 16.2 mEq elemental magnesium) four times a day until serum magnesium is within normal limits" (16). While the "1 to 2 grams of a 50% solution" is confusing (does this really mean to weigh out 1 to 2 grams of a 50% solution?), the presence of specific information, 8.1 to 16.2 mEq of elemental magnesium, allows the physician and pharmacist to figure out precisely what is intended. It does require that the practitioner know how to convert between milliequivalents and grams. For this example, let us assume that 1 to 2 grams of a 50% solution really means 1 to 2 grams of magnesium sulfate heptahydrate ($MgSO_4$ hh) in a 50% solution; we can validate this assumption by performing the following calculation:

$$\left(\frac{2\ mEq\ Mg^{+2}}{mmol\ MgSO_4\ hh} \right) \left(\frac{mmol\ MgSO_4\ hh}{246\ mg\ MgSO_4\ hh} \right) \left(\frac{1000\ mg}{1\ g} \right) \left(\frac{1-2\ g\ MgSO_4\ hh}{} \right) = 8.1-16.2\ mEq\ Mg^{+2}$$

2. The *USP* has partly addressed this issue with a formula for making adjustments based on salt or complex form, hydrate form, and moisture content in the Certificate of Analysis that accompanies some pure drugs and chemicals for compounding. The formula and explanation can be found either in a former revision of Chapter ⟨795⟩"Pharmacy Compounding—Nonsterile Preparations," or in a new Chapter ⟨1060⟩ "Pharmaceutical Calculations in Prescription Compounding" that has been proposed in the *Pharmacopeial Forum* for addition to the *USP*. The formula gives one method of handling this problem; however, to use the formula, the pharmacist must know the intent of the prescriber.

3. One must be aware of these issues because then appropriate steps can be taken when calculating amounts and concentrations of drugs and chemicals used in drug products and preparations for patients.

References

1. Summary of Information Submitted to MedMARχ in the Year 2000: Charting a Course for Change, Rockville, MD. The United States Pharmacopeial Convention, Inc., 2002;1.
2. Scatchard, G, Hamer WG, Wood SE. Isotonic solutions. I. The chemical potential of water in aqueous solutions of sodium chloride, potassium chloride, sulfuric acid, sucrose, urea, and glycerol at 25°. J Am Chem Soc. 1938; 60: 3061–70.
3. The United States Pharmacopeia 25/National Formulary 20, Rockville, MD. The United States Pharmacopeial Convention, Inc., 2001; 11.
4. Stoklosa MJ, Ansel HC. Pharmaceutical calculations, 11th ed. Baltimore: Lippincott Williams & Wilkins, 2001; 120.
5. The United States Pharmacopeia 25/National Formulary 20, Rockville, MD. The United States Pharmacopeial Convention, Inc., 2001; 5.
6. The United States Pharmacopeia 25/National Formulary 20, Rockville, MD. The United States Pharmacopeial Convention, Inc., 2001; 10.
7. Urdang A, Leuallen EE. The effect of pH upon the solubility of phenobarbital in alcohol-aqueous solutions. J APhA Sci Ed 1956; 40: 526.
8. Krause GM, Cross JM. Solubility of phenobarbital in alcohol-glycerin-water systems. J APhA Sci Ed 1951; 40: 139.

9. The United States Pharmacopeia 25/National Formulary 20, Rockville, MD. The United States Pharmacopeial Convention, Inc., 2001; 42.

10. Reynolds JEF, ed. Martindale the extra pharmacopoeia, 28th ed. London: The Pharmaceutical Press, 1982; 784.

11. Parfitt K, ed. Martindale the complete drug reference, 32d ed. London: Pharmaceutical Press, 1999; 1329.

12. Budavari S, ed. The Merck Index, 11th ed. Rahway, NJ: Merck & Co., Inc., 1989; 662.

13. Horn DW, Osol A. Fumigation with formaldehyde. Am J Pharm 1929; 101: 742.

14. Parfitt K, ed. Martindale the complete drug reference, 32d ed. London: Pharmaceutical Press, 1999; 1113.

15. The United States Pharmacopeia 25/National Formulary 20. Rockville, MD: The United States Pharmacopeial Convention, Inc., 2001; 1043.

16. USP/DI, 22nd ed. Greenwood Village, CO: MICROMEDEX Thomson Healthcare, 2002; 1948.

CHAPTER 8

Evaluating Dosage Regimens

INTRODUCTION

As stated in Chapter 7, an essential function of the pharmacist is to ensure that patients get the intended drug in the correct amount. Chapter 7 discussed the various units or dimensions of quantity and of concentration that form the basis for our expressions of dose. The current chapter examines the various accepted methods of expressing doses and dosage regimens and shows some sample dosing calculations. Special attention will then be given to several types of cases that require consideration of additional factors. In all instances of providing patients with drug products, whether they be manufactured dosage forms or preparations specially formulated by the pharmacist, the dose and dosage regimen must always be verified for accuracy and appropriateness.

II. **DOSES**

   A. Individual doses are expressed using one of the following formats:
     1. Quantity of drug; for example, 25 mg drug
      (See Chapter 7 for the various units or dimensions used in pharmacy and medicine for expressing quantity of drug.)
     2. Quantity of drug per kilogram of patient body weight; for example, 5 mg drug/kg body weight
     3. Quantity of drug per square meter of patient body surface area; for example, 10 mg drug/m^2 of body surface area (BSA)

   B. For topical products and preparations, doses are expressed as concentrations. This makes conceptual sense since the concentration gradient is the driving force for transfer of drug across the skin or membrane barrier. See Chapter 7 for accepted methods of expressing concentrations and related sample calculations.

   C. The methods for individual doses that are based on the patient's body size (weight or BSA) are often used for pediatric doses, but they are also important when determining adult doses for drugs that have narrow therapeutic indices. BSA is used routinely for dosing chemotherapy agents.
     1. Body weight
      a. Usually actual body weight (ABW) is used for calculating doses based on body weight. When a prescription or medication drug order is written in terms of a

quantity (mcg, mg, g, etc.) per kilogram or pound of body weight, the pharmacist must ascertain the ABW, either from the prescriber or the patient or patient caregiver, and use this in calculating the intended dose.

b. In some situations, the order is written in terms of quantity (e.g., mcg, mg, or g) of drug, but the drug information references give the dose in a quantity/kg body weight basis. In this case, the pharmacist needs to know the approximate ABW to check the prescribed dose for appropriateness. Again the pharmacist may ascertain the ABW either from the prescriber or the patient or patient caregiver.

c. For pediatric patients, initial dosing checks can be done without ABW if the child's age is known by using an estimate of the body weight from one of the percentile charts of body weight versus age. Percentile weight–height measurements based on ages for infants and children are given in Appendices F and G. The charts in Appendix G are also available on the Centers for Disease Control (CDC) Internet site at www.cdc.gov.growthcharts. Although charts like this are handy for initial checking of dosage ranges, the pharmacist should always verify the dose based on the child's ABW.

d. For some types of therapy, dosing is based on estimated ideal body weight (IBW), also referred to as lean body weight (LBW). The following equations are used to calculate estimated IBW in kilograms. Several methods are shown to calculate IBW for children. The equations for children given below in item 3 are based on CDC data for the 50th percentile for a given height, so the charts in Appendices F and G could also be used to determine an IBW for a child of a given height by choosing the weight at the 50th percentile for that height [1].

Adult Males:

$IBW_{(kg)} = 50 + (2.3 \times$ height in inches over 5 feet$)$

Adult Females:

$IBW_{(kg)} = 45.5 + (2.3 \times$ height in inches over 5 feet$)$

Children:

1. Children less than 5 feet tall [2]

$$IBW_{(kg)} = \frac{height^2_{(cm)} \times 1.65}{1000}$$

2. Children 5 feet and taller [2]

Males: $IBW_{(kg)} = 39 + (2.27 \times height_{(in)}$ over 5 feet$)$

Females: $IBW_{(kg)} = 42.2 + (2.27 \times height_{(in)}$ over 5 feet$)$

3. Ages 1–17 years [1]

$$IBW_{(kg)} = 2.396e^{0.01863(height)}; \ height \ is \ in \ cm.$$

2. Body Surface Area (BSA)

a. Drug dosage may also be based on estimated BSA of the patient. This method is commonly used for pediatric dosing, and as stated above, many cancer drug protocols base dosage on BSA. When a prescription or medication drug order is written in terms of a quantity (mcg, mg, g, etc.) per m^2 of BSA, the pharmacist must determine the BSA using the weight and height (or length for an infant) of the patient, and use this in calculating the intended dose.

b. BSA nomograms for adults and children are shown in Appendix E. They are used as follows:

1. Find the patient's weight in pounds or kilograms on the right-hand side of the nomogram.

2. Find the patient's height in inches or centimeters on the left-hand side of the nomogram.

3. Draw a straight line connecting these two points and read the BSA in m^2 at the point where the line intersects with the middle BSA line.

    c. BSA can also be calculated using one of the equations given below (3,4).

        1. Using weight in pounds and height in inches:

$$BSA(m^2) = \sqrt{\frac{Ht\,(in) \times Wt\,(lb)}{3131}}$$

        2. Using weight in kilograms and height in centimeters:

$$BSA(m^2) = \sqrt{\frac{Ht\,(cm) \times Wt\,(kg)}{3600}}$$

III. DOSAGE REGIMENS

A. Dosage regimens combine the name and quantity or dose of the drug with a frequency of administration or use. As with doses, dosage regimens can be written in different formats. It is extremely important for the pharmacist to be attentive when reading and checking dosage regimens, because slight changes in wording can mean significant differences in intended dosing.

B. Formats for dosage regimens
    1. Name and quantity of drug with frequency of use or administration
        For example,
            Diazepam 1 mg three times a day
            or
            Diazepam 3 mg per day in 3 divided doses
        Note: Use great caution when doses are expressed in the second way because it has been misread as 3 mg/dose to be given 3 times a day rather 3 mg total per day—in this case a 3-fold error!
    2. Name and concentration of drug with frequency of use or application
        For example,
            Hydrocortisone Lotion 1% apply q.i.d.
    3. Name and quantity of drug per kilogram of body weight with frequency of use or administration
        For example,
            Diazepam 40 mcg per kg 3 times a day
            or
            Diazepam 120 mcg per kg per day in 3 divided doses
        Note: Again, use great caution with this equivalent expression because it has been misread.
    4. Name and quantity of drug per square meter of body surface area with frequency of use or administration
        For example,
            Diazepam 1.17 mg/m^2 BSA 3 times a day
            or
            Diazepam 3.51 mg per m^2 BSA per day in 3 divided doses
        Note: Again, use great caution with this equivalent expression because it has been misread.

IV. SPECIAL CASES

A. Use of pharmacokinetic parameters and laboratory values to set and adjust dosage levels
    1. For some therapeutic classes and certain patient populations, pharmacokinetic parameters are used to adjust dose quantities and dosage regimens. An example is the use of creatinine clearance for initial maintenance dosing of aminoglycosides.

2. There are numerous examples of using laboratory values to set and adjust dose and dosage regimens. Common examples include anticoagulants, electrolyte therapy, and theophylline.
3. Discussion of these topics, while extremely important, is beyond the scope of this text.

B.   Geriatric Patients

1. Geriatric patients may require special consideration when designing dosage regimens. Often the organ systems of these patients are not functioning at top efficiency because of the aging process or disease. Because some clinical conditions, such as liver impairment and kidney dysfunction, that are important to the metabolism and elimination of drugs are more prevalent in the elderly, it is essential for the pharmacist to have medical histories of these patients.
2. With geriatric patients, modifications in dosing regimen are often given, when applicable, in drug information references such as the *USP/DI, Drug Facts and Comparisons, Drug Information Handbook, AHFS Drug Information,* and product package inserts.

C.   Pediatric Patients

1. One obvious difference between adults and pediatric patients is size, but it is important to remember that infants and children are not just little adults. Their physiologic systems often are not fully developed, and this must be considered in dosing these patients. Furthermore, there are differences in metabolism and excretion capabilities as children progress from birth to adulthood. When these factors are significant in drug dosing, this information is usually given in drug references and product package inserts. To use this information, it is helpful to know the accepted descriptive terms for the stages of childhood. Below is given a scheme in common use.
   a. Neonate or newborn: birth to 1 month
   b. Infant: 1 month to 1 year
   c. Early childhood: 1 year through 5 years
   d. Late childhood: 6 years through 12 years
   e. Adolescence: 13 years through 17 years (5)
      Another more recently published system has slight changes in the descriptive terms and ages for childhood through adolescence. They are: early childhood—1 year through 4 years; middle childhood—5 years through 10 years; and adolescence—11 years through 17 years (6).
2. As with geriatric patients, references such as the *USP/DI, Drug Facts and Comparisons, Drug Information Handbook, AHFS Drug Information,* and product package inserts sometimes give modifications in dosing regimens for pediatric patients. Unfortunately this information is often limited or unavailable, and the reference will state that safety and efficacy have not been established. Because of the importance of this topic and the potential danger to infants and children caused by the absence of well-documented pediatric dosing information, the FDA has recently been encouraging pharmaceutical manufacturers to perform more studies in pediatric populations.
4. In the absence of specific pediatric dosing information, there are general rules for calculating an infant's or child's dose of medication when given the age, weight, or BSA of the patient and the normal adult dose. **The general rules are not drug-specific and should be used only in the absence of more complete information.** It is the duty of the pharmacist to be knowledgeable about the limitations of using set formulas or rules for calculating pediatric doses. In the absence of specific pediatric dosing information, always be conservative in dosing these patients, particularly neonates and infants.
5. Sample calculations for pediatric dosing are given below.

➤ *EXAMPLE 8.1:*
   Dosing based on specific information in the *USP/DI* or similar references:
   D. A. is a 5-year-old male patient. He weighs 42 pounds and is 43 inches tall. The prescriber wants to give Diazepam to D. A. What is an acceptable dose of Diazepam for D. A.?

USP/DI:

"Usual pediatric dose: Children 6 months of age and over—Oral, 1 to 2.5 mg, 40 to 200 mcg (0.04 to 0.2 mg) per kg of body weight, or 1.17 to 6 mg per square meter of body surface, three to four times a day, the dosage being increased gradually as needed and tolerated" (7).

1. What is the dosage regimen of Diazepam for D. A. based on the **quantity** given in the *USP/DI?*

    1–2.5 mg given 3 to 4 times a day

2. What is the dose regimen of Diazepam for D. A. based on the **mg/kg** dose given in the *USP/DI?*

    a. Calculation of kg weight of DA:

    $$\frac{2.2\ lbs}{1\ kg} = \frac{42\ lbs}{x\ kg}; x = 19.1\ kg$$

    b. Calculation of dose:

    $$\left(\frac{0.04 - 0.2\ mg}{kg}\right)\left(\frac{19.1\ kg}{}\right) = 0.76 - 3.82\ mg$$

    c. Dosage regimen: 0.76–3.82 mg given 3 to 4 times a day

3. What is the dosage regimen of Diazepam for D. A. based on the **mg/m² BSA** dose given in the *USP/DI?*

    a. Determine the BSA of D. A. from the pediatric nomogram found in Appendix E:

    Answer: BSA = 0.76 m²

    b. Calculation of dose:

    $$\left(\frac{1.17 - 6\ mg}{m^2}\right)\left(\frac{0.76\ m^2}{}\right) = 0.89 - 4.56\ mg$$

    c. Dosage regimen: 0.89–4.56 mg given 3 to 4 times a day

Notice there is some variation in dosage range based on the various methods used to calculate dose.

➤ *EXAMPLE 8.2:*

Dosing for a child calculated using a normal adult dose and "rules" for pediatric doses based on the child's age, weight, and BSA

For the following examples, Diazepam doses are calculated for D. A. using one of the so-called "rules" for pediatric dosing. A variety of these rules are given in Table 8.1. The numbers for the example below are based on the age/weight/height information for D. A. given in the above example and on the adult dose information given in the *USP/DI* for Diazepam for similar therapeutic indications. This adult dose is given as:

"Oral, 2 to 10 mg two to four times a day" (7).

In each case given below, the calculated dose would be given 2 to 4 times a day.

1. Using Young's Rule, what is the dose of Diazepam for D. A. based on the normal adult dose and D. A.'s **age?**

$$\frac{Age}{Age + 12} \times Adult\ dose = Dose\ for\ child$$

$$\frac{5}{5 + 12} \times 2 - 10\ mg = 0.59 - 2.94\ mg$$

2. Using Clark's Rule, what is the dose of Diazepam for D. A. based on the normal adult dose and D. A.'s **weight**?

$$\frac{Weight\ (lbs)}{150} \times Adult\ dose = Dose\ for\ child$$

$$\frac{42\ lbs}{150} \times 2 - 10\ mg = 0.56 - 2.8\ mg$$

3. What is the dose of Diazepam for D. A. based on the normal adult dose and D. A.'s **BSA**?

Note: This is based on the BSA of an "average" adult of 1.73 m².

$$\frac{BSA\ m^2}{1.73\ m^2} \times Adult\ dose = Dose\ for\ child$$

$$\frac{0.76\ m^2}{1.73\ m^2} \times 2 - 10\ mg = 0.87 - 4.39\ mg$$

Notice that in each case, the doses of Diazepam for D. A. are similar. At stated above, Table 8.1 lists several other equations for calculating pediatric doses from established adult doses. While these so-called rules may be helpful as a starting point in determining a pediatric dose in the absence of specific information, the following example shows the danger inherent in using this generalized approach.

REMEMBER: INFANTS AND CHILDREN ARE NOT LITTLE ADULTS.

TABLE 8.1 Formulas for Pediatric Dosage Calculations

Rule Name	Equation	Examples*
Drug-Specific Calculation Based on Weight:	$\dfrac{Dose}{kg\ of\ body\ weight} \times Weight\ (kg) = Dose\ for\ child$	$\left(\dfrac{0.04 - 0.2\ mg}{kg}\right)\left(\dfrac{19.1\ kg}{}\right) = 0.76 - 3.82\ mg$
Drug-Specific Calculation Based on BSA:	$\dfrac{Dose}{BSA\ m^2} \times BSA\ (m^2) = Dose\ for\ child$	$\left(\dfrac{1.17 - 6\ mg}{m^2}\right)\left(\dfrac{0.76\ m^2}{}\right) = 0.89 - 4.56\ mg$
General Rule Based on Weight: Clark's Rule	$\dfrac{Weight\ (lbs)}{150} \times Adult\ dose = Dose\ for\ child$	$\dfrac{42\ lbs}{150} \times 2 - 10\ mg = 0.56 - 2.8\ mg$
General Rule Based on BSA:	$\dfrac{BSA\ m^2}{1.73\ m^2} \times Adult\ dose = Dose\ for\ child$	$\dfrac{0.76\ m^2}{1.73\ m^2} \times 2 - 10\ mg = 0.87 - 4.39\ mg$
General Rules Based on Age: Young's Rule	$\dfrac{Age}{Age + 12} \times Adult\ dose = Dose\ for\ child$	$\dfrac{5}{5 + 12} \times 2 - 10\ mg = 0.59 - 2.94\ mg$
Cowling's Rule	$\dfrac{Age\ at\ next\ birthday\ (in\ years)}{24} \times Adult\ dose = Dose\ for\ child$	$\dfrac{6}{24} \times 2 - 10\ mg = 0.5 - 2.5\ mg$
Bastedo's Rule	$\dfrac{Age\ in\ years + 3}{30} \times Adult\ dose = Dose\ for\ child$	$\dfrac{8}{30} \times 2 - 10\ mg = 0.53 - 2.67\ mg$
Dilling's Rule	$\dfrac{Age\ (in\ years)}{20} \times Adult\ dose = Dose\ for\ child$	$\dfrac{5}{20} \times 2 - 10\ mg = 0.5 - 2.5\ mg$
Fried's Rule for Infants	$\dfrac{Age\ (in\ months)}{150} \times Adult\ dose = Dose\ for\ infant$	$\dfrac{0.5}{150} \times 25\ mg = 0.083\ mg\ *$

*Note: These examples use the data from the text on patient DA with the drug and dosage information for Diazepam except for the final example for Fried's Rule for Infants; that example uses the data for the two-week old infant JA and dosing for Captopril.

➤ *EXAMPLE 8.3:*

Dosing for an infant based on normal adult dose and "rules" for pediatric dosing

J. A. is a 2-week-old infant who weighs 8 pounds. The prescriber wants to give Captopril to J. A. What is an acceptable dose of Captopril for J. A.?

USP/DI:

"Usual adult and adolescent dose"

Antihypertensive—Initial: Oral, 25 mg two or three times a day, the dosage being increased if necessary...." (8)

"Usual pediatric dose

Newborns—

Initial: Oral, 10 mcg (0.01 mg) per kg of body weight two or three times a day, the dosage being adjusted as needed and tolerated" (8).

1. What is the dose of Captopril for J. A. based on the **mg/kg** dose given in the *USP/DI?*

   a. Calculation of kg weight of J. A.:

$$\frac{2.2 \ lbs}{1 \ kg} = \frac{8 \ lbs}{x \ kg} ; x = 3.6 \ kg$$

   b. Calculation of dose:

$$\left(\frac{0.01 \ mg}{kg}\right)\left(\frac{3.6 \ kg}{}\right) = 0.036 \ mg$$

2. Using Clark's Rule, what is the dose of Captopril for J. A. based on normal adult dose and J. A.'s **weight**?

$$\frac{8 \ lbs}{150} \times 25 \ mg = 1.33 \ mg$$

This method was not so successful—nearly 20 times the recommended dose!

ALWAYS USE DRUG-SPECIFIC PEDIATRIC DOSES WHEN THESE ARE AVAILABLE.

References

1. Traub SL, Kitchen L. Estimating ideal body mass in children. Am J Hosp Pharm 1983; 40: 107-110.
2. Traub SL, Johnson CE. Comparison of methods of estimating creatinine clearance in children. Am J Hosp Pharm 1980; 37: 195-201.
3. Mosteller RD. Simplified calculation of body surface area. N Engl J Med 1987; 317: 1098.
4. Lam TK, Leung DT. More on simplified calculation of body surface area. N Engl J Med 1988; 318: 1130.
5. Berkow R, ed. The Merck Manual, 15th ed. Rahway, NJ: Merck & Co., Inc., 1987; 1798-1799.
6. Berkow R, Beers MH, ed. The Merck Manual, 17th ed. West Point, PA: Merck & Co., Inc., 1999; 2076-2077.
7. USP DI, Vol. I, 22d ed. Greenwood Village, CO: MICROMEDEX Thomson Healthcare, 2002; 587.
8. USP DI, Vol. I, 22d ed. Greenwood Village, CO: MICROMEDEX Thomson Healthcare, 2002; 209-210.

CHAPTER 9

Aliquots Calculations

I. GENERAL PRINCIPLES

A. In pharmacy we often deal with potent drug substances that require accurate measurement when preparing drug delivery systems for our patients. When the quantity of drug desired requires a degree of precision in measurement that is beyond the capability of the available measuring devices, the pharmacist may use the aliquot method of measurement.

B. Aliquot means "contained an exact number of times in something else." Therefore, 5 is an aliquot part of 15 because 5 is contained exactly 3 times in 15.

C. When aliquots are used in pharmacy, the general procedure is as follows:
  1. Weigh or measure an amount of the desired drug that is within the degree of accuracy provided by the measuring device.
  2. Weigh or measure a compatible, inert diluent. For solid aliquots, lactose is a common diluent. For liquid aliquots, water is used if possible, but alcohol or another pharmaceutical solvent may also be used when solubility or miscibility dictates this.
  3. Add the diluent to the drug with adequate mixing to give a homogeneous mixture or solution. In all cases when combining powders, use geometric dilution and mix thoroughly using trituration in a glass mortar. (Note: A description of geometric dilution is given in Chapter 24, Powders, the section "Principles of Compounding for Powders.")
  4. Weigh or measure an aliquot part of the mixture that contains exactly the desired amount of drug.

D. How are the numbers for aliquot parts determined?
  1. Examples are given below showing several commonly used methods. Any method is satisfactory as long as the correct amount of drug is obtained. Use a system that makes sense to you because this usually means that there is less potential for error.
  2. Because aliquots usually are used for potent drugs, it is always best, when possible, to have a colleague independently check the amounts calculated.
  3. For the examples given below, the following assumptions were made: 1) the available balance had a minimum weighable quantity (MWQ) of 120 mg; 2) the smallest graduate available had a capacity of 10 mL with a minimum measurable quantity (MMQ) of 2 mL (20% of the graduated cylinder capacity); 3) the smallest syringe or micropipette available had an MMQ of 0.2 mL; 4) lactose could be used as the inert diluent for the solid-solid aliquots; and 5) water could be used as the inert diluent for liquid aliquots.

▊▊ **II. SIMPLE SOLID-SOLID ALIQUOTS**

A. Method 1

   1. This method is the simplest.

     a. An amount of drug is weighed that is within the degree of accuracy provided by the balance. For economic reasons the amount chosen is usually the MWQ.

     b. The drug is diluted with an arbitrary amount of diluent using geometric dilution when appropriate.

     c. The amount of the dilution that will give the desired amount of drug is calculated, and this amount is weighed.

   2. Method 1 is usually the easiest aliquot method to use when the amount of drug being weighed is restricted to a given value, such as the MWQ. This is true when the desired drug is a controlled substance because only minimum waste is allowed for controlled substances. Using the MWQ is also preferred when the drug is expensive.

   3. Method 1 is illustrated with several examples. The first example (9.1), Trial #1, starts with the basic necessary steps. Trial #1 is then analyzed and the method is refined. Trial #2 shows the results of these modifications. A final analysis is then given to show additional possibilities. The objective of presenting the method in this way is to show a pattern of possible thought processes that can be used in a general sense for developing methods of problem solving when dealing with pharmaceutical calculations.

➤ *EXAMPLE 9.1:* drug/amount desired: Codeine 20 mg

   1. Trial #1: Basic steps

     a. Weigh the MWQ of Codeine: 120 mg.

     b. Weigh an arbitrary amount of lactose that is ≥ the MWQ: 300 mg.

     c. Mix the two powders thoroughly by triturating in a mortar.

     d. Calculate the total weight of the dilution: 120 mg + 300 mg = 420 mg.

     e. Calculate the number of milligrams of dilution that contain the desired 20 mg of Codeine.

   By proportion:

$$\frac{120\ mg\ Codeine}{420\ mg\ dilution} = \frac{20\ mg\ Codeine}{x\ mg\ dilution};\ x = 70\ mg\ dilution$$

   By dimensional analysis:

$$\left(\frac{420\ mg\ dilution}{120\ mg\ Codeine}\right)\left(\frac{20\ mg\ Codeine}{}\right) = 70\ mg\ dilution$$

     f. Weigh this calculated amount of the dilution, 70 mg, to get the desired 20 mg of Codeine.

   2. Analysis of Trial #1

   Analysis of these calculations reveals that some judgment is required in selecting the quantity of diluent to add to the drug. In this case, the required amount of the aliquot was calculated to be 70 mg, which is below the MWQ. The following are general guidelines for selecting the amount of diluent to use:

     a. Pick a quantity of diluent that will give aliquots that are at or above the MWQ. In this case, it is obvious that 300 mg of lactose is not enough diluent when the desired amount of drug is 20 mg. The 70 mg of the dilution, which is the amount needed to give 20 mg of Codeine, is below the MWQ of 120 mg and cannot be weighed with the desired level of accuracy.

     b. When possible, pick convenient amounts of diluent to make the mathematics easy. It is always best to use simple numbers, or amounts that reduce to simple numbers, because it is then easier to spot errors. In this case, if the amount of diluent is chosen to be a multiple of 120 mg (the amount of Codeine weighed), then the number that is multiplied times the 20 mg of Codeine reduces to a simple number. The example below illustrates this principle.

3. Trial #2 Revised steps

   Below is a repeat of the above problem using a more "convenient" quantity of diluent that will give an aliquot $\geq$ the MWQ.

   a. Weigh the MWQ of Codeine: 120 mg.

   b. Weigh a convenient amount of lactose (that is, a multiple of 120 mg) that will give an aliquot $\geq$ the MWQ: 600 mg is selected

   c. Add the lactose to the Codeine using geometric dilution and mix the two powders thoroughly by triturating in a mortar.

   d. Calculate the weight of the dilution: 120 mg + 600 mg = 720 mg.

   e. Calculate the number of milligrams of dilution that contain the desired 20 mg of Codeine.

   By proportion:

   $$\frac{20\ mg\ Codeine}{720\ mg\ dilution} = \frac{20\ mg\ Codeine}{x\ mg\ dilution};\ x = 120\ mg\ dilution$$

   By dimensional analysis:

   $$\left(\frac{720\ mg\ dilution}{120\ mg\ Codeine}\right)\left(\frac{20\ mg\ Codeine}{}\right) = 120\ mg\ dilution$$

   f. Weigh this calculated amount of the dilution to get the desired 20 mg of Codeine.

4. Analysis of Trial #2

   a. As you can see, 720 is a multiple of 120 (6 × 120 = 720), so the mathematics becomes a simple matter of multiplying 20 mg of Codeine by 6 to get 120 mg of dilution.

   $$\frac{\overset{1}{\cancel{120}}\ mg\ Codeine}{\underset{6}{\cancel{720}}\ mg\ dilution} = \frac{20\ mg\ Codeine}{x\ mg\ dilution};\ x = 120\ mg\ dilution$$

   Even though most of us use calculators for math operations, it is important to look at the answers we get to see if they seem reasonable. This sort of inspection is much easier to do if the numbers are simple.

   b. In using this method, you may wonder: What is the best way to pick the quantity of diluent so that the amount of dilution needed is at least the MWQ, but the amounts are not so large as to waste ingredients or give an aliquot that is excessively bulky? There are several ways in which this may be accomplished.

      (1) Pick any reasonable amount, do the math, and, if the amount of dilution calculated is too little or too much, pick a different amount. While simple, this can be tedious.

      (2) In picking amounts, notice that the amount of diluent needed is not completely arbitrary. An inspection of the calculations given above reveals that the smaller the amount of drug needed (20 mg in this case), the larger the amount of diluent needed to give a minimum amount of dilution to weigh.

      (3) Further inspection of the equations in Trial #2 reveals that instead of picking the amount of the diluent and solving for the amount of the aliquot, you may also set up the equation by picking the amount of the aliquot and solving for the amount of the dilution. For example, if you want 120 mg for the aliquot, set up the equation as shown here:

      $$\frac{120\ mg\ Codeine}{x\ mg\ dilution} = \frac{20\ mg\ Codeine}{120\ mg\ dilution};\ x = 720\ mg\ dilution$$

You will need to remember that the 720 mg is the total amount of the dilution (that is, drug plus diluent). To determine the amount of diluent, subtract the quantity of drug weighed from this total to obtain the amount of the diluent. In this case,

720 mg dilution—120 mg drug = 600 mg diluent

(4) For pharmacists who like formulas, the formula given below may be useful:

$$\frac{Amount\ of\ drug\ desired}{Amount\ of\ drug\ weighed} = \frac{Amount\ of\ dilution\ weighed}{Total\ amount\ of\ dilution}$$

To use this formula, fill in the desired quantities for Amount of drug desired, Amount of drug weighed, and Amount of dilution weighed. Then, solve for Total amount of dilution. In the example above:

$$\frac{20\ mg}{120\ mg} = \frac{120\ mg}{x};\ x = 720\ mg$$

As with the previous example, remember that the 720 mg is the total amount of the dilution (that is, drug plus diluent). To determine the amount of diluent, subtract the quantity of drug weighed from this total to obtain the amount of the diluent. Although formulas may simplify solving pharmaceutical calculations, the problem with using a formula is that you have to remember it—unless, of course, it is intuitive to you.

(5) You may wish to perform the calculations for aliquots for a variety of drug weights and construct a table of values like the one shown in Table 9.1. Using a table like this is easy.

(a) Determine the amount of drug needed: 20 mg.

(b) Weigh 120 mg of the drug. (This amount is always the same; usually 120 mg, the MWQ, is chosen.)

(c) Determine the weight range for the amount of drug needed from column (a), 12–29 mg, and read off the amount of lactose or other diluent from column (c), 1,080 mg. The combined weight of the dilution is shown in column (d), 1,200 mg.

(d) Calculate the amount of dilution to weigh that will contain the desired amount of drug.

$$\frac{\overset{1}{\cancel{120}}\ mg\ Codeine}{\underset{10}{\cancel{1200}}\ mg\ dilution} = \frac{20\ mg\ Codeine}{x\ mg\ dilution};\ x = 200\ mg\ dilution$$

(e) Alternatively you may read the appropriate dilution factor given in column (e), which in this case is 10, and multiply the dilution factor times the amount of drug needed to get the amount of aliquot to weigh.

10 × 20 mg = 200 mg

When using this approach, it is always best to check the values obtained for accuracy by completing a full calculation using the chosen numbers, as shown in the calculation in part (d) above.

TABLE 9.1 Determination of Solid–Solid Aliquot Amounts

Amount of Drug Needed (a)	Amount of Drug Weighed (b)	Amount of Diluent (lactose) (c)	Amount of Dilution (d)	Dilution factor (d) ÷ (b) (e)
60–120 mg	120 mg	120 mg	240 mg	2
30–59 mg	120 mg	360 mg	480 mg	4
12–29 mg	120 mg	1080 mg	1200 mg	10
3–11 mg	120 mg	4680 mg	4800 mg	40
1.2–2.9 mg	120 mg	11,880 mg	12,000 mg	100

B. Method 2

1. This method is useful when there is more flexibility in the amount of drug that may be weighed; for example, you are not required to use the MWQ.

2. This method consists of the following steps:

    a. The quantity of drug to be weighed is determined by multiplying the amount of drug needed by an appropriately determined factor, called the multiple factor.

    b. An arbitrary amount of diluent is weighed and added.

    c. The amount of dilution needed is determined by multiplying the weight of the dilution by the inverse of the multiple factor. Multiple factors are usually chosen to be whole numbers.

➤ *EXAMPLE 9.2:* drug/amount desired: Codeine 20 mg

1. Trial #1

    a. Select a multiple of the amount of drug needed that will give a quantity which is ≥ the MWQ. Weigh this amount. In this case the multiple may be anything ≥6 because 6 × 20 mg = 120 mg.

    b. Weigh a convenient amount of lactose that will give an aliquot ≥ the MWQ: 600 mg is selected

    c. Mix the two powders thoroughly by triturating in a mortar.

    d. Calculate the total weight of the dilution: 120 mg + 600 mg = 720 mg.

    e. Calculate the aliquot part of the dilution that contains the 20 mg of Codeine by multiplying the total weight of the dilution by the inverse of the multiple factor, 1/6 in this case: 1/6 × 720 mg = 120 mg.

    f. Weigh this calculated amount of the dilution to get the desired 20 mg of Codeine.

2. Analysis of Trial #1

    a. Once again there is the problem of selecting an appropriate amount of diluent. Fortunately, in the example above, 600 mg was sufficient to give an aliquot that is ≥ the MWQ.

    b. With this method, because the aliquot part is determined by multiplying the weight of the total dilution by the inverse of the multiple factor, the easiest way to determine the minimum amount of dilution is to set up and solve the following equation:

$$\left(\frac{1}{multiple\ factor}\right)x = 120\ mg\ (or\ desired\ weight\ of\ aliquot)$$

where x is the total amount of the dilution.
In the sample above:

$$\left(\frac{1}{6}\right)x = 120\ mg;\ x = 720\ mg$$

    c. As was mentioned above, the multiple factors chosen are usually whole numbers. This means that the only time the amount of drug weighed may be calculated to be a specified quantity, such as 120 mg, is when the weight of drug needed is a factor of that specified quantity.

    d. Method 2 becomes more difficult when you are restricted to weighing a certain amount of drug, such as the MWQ. In this case, the multiple factor must be calculated in the following fashion:

    multiple factor × amount of drug needed = 120 mg

    For example, if the amount of drug needed is 14 mg,

    multiple factor × 14 mg drug needed = 120 mg drug weighed

    Solving for the multiple factor:

    multiple factor = 120 mg /14 mg = 8.57

    The value 8.57 is a rounded value, so the calculated amounts are somewhat imprecise.

e. Once the multiple factor is determined, the amount of the dilution can then be calculated just as was done in the example above:

$$\left(\frac{1}{8.57}\right) x = 120 \ mg; \ x = 1028 \ mg$$

For this example, 120 mg of drug and 908 mg of lactose are weighed (908 mg lactose + 120 mg drug = 1,028 mg dilution). These are triturated together and 120 mg of the dilution is weighed to give 14 mg of drug. This should always be verified.

By proportion:

$$\frac{120 \ mg \ Codeine}{1028 \ mg \ dilution} = \frac{14 \ mg \ Codeine}{x \ mg \ dilution}; \ x = 119.9 \ mg \ dilution$$

By dimensional analysis:

$$\left(\frac{1028 \ mg \ dilution}{120 \ mg \ Codeine}\right)\left(\frac{14 \ mg \ Codeine}{}\right) = 119.9 \ mg \ dilution$$

f. When circumstances dictate that the multiple factor must be calculated, Method 2 becomes cumbersome. This occurs when the amount of drug to be weighed is restricted to a specified amount, such as when an aliquot must be made for a controlled substance.

III. SOLID–SOLID SERIAL DILUTIONS

A. Notice that in the table of values given in part (5) above, the minimum amount given in the "Amount of Drug Needed" column is 1.2 mg. This is because, as a general rule, an amount of drug requiring a dilution of greater than 100 to 1 is usually not done with a single dilution because homogeneous mixing at this level is difficult. Furthermore, the amount of diluent needed becomes unreasonably large. When very small quantities of drug are needed (e.g., <1 mg), a serial dilution is usually used. This method is avoided when possible because the mathematics is more difficult, and it is easy to get confused.

B. Determine the necessity of a serial dilution

➤ **EXAMPLE 9.3:** drug/amount desired: Hyoscine HBr 0.35 mg
  1. Notice in the table above that 0.35 mg of drug requires a dilution of greater than 100 to 1 (greater than 12,000 mg dilution to 120 mg drug).
  2. Refer back to Example 9.1, the Analysis of Trial #2. Notice that there are two methods that could be used to calculate the amount of dilution needed for a single aliquot to measure 0.35 mg of drug.
    a. A calculation like that described in part (3) could be used:

$$\frac{120 \ mg \ Hyoscine}{x \ mg \ dilution} = \frac{0.35 \ mg \ Hyoscine}{120 \ mg \ dilution}; \ x = 41,143 \ mg \ dilution$$

    b. The equation given in part (4) could also be used:

$$\frac{Amount \ of \ drug \ desired}{Amount \ of \ drug \ weighed} = \frac{Amount \ of \ dilution \ weighed}{Total \ amount \ of \ dilution}$$

$$\frac{0.35 \ mg}{120 \ mg} = \frac{120 \ mg}{x}; \ x = 41,143 \ mg \ dilution$$

The amount of dilution needed is 41,143 mg (120 mg Hyoscine plus 41,023 mg of lactose). This represents a ratio of 41,023 to 120, or 342:1.

C.   Perform a serial dilution using the following steps.

➤ *EXAMPLE 9.4:* drug/amount desired: Hyoscine HBr 0.35 mg
1. Weigh the MWQ of Hyoscine 120 mg.
2. Weigh an arbitrary amount of lactose that is ≥ the MWQ. In this case, because we need such a small quantity of drug, choose a larger quantity of lactose: 3,000 mg is selected
3. Thoroughly mix the two powders by triturating in a mortar. Remember to use geometric dilution.
4. Calculate the total weight of the dilution: 120 mg + 3,000 mg = 3,120 mg dilution A.
5. Weigh the MWQ, 120 mg, of dilution A.
6. Calculate the number of milligrams of Hyoscine that will be contained in 120 mg of dilution A.
   By proportion:

$$\frac{120 \; mg \; Hyoscine}{3120 \; mg \; dilution \; A} = \frac{x \; mg \; Hyoscine}{120 \; mg \; dilution \; A}; \; x = 4.6 \; mg \; Hyoscine$$

By dimensional analysis:

$$\left(\frac{120 \; mg \; Hyoscine}{3,120 \; mg \; dilution \; A}\right)\left(\frac{120 \; mg \; dilution \; A}{}\right) = 4.6 \; mg \; Hyoscine$$

7. Weigh a second amount of lactose that is ≥ the MWQ. Again, because we need such a small quantity of drug, choose a moderate quantity of lactose: 3,000 mg is selected
8. Thoroughly mix the 120 mg of dilution A with the 3,000 mg of lactose by triturating in a mortar.
9. Calculate the total weight of this second dilution: 120 mg + 3,000 mg = 3,120 mg dilution B.
10. Calculate the number of milligrams of dilution B that contains the desired 0.35 mg of Hyoscine. (Remember that although you weighed 120 mg of dilution A, it only contained 4.6 mg of Hyoscine.)
    By proportion:

$$\frac{4.6 \; mg \; Hyoscine}{3120 \; mg \; dilution \; B} = \frac{0.35 \; mg \; Hyoscine}{x \; mg \; dilution \; B}; \; x = 237 \; mg \; dilution \; B$$

By dimensional analysis:

$$\left(\frac{3,120 \; mg \; dilution \; B}{4.6 \; mg \; Hyoscine}\right)\left(\frac{0.35 \; mg \; Hyoscine}{}\right) = 237 \; mg \; dilution \; B$$

11. Weigh this calculated amount of dilution B to get the desired 0.35 mg of Hyoscine.

If the amount of dilution B is calculated to be less than the MWQ, larger amounts of lactose need to be chosen. If you do calculations of this sort frequently, you may wish to do an analysis like that done above for simple dilutions, or you may want to make a table similar to Table 9.1.

IV.   **SOLID-LIQUID ALIQUOTS**

A.   When a quantity of drug is needed that is below the MWQ, and the drug is to be incorporated into a liquid product, such as a solution, an emulsion, or a suspension, it is usually better to make a solid-liquid aliquot. This can be done only if the drug or chemical is soluble in a suitable solvent, such as water or alcohol, that is compatible with the product. Solid-liquid aliquots are preferred because: 1) they are easier to make—dissolving a drug in a solvent is less time-consuming than triturating a drug with a powdered diluent; and 2) complete homogeneity of the dilution is achieved with the solutions obtained using solid-liquid aliquots, so there is not the concern about uniform mixing; which is a possible problem with solid-solid aliquots.

B. Method 1

➤ *EXAMPLE 9.5*: drug/amount desired: Hydromorphone HCl 8 mg
   1. Basic steps
      a. Weigh the MWQ of Hydromorphone HCl: 120 mg.
      b. Check the solubility of Hydromorphone HCl in the chosen solvent, water: 1 g/3 mL.
      c. Dissolve the Hydromorphone in a convenient volume of water: 12 mL.
      d. Calculate the concentration of the drug in solution:

$$120 \text{ mg}/12 \text{ mL} = 10 \text{ mg/mL}$$

      e. Calculate the number of milliliters of dilution that contain the desired 8 mg of Hydromorphone.
      By proportion:

$$\frac{10 \text{ mg Hydromorphone}}{1 \text{ mL solution}} = \frac{8 \text{ mg Hydromorphone}}{x \text{ mL solution}}; \ x = 0.8 \text{ mL solution}$$

      By dimensional analysis:

$$\left(\frac{1 \text{ mL solution}}{10 \text{ mg Hydromorphone}} \right) \left(\frac{8 \text{ mg Hydromorphone}}{} \right) = 0.8 \text{ mL solution}$$

      f. Measure this calculated amount of the solution to get the desired 8 mg of Hydromorphone.
   2. Analysis
      a. When using 120 mg of the drug, 12 mL and 120 mL are convenient quantities of diluent since they give concentrations of 10 mg/mL (120 mg/12 mL) and 1 mg/mL (120 mg/120 mL), respectively. Concentrations like these make the mathematics relatively easy.
      b. The amount of diluent chosen depends on the solubility of the drug, the amount of liquid that can be accommodated in the preparation, and the minimum measurable quantity (MMQ) of the available measuring device.
      c. In the example above, the amount of solution to be measured is 0.8 mL. This quantity can be measured accurately in a 1- or 3-mL syringe. If syringes or micropipettes are not accessible and the smallest graduate available has a capacity of 10 mL, a different aliquot would be necessary. Because the MMQ is 20% of the capacity of a graduate, 2 mL would be the MMQ for a 10-mL graduate. In this case, the drug could be dissolved in 120 mL of water, giving a concentration of 1 mg/mL. The volume needed for 8 mg would be 8 mL. Other intermediate dilutions could be used as the circumstances dictate.

C. Method 2

➤ *EXAMPLE 9.6*: drug/amount desired: Hydromorphone HCl 8 mg
   1. Basic steps
      a. Select a multiple of the amount of drug needed that gives an amount which is ≥ the MWQ and weigh this amount:

$$15 \times 8 \text{ mg} = 120 \text{ mg}$$

      b. Check the solubility of Hydromorphone HCl in the chosen solvent, water: 1 g/3 mL

c. Dissolve the Hydromorphone in a convenient volume of water: 15 mL

d. Calculate the aliquot part of the dilution that contains the 8 mg of Hydromorphone by multiplying the solution volume by the inverse of the multiple, 1/15 in this case: $1/15 \times 15$ mL $= 1$ mL.

e. Measure this volume of the solution to get the desired 8 mg of Hydromorphone.

2. Analysis

a. Again, the amount of diluent chosen depends on the solubility of the drug, the amount of liquid that can be accommodated in the preparation, and the MMQ of the available measuring device.

b. In the case above, the multiple factor may not be chosen at random. It must be 15 because 15×8 mg $= 120$ mg. Hydromorphone is a controlled substance that requires no extra waste. As was illustrated in the section on solid-solid aliquots, the multiple factor can be calculated using the following equation:

$$(multiple\ factor)\ (amount\ of\ drug\ needed) = 120\ mg$$

As was illustrated in the discussion on solid-solid aliquots, this method is not as convenient when a specified weight of drug must be measured, such as 120 mg, and the amount of drug needed is not a factor of this weight. For our example, 8 is a factor of 120, so a convenient integer, 15, is calculated for the multiple factor. If the amount of drug needed was 9 mg, the multiple factor would be a less convenient 13.33.

c. In choosing the amount of solution to make, 15 mL was chosen as a convenient volume. Any volume that is a multiple (may be a whole number or a decimal) of the multiple factor is a convenient amount. This is because the volume of the aliquot is determined by multiplying the volume of solution by the inverse of the multiple factor. Any volume that is a multiple of the multiple factor gives an aliquot that has a non-rounded volume.

d. In the example above, the amount of solution to be measured is 1 mL. This quantity can be measured accurately in a 1- or 3-mL syringe. If syringes or micropipettes are not accessible and the smallest graduate available has a capacity of 10 mL, a different aliquot would be necessary. Because the MMQ is 20% of the capacity of a graduate, 2 mL would be the MMQ for a 10-mL graduate. In this case, the drug could be dissolved in 30 mL of water. A 1/15 aliquot needed to obtain 8 mg would then be 2 mL. Other dilutions could be used as the circumstances dictate.

V. LIQUID–LIQUID ALIQUOTS

A. Liquid–liquid aliquots can be required of two different types of liquids: a pure liquid or a concentrated solution of a drug. Aliquots of pure liquids are relatively uncommon because few drugs are liquid in their pure state. Aliquots involving concentrated solutions are more common. Examples of both are given here.

B. Pure Liquid

1. Method 1

Use direct volumetric measurement if appropriate equipment is available.

➤ **EXAMPLE 9.7:** drug/amount desired: Glacial Acetic Acid 0.2 mL

If a 1-mL syringe or a micropipette is available, measure 0.2 mL directly.

2. Method 2

If appropriate equipment is not available for direct measurement, you may use an aliquot method that is based on the MMQ for your smallest measuring device.

➤ **EXAMPLE 9.8:** drug/amount desired: Glacial Acetic Acid 0.2 mL

1. The smallest volumetric device available is a 10-mL graduate.

2. Measure the MMQ (20% of the graduated cylinder capacity) in a 10-mL graduate: 2 mL.
3. Completely transfer the liquid to a graduate of adequate size: a 25-mL graduate is selected.
4. Q.s. with water to a convenient amount: 20 mL.

Note: In this case, because Glacial Acetic Acid is a concentrated acid for which the normal procedure is to add acid to water, you would put some of the water in the 25-mL graduated cylinder, transfer the Glacial Acetic Acid, and then q.s. to the final volume with water.

5. Calculate the volume of the solution needed to give the 0.2 mL of Glacial Acetic Acid:

By proportion:

$$\frac{2 \ mL \ Gl. \ Acetic \ Acid}{20 \ mL \ solution} = \frac{0.2 \ mL \ Gl. \ Acetic \ Acid}{x \ mL \ solution}; \ x = 2 \ mL \ solution$$

By dimensional analysis:

$$\left(\frac{20 \ mL \ solution}{2 \ mL \ Gl. \ Acetic \ Acid}\right)\left(\frac{0.2 \ mL \ Gl. \ Acetic \ Acid}{}\right) = 2 \ mL \ solution$$

6. Measure this calculated amount of the solution to get the desired 0.2 mL of Glacial Acetic Acid.

3. Method 3

If appropriate equipment is not available for direct measurement, you may use an aliquot method that is based on a multiple of the quantity desired.

➤ **EXAMPLE 9.9**: drug/amount desired: Glacial Acetic Acid 0.2 mL
1. The smallest volumetric device available is a 10-mL graduate, which has a MMQ of 2 mL.
2. Select a multiple of the volume of drug needed that gives an amount that is ≥ the MMQ for your smallest measuring device and measure this amount:

$$10 \times 0.2 \ mL = 2 \ mL$$

3. Transfer the liquid to a graduate of adequate size: a 25-mL graduated cylinder is selected.
4. Q.s. with water to a convenient amount: 20 mL.

Note: Again with this case, because Glacial Acetic Acid is a concentrated acid for which the normal procedure is to add acid to water, you would put some of the water in the 25-mL graduated cylinder, transfer the Glacial Acetic Acid, and then q.s. to the final volume with water.

5. Calculate the aliquot part of the dilution that contains the 0.2 mL of Glacial Acetic Acid by multiplying the solution volume by the inverse of the multiple factor, 1/10 in this case:

$$1/10 \times 20 \ mL = 2 \ mL$$

6. Measure this volume of the solution to get the desired 0.2 mL of Glacial Acetic Acid.

C. Concentrated Solutions

1. Determine if the volume can be measured directly:

➤ **EXAMPLE 9.10**: drug/amount desired: Benzalkonium Chloride 1.5 mg
Benzalkonium Chloride (BAC) is available as a 17% w/v concentrated solution.
By proportion:

$$\frac{17 \ g \ BAC}{100 \ mL \ solution} = \frac{0.0015 \ g \ BAC}{x \ mL \ solution}; \ x = 0.0088 \ mL \ solution$$

By dimensional analysis:

$$\left(\frac{100\ mL\ solution}{17\ g\ BAC}\right)\left(\frac{0.0015\ g\ BAC}{}\right) = 0.0088\ mL\ solution$$

The volume 0.0088 mL is too small to measure, even with a syringe. An aliquot method must be used.

2. Aliquot method

For this situation, if appropriate equipment is not available for direct measurement, it is easiest to use an aliquot method that is based on the MMQ for your smallest measuring device.

➤ **EXAMPLE 9.11**: drug/amount desired: Benzalkonium chloride 1.5 mg

Benzalkonium Chloride (BAC) is available as a 17% w/v concentrated solution.
1. Measure the MMQ in a 1-mL syringe: 0.2 mL.
2. Calculate the amount of BAC in the 0.2 mL:

By proportion:

$$\frac{17\ g\ BAC}{100\ mL\ solution} = \frac{x\ g\ BAC}{0.2\ mL\ solution};\ \ x = 0.034\ g = 34\ mg\ BAC$$

By dimensional analysis:

$$\left(\frac{17\ g\ BAC}{100\ mL\ solution}\right)\left(\frac{0.2\ mL\ solution}{}\right) = 0.034\ g = 34\ mg\ BAC$$

3. From the quantity calculated above, determine a convenient volume of solution for the dilution: 34 mL is selected.
4. Transfer the 0.2 mL of concentrated BAC to an appropriate-sized graduated cylinder (e.g., 50 mL) and q.s. with water to the volume determined above: 34 mL.
5. Calculate the concentration of the drug in the solution: 34 mg/34 mL = 1 mg/mL.
6. Calculate the volume of the solution needed to give the 1.5 mg of BAC:

By proportion:

$$\frac{1\ mg\ BAC}{1\ mL\ solution} = \frac{1.5\ mg\ BAC}{x\ mL\ solution};\ \ x = 1.5\ mL\ solution$$

By dimensional analysis:

$$\left(\frac{1\ mL\ solution}{1\ mg\ BAC}\right)\left(\frac{1.5\ mg\ BAC}{}\right) = 1.5\ mL\ solution$$

7. Measure this calculated amount of the solution to get the desired 1.5 mg of BAC.

3. Analysis

a. The mathematics are easiest if the amount of the aliquot solution is chosen to give a convenient concentration of the drug in solution. This is done by first calculating the amount of drug or chemical in the measurable volume of the concentrate and then matching the volume of the aliquot solution to this quantity. In this case, the measurable volume of 0.2 mL of the BAC concentrate gives 34 mg of BAC. Therefore, 34 mL was chosen for the aliquot volume to give a convenient concentration of 1 mg/mL. Convenient numbers like these make it easier to check your answers to be sure that they are reasonable.

b. Once again, the amount of diluent chosen depends on the amount of liquid that can be accommodated in the final product.

CHAPTER 10

Isotonicity Calculations

I. GENERAL PRINCIPLES

A. Pharmaceutical solutions are sometimes applied to the sensitive membranes of the eye or nasal passages, or they may be injected into muscles, blood vessels, organs, tissue, or lesions. These solutions should be adjusted to have approximately the same osmotic pressure as that of body fluids because solutions that have the same osmotic pressure as cell contents do not cause a net movement of fluid into or out of the cells and therefore do not cause tissue damage or discomfort when placed in contact with cells. Solutions that exert the same osmotic pressure are called isoosmotic; solutions that exert the same osmotic pressure as a body fluid are termed isotonic, meaning of equal tone.

B. Osmotic pressure, like vapor pressure, freezing point, and boiling point, is a colligative property. Colligative properties depend not on the weight or the nature of the solute present in solution but only on the number of solute particles per given volume of solution. For example, one mole of dextrose (180 grams), when dissolved in one liter of solution, has the same effect on the osmotic pressure as does one mole per liter of sucrose (342 grams). Both of these substances are nonelectrolytes, and one mole of each gives an equal number of solute particles (Avogadro's number—6.02×10^{23}) when dissolved in water. In contrast, one mole of a univalent–univalent electrolyte, such as sodium chloride (58.5 grams), has twice the effect on osmotic pressure when dissolved in a liter of water because each sodium chloride gives two particles, a Na^+ ion and a Cl^- ion, when this salt is dissolved in water.

C. Although for pharmaceutical solutions we are interested in the changes in osmotic pressure caused by drugs and chemicals, we usually measure changes in freezing point caused by these substances. This is because osmotic pressure is difficult to measure directly, whereas freezing points are determined rather easily. Because both osmotic pressure and freezing point are colligative properties, freezing point depression can be used as a measure of change in osmotic pressure caused by dissolved drug or solute.

D. The fundamental expression relating freezing point depression and concentration of solute in solution is given by the equation: $\Delta T_f = K_f m$ where ΔT_f is the freezing point depression, K_f is the molal depression constant, and m is the molal concentration of the solute in solution. For water, K_f is 1.86 and the freezing point depression, ΔT_f, for a 1-m aqueous solution is $-1.86°C$.

E. Experimentally, the above equation holds true only for nonelectrolytes in dilute solution. Known concentrations of various drugs and chemicals have been dissolved in water and the freezing points of the solutions measured and compared to the normal freezing point of water, which is 0°C at normal atmospheric pressure of 1 atm. Although the freezing point depression of a 1-molal solution of a nonelectrolyte is approximately −1.86°C, electrolytes give larger molal freezing point depressions, the amount dependent on the number of ions generated per molecule, the degree of dissociation, and the degree of attraction of ions for the solvent. If a univalent–univalent solute like sodium chloride were completely dissociated in water, and if the molecules behaved ideally, a 1-molal aqueous solution of sodium chloride would have a freezing point of 2 × −1.86° = −3.72°C. Because molecules do not behave ideally in solution, the actual freezing point depression is somewhat less, approximately −3.35°C. (This discrepancy is an experimental measure of the extent of nonideal behavior.) The van't Hoff equation takes these factors into account with the equation $\Delta T_f = iK_f m$ where i, the van't Hoff factor, is the ratio of the colligative effect produced by a given concentration of electrolyte divided by the effect observed for the same concentration of nonelectrolyte. This expression has been further modified for the dilute aqueous solutions encountered at isotonic concentrations to give the useful equation:

$$\Delta T_f = L_{iso}\, c$$

where c is the molar (rather than the molal) concentration of solute in aqueous solution and L_{iso} is the experimentally determined iK_f, the molar freezing point depression at isotonic concentration, of the various ionic types (e.g., nonelectrolytes, univalent-univalent electrolytes, univalent-divalent electrolytes, and so on). Table 10.1 gives average L_{iso} values for various ionic types (1). The above equation and the values in Table 10.1 can be used to estimate freezing point depression for solutes in aqueous solution for which there are no published values of freezing point depression for that solute. For more information on this

TABLE 10.1 Average L_{iso} values by ionic type (1)

Ionic Type	Average L_{iso} Value	Examples
Nonelectrolytes: Substances that do not dissociate in aqueous solution	1.9	sucrose, dextrose, camphor, glycerin
Weak electrolytes: Substances that dissociate very slightly in solution	2.0	weak acids such as boric acid and citric acid, amine bases such as ephedrine and codeine
Divalent-divalent electrolytes: Substances that dissociate into two ions, the anion polyvalent	2.0	magnesium sulfate, zinc sulfate
Univalent-univalent electrolytes: Substances that dissociate into two ions, the anion univalent	3.4	sodium chloride, silver nitrate, cocaine hydrochloride, pilocarpine hydrochloride, acyclovir sodium
Univalent-divalent electrolytes: Substances that dissociate into three ions, the anion polyvalent	4.3	atropine sulfate, sodium carbonate, dibasic sodium phosphate (Na_2HPO_4), physostigmine sulfate
Divalent-univalent electrolytes: Substances that dissociate into three ions, the anion univalent	4.8	calcium chloride, calcium gluconate, zinc chloride, magnesium chloride,
Univalent-trivalent electrolytes: Substances that dissociate into four ions, the anion polyvalent	5.2	sodium citrate, potassium citrate
Trivalent-univalent electrolytes: Substances that dissociate into four ions, the anion univalent	6.0	aluminum chloride, ferric chloride
Tetraborates	7.6	sodium borate, potassium borate

subject, consult a book on physical pharmacy or the applicable chapters in *Remington: The Science and Practice of Pharmacy.*

II. FREEZING POINT DEPRESSION METHOD

A. Scientists have accurately measured the freezing points of the two critical body fluids, blood and tears, and have found these to be approximately the same namely, –0.52°C. For drug solutions to be isotonic with these fluids, they must have this same freezing point.

B. The freezing point depressions of many drugs in various concentrations in water have been measured and published in tables like those shown in Appendix H, where the values in the column marked $\Delta T_f^{1\%}$ are the freezing point depressions of 1% solutions of the drug or chemical in water. Because freezing point depression is additive, pharmacists can use these data to calculate the amount of solute to add in making isotonic solutions (that is, in making solutions with the same freezing point as blood or tears). This method of adjusting the tonicity of solutions using freezing point depression is shown below. The values for the example are taken from Appendix H. This table gives values for many common drugs; more complete tables of values can be found in *Remington: The Science and Practice of Pharmacy,* and in the miscellaneous tables section in the back of *The Merck Index.*

C. Basic Steps of the Freezing Point Depression Method
   1. Determine the percent concentration of the drug in solution.
   2. Read from Appendix H the freezing point depression caused by a 1% concentration of the drug in solution.
   3. Calculate the freezing point depression caused by the calculated concentration of drug in solution.
   4. Subtract this from the desired freezing point depression of 0.52°.
   5. Decide on an appropriate solute for adjusting the tonicity of the solution.
   6. Using the table, determine the freezing point depression caused by a 1% concentration of this solute in solution.
   7. Calculate the concentration of solute needed to give the remaining freezing point depression.
   8. Calculate the weight of solute in grams needed for the desired quantity of solution.

➤ **EXAMPLE 10.1:**

℞   Atropine Sulfate   2%
       Make isotonic with Boric Acid
       Purified Water q. s. ad   15 mL

   1. Determine the percent concentration of the drug in solution: 2%.
   2. Read from Appendix H the freezing point depression caused by a 1% concentration of the drug in solution: 0.07°.
   3. Calculate the freezing point depression caused by the calculated concentration of drug in solution.

$$\frac{1\%}{0.07°} = \frac{2\%}{x}; \; x = 0.14°$$

   4. Subtract this from the desired freezing point depression of 0.52°.

$$0.52 - 0.14° = 0.38°$$

   5. Decide on an appropriate solute for adjusting the tonicity of the solution.
      Boric Acid
   6. Using the table, determine the freezing point depression caused by a 1% concentration of this solute in solution: 0.29°.

7. Calculate the concentration of solute needed to give the remaining freezing point depression.

$$\frac{1\%}{0.29°} = \frac{x\%}{0.38°}; \ x = 1.3\%$$

8. Calculate the weight of solute in grams needed for the desired quantity of solution.

1.3% × 15 mL = 0.195 g Boric Acid

III. SODIUM CHLORIDE EQUIVALENT METHOD

A. Pharmaceutical scientists decided it would be convenient to have an easier way of calculating the amount of solute to add in adjusting the tonicity of solutions. In 1936 Mellen and Seltzer devised a system to compare the freezing point depression caused by sodium chloride to that of common drugs (2). Sodium chloride was chosen because it is the most common solute used for tonicity adjustment.

B. Mellen and Seltzer developed a factor, called the Sodium Chloride Equivalent, which is the weight in grams of sodium chloride that will give an equivalent osmotic effect to that of 1 gram of the designated drug.

C. Sodium Chloride Equivalents for a large number of drugs have been published. Values for many common drugs and chemicals are shown in Appendix H in the column marked $E_{NaCl}{}^{1\%}$. Some references use the designation "E" (for Equivalent) to designate the Sodium Chloride Equivalents.

D. The Sodium Chloride Equivalent method is based on the fact that a 0.9% concentration of sodium chloride in water gives an isotonic solution. This isotonic solution is also known as normal saline, isotonic saline, or isotonic sodium chloride. It is often abbreviated NSS for normal saline solution or NS for normal saline. The Sodium Chloride Equivalent method is illustrated below.

E. Basic Steps of the Sodium Chloride Equivalent Method
1. Calculate the number of grams of drug in the solution.
2. Read from Appendix H the Sodium Chloride Equivalent for the drug (that is, the weight in grams of sodium chloride that is equivalent to one gram of drug).
3. Calculate the weight in grams of sodium chloride that is equivalent to the weight in grams of the drug in this solution.
4. Calculate the number of grams of sodium chloride needed to make the desired volume of the drug solution isotonic if no other solute were present.
5. Subtract the weight in grams of sodium chloride that is equivalent to the weight of the drug from the weight of sodium chloride that would be needed to make the solution isotonic.
6. Add this amount of sodium chloride to the solution.

➤ *EXAMPLE 10.2:*

R̸	Atropine Sulfate	2%
	Make isotonic with Sodium Chloride	
	Purified Water q. s. ad	15 mL

1. Calculate the number of grams of drug in the solution.

2% × 15 mL = 0.3 g Atropine Sulfate

2. Read from Appendix H the Sodium Chloride Equivalent for the drug.
   0.13 (that is, 0.13 g NaCl is equivalent to 1 g Atropine Sulfate)

3. Calculate the weight in grams of sodium chloride that is equivalent to the weight in grams of the drug in this solution.

$$\frac{0.13 \ g \ NaCl}{1 \ g \ Atropine \ Sulfate} = \frac{x \ g \ NaCl}{0.3 \ g \ Atropine \ Sulfate}; \ x = 0.039 \ g \ NaCl$$

4. Calculate the number of grams of sodium chloride needed to make the desired volume of the drug solution isotonic if no other solute were present.

$$0.9\% \times 15 \ mL = 0.135 \ g \ NaCl$$

5. Subtract the weight in grams of sodium chloride that is equivalent to the weight of the drug from the weight of sodium chloride that would be needed to make the solution isotonic.

$$0.135 \ g - 0.039 \ g = 0.096 \ g \ NaCl \ needed$$

6. Add this amount of sodium chloride to the solution.

If the sodium chloride is available as sterile normal saline solution (NSS), the amount of this solution needed for isotonicity can be determined easily:

$$\frac{0.9 \ g \ NaCl}{100 \ mL \ NSS} = \frac{0.096 \ g \ NaCl}{x \ mL \ NSS}; \ x = 10.7 \ mL \ NSS$$

In this case, the solution would be made by dissolving the 0.3 g of Atropine Sulfate in 10.7 mL of NSS and then q.s. ad 15 mL with Sterile Water.

➤ **EXAMPLE 10.3:**

As you can see, this method is fairly simple if the tonicity adjustor is sodium chloride. It becomes more difficult if you want to use a different solute to adjust tonicity, such as the Boric Acid, which was used in the first example. In that case, another set of calculations is necessary to convert the amount of sodium chloride needed to an equivalent amount of the other solute. From Appendix H, the Sodium Chloride Equivalent for boric acid is 0.5. Therefore:

$$\frac{0.5 \ g \ NaCl}{1 \ g \ Boric \ Acid} = \frac{0.096 \ g \ NaCl}{x \ g \ Boric \ Acid}; \ x = 0.192 \ g \ Boric \ Acid$$

As you can see, the answer of 0.192 g of Boric Acid is very close to the 0.195 g of Boric Acid that was calculated using the freezing point depression method.

IV. USP METHOD (ALSO KNOWN AS THE WHITE–VINCENT METHOD OR THE SPROWLS METHOD)

A. The example shown above using Boric Acid is somewhat common because buffering agents are sometimes desired in isotonic ophthalmic solutions, and they can serve the dual purpose of buffering and tonicity adjustment. When several solutes are being added to a solution, such as when Sorensen's Buffer is used, the mathematics in using the Sodium Chloride Equivalent method become cumbersome.

B. In 1947 White and Vincent developed a simple and easy system to handle these situations (3). They made use of the fact that colligative effects are additive, so when one isotonic solution is added to another isotonic solution, you get an isotonic solution. They reasoned that the easiest way to make an isotonic solution would be to add sufficient water to the drug to make an isotonic solution and then q.s. to the desired volume with an isotonic diluting solution, either normal saline or an isotonic buffer.

C. White and Vincent developed this equation:

$$V = w \times E \times 111.1$$

where V = the volume in milliliters of isotonic solution that may be prepared by mixing the drug with water

w = the weight in grams of the drug

E = the sodium chloride equivalent of the drug and *111.1* is the volume in milliliters of the isotonic solution obtained when dissolving 1 g of sodium chloride in water.

Note: The value 111.1 is calculated from the 0.9% w/v concentration of sodium chloride in water, which gives an isotonic solution:

$$\frac{0.9 \; g \; NaCl}{100 \; mL \; isotonic \; solution} = \frac{1 \; g \; NaCl}{x \; mL \; isotonic \; solution}; x = 111.1 \; mL \; isotonic \; solution$$

The validity of the White-Vincent equation can be verified using dimensional analysis:

$$\left(\frac{w \; g \; of \; drug}{} \right) \left(\frac{E \; g \; NaCl}{1 \; g \; drug} \right) \left(\frac{111.1 \; mL \; isotonic \; sol'n}{1 \; g \; NaCl} \right) = w \times E \times 111.1 \; mL \; isotonic \; sol'n$$

D.   In 1949 Sprowls published a paper on the use of this type of system for making isotonic solutions in the pharmacy.

   1. The paper, "A Further Simplification in the Use of Isotonic Diluting Systems," appeared in *The Journal of the American Pharmaceutical Association, Practical Pharmacy Edition,* and included a list of calculated V values, the number of milliliters of water that will make given weights of various drugs isotonic (4).

   2. Sprowls' list gave the volume of water to make 0.3 g of drug isotonic. This weight was chosen because 0.3 g is the weight of drug for 1 oz or 30 mL of a 1% solution, a common situation with ophthalmic solutions. Some later tables of V values list the volumes for 1 g of drug. Column V^{1g} in Appendix H uses this later convention.

E.   It should be noted that the V values are not experimentally determined; they are derived values calculated from published Sodium Chloride Equivalents.

F.   Although the published tables of V values state that these are volumes of **water** needed to make a given weight of drug isotonic, the calculated volumes are really volumes of isotonic **solutions.** Furthermore, the assumption is made that the drug and sodium chloride have the same powder volume. Because isotonic solutions are dilute, the errors introduced by these approximations are small and insignificant for the intended purpose.

G.   This method is sometimes called the USP method because the USP published tables with these values and explained this method of making isotonic solutions. This method is illustrated below.

H.   Basic Steps in the USP Method

   1. Calculate the number of grams of drug in the solution.

   2. Read from Appendix H the number of milliliters of water needed to make 1 g of drug isotonic.

   3. Calculate the number of milliliters of water needed to make the desired weight of drug isotonic.

   4. Make this solution.

   5. Q.s. to the final desired volume with any isotonic solution.

➤ **EXAMPLE 10.4:**

℞	Atropine Sulfate	2%
	Make isotonic	
	Purified Water q. s. ad	15 mL

1. Calculate the number of grams of drug in the solution.
$$2\% \times 15\ mL = 0.3\ g$$
2. Read from Appendix H the number of milliliters of water needed to make 1 g of drug isotonic.
$$14.3\ mL$$
3. Calculate the number of milliliters of water needed to make the desired weight of drug isotonic.
$$\frac{1\ g\ Atropine\ sulfate}{14.3\ mL\ water} = \frac{0.3\ g\ Atropine\ sulfate}{x\ mL\ water}; \ x = 4.29\ mL\ water$$

4. Make this solution.
5. Q.s. to the final desired volume with any isotonic solution: 0.9% Sodium Chloride, 1.9% Boric Acid solution, Sorensen's Modified Buffer, and so on.

Notice that the 4.3 mL of water calculated in this part plus the 10.7 mL of isotonic saline calculated in the section on sodium chloride equivalents add up to the 15 mL of total solution needed.

J. If you prefer to use a system like this but you do not have V values, you can calculate them easily using published Sodium Chloride Equivalents and the equation of White and Vincent. They also can be calculated from the percent concentration of isotonic sodium chloride solution and the Sodium Chloride Equivalent for the drug. Sample calculations for both methods are shown here using the Atropine Sulfate example:

$$V = \left(\frac{0.3\ g\ Atropine}{1\ g\ Atropine}\right)\left(\frac{0.13\ g\ NaCl}{1\ g\ Atropine}\right)\left(\frac{111.1\ mL\ isotonic\ sol'n}{1\ g\ NaCl}\right) = 4.3\ mL$$

$$\left(\frac{100\ mL\ isotonic\ sol'n}{0.9\ g\ NaCl}\right)\left(\frac{0.13\ g\ NaCl}{1\ g\ Atropine}\right)\left(\frac{0.3\ g\ Atropine}{}\right) = 4.3\ mL$$

IV. L$_{iso}$ METHOD

A. As was discussed in the introduction to this chapter, the equation $\Delta T_f = L_{iso}\ c$ can be used to estimate freezing point depressions for solutes in aqueous solution when isotonicity values for freezing point depression or Sodium Chloride Equivalents are not available. It is possible that this will become more common in coming years. For nearly 30 years, two pharmaceutical scientists, Dr. E. R. Hammarlund and Dr. Kaj Pedersen-Bjergaard, were responsible for determining freezing point depression and Sodium Chloride Equivalent values for many drugs and chemicals, and together or individually they published these values in pharmaceutical journals from 1958 until 1989. As new drugs become available, the needed values may not be available for pharmacists to use in making the above calculations, and it will be necessary to rely on estimates based on the general L_{iso} equation.

B. Basic Steps of the L$_{iso}$ Method
1. Look up the MW of the drug and determine the molar concentration of the drug in solution.
2. From the chemical structure of the drug, determine its ionic type.
3. Read from Table 10.1 the L$_{iso}$ for the ionic type of the drug.
4. Calculate the freezing point depression caused by the calculated molar concentration of drug in solution.
5. Subtract this from the desired freezing point depression of 0.52°.
6. Decide on an appropriate solute for adjusting the tonicity of the solution.
7. Using the table in Appendix H, determine the freezing point depression caused by a 1% concentration of this solute in solution.

8. Calculate the concentration of solute needed to give the remaining freezing point depression.
9. Calculate the weight of solute in grams needed for the desired quantity of solution.

➤ **EXAMPLE 10.5:**

For ease of comparison with results obtained from published freezing point depression values, we will use the same prescription order as was given in Example 10.1.

Rx   Atropine Sulfate   2%
            Make isotonic with Boric Acid
            Purified Water q. s. ad   15 mL

1. Look up the MW of the drug and determine the molar concentration of the drug in solution.

Atropine Sulfate is available as the monohydrate with a MW = 695.

$$\left(\frac{mol\ Atr.\ Sulfate}{695\ g\ Atr.\ Sulfate}\right)\left(\frac{2\ g\ Atr.\ Sulfate}{100\ mL\ solution}\right)\left(\frac{1000\ mL}{L}\right) = 0.0288\ mol/L$$

2. From the chemical structure of the drug, determine its ionic type.

Atropine Sulfate is a univalent-divalent electrolyte

3. Read from Table 10.1 the L_{iso} for the ionic type of the drug.

4.3

4. Calculate the freezing point depression caused by the calculated molar concentration of drug in solution.

$$\Delta T_f = L_{iso}\ c = 4.3\ (0.0288) = 0.12$$

5. Subtract this from the desired freezing point depression of 0.52°.

$$0.52 - 0.12° = 0.40°$$

6. Decide on an appropriate solute for adjusting the tonicity of the solution.

Boric Acid

7. Using the table, determine the freezing point depression caused by a 1% concentration of this solute in solution: 0.29°.

8. Calculate the concentration of solute needed to give the remaining freezing point depression.

$$\frac{1\%\ Boric\ Acid}{0.29°} = \frac{x\%\ Boric\ Acid}{0.38°}; \ x = 1.4\%\ Boric\ Acid$$

9. Calculate the weight of solute in grams needed for the desired quantity of solution.

$$1.4\% \times 15\ mL = 0.21\ g\ Boric\ Acid$$

As is apparent from the results in this example, the estimate of required Boric Acid from the L_{iso} method is very close to that calculated from experimentally determined freezing point depression values. The answer is well within the range that is considered useful for the purpose of making isotonic solutions.

References

1. Wells JM. Rapid method for calculating isotonic solutions. J Am Pharm Assoc Prac Ed 1944; 5: 99–106.
2. Mellen M, Seltzer LA. A ready method for the extemporaneous preparation of isotonic collyria. J Am Pharm Assoc Sci Ed 1936; 25: 759–763.
3. White AI, Vincent HC. Diluting solutions in preparation of adjusted solutions. J Am Pharm Assoc Prac Ed 1947; 8: 406–411.
4. Sprowls JB. A further simplification in the use of isotonic diluting solutions. J Am Pharm Assoc Prac Ed 1949; 10: 348–351.

PART 3

COMPOUNDING DRUG PRODUCTS

CHAPTER 11

General Guidelines For Preparing Compounded Drug Preparations

I. DEFINITIONS

A. The following are definitions of compounding and manufacturing from the *National Association of Boards of Pharmacy (NABP) Model State Pharmacy Act*. They are also included in the NABP *Good Compounding Practices Applicable to State Licensed Pharmacies*. (The complete text of the latter document can be accessed on the CD that accompanies this book.)

    1. "**Compounding**–the preparation, mixing, assembling, packaging, or Labeling of a Drug or Device (i) as the result of a Practitioner's Prescription Drug Order or initiative based on the Practitioner/patient/pharmacist relationship in the course of professional practice, or (ii) for the purpose of, or as an incident to, research, teaching, or chemical analysis and not for sale or Dispensing. Compounding also includes the preparation of Drugs or Devices in anticipation of Prescription Drug Orders based on routine, regularly observed prescribing patterns" (1).

    2. "**Manufacturing**–the production, preparation, propagation, conversion, or processing of a Drug or Device, either directly or indirectly, by extraction from substances of natural origin or independently by means of chemical or biological synthesis, and includes any packaging or repackaging of the substance(s) or Labeling or relabeling of its containers, and the promotion and marketing of such Drugs and Devices. Manufacturing also includes the preparation and promotion of commercially available products from bulk compounds for resale by pharmacies, Practitioners, or other Persons" (1).

B. There are other definitions that communicate the essence of drug compounding.

    1. In a 2002 U.S. Supreme Court decision that dealt with the application of federal law to pharmacy compounding, Justice O'Connor, in the opinion of the Court, described compounding as follows:

    "Drug compounding is a process by which a pharmacist or doctor combines, mixes, or alters ingredients to create a medication tailored to the needs of an individual patient" (2).

2. In background information of a 2002 FDA study, "Survey of Drug Products Compounded by a Group of Community Pharmacies: Findings from a Food and Drug Administration Study," compounding is defined as:

"Combining, mixing, or altering of ingredients by a licensed pharmacist to create a customized drug (e.g., removal of a dye due to patient allergy, conversion to a different dosage form for ease of administration) for a patient based on the receipt of a valid prescription or in anticipation of prescriptions based on an order history from pharmacist-physician-patient relationship. Excludes: mixing, reconstituting, or other acts in accordance with directions in FDA approved labeling" (3).

II. EVOLUTION AND CURRENT STATUS OF COMPOUNDING IN PHARMACY PRACTICE

A. Although compounding drug dosage forms has been an integral part of the profession of pharmacy since antiquity, over the last 70 or 80 years, with the birth and growth of the pharmaceutical industry, there has been a significant decline in compounding by pharmacists. Estimates vary on the number of compounded prescriptions that are dispensed by pharmacies: a 1994 survey of U.S. pharmacies showed that number to be less than 1% (4); a 2002 FDA estimate places that number at approximately 250 million compounded prescriptions per year, between 1% and 8% of total prescriptions dispensed (3).

B. Relatively recently, primarily over the last 20 years, compounding of customized drug preparations by pharmacists has increased. The reasons for this are varied.

1. This increase has been due partly to a shift of interest on the part of the profession from merely "dispensing" drugs to an intensified concern for patients and their individual drug therapy needs—the pharmaceutical care movement. The commonly used definition of pharmaceutical care promulgated by Hepler and Strand, "the responsible provision of drug therapy for the purpose of achieving definite outcomes that improve a patient's quality of life" (5), carries with it the tacit requirement for considering individualized dosage and drug delivery systems.

2. There is a renewed awareness that individual patient therapy needs cannot always be met by drug products from the pharmaceutical industry, which has constraints imposed upon it by mass production and market-share requirements.

   a. This is manifested in several ways: specialty and projected low-profit items are never introduced by a manufacturer, low-volume products are discontinued, and there are periodic shortages (sometimes for considerable lengths of time) for some products.

   b. The latter has become such a difficult and common problem that in 2001, the American Society of Health-System Pharmacists (ASHP) published the document *ASHP Guidelines on Managing Drug Product Shortages*. ASHP also has maintained a update service for its members that attempts to help pharmacies with this chronic problem, and the FDA has a web site for posting availability of medically necessary products that are in short supply: www.fda.gov/cder/drug/shortages (Accessed December 2002).

   c. One obvious alternative for dealing with these problems is for the pharmacist to compound needed drug preparations when they are either temporarily or permanently not available from commercial sources.

3. Another factor that has contributed to an increase in drug compounding has been the trend toward home health care. For various reasons, including cost containment and patient comfort, patients' who previously would have been concentrated for treatment in hospitals and medical centers' are being treated at home. These patients often require individualized infusion therapy and other treatment modalities. This has created the need for a whole new type of pharmacy practice in which pharmacists in retail settings are required to prepare custom sterile and nonsterile dosage forms.

4. The expansion of custom-compounded drug preparations has been made possible in recent years partly because of the availability of new and useful items of equipment, packaging and labeling materials, excipients, and drugs and chemicals. New companies have been established and older existing companies have expanded that specialize in marketing these needed compounding supplies.

5. Needed information on compatibility and stability of compounded drug preparations has become available and more widely disseminated.

   a. New books, journals, and technical support from the vendors of pharmacy supplies have played an important role in enabling compounding to modernize and flourish. The recent addition to the pharmaceutical literature of the book *Trissel's Stability of Compounded Formulations*, and the journal *The International Journal of Pharmaceutical Compounding* are two prime examples.

   b. The United States Pharmacopeia (USP), which has for many years provided standards for purity and stability of manufactured drug products, has taken the initiative to develop and publish monographs for compounded drug preparations with tested formulations and stability information.

C. The present status of compounding in pharmacy practice can be judged in part by its inclusion in current written standards of practice, in published national competencies for pharmacist licensure, and in laws, court decisions, and FDA compliance guidelines on compounding. It is the responsibility of the pharmacist to be knowledgeable about these standards.

   1. The National Association of Boards of Pharmacy (NABP) have several Model Rules that address compounding. (The complete texts of the documents listed here are in the Appendices section of the CD that accompanies this book.)

      a. *Model Rules for Pharmaceutical Care*

         (1) In Section 1, Facility, Part A. Minimum Requirements for a Pharmacy, it states, "Each pharmacy shall be of sufficient size to allow for the safe and proper storage of Prescription Drugs and for the safe and proper Compounding and/or preparation of Prescription Drug Orders" (6).

         (2) In Section 5, Unprofessional Conduct, included as an act of unprofessional conduct is "Unreasonably refusing to Compound or Dispense Prescription Drug Orders that may be expected to be Compounded or Dispensed by Pharmacies or Pharmacists" (6).

      b. *Good Compounding Practices Applicable to State Licensed Pharmacies*

      c. *Model Rules on Sterile Preparations*

   2. ASHP has developed a number of Guidelines and Technical Assistance Bulletins that address compounding. These are listed here; the complete documents can be accessed on the ASHP web site at www.ashp.org.

      a. ASHP has two published guidelines that set minimum standards for pharmacies and pharmaceutical services: *ASHP Guidelines: Minimum Standard for Pharmacies in Hospitals* and *ASHP Guidelines: Minimum Standard for Pharmaceutical Services in Ambulatory Care.* Each has similar standards for extemporaneous compounding and sterile products. As an example, the wording of the standards for ambulatory care are given here.

      "***Extemporaneous Compounding.*** Drug formulations, dosage forms, strengths, and packaging that are not available commercially but deemed necessary for patient care should be prepared by appropriately trained personnel in accordance with applicable standards and regulations (e.g., FDA, U.S.P., state board of pharmacy). Adequate quality control and quality assurance procedures should exist for these operations. Commercially available products should be used to the maximum extent possible.

      Sterile Products. All sterile medications for use in the ambulatory care facility or for use by patients in the home should be prepared in a suitable environment by appropriately trained personnel and labeled appropriately for the user. Quality control and quality assurance procedures for the preparation of sterile products should exist, including periodic assessment of personnel on aseptic technique" (7).

    b. *ASHP Technical Assistance Bulletin on Compounding Nonsterile Products in Pharmacies*

    c. *ASHP Technical Assistance Bulletin on Quality Assurance for Pharmacy-prepared Sterile Products*

    d. *ASHP Technical Assistance Bulletin on Handling Cytotoxic Hazardous Drugs*

    e. *ASHP Technical Assistance Bulletin on Pharmacy-prepared Ophthalmic Products*

3. USP has developed and published General Chapters on compounding and monographs for compounded drug preparations.

    a. In November 1996, Chapter ⟨1161⟩ Pharmacy Compounding Practices was published in the 5th Supplement to *USP 23–NF18*. This chapter has subsequently been renumbered as Chapter ⟨795⟩, which places it in that section of the *USP* that gives it status as a potentially legally enforceable standard.

    b. General Information Chapter ⟨1206⟩ Sterile Drug Products for Home Use is current as of *USP 26–NF 21*, but changes to this chapter have been proposed in the *Pharmacopeial Forum*, including a change in chapter number to ⟨797⟩, which would also put this in the section of potentially legally enforceable chapters.

    c. Additional General Information Chapters on topics such as calculations for compounding, good compounding practices, and others are currently being drafted and discussed and will be added to the *USP*.

    d. The first 4 modern compounding monographs became official with the 9th Supplement to *USP 23–NF18*, 15 were included in *USP 24–NF19*, and the number of compounding monographs continues to grow.

4. The International Academy of Compounding Pharmacists (IACP) was founded in 1991 as a not-for-profit association of compounding pharmacists. With a membership of over 1,000 pharmacists, the organization works to promote the practice of pharmacy compounding by lobbying efforts at the state and national level. It provides a monthly newsletter and serves its members by providing a network of pharmacists with a common interest in compounding. Information about IACP is available at its web site at www.iacprx.org.

5. The competency statements listed for NAPLEX®, the national pharmacist licensing exam, include sections on compounding.

    a. 2.1.0 Perform calculations required to compound, dispense, and administer medication.

    b. 2.1.1 Calculate the quantity of medication to be compounded or dispensed, reduce and enlarge formulation quantities, and calculate the quantity or ingredients needed to compound the proper amount of the preparation.

    c. 2.3.0 Prepare and compound extemporaneous preparations and sterile products

    d. 2.3.1 Identify and describe techniques and procedures related to drug preparation, compounding and quality assurance.

    e. 2.3.2 Identify and use equipment necessary to prepare and extemporaneously compound medications.

    f. 2.3.3 Identify the important physicochemical properties of a preparation's active and inactive ingredients; describe the mechanism of, and the characteristic evidence of, incompatibility or degradation; and identify methods for achieving stabilization of the preparation (8).

6. Federal law and Food and Drug Administration Guidances

    a. In November 1997, Congress passed Public Law 105-115, Section 127, Application of Federal Law to Practice of Pharmacy Compounding. This law was part of the Food and Drug Administration Modernization Act of 1997 (FDAMA). It added a section, Sec. 503 A, Pharmacy Compounding, to the Federal Food, Drug and Cosmetic Act. This new provision supported the right of licensed pharmacists and physicians to compound drug products. Although this law was later found to be unconstitutional due to one of its provisions that restricted free speech, the Supreme Court opinion supported the general concept of extemporaneous compounding of drug products by pharmacists and physicians.

    b. In its most recent compliance policy guidance on pharmacy compounding, the FDA stated that it recognizes that pharmacists traditionally have extemporaneously compounded and manipulated drug products upon receipt of a valid prescription (9).

D. Historical perspective

Over the last century, changes in the methods used to produce and furnish drug products to patients have been accompanied by "growing pains" in the pharmaceutical industry, in the practice of pharmacy, and in federal and state regulatory bodies.

    1. As the pharmaceutical industry became established and grew, there were problems with quality control issues, unsubstantiated therapeutic claims, and questions of safety for industry-prepared drug products. In response, the federal government passed legislation and established administrative bodies aimed at providing the public with safe and reliable drug products. A brief chronological outline of the federal regulations enacted since 1900 is given in Table 11.1.

    2. Some of the same problems that have plagued the pharmaceutical industry are shared by pharmacists in professional practice, and pharmacy-prepared products have not been free from quality control problems. Several serious compounding incidents occurred in 1990 that alerted pharmacists, the FDA, and the public to some of these problems. These accidents illustrated what can happen when proper compounding procedures and controls are not used.

        a. In one case, a pharmacist prepared indomethacin ophthalmic drops that were not properly sterilized and preserved. The result was 12 patients who had eye infections and 2 patients who had to have an eye surgically removed (12,13).

        b. The second case also involved lack of sterility for preparations that were intended to be sterile. In this case, solutions prepared for use in a surgical unit were contaminated, and two patients died (12,13).

        c. In November 1990 the FDA issued an Alert Letter informing pharmacists about these incidents and warning them to use proper procedures and control measures for batch production of drug products that are intended to be sterile (12).

    3. These incidents caused the FDA, with its role in protecting public health, to consider ways of addressing these problems, but in each of the above cases, the drug product was made by compounding in a pharmacy, and compounding is a part of professional practice, a function regulated primarily by state laws with enforcement by state government agencies. In contrast, the FDA regulates pharmaceutical manufacturing through the Federal Food, Drug and Cosmetic Act; the FDA has lacked jurisdiction over professional practice unless misbranding or adulteration is involved.

    4. Unfortunately, the line between compounding and manufacturing is fuzzy. In fact, the controversy over what constitutes compounding and what constitutes manufacturing has yet to be resolved. While the debate continues, there are continuing initiatives aimed at finding a resolution that will protect all parties, most importantly the patients being served. Although a full exploration of all the issues is beyond the scope of this book, a chronology of recent events and initiatives is given here.

        a. At the time of the incidents mentioned above, the status of pharmacy-prepared drug products was vulnerable because there were cases of pharmacies/pharmacists who were engaged in manufacturing drug products under the guise of compounding. At an annual meeting of the American Pharmaceutical Association, then FDA Commissioner David Kessler reported, "Some of these operators [persons not registered with the FDA, but holding state pharmacy licenses] have their own detail persons, marketing consultants, and promotion departments. They buy unapproved drug substances in bulk quantities and manufacture products on a large scale. They operate like big manufacturers or wholesalers, but without the stringent safety and quality controls of legitimate pharmaceutical companies" (13). Obviously this type of activity would not and could not be tolerated.

        b. As a result, the FDA, through its field representatives and district offices, began to assert that it had both the right and responsibility to regulate drug products

TABLE 11.1   Historical Perspective on Regulation of Drug Quality

1906—Pure Food and Drug Act of 1906

1. The Act prohibited adulteration and misbranding of foods and drugs in interstate commerce.
2. It was originally administered by the Chemistry Bureau in the US Department of Agriculture; the Food and Drug Administration (FDA) evolved from this Bureau and by 1930 it was known by its present name. In 1940 it was transferred from the Department of Agriculture to the Federal Security Agency, the forerunner to the current Department of Health and Human Services (10).
3. When the Act was amended in 1912 to prohibit false or fraudulent efficacy claims, drug companies were able to circumvent prosecution by omitting all directions for use, etc. (10).
4. The USP and NF were already being published and were the official standards.
5. Drugs available at this time: many of the natural plant alkaloids such as codeine, morphine, cocaine, atropine, scopolamine, caffeine, colchicine, strychnine, etc; aspirin and salicylic acid; digitalis compounds; phenol; epinephrine; benzocaine; arsenic compounds and many other inorganic compounds such as Epsom salts ($MgSO_4$) and Glaubers salts (Na_2SO_4).

1938—Federal Food, Drug and Cosmetic Act

1. This Act required premarket documentation of **safety** of *new drugs*, that is, drugs not commonly used before 1938. All those listed above plus phenobarbital and digoxin were exempted by a "grandfather clause". As any of these *old drugs* came off patent, other firms could market them without FDA clearance (10).
2. This Act was passed in response to the sulfanilamide elixir tragedy in which over 100 people died as the result of taking an elixir which was made with a toxic solvent, diethylene glycol (antifreeze).
3. New Drug Applications, or NDAs, were used as the screening mechanism for drug safety, but the 1938 Act did not require proof of efficacy or therapeutic effectiveness (10).
4. Examples of drugs marketed after 1938 but before 1962, which were governed solely by the safety requirement, include hydrocortisone, prednisone, many antibiotics such as penicillin and tetracycline, many antihistamines such as chlorpheniramine and diphenhydramine, warfarin, chlorpromazine, chlorothiazide, and isoniazid.

1962—Federal Food, Drug and Cosmetic Act Amended

1. The Amended Act requires premarket proof of **safety and efficacy** of new drugs (10). The efficacy requirement brings with it the necessity of bioavailability testing.
2. The grandfather clause for drugs marketed prior to 1938 was left intact.
3. Congressional mandate required that drugs approved between 1938 and 1962 solely on safety be re-evaluated on efficacy. Any drug not recognized as effective would be considered a *new drug* subject to all regulations and requiring an NDA.

1967—Drug Efficacy Study Implementation (DESI)

1. FDA contracted with the National Academy of Science/National Research Council to do evaluations of the 1938–1962 drugs.
2. Thirty panels basically completed their work by mid-1969, but there are still some products in study and litigation. These are classified as "less than effective."

1970—Abbreviated New Drug Applications (ANDA) for DESI drugs

1. FDA introduced ANDA's for new products of 1938–1962 drugs that had cleared a DESI panel as efficacious. These required bioequivalence testing but no clinical testing for efficacy.

(Continued)

compounded by pharmacists. In one case involving a Georgia community pharmacist who was engaged in limited compounding for patients needing unique dosage forms, the director of the FDA's Atlanta district office wrote, "In simple terms, the practice of pharmacy does not include the compounding or dispensing of an unapproved new drug. Stating it another way, a drug product compounded in a pharmacy without FDA's approval is an unapproved new drug subject to all provisions" of the Food, Drug and Cosmetic Act (13). Fortunately this expanded interpretation of a *new drug* was not upheld, partly for practical reasons—there is an obvious need for unique dosage forms and the industry does not and cannot make doses or dosage forms uniquely.

   c. In March 1992, the FDA issued FDA Compliance Policy Guide 77132.16, Chapter 32, "Drugs General—Manufacture, Distribution, and Promotion of Adulter-

TABLE 11.1 Continued

2. Manufacturers of new generic products for drugs which were introduced after 1962 had to complete a "paper NDA" which gave literature citations on efficacy plus bioequivalence testing.

1974—Congress set up panels to study problems of chemical-therapeutic equivalence

1. The Office of Technology Assessment (OTA) of the U.S. Congress set up a panel of nine experts to review the relationship between chemical and therapeutic equivalence and the ability of current technology to determine this.

1977—First published list "Therapeutically Equivalent Drugs"

1. This list gave currently marketed drug products with their manufacturers that have complied with NDA or ANDA requirements.
2. Drugs not expected to have bioequivalence problems were given the designation "A" and those with documented or potential problems were given a "B" rating.

1978—Current Good Manufacturing Practice in Manufacture, Processing, or Holding of Human and Veterinary Drugs (CGMP or GMP)

1. FDA issued these regulations to aid them in assuring the public of safe, pure, and high quality drug products which have the appropriate identity, strength, quality and purity at the time of use (11).
2. It gives FDA the authority to do inspections of manufacturing facilities and it requires manufacturers to have written quality control procedures and stability testing programs.

1980—First annual *Approved Drug Products with Therapeutic Equivalence Evaluations* ("Orange Book") published

1. This update of FDA's "Therapeutically Equivalent Drugs" includes definitions of terms such as pharmaceutical and therapeutic equivalents, bioavailability, and bioequivalent drug products.
2. Published annually, this book of bioequivalence ratings of drug products becomes the basis for generic product evaluation and selection by pharmacists.

1984—Drug Price Competition and Patent Term Restoration Act

1. Eliminated "paper NDA" and allowed generic equivalents of post-1962 drug products coming off patent to be marketed using ANDA's. This made it easier to market generic products.
2. Innovator drug firms are compensated by being assured of a certain length of time to market new products under patent.

1997—Food and Drug Administration Modernization Act (FDAMA) of 1997

1. Sec. 503 A. Pharmacy Compounding was added to the Federal Food, Drug, and Cosmetic Act.
2. This addition to the Act codifies the right of pharmacists (and physicians) to compound drug preparations.

2002—Sec. 503 A. for FDAMA declared invalid by the U.S. Supreme Court

1. On a 5–4 decision the U.S. Supreme Court upheld a ruling by the 9th Circuit Court that the advertizing regulation of Sec. 503 A. is a violation of the First Amendment and an unconstitutional restriction of commercial free speech.
2. The Supreme Court also held that the restrictions on advertizing and solicitation in Sec. 503 A. could not be separated from the main part of the law and therefore the entire compounding provisions of FDAMA are declared invalid.

ated, Misbranded, or Unapproved New Drugs of Human Use by State-licensed Pharmacies." Briefly, it stated the following:

(1) FDA recognizes the right of pharmacists to compound drug products for individual patients when a prescription order has been received.

(2) Retail pharmacies are exempt from the biennial inspections to which manufacturers are subject provided they are licensed by their state and are operating within the scope of practice for pharmacies and are not manufacturing.

(3) FDA will usually defer the regulation of professional practice to state and local officials.

(4) FDA may exercise its enforcement prerogative if it deems that a pharmacy's activities are manufacturing. The Compliance Policy Guide lists nine possible acts that it will consider when making a decision about intervention. The list included such things as advertising and soliciting business for specific compounded products, making large amounts of products, using commercial-scale manufacturing equipment, and so on (14).

d. On May 26, 1993, at its 89th Annual Meeting, the National Association of Boards of Pharmacy approved *Good Compounding Practices Applicable to State Licensed Pharmacies*. This document distinguishes between compounding and manufacturing, and, as its name implies, it concisely defines good compounding practices. A primary difference in the interpretation of compounding as stated in the 1992 FDA Compliance Policy Guide and the NABP Good Compounding Practices concerns FDA's omission and NABP's acceptance of anticipatory compounding (that is, the preparation of drug products in anticipation of prescription orders based on regularly encountered prescribing patterns in the pharmacy).

e. In September 1995, at the annual meeting between representatives of FDA and NABP, improved communication and cooperation between the federal and state officials regarding enforcement of laws on manufacturing of drug products was discussed. A joint letter was drafted and sent to FDA district directors and state boards of pharmacy that reiterated basic policy on the issues.

  (1) The letter stated in part, "The basic policy that FDA will generally defer to state and local officials for the regulation of the day-to-day practice of retail pharmacy and related activities has not changed. The FDA does not intend to interfere with extemporaneous compounding and manipulation of reasonable quantities of drugs by licensed pharmacists based on valid prescriptions written for individual patients by licensed practitioners. However, both FDA and state officials continue to have significant concerns about commercial amounts of drugs being manufactured under the guise of compounding" (15).

  (2) The letter designated contact persons at FDA district offices and state pharmacy boards who could answer questions on these issues. A pharmacist with questions could contact his or her state pharmacy board for the designated persons in the state and district.

f. On Nov. 9, 1997, Congress passed Public Law 105-115, Section 127, Application of Federal Law to Practice of Pharmacy Compounding.

  (1) This law was part of the FDAMA. It added a section, Sec. 503 A, Pharmacy Compounding, to the Federal Food, Drug and Cosmetic Act. The new law took effect 1 year later on Nov. 21, 1998.

  (2) Although the new law supported the right of licensed pharmacists and physicians to compound drug products, it did establish certain restrictions.

  (3) Some of the provisions of FDAMA, as they apply to pharmacists (and physicians) who compound drug products, are briefly summarized here (16).

    (a) There must be a valid prescription based on an established relationship between the patient, an authorized prescribing practitioner, and the pharmacist.

    (b) Compounded quantities are limited to those for a patient on an individual prescription and based on a history of such valid prescriptions (that is, limited anticipatory compounding is allowed).

    (c) The substances used in compounding must either 1) comply with standards for *USP–NF* monographs and the *USP* chapter on pharmacy compounding, or 2) be a component of an FDA-approved product, or 3) be on a list of substances approved by a committee of the FDA.

    (d) Substances used in compounding cannot be on a list published in the Federal Register by the FDA that have been removed from the market because they have been found to be unsafe or not effective.

    (e) Drug products that are copies of commercially available products may not be compounded regularly or in inordinate amounts.

    (f) Drug products may not be compounded if they have been identified by the FDA as too difficult to compound so that they may not be safe or may be ineffective when compounded.

(g) The drug product must be compounded either 1) in a state that has a memorandum of understanding with the FDA concerning inordinate amounts of compounded drug products distributed outside the state, or 2) the amount sent outside of state by the compounder may not exceed 5% of the total prescriptions dispensed by that pharmacy.

(h) The compounding pharmacist may not advertise or promote the compounding of a particular drug or class of drugs (16).

g. In 1998 a group of pharmacists (Western States Medical Center *v*. Shalala) challenged that section of the new law that restricted their right to advertise, asserting that this violated their First Amendment right to free speech. The case was originally heard in the U.S. District Court in Nevada, which found for the plaintiffs. This was appealed by the federal government to the 9th U.S. Circuit Court of Appeals. Although both courts held that the advertising restriction of the law violated the plaintiffs' right to commercial free speech, the Court of Appeals also held that the restriction on advertising and solicitation in Section 127 could not be separated from the main part of the law, and therefore found the entire compounding provisions of Section 127 of FDAMA invalid.

h. On Feb. 26, 2002, in Thompson, Secretary of Health and Human Services, et al. *v*. Western States Medical Center et al., the federal government appealed the Circuit Court decision to the U.S. Supreme Court. On April 29, 2002, in a 5–4 decision, the Supreme Court upheld the decision of the Circuit Court of Appeals. In the opinion of the court, written by Justice O'Connor, it was found that the restrictions on speech were more extensive than necessary, and that the government could rather use other restrictions such as prohibiting compounding pharmacists from using commercial-scale manufacturing or testing equipment, or limiting the amount that can be compounded to that for prescriptions already received, or banning compounded drug products from being sold at wholesale to other state-licensed entities. This ruling rendered all of section 503A invalid (2). (The entire court decision, including the dissenting opinion, can be accessed in the Appendices section of the CD that accompanies this book.)

i. New FDA Compliance Policy Guides Manual

(1) In May 2002, in response to the Supreme Court decision, the FDA issued a new Compliance Policy Guides Manual, Sec. 460.200, Pharmacy Compounding. This guidance, while it does not have the force of law, is intended to inform both FDA staff and the individuals involved with compounding about FDA's current views on the topic of pharmacy compounding and the sort of practices that FDA will consider to be violations of the Federal Food, Drug and Cosmetic Act. The introductory paragraph in the discussion begins as follows:

"FDA recognizes that pharmacists traditionally have extemporaneously compounded and manipulated reasonable quantities of human drugs upon receipt of a valid prescription for an individually identified patient from a licensed practitioner. This traditional activity is not the subject of this guidance" (9).

(2) The guidance describes those activities of pharmacies that the FDA contends puts them in the ranks of manufacturers rather than compounding pharmacies. These include such things as buying and using large quantities of bulk drug substances, making substantial quantities of drug products in advance of receiving a valid prescription for the product, and selling the products to patients and physicians with only a remote professional relationship (9).

(3) The FDA states that it will continue to defer to state boards regarding "less significant" violations associated with compounding by pharmacies and will work with states concerning investigations and enforcement of applicable regulations (9).

(4) If the range of compounding activities of the pharmacy places it more in the category of a manufacturer, and there are significant violations of the new drug, adulteration, or misbranding regulation of the Food, Drug and Cosmetic Act, FDA will consider federal enforcement of that pharmacy practice. The Guidance lists nine items that it will consider in making this determination. Interestingly, some of the items listed use the same or similar language as was used by Justice O'Connor in her Supreme Court opinion described above (e.g., "Using commercial-scale manufacturing or testing equipment for compounding drug products") (2). Other items are the same or similar to those in FDAMA Section 127. The Guidance includes the list of drugs, compiled under FDAMA, that should not be compounded because they have been removed from the market for safety reasons (9).

(5) The FDA asked for comments about the new Guidance, and several groups such as the International Academy of Compounding Pharmacists have issued their critiques of the document.

(6) The full text of this document is given in the Appendices section of the CD that accompanies this book.) It is also available from the Division of Compliance Policy (HFC-230, Food and Drug Administration, 5600 Fishers Lane, Rockville, MD 20857 or on the Internet at: www.fda.gov/ora/compliance_ref/cpg/ default.htm. Because this Guidance is subject to revision, it would be best to make sure that you have the most current version.

j. It would seem that compounding accidents and incidents would be a rarity as we progress into the 21st century. Surely with news media stories of accidents and well-researched and widely distributed reports such as the Institute of Medicine's *To Err is Human*, there should be a heightened awareness of potential problems concerning patient safety. Furthermore, especially since the early 1990s, there has been increased activity in published standards of practice, guidelines, and federal guidances plus a great variety of readily available information on acceptable techniques, processes, and formulations. Unfortunately, problems with unacceptable compounded preparations continue to be reported.

(1) In a June 23, 2002, story in the *San Francisco Chronicle*, the investigative reporters related a list of recent compounding accidents: 4,200 cancer patients in the Kansas City, Missouri area who received diluted chemotherapy agents; four patients in Atlanta who were hospitalized after taking a compounded thyroid preparation that was 1,000 times its intended potency; eight patients in Memphis who had neurological damage due to a drug error in an implanted pump; and two separate incidents with *Serratia* contamination in drug solutions that were intended to be sterile—with one of the incidents, 38 patients received contaminated spinal injections, and 3 of these patients died (17).

(2) In October 2002 the FDA reported on a study that it had just conducted on compounded preparations it obtained from 12 pharmacies. The pharmacies were selected because they furnished compounded medicines ordered through the Internet. Of the 29 formulations tested, 9 were subpotent when measured against USP standards; 5 had 70% or less of the required active ingredient. One injectable product had an unacceptable level of endotoxins (3).

(3) In December 2002, the Centers for Disease Control and Prevention (CDC) reported that a compounding pharmacy in South Carolina had made and dispensed injectable methylprednisolone acetate suspensions that were contaminated with the fungal agent *Exophiala dermatitidis*. The injections had been distributed in 11 states. The report described five cases of infection caused by these injections; one patient had died. An inspection of the pharmacy showed an autoclave that did not perform properly and a series of practices that did not meet the ASHP guidelines for pharmacy-prepared sterile products, including lack of sterility testing and inadequate cleanroom procedures (18).

k. While we all know that accidents do happen (e.g., *To Err is Human*), the above pattern of incidents is clearly unacceptable. As pharmacists we can and should do better; in fact, **we must do better**. In analyzing compounding medication accident cases, they occur for a variety of reasons. While most incidents are truly accidents, the Kansas City case described above was an exception in that increased profit was the motive behind the pharmacist's intentionally dispensing subpotent antineoplastic products. In some cases, there is either inadequate training or lack of knowledge of the accepted standards, while other times the pharmacist is aware of the guidelines but thinks that the standards are too stringent and/or too costly and disregards them. For example, in one of the *Serratia* contamination cases identified above, there are published standards for sterile products in Risk Level 3 (see Chapter 32, Parenteral Products), but for some reason these standards were not followed. In other cases, there are mathematical, weighing and measuring, ingredient selection, or compounding procedure errors. Often these mistakes could have been avoided by using well-documented procedures, independent colleague verification, and/or the triple-check systems that have been advocated for many years.

In summary, pharmacists need to be both knowledgeable and careful. They need a solid pharmacy education followed by life-long learning, and they need to know their limitations. If embarking on a new or specialty area of practice, such as sterile products, the pharmacist should read and study available literature, guidelines, and standards, get training from well-respected sources, network with a diverse set of colleagues, obtain information from a variety of professional organizations and governmental agencies, and use both basic science knowledge and critical thinking skills to make good judgments, always in the best interests of the patient.

IV. BASIC STEPS TO FOLLOW IN COMPOUNDING DRUG PRODUCTS

A. The chapters that follow in this book were written to give guidance on extemporaneous compounding.

1. Information is given on the selection and use of compounding ingredients, equipment, and pharmaceutical necessities.

2. In chapters 24 through 33, the various dosage forms are described, and information is presented that is specific to each dosage form. In each case, sample prescription or medication orders are given with a sample evaluation of stability and compatibility for the formulation, calculations of dose and quantities, compounding procedure, basic quality assessment of the preparation, and labeling; a sample patient consultation is given for prescription orders for ambulatory patients. The calculations portions of the samples build on the basic calculations given in chapters 7 through 10. For the non-parenteral sample prescriptions, the scenarios are those of an individual prescription for a customized drug preparation being presented by a patient or caregiver to a pharmacist, a situation that could occur in almost any pharmacy practice setting. Those sample medication orders for parenteral medications would be typical of those seen in an institutional setting.

3. Sample compounding formula sheets and sample control sheets are given in this chapter. Samples of some basic standard operating procedures (SOP), such as those needed for testing balances and capsule weights, are given in the applicable chapters. Other SOPs are beyond the scope of this text, but samples are readily available through sources such as the *International Journal of Pharmaceutical Compounding*.

4. Finally, material, applicable to all dosage forms, on compatibility and stability of drugs, chemicals, and drug preparations is discussed in Chapter 34.

B. The following are basic steps to use when compounding any drug preparation.

1. Carefully read and interpret the prescription or medication order. It may be necessary or helpful to consult with the prescriber and the patient about the intent of the drug preparation and preferences or limitations of the patient.

2. Note any missing or confusing information; clarify, gather, and add this information to the drug order.

3. Check the dose, dosage regimen, dosage form, and route of administration for appropriateness.

4. Check compatibility and stability information for the individual ingredients and the ingredient combination in the formation, and determine a beyond-use date. If there are any problems in this regard, consult with the prescriber to resolve the issues.

5. Determine a preliminary compounding procedure based on the available ingredients and the prescribed dosage form.

6. Perform necessary calculations. If possible, have a colleague check the calculations for appropriateness and accuracy.

7. Select the required ingredients.

8. Choose appropriate compounding equipment.

9. Using recommended techniques, prepare the product.

10. Perform quality control procedures.

    a. Visual inspection of the preparation should always be done and documented on the prescription order or record of compounding.

    b. Make measurements when this is possible and appropriate (e.g., capsule weights, pH measurements, final weight or volume compared to the theoretical values, etc.).

    c. In all cases, the user-patient should be instructed to watch for any change in the preparation that may indicate that physical instability, chemical degradation, or microbial growth has occurred; the patient should be told to contact the pharmacist if there are questions.

11. Choose an appropriate container and package the preparation.

12. Label the container, including recommended auxiliary labels.

13. Recheck all work.

14. Document the compounding process. This includes adding additional information to the prescription document or making a quality control record. As indicated above, a sample compounding formula sheet is shown in Figure 11.1 and a sample compounding record sheet is shown in Figure 11.2.

15. Deliver the product to the patient or caregiver with appropriate consultation, and check for understanding of use of the product.

■ **Figure 11.1** Sample compounding formula sheet.

COMPOUNDING FORMULA

Name and Strength of Product:_____

Quantity:_____
(Number of units, volume, weight, etc.)

Therapeutic Use/Category:

Route of Administration:

Formula:

Ingredient	Quantity	Physical Description	Solubility	Function

Method of Preparation:

Calculations:

Theoretical Information (Literature Search):
(Information on compatibility, stability, and special processing procedures)

Specialized Equipment (If needed):

Description of Finished Product:

Quality Control Tests:

Recommended Storage Conditions:

Packaging:

Stability/Beyond-Use Date:
(with references when available)

Labeling Information:
(Product content and auxiliary labels)

Patient/Caregiver/Staff Instructions:

■ **Figure 11.2** Sample compounding record sheet.

COMPOUNDING RECORD

Control # _____

Name and Strength of Product: _____

Quantity Made: _____
(Number of units, volume, weight, etc.)

Ingredient	Manufacturer/Lot #	Quantity

Prepared by: _____ **Checked by:** _____

Quality Control Data:

Date Prepared:_____ **Beyond-use Date:** _____

References

1. National Association of Boards of Pharmacy Good Compounding Practices Applicable to State Licensed Pharmacies. National Association of Boards of Pharmacy. Park Ridge, IL, 2001; 151.

2. Thompson, Secretary of Health and Human Services, et al. *v.* Western States Medical Center et al. 535 U.S. 2 (2002).

3. Subramaniam V, Sokol G, Zenger V, et al. Survey of Drug Products Compounded by a Group of Community Pharmacies: Findings from a Food and Drug Administration Study. Rockville, MD: Food and Drug Administration, www.fda.gov/cder/pharmcomp/communityPharmacy/default.htm Accessed December 2002.

4. Geesman J, Huffman DC. NARD-Lilly Digest. Alexandria, VA: NARD Foundation, 1994.

5. Hepler CD, Strand LM. Opportunities and responsibilities in pharmaceutical care. Am J Hosp Pharm 1990; 47: 533–543.

6. National Association of Boards of Pharmacy Model Rules for Pharmaceutical Care. National Association of Boards of Pharmacy. Park Ridge, IL, 2001; 71, 95.

7. American Society of Health-System Pharmacists. ASHP guidelines: minimum standard for pharmaceutical services in ambulatory care. Am J Health-Syst Pharm 1999: 56: 1744-1753.

8. Area II Assure safe and accurate preparation and dispensing of medicines. NAPLEX® Candidate's Review Guide 5.0, Park Ridge, IL. National Association of Boards of Pharmacy, www.nabp.org Accessed December 2002.

9. Guidance for FDA staff and industry, Compliance policy guides manual, Sec. 460.200 Pharmacy compounding. Rockville, MD: Food and Drug Administration Center for Drug Evaluation and Research, May 2002, www.fda.gov/ora/compliance_ref/cpg/default.htm. Accessed December 2002.

10. Fink JL, Marquardt KW, Simonsmeier LM, eds. Pharmacy Law Digest, 26th rev. St. Louis: Facts and Comparisons, Inc., 1995; DC-3–DC-4.

11. Vadas EB. Stability of pharmaceutical products. In: Gennaro AR, ed. Remington: The science and practice of pharmacy, 19th ed. Easton, PA: Mack Publishing Co., 1995; 639.

12. Bloom MZ. Compounding in today's practice. Am Pharm 1991; 31: 31–37.

13. Conlan MF. Compounding versus manufacturing. Where is the line? Drug Topics 1992; 136: 46–51.

14. FDA Compliance Policy Guide 77132.16. Chapter 32–Drugs General—Manufacture, Distribution, and Promotion of Adulterated, Misbranded, or Unapproved New Drugs of Human Use by State-licensed Pharmacies. Rockville, MD: U.S. Department of Commerce, National Technical Information Service, March 1992.

15. NABP/FDA Annual Meeting. Initiatives Support Federal-State Cooperation. NABP Newsletter, December 1995: 135, 142.

16. Public Law 105-115. Section 127. Application of Federal Law to Practice of Pharmacy Compounding.

17. Hallissy E, Russell S. Who's mixing your drugs? Bad medicine: Pharmacy mix-ups a recipe for misery; some drugstores operate with very little oversight. *San Francisco Chronicle* June 23, 2002: A-1.

18. *Exophiala* infection from contaminated injectable steroids prepared by a compounding pharmacy—United States, July–November 2002. Centers for Disease Control and Prevention. MMWR 2002; 51: 1109–1112.

CHAPTER 12

Selection, Storage, and Handling of Compounding Equipment and Ingredients

I. COMPOUNDING EQUIPMENT

A. The minimum requirements for compounding equipment for pharmacies usually are set by state pharmacy practice acts. Consult your state statutes for this information.

B. The following is a modest list of equipment that will serve most extemporaneous compounding needs. Where appropriate, descriptions, uses, and limitations are also given.
   1. Balances
   For detailed descriptions of balances, their specifications, and proper care and use, see Chapter 13, Weighing and Measuring.
   2. Volumetric apparatus
   For specifications and descriptions of graduated cylinders and other volumetric apparatus, see Chapter 13, Weighing and Measuring.
   3. Mortars and pestles
      a. Wedgewood mortars are heavy-duty, durable mortars available in various sizes, 2 oz, 4 oz, 8 oz, 16 oz, and 32 oz. They are made with rough interior surfaces, making them ideal for particle size reduction and for making emulsions, where efficient shear is desirable. Because of their porous interiors, Wedgewood mortars should not be used for drugs that stain, for drugs present in small quantities, or for very potent drugs. The rough surfaces of Wedgewood mortars do become smooth with continued use. When this occurs, some pharmacists triturate washed sand in the mortar in an effort to re-roughen the surfaces, but this procedure has limited success.
      b. Porcelain mortars are similar to Wedgewood mortars but are usually smaller and somewhat less durable.
      c. Ceramic mortars are similar to Wedgewood mortars with abradant interior working surfaces, and therefore have similar uses and precautions. They are available in sizes ranging from 2 oz to 16 oz. They are less expensive but also less durable than Wedgewood mortars.

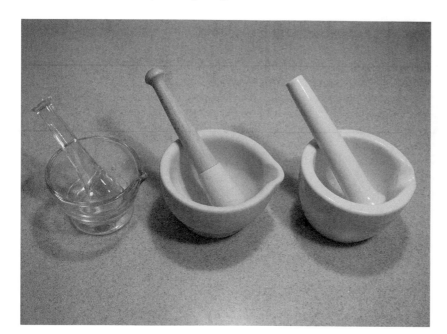

Mortars and pestles (glass, Wedgewood, and ceramic)

    d. Clear glass mortars have smooth, nonporous interior surfaces, making them useful for triturating drugs that stain. They are also preferred for triturating highly potent drugs. Because of their smooth sides, glass mortars are not as efficient as Wedgewood or ceramic mortars in reducing particle size of powders. They are also not preferred for making emulsions because adequate shear is difficult to achieve with a glass mortar and pestle. Like Wedgewood mortars, they are available in sizes ranging from 2 oz to 32 oz.

4. Spatulas

    a. Stainless steel spatulas with wooden or hard plastic handles are available in various sizes, with blades from 3 to 12 inches in length. It is important to use the appropriate size and type for the task.

        (1) The small sizes are used for handling dry chemicals, for scraping materials from other spatulas and from the sides of small mortars and pestles, and for levigating small quantities of drugs and chemicals on ointment pads or slabs.

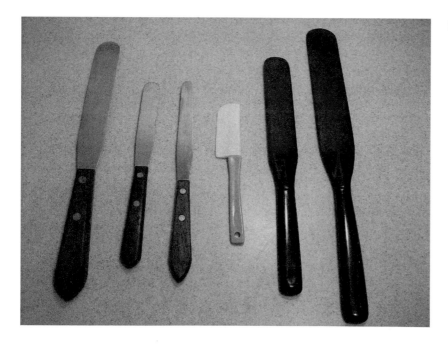

Spatulas

    (2) The larger sizes are used for handling larger quantities of materials. Spatulas with 8- to 12-inch blades are preferred for levigating moderate to large quantities of drugs and for mixing or spatulating ointments.

    (3) Special spatulas of this type with angled blades are also available.

  b. Small, double-bladed, nickel-stainless steel spatulas, sometimes called micro spatulas, are useful for withdrawing small amounts of chemicals and drugs from their containers. They are not used for levigation.

  c. Hard rubber or Teflon®-coated stainless steel spatulas, 4 and 6 inches, are **special purpose only:** they are used in handling drugs and chemicals, such as iodine, that react with metal. In general, they lack the flexibility needed for levigating and spatulating ointments.

  d. Flexible rubber spatulas, sometimes called rubber policemen or rubber scrapers, have broad, rectangular, flexible, rubber, silicone, or plastic scrapers with wooden or plastic handles. These spatulas are very useful for scraping material from the inside surface of mortars when transferring a preparation from the mortar to a packaging container.

5. Glass and plastic funnels come in various sizes: 2 oz, 4 oz, 8 oz, 16 oz, and 32 oz. They are used for transferring solutions from one vessel or bottle to another. These are also used with filter papers in filtering solutions. **Do not try to use them for transferring suspensions or emulsions from a mixing vessel to a prescription bottle—** the bore on the glass stem will generally get clogged and you will have a mess!

6. Ointment slabs and pads

  a. Ointment slabs

    (1) Although these are called *ointment* slabs because of their use as a surface for levigation and spatulation in compounding ointments, an ointment slab may also be used as a clean, hard surface for holding powders when punching capsules, and as a surface for rolling semi-solid materials when marking hand-rolled suppositories or troches.

    (2) Some ointment slabs have a rough surface on one side to facilitate particle size reduction when levigating powders for ointments. Care must be exercised to avoid getting water-insoluble materials (dyes, tars) in the pores on this rough side because this surface is difficult to clean and residues may contaminate future products.

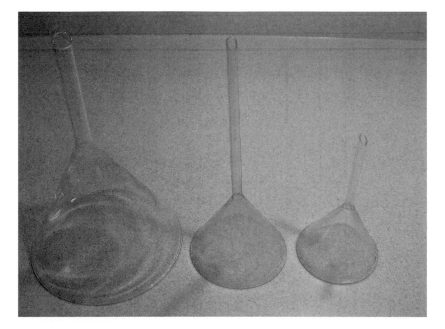

Glass funnels

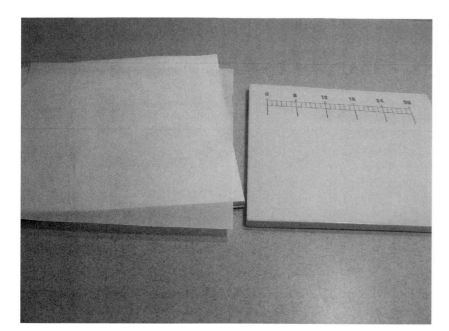

Ointment pad and
ointment slab

    b. Ointment pads

       (1) Ointment pads are convenient because the top sheet is used and then torn off and discarded when the job is completed—a great time-saver.

       (2) They do have some limitations. They soak up liquids, including the water phase of creams, aqueous solutions to be incorporated into ointment bases, and even thick tar-like ingredients; ointment slabs are preferred over pads in these situations.

7. Glass stirring rods are useful for stirring liquid preparations. Spatulas are not to be used as stirring rods.

8. Pyrex® or other heat-resistant beakers: 50 mL, 100 mL, 150 mL, 250 mL, 400 mL, 600 mL, and 1,000 mL. These are described in Chapter 13, Weighing and Measuring.

9. Crucibles and evaporating dishes are handy for heating suppository and ointment bases. They can also be used as the water vessel for a hot-water bath.

10. Suppository and troche molds

    a. Aluminum and plastic disposable suppository molds are needed for making suppositories by fusion. These are described and pictured in Chapter 31, Suppositories.

    b. Plastic disposable troche molds are described and pictured in Chapter 25, Capsules, Lozenges, and Other Solid Dosage Forms.

11. Filter papers, various sizes

12. Cutting devices, such as scissors and single-edge razor blades

13. Laboratory thermometer

14. Wax or other marking pen

15. Brushes of various sizes and shapes for cleaning graduates and funnels

16. Heating devices

    a. Microwave oven

       (1) As a heating device, a microwave oven is convenient, safe, and fast.

       (2) Because microwave ovens work on the principle of alternating polarity, they do not heat non-polar substances such as white petrolatum or waxes. This disadvantage can be overcome by using the microwave oven to heat water in a crucible or beaker; this may then be used as a hot-water bath for heating or melting nonpolar items.

       (3) Microwave ovens can develop "hot spots" that may cause overheating and degradation of ingredients.

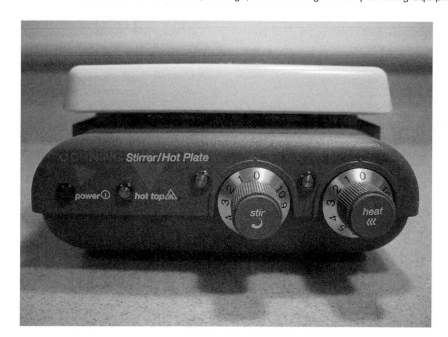

Hot-plate with magnetic stirrer

b. Hot-plate

(1) Hot-plates offer fast and direct sources of heat, but they require careful monitoring to avoid overheating or scorching of ingredients. When heating a preparation that must have a carefully controlled temperature, and the desired temperature is 100°C or less, a hot-water bath may be the preferred heating device.

(2) Some hot plates are available with magnetic stirring devices, which can be very handy.

c. Hot-water bath

A hot-water bath can be improvised by using two Pyrex® beakers or similar vessels of different sizes. Water is added to the larger beaker, and this is heated to the desired temperature either on a hot-plate or in a microwave oven. The material to be heated is placed in the smaller beaker and the smaller beaker is then floated in the hot water in the larger beaker.

17. Refrigerator (including a freezing compartment) that will maintain temperatures as specified in the *USP*

18. A sink with hot and cold tap water, hand soap and dish detergent, and air dryer or single-use towels to be used for washing hands and for washing glassware and other compounding equipment

a. Potable (tap) water is acceptable for washing hands, glassware, and compounding equipment, but it is not to be used as an ingredient in making drug preparations.

b. Potable water should meet the requirements of the Environmental Protection Agency's (EPA) National Primary Drinking Water Regulations as given in 40 CFR Part 141 (1).

c. **Do not** dispose of insoluble powders or water-immiscible liquids in sinks.

19. A source of Purified Water

USP Chapter ⟨795⟩ states that Purified Water must be used in the following instances (1):

a. When water is called for as an ingredient in the compounding of non-sterile drug preparations

b. For rinsing compounding equipment and utensils

20. If sterile products are made, special equipment, including either a laminar airflow hood or a barrier isolator, is required. The equipment and the specialized environment needed for this sort of practice are discussed in Chapter 32, Parenteral Products.

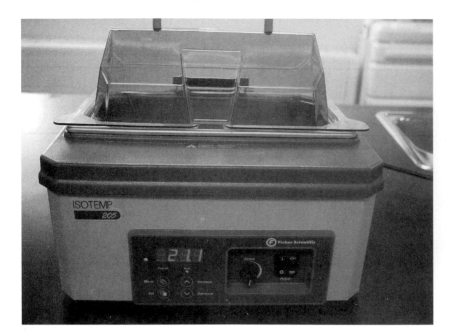

Thermostatically controlled hot water bath

21. A wide variety of other useful pieces of equipment is available. Decisions on the purchase and use of particular equipment depend on the amount and type of compounding performed and the economic circumstances of the professional practice. Several examples of other types of equipment are listed here.

a. A source of homogenization, such as a hand-homogenizer or a blender

b. A magnetic stirring device. A combination hot-plate and magnetic stirrer is more versatile but also more expensive.

c. Sieves, both individual and as sets with various mesh sizes, are available at a modest cost. These are useful when powders of a particular size are needed for product uniformity or comfort.

d. Capsule-filling machines, ranging from very simple devices at approximately $20 to motorized machines for over $5,000, can be purchased from pharmacy supply vendors.

e. Electric mixer

f. Thermostatically controlled hot water baths offer convenience, especially if formulations are made that require carefully controlled constant temperatures. These water baths have the disadvantage of being expensive.

g. Ointment mills make very fine ointments, but this piece of equipment is quite expensive, usually several thousand dollars, so you need to make a lot of ointments for this sort of equipment to make economic sense.

II. INGREDIENTS

A. Definitions

1. Active Ingredients: *USP* Chapter ⟨795⟩ states that the term *active ingredient(s)* "usually refers to chemicals, substances, or other components of articles intended for use in the diagnosis, cure, mitigation, treatment, or prevention of diseases in humans or other animals or for use as nutritional supplements" (1).

2. Added Substances: Also called inactive ingredients, excipients, pharmaceutic ingredients, and pharmaceutical necessities, these ingredients are necessary for preparing dosage forms or for enhancing the stability of finished preparations; they should not give a therapeutic response if given alone in the concentration present in the dosage form (1).

B. Ingredients that may be used in compounding

1. Section 503A of the Food and Drug Administration Modernization Act of 1997 (FDAMA) specified the classes of bulk drug substances (i.e., active ingredients) and other ingredients (i.e., added substances) that could be used in compounding. These included substances that:

   a. Comply with a *USP/NF* monograph and the *USP* chapter on pharmacy compounding

   b. Are components of an FDA-approved product

   c. Appear on a list of approved substances that is compiled by a committee appointed by the FDA

   d. Do not appear on a list of substances that have been withdrawn or removed from the market for safety reasons

2. When Section 503A of FDAMA was declared invalid by the U.S. Supreme Court (see the historical perspective section of Chapter 11), the FDA issued a new Compliance Policy Guide for Pharmacy Compounding that addressed the issue of allowed ingredients for compounding. The list is similar to the one given above except that it does not mention the compiled list of extra approved substances (2).

   a. A list of extra approved substances was proposed, but it was not finalized before the Supreme Court decision, so that list has questionable legal status. Fortunately, many of the drug substances on the list have subsequently had monographs approved for inclusion in the *USP/NF*.

   b. The list of drug substances (as of May 2002) that may not be used in compounding because they have been withdrawn or removed from the market for safety reasons is available as Appendix A of the Compliance Policy Guide for Pharmacy Compounding (2). Because this list is updated from time to time, the most current list should be consulted. (The FDA Compliance Policy Guide for Pharmacy Compounding can be accessed in the Appendices section of the CD that accompanies this book and is available on the Internet site given here: www.fda.gov/ora/compli-cance_ref/cpg/ cpgdrg/cpg460-200.htm, accessed December 2002).

C. Grades and standards for bulk ingredients

1. It is the responsibility of the pharmacist to choose appropriate, quality ingredients for compounded drug products.

   a. The **preferred grade for compounding is USP or NF.**

   b. If an official USP or NF ingredient is not available, the pharmacist should use professional judgment in the selection of an alternative source so that the safety and purity of the ingredient is ensured. Recommended grades include AR, ACS, and FCC (1); these grades are described below.

   c. In general, drug substances used for compounding should be made in an FDA-registered facility.

      (1) Many vendors of drugs and chemicals for compounding now state in their catalogs that their products conform to the requirements of cGMPs (current Good Manufacturing Practices) and that their facilities are inspected by and registered with FDA.

      (2) This does not mean that a pharmacist who is extemporaneously compounding a drug preparation for an individual patient cannot use a food item such as sucrose or chocolate syrup in the preparation. As the FDA Compliance Policy Guideline states, "FDA recognizes that pharmacists traditionally have extemporaneously compounded and manipulated reasonable quantities of human drugs upon receipt of a valid prescription for an individually identified patient from a licensed practitioner. This traditional activity is not the subject of this Guidance" (2).

      (3) Pharmacies that do a significant amount of compounding should, when possible, use ingredients that are made in an FDA-registered facility.

   d. *USP* Chapter ⟨795⟩ states, "For any substance used in compounding not purchased from a registered drug manufacturer, the pharmacist should establish purity and safety by reasonable means, which may include lot analysis, manufacturer reputation, or reliability of source" (1). This may include requesting a certificate of analysis from the supplier.

2. The various grades of ingredients are as follows:
   a. USP: The ingredient is certified to meet or exceed the specifications prescribed in the current edition of the *USP*.
   b. NF: The ingredient is certified to meet or exceed the specifications prescribed in the current edition of the *NF*.
   c. FCC: The ingredient is certified to meet or exceed the specifications listed in the current edition of the *Food Chemical Codex*.
   d. ACS: The ingredient is certified to meet or exceed the specifications listed in the current edition of *Reagent Chemicals*, which is published by the American Chemical Society.
   e. AR: Also known as analytical reagent grade, this is the grade assigned to chemicals of high purity that are suitable for analytic laboratory work.
   f. Purified: A designation given to chemicals of superior quality for which there is no official standard.
   g. CP: Also known as chemically pure, this designation is applied to chemicals which are more refined than technical grade, but for which only partial analytic information is available.
   h. Technical: Also called commercial grade, this grade is assigned to chemicals of commercial or industrial quality.
   i. Food Grade: This grade is assigned to chemicals that have clearance for use in foods.
   j. Cosmetic Grade: This designation can be given to chemicals approved for use in cosmetics.

D. Manufactured drug products as compounding ingredients

Manufactured drug products, such as tablets, capsules, or injections, are often used as sources of ingredients for compounded preparations. This is illustrated with sample prescriptions in Chapter 24, Powders (Sample Prescriptions 24.5 and 24.6), Chapter 25, Capsules, Lozenges and Other Solid Oral Dosage Forms (Sample Prescriptions 25.2, 25.3, 25.4, and 25.8), and Chapter 28, Suspensions (Sample Prescriptions 28.5 and 28.6).

1. To be used as an ingredient in compounding, the manufactured drug product must contain a batch control number, and the product must be within its stated expiratory date (1).
2. Certain solid dosage forms should not be crushed and used as ingredients for compounding.
   a. Controlled-release and enteric-coated products are specially formulated or coated to give certain desired or required release characteristics. These features may be destroyed by crushing the product.
   b. Some drugs are put in capsules or are formulated into tablets that are sugar- or film-coated to mask their unpleasant taste, to protect the mouth or throat from irritation, or to protect the teeth from staining. Crushing the tablets or emptying the contents of the capsules to use these as compounding ingredients destroys this protection.
   c. Sublingual or buccal tablets may contain drugs that require this special route of administration for therapeutic activity.
   d. The journal *Hospital Pharmacy* periodically publishes a list of oral solid dosage forms that should not be crushed. This list is reproduced each year in *American Drug Index*. Consult one of these sources for a current comprehensive list of drug products that should not be crushed. Often the product package insert for the particular product also contains information of this sort.
3. Special care must be exercised when manipulating chemotherapy drug products as ingredients for compounding. For example, when crushing oral solid dosage forms of cytotoxic drugs, the dosage form should be placed in a sealable plastic bag and crushed with the back of a spoon or with a pestle, taking care not to puncture the bag. This is illustrated with Sample Prescription 24.6 in Chapter 24.

4. Care must be exercised when selecting injectable products as ingredients for other routes of administration.

    a. Some injectable products use prodrugs to enhance the solubility of the active ingredient. These prodrugs may or may not be therapeutically active when used by other routes of administration. For example, if the prodrug is an ester, esterases must be present at the site of administration for the drug to be active.

    b. Some drugs that are efficacious when given parenterally may not be therapeutically active orally or topically. This can be caused by factors such as loss by first-pass effect; degradation in the gastrointestinal tract or lack of absorption in the gut when the drug product is given orally; or lack of absorption through the skin or mucous membranes when given topically.

5. The pharmacist should consider all these factors when deciding to use a manufactured drug product as an ingredient for a compounded drug preparation. The product package insert should always be consulted for helpful information from the product's manufacturer.

III. STORAGE OF DRUG PRODUCTS AND INGREDIENTS

A. All drugs, chemicals, and drug products should be stored and distributed under conditions that meet or exceed *USP-NF* or manufacturer's specifications. This includes shipment of these articles to the consumer (3).

B. Definitions of storage temperatures

Storage temperatures are defined in the General Notices of the *USP* (3). These are given below. Where a place, such as a refrigerator, is indicated, the definition states that this place must be thermostatically controlled within the given temperature range. The Centigrade temperatures are given first, with the Fahrenheit temperatures following in parentheses.

    1. Freezer: –25° to –10° (–13° to 14°)

    2. Cold: Not exceeding 8° (46°)

    3. Refrigerator: 2° to 8° (36° to 46°)

    4. Cool: 8° to 15° (46° to 59°)

    Note: An article that is to be stored in a cool place may be stored and distributed in a refrigerator unless otherwise specified.

    5. Room Temperature: The ambient temperature in the room

    6. Controlled Room Temperature: 20° to 25° (68° to 77°)

    Note: An article that is to be stored at controlled room temperature may be stored and distributed in a cool place unless otherwise specified.

    See additional information below.

    7. Warm: 30° to 40° (86° to 104°)

    8. Excessive Heat: Above 40° (104°)

    9. Protection from Freezing: Store above 0° (32°)

    10. Dry place: Controlled room temperature with average relative humidity (RH) not exceeding 40% or equivalent humidity at other temperatures. The determination of temperature–relative humidity can be based on actual measurement in the storage place or reported climatic conditions. It is based on not less than 12 equally spaced measurements during a season, a year, or the length of storage of the article. Relative humidity values can be up to 45% RH as long as the average RH is 40% or less (4).

    11. When no storage conditions are given for an article, it should be stored in an environment where it is protected from moisture, freezing, and excessive heat.

C. Controlled Room Temperature (CRT) and Mean Kinetic Temperature (MKT)

    1. The definition of CRT has recently been refined to include the concept of MKT. This was the result of studies conducted by USP and discussions and conferences held during the late 1990s following reports of drug product degradation resulting from improperly controlled warehouse or shipment conditions (including mailing of prescription products to patients). The exact new definition of CRT is quoted here from the General Notices of *USP 2002*:

"*Controlled Room Temperature*—A temperature maintained thermostatically that encompasses the usual and customary working environment of 20° to 25° (68° to 77°F); that results in a mean kinetic temperature calculated to be not more than 25°; and that allows for excursions between 15° and 30° (59° and 86°F) that are experienced in pharmacies, hospitals, and warehouses. Provided the mean kinetic temperature remains in the allowed range, transient spikes of up to 40° are permitted as long as they do not exceed 24 hours. Spikes above 40° may be permitted if the manufacturer so instructs" (3).

2. The MKT (or T_k) is a single calculated temperature that gives approximately the same drug product degradation as would occur if the product were subjected to various temperatures. It is calculated using an equation derived from the Arrhenius equation and gives a value that is slightly higher than a simple arithmetic mean. The equation for MKT is given in the *USP* General Information Chapter ⟨1151⟩ Pharmaceutical Dosage Forms and is shown here.

$$T_k = \frac{\Delta H / R}{-\ln\left(\dfrac{e^{-\Delta H / RT_1} + e^{-\Delta H / RT_2} + ... + e^{-\Delta H / RT_n}}{n}\right)}$$

where: T_k = mean kinetic temperature in °K (Kelvin)
   ΔH = heat of activation (83.144 kJ mol^{-1})
   R = universal gas constant (0.0083144 kJ mol^{-1} deg^{-1})
   T_1 = ave. temperature in °K for period 1 (e.g., week)
   T_n = ave. temperature in °K for the nth period
   n = the total number of storage temperatures recorded during the annual observation period (minimum of 52 weekly entries)

3. The MKT equation is used as follows. Refer to Table 12.1 for sample data.
   a. The temperature in the pharmacy or storage area is monitored and recorded. The easiest method is to use an automated recording device that gives a tracking of temperatures measured at specified intervals (e.g., every 30 minutes) or gives a high and low temperature for the period. For example, each week at the same time, the pharmacist checks the temperature monitor, notes the recorded high and low temperatures for the previous week, and calculates an arithmetic mean of the high and low temperature. This temperature, when expressed in °K, is T_n for that week.
   b. This procedure is repeated weekly and average temperatures are calculated for a minimum of 52 equally spaced periods over a year.

TABLE 12.1   Mean kinetic temperature (MKT) sample control sheet

Week	Date/Time	High Temp. °C	Low Temp. °C	Average Temp. T_n °C	Average Temp. T_n °K	$-\Delta H/RT$	$e^{-\Delta H/RT}$
1	1/01/00 0900	17	25	21	294.1	−34.0020	1.7104×10^{-15}
2	1/08/00 0900	19	27	23	296.1	−33.7724	2.1520×10^{-15}
3	1/15/00 0900	20	24	22	295.1	−33.8868	1.9193×10^{-15}
4	1/22/00 0900	22	28	25	298.1	−33.5458	2.6993×10^{-15}
5	1/29/00 0900	23	29	26	299.1	−33.4336	3.0197×10^{-15}
6–52							
Totals				117	1482.5		11.5007×10^{-15}
Means				23.4	296.7		2.3001×10^{-15}

c. Using the equation above, the pharmacist uses the T_1 through T_n values for all weeks monitored to calculate the MKT for the storage space. Because of the numerical values for ΔH and R, the MKT equation is easier to use than it would appear. A sample calculation using data in Table 12.1 is shown below.

(1) The numerator of the equation, $\Delta H/R$, is simply $10,000°K$, as can be seen here:

$$\Delta H / R = \frac{83.144 \; kJ \; mol^{-1}}{0.0083144 \; kJ \; mol^{-1} \; deg^{-1}} = 10,000 \; deg$$

(2) In the denominator, the exponent of e for each time period is simply $-10,000$ divided by the temperature (in $°K$) for that time period. For example, if the average temperature for a given week is $21°C$, the average temperature in $°K$ is calculated to be $21° + 273.1° = 294.1°K$ (recall that you add 273.1 to the Centigrade temperature to convert it to degrees Kelvin). The exponent of e for that week is calculated to be:

$$-\Delta H / RT_1 = -10,000 / 294.1 = -34.0020$$

(3) With the value of the exponent known, calculating the value of e taken to that exponent is a simple matter on a hand-held calculator that has logarithmic functions: enter the number, -34.0020 in this case, and use of operation key e^x. In this case the answer is 1.7104×10^{-15}.

(4) These numbers for all the periods are then summed. An example of this is shown in Table 12.1, where, for simplicity, data for just five time periods are shown. In this case the sum is 11.5007×10^{-15}.

(5) This sum for all the periods is then divided by the number of periods. For the example in Table 12.1, the sum 11.5007×10^{-15} is divided by 5 to give 2.3001×10^{-15}.

(6) Using a calculator or spreadsheet program, take the $-\ln$ of this number. For this example,

$$-\ln 2.3001 \times 10^{-15} = 33.7058$$

(7) This answer is then divided into 10,000 to get the MKT in $°K$. In this case the MKT is $296.7°K$ or $23.6°C$. This calculation is shown here for these sample data:

$$T_k = \frac{10,000 \; deg}{-\ln\left(\frac{11.5007 \times 10^{-15}}{5}\right)} = \frac{10,000 \; deg}{-\ln(2.3001 \times 10^{-15})} = \frac{10,000 \; deg}{33.7058} = 296.7 \; °K = 23.6 \; °C$$

d. This information is used to make any necessary adjustments in the temperature-controlling equipment for the pharmacy or storage space.

e. If the temperature in the storage space is consistently maintained below 25°C, the MKT need not be calculated.

IV. CONTAINERS

A. The General Notices of the *USP* give instructions for containers used for drugs, chemicals, and drug products. Some of these are common sense: for example, the container should be clean, and the container should not interact physically or chemically with the article placed in it (3).

B. When container specifications are given in official monographs, these apply not only to those products produced by manufacturers but also to these same drug products dispensed by the pharmacist.

C. Definitions are given for certain types of containers.

    1. Light-resistant Container: These containers protect the article or product from the effects of light. While the specifications for light-resistant containers are spelled out in detail in *USP* Chapter ⟨661⟩ Containers, the pharmacist does not need to be an expert on these specifications. Companies that sell containers for drug products specify if a particular container is light-resistant. Be watchful of these specifications. Also be knowledgeable about the storage specifications for all products stored in the pharmacy. When an opaque outer wrapper or carton is used by the manufacturer as part of the container for protecting the product from light, this wrapper must not be removed when storing the drug product in the pharmacy.

    2. Well-closed Container: A well-closed container merely provides protection from extraneous solids getting in or the contents of the container getting out under normal conditions.

    3. Tight Container: Most drugs, chemicals, and drug products are stored in tight containers. The *General Notices* of the *USP* define a tight container as one that provides protection from "contamination by extraneous liquids, solids, or vapors, from loss of the article, and from efflorescence, deliquescence, or evaporation under ordinary or customary conditions of handling, shipment, storage, and distribution, and is capable of tight re-closure" (3).

    4. Hermetic Container: This is the most secure container type. It is impervious to air or any other gas under normal conditions.

    5. The moisture permeation specifications for well-closed and tight containers used for dispensing are spelled out in detail in the *USP* Chapter ⟨671⟩ Containers–Permeation.

        a. The introduction to this chapter states:
The tests that follow are provided to determine the moisture permeability of containers utilized for drugs being dispensed on prescription and containers utilized by manufacturers or distributors for products that are repackaged by the dispenser prior to distribution or sale (5).

        b. Chapter ⟨671⟩ sets the moisture permeation standards for multiple-unit containers and single-unit and unit-dose dispensing containers for tablets and capsules. A manufacturer's unopened container is exempt from the requirements in this chapter.

        c. For normal dispensing of tablets and capsules in multiple-unit containers, the pharmacist does not need to be an expert on the details of these specifications because the companies that sell these containers specify their type. It is important to purchase dispensing containers from reliable sources.

        d. If a pharmacy is repackaging drug products or contracting for repackaging, it is important that the pharmacist be knowledgeable about the packaging standards for the types of containers used. In addition to *USP* chapters ⟨661⟩ and ⟨671⟩, a new chapter, ⟨1146⟩ Packaging Practice—Repackaging a Single Solid Oral Drug Product into a Unit-dose Container, should be consulted (6). The details of repackaging standards is beyond the scope of this text.

V. LEGAL REQUIREMENTS FOR HANDLING HAZARDOUS MATERIALS IN THE PHARMACY

A. The Occupational Safety and Health Administration (OSHA) of the federal government is charged with protecting the health and safety of all workers. One way in which it does this for employees of pharmacies, hospitals, health care work environments, laboratories in colleges of pharmacy, and so on is by setting and enforcing the Hazard Communication Standard (HCS).

B. The following information is taken from a document prepared by the Virginia Commonwealth University Office of Environmental Health and Safety and edited by the former laboratory director of the Pharmacy Skills Lab at the VCU School of Pharmacy (7). It will help you to understand the HCS, and it will give a guideline for the sort of information you, as a pharmacist, are required to furnish to employees under your supervision.

Under the Occupational Safety and Health Administration (OSHA) Hazard Communication Standard, all workers and students are guaranteed the right to know about possible hazards associated with chemical substances found in their work environment and be trained in the proper use of chemical hazards. Please review this information carefully because it could help prevent serious injury to you or a colleague.

1. Chemicals and Our Environment

    There are more than a half-million different chemicals currently used in this country every day. Many more are introduced every year. Such chemicals enhance our lives and become an integral part of our lifestyles. Chemicals are found in nearly every area of our environment. Some are as commonplace as correction fluid, but in a pharmacy or research university some chemicals are complex and highly toxic. Therefore, it is necessary to become familiar with all of the chemical substances present in your environment, the proper precautions required to handle them safely, and first aid procedures unique to those substances should an accident occur.

2. Routes of Entry Into the Body

    There are three basic ways in which an environmental chemical can enter the body:

    a. Inhalation—The most common way that a chemical substance can enter the body is by inhaling a chemical that is mixed in the surrounding air. The lungs readily absorb particles and gases in the same way as oxygen. For example, mercury from a broken thermometer can be toxic when inhaled. Hazardous chemicals that can be made airborne should only be used in well-ventilated areas or while using proper respiratory protection.

    b. Ingestion—The second way that chemicals enter the body is through the mouth. Ingestion of chemicals is usually done unknowingly and unintentionally. Occasionally, a person ingests a chemical they mistake for a food or beverage. More likely, however, chemical ingestion occurs when an individual eats or drinks contaminated food or beverages. Therefore, eating and/or drinking should not be permitted in the laboratory or pharmacy. Lab coats or other protective clothing should be worn in the lab or pharmacy, and hands should be washed thoroughly before leaving the lab or pharmacy.

    c. Absorption—The third way that environmental chemicals enter the body is through the skin. Chemicals such as organic solvents can be absorbed directly through the skin. Some chemicals cause damage to the protective layers of the skin and are then readily absorbed. To protect yourself from accidental absorption, wear appropriate personal protective clothing such as gloves and lab coats.

3. The Hazard Communication Standard

    Through the Hazard Communication Standard (HCS), OSHA mandates the following items for laboratories and pharmacies:

    a. Pharmacies and labs must maintain a comprehensive inventory of all hazardous materials in the workplace.

    b. Material Safety Data Sheets (MSDS) must be maintained and must be accessible to all employees.

    c. All containers of hazardous chemicals must be labeled with the appropriate warning information, including the potential hazards of the product. The HCS provides exemptions for several types of chemicals found in pharmacies:

        (1) Drugs in a retail setting that are packaged for sale to consumers

        (2) Drugs intended for personal consumption by employees in the workplace

        (3) Any drug, when it is in solid final form, for direct administration to a patient

    d. A written program to describe how the pharmacy or laboratory will comply with the HCS must be available to employees.

    e. Students and pharmacy employees must be informed of the chemical hazards in their workplace and how to protect themselves from these hazards.

    f. Students and employees of pharmacies must be informed of the elements of the HCS.

4. Material Safety Data Sheets
   a. OSHA requires that manufacturers of chemical products provide the consumers of those products with Material Safety Data Sheets (MSDS).
   b. As stated previously, facilities using chemical products are required to have MSDS accessible to all employees. In the past, these sheets were kept physically in a file, but more recent OSHA standards also allow access to be through electronic files on a computer. Many vendors of pharmacy supplies offer access to MSDS in three ways: printed copies available on request either by mail or by fax or computer access through their Internet site.
   c. Students and employees are encouraged to review these sheets, especially before handling a particular drug or chemical.
   d. An MSDS must provide the following information:
      (1) Physical and chemical characteristics of each hazardous chemical
      (2) Known acute or chronic health effects
      (3) Exposure limits
      (4) Whether or not the chemical is known to be a carcinogen (cancer-causing)
      (5) Precautionary measures to take in handling the chemical safely
      (6) Emergency and first aid procedures
      (7) The identity of the organization that prepared the MSDS

5. Labels and other forms of warning
   a. OSHA requires that manufacturers of chemicals label their products with the following information:
      (1) Identity of the hazardous chemical
      (2) Appropriate hazard warnings
      (3) The name, address, and phone number of the manufacturer
   b. If chemicals are transferred to other containers, these containers must be labeled with the identity of the chemical and the appropriate hazard warning information.
   c. Because of the diversity and quantities of chemical substances in laboratories and pharmacies, the responsibility of preparing a chemical inventory lies with the lab supervisor or pharmacist-in-charge. They have the responsibility to ensure that all students and employees are made fully aware of chemical hazards they may encounter. It is advisable to document this training or instruction and keep it on file.

6. Chemical effects
   Chemical substances can have different effects on the body.
   a. Some chemicals cause *acute* problems that you feel right away, such as breathing difficulties, burns, and rashes.
   b. Other chemicals cause *chronic* problems in which the effects of exposure may not be evident for months or even years.

7. Types of chemical substances
   a. Fumes, mists, and dusts
      (1) All of these substances are carried in the air and may be inhaled; they can cause breathing problems and may also cause burning and stinging of the eyes, nose, throat, or lungs.
      (2) Adequate ventilation and proper protective equipment will limit exposure to these substances. An example of such a chemical is salicylic acid powder. Use caution when handling this powder and do not "smell" it.
   b. Solvents
      (1) These products are used both as ingredients in formulations and as solvents for cleaning glassware and equipment. Common examples include acetone and alcohol.
      (2) These products commonly affect the skin, causing drying and cracking. Use techniques or protective coverings such as gloves to minimize contact with the skin.
      (3) The fumes or vapors from these products may also cause breathing problems. Work in well-ventilated areas. When working with ether-containing products (Flexible Collodion), keep the solvents contained in closed containers and, if possible, work with these products in a vented hood.

(4) Use caution when handling flammable solvents. Do not use near an open flame or lighted smoking materials.

c. Acids and caustic substances

(1) These products damage the skin and burn the eyes. Examples include Hydrochloric Acid, Glacial Acetic Acid, Phenol, and Menthol.

(2) Protection from acids and caustics includes protective clothing, such as lab coats, gloves, and safety glasses or goggles. If one of these compounds gets on the skin or eyes, flush immediately with water and contact a supervisor. Medical attention may be required.

d. Cytotoxic agents

(1) Special procedures for handling cytotoxic agents, such as drugs used for chemotherapy, have been spelled out in detail in various government documents and professional bulletins.

(2) OSHA Technical Manual Section VI, Chapter 2, Controlling Occupational Exposure to Hazardous Drugs, replaces the 1986 OSHA document Guideline for Antineoplastic (Cytotoxic) Drugs. This chapter is a very complete and well-referenced document that deals with both cytotoxic and other hazardous drugs. It is available through OSHA's Internet site at: www.osha.gov/dts/osta/otm/otm_vi/otm_vi_2.html (accessed December 2002)

(3) The American Society of Health-System Pharmacists has an excellent resource, *Technical Assistance Bulletin on Handling Cytotoxic and Hazardous Drugs.* As with all of ASHP's practice guidelines, this is available on their Internet site at: www.ashp.org.

(4) Additional publications by the U.S. Public Health Service, the American Medical Association, and others can be found using the reference section for either the OSHA or ASHP documents listed above.

(5) Special training is required before a student or employee handles any cytotoxic drug product.

VI. SOURCES OF SUPPLY FOR DRUGS AND CHEMICALS, COMPOUNDING EQUIPMENT, PACKAGING AND LABELING MATERIALS, AND COMPOUNDING INFORMATION

A. Compounding of custom drug preparations has expanded in recent years, partly because of the availability of new and useful items of equipment, packaging and labeling materials, excipients, drugs, and chemicals. Vendors such as those listed below specialize in marketing these supplies:

1. Apothecary Products, Inc. (1-888-770-8767; www.apothecaryproducts.com)
2. B & B Pharmaceuticals, Inc. (1-800-499-3100; www.bandbpharmaceuticals.com)
3. Fisher Scientific (1-800-766-7000; www.fishersci.com)
4. Gallipot, Inc. (1-800-423-6967; www.gallipot.com)
5. Kalchem International Chemicals and Compounding Supplies (1-888-298-9905; www.kalcheminternational.com)
6. The Letco Companies (1-800-239-5288)
7. Mallinckrodt Pharmaceuticals (1-800-325-8888)
8. Medisca (1-800-932-1039; www.medisca.com)
9. Paddock Laboratories, Inc. (1-800-328-5113; www.paddocklabs.com)
10. Ruger Chemical Co., Inc. (1-800-274-2636; www.rugerchemical.com)
11. Spectrum Pharmacy Products (1-800-791-3210; www.spectrumRx.com)

B. In addition to selling drugs and chemicals, equipment, and supplies, some companies provide technical support for compounding problems. The following are just a few examples:

1. Paddock Laboratories offers technical support on compounding to pharmacists. Their newsletter *Secundum Artem* was first published in 1988; provided as a service to phar-

macists, it gives current and practical information on compounding. Paddock pharmacists and chemists provide technical support and advice on compounding by telephone, and more recently the company has developed an excellent web site that has a vast array of information on formulations and compounding methods.

2. Gallipot is another company that has for many years offered free technical support from their staff of consulting pharmacists. Other companies such as Spectrum Pharmacy Products and Medisca advertise technical support to pharmacists in buying and using their compounding products. Some of these companies also provide training and continuing education opportunities.

3. Professional Compounding Centers of America, Inc. (1-800-331-2498; www.pccarx.com) offers its members technical advice, marketing support, training and continuing education opportunities, and access to a wide variety of compounding drugs, chemicals, and supplies. It operates with a membership fee, and its services are targeted to pharmacists who have practices that specialize in pharmacy compounding.

C. Various specialty companies cater to particular compounding needs:

1. Baxa Corporation (1-800-525-9567) specializes in sterile product supplies and oral liquid medication needs for hospitals and providers of home health care.

2. Pharma-Tek (1-800-645-6655; www.pharma-tek.com) specializes in steroid and antibiotic powders and offers technical support on their use.

3. Q.I. Medical, Inc. (1-800-837-8361; www.qimedical.com) supplies technical support on sterile product testing and markets validation supplies.

4. Liberty (1-800-828-5656), Laminaire Corporation (1-800-777-4500), Germfree Laboratories, Inc. (1-800-888-5357), and Baker (1-800-992-2537) are vendors of laminar flow hoods, IV prep rooms, and cleanroom supplies.

5. There are also companies that specialize in packaging equipment, computer software for standard operating procedures and record-keeping, and quality control, analysis, and sterility testing for compounded preparations.

D. For more information on these services and supply catalogs, call the 800 numbers listed or access information on the Internet.

E. For further information on vendors of compounding equipment and supplies, consult the advertisements in current professional journals such as the *International Journal of Pharmaceutical Compounding, American Journal of Health-System Pharmacists,* or the *Journal of the American Pharmaceutical Association.* The International Academy of Compounding Pharmacists (www.iacprx.org 1-800-927-4227) is also a good source of information.

References

1. The 2002 United States Pharmacopeia 25/National Formulary 20. Rockville, MD: The United States Pharmacopeial Convention, Inc., 2001; 2053–2057.
2. Compliance Policy Guidance for FDA Staff and Industry, Chapter 4, Subchapter 460, Section 460.200 Pharmacy Compounding. U.S. Department of Health and Human Services, Food and Drug Administration, Office of Regulatory Affairs, Center for Drug Evaluation and Research, May 2002; *www.fda.gov/ora/compliance_ref/cpg/cpgdrg/cpg460-200.htm.*
3. The 2002 United States Pharmacopeia 25/National Formulary 20. Rockville, MD: The United States Pharmacopeial Convention, Inc., 2001; 9.
4. The 2002 United States Pharmacopeia 25/National Formulary 20, First Supplement. Rockville, MD: The United States Pharmacopeial Convention, Inc., 2001; 2712.
5. The 2002 United States Pharmacopeia 25/National Formulary 20. Rockville, MD: The United States Pharmacopeial Convention, Inc., 2001; 2005–2006.
6. The 2002 United States Pharmacopeia 25/National Formulary 20, First Supplement. Rockville, MD: The United States Pharmacopeial Convention, Inc., 2001; 2791–2795.
7. Kirkpatrick MA. The Hazard Communication Standard. Virginia Commonwealth University Pharmacy Skills Lab Manual, 1997.

CHAPTER 13

Weighing and Measuring

I. GENERAL PRINCIPLES

To prepare accurate dosage forms, the pharmacist must use weighing and measuring apparatus with care and understanding and must be conscious of the following general principles:

A. Select weighing equipment and measuring devices appropriate for the intended purpose.

B. Use the devices and operate the equipment with recommended techniques that ensure accuracy of measurement.

C. Maintain the equipment so that it is clean and free of chemical contamination and retains the prescribed tolerances.

II. STANDARD-SETTING AGENCIES FOR BALANCES, WEIGHTS, AND VOLUMETRIC DEVICES

In understanding the standards for balances, weights, and volumetric devices and in obtaining information on these standards, it is useful to know the organizations and agencies that have responsibility for these areas. In the United States this is a patchwork of state and federal agencies and not-for-profit organizations. You will notice the initials of these organizations in the equipment standards that follow in this chapter. The organizations are identified briefly here, but contact information (as of December 2002) and Internet sites are given where more complete information is available.

A. The National Institute for Standards and Technology (**NIST**), formerly the National Bureau of Standards (**NBS**), was established by Congress in 1901 to "serve as a national scientific laboratory in the physical sciences, and to provide fundamental measurement standards for science and industry" (1).

  1. This agency, which is under the Department of Commerce, is charged with working with the states to develop laws, codes, and procedures to secure uniformity of weights and measures and methods of inspection.

  2. Since 1949 NIST has published annually the guidebook known as *Handbook 44.* The standards in this book are reviewed, revised, amended, and adopted each year by state weights and measures officials at the Annual Meeting of the National Conference on Weights and Measures (NCWM). The full texts of the recent editions of *Handbook 44* are available on the Internet in Adobe Acrobat Format (pdf) and Word Perfect 7.0 Format. The 2002 edition has the following Internet address: http://ts.nist.gov/ts/htdocs/230/235/h442002.htm

3. Contact information: The Weights and Measures Division of NIST has the following contact information: Weights and Measures Division, NIST, 100 Bureau Drive, Stop 2600, Gaithersburg, MD 20899-2600; phone: (301) 975-4004; e-mail: *owm@nist.gov;* Internet site: www.nist.gov.

B. The National Technical Information Service (**NTIS**) is also an agency of the U S Department of Commerce. Because its name and initials are so close to that of NIST, it can be confusing when either of these agencies is referenced by its initials.
1. NTIS serves as the repository and disseminator of information by the federal government. For example, you may purchase copies of *Handbook 44* through NTIS.
2. In 1992 NTIS developed a web site as a "gateway" to government information. Called FedWorld.gov (www.fedworld.gov), this site gives access to everything from Supreme Court decisions to federal government jobs, to government R & D reports, and documents such as *Handbook 44.*
3. Contact information: National Technical Information Service, Springfield VA 22161; phone: (703) 605-6000; Internet site: www.ntis.gov

C. ASTM International, formerly **ASTM** or the American Society for Testing and Materials, is a not-for-profit organization that develops and publishes voluntary standards for materials, products, systems, and services.
1. The "Standard Specifications for Laboratory Weights and Precision Mass Standards" (E617–97), which specifies our classes of weights, is a publication of ASTM.
2. Contact information: ASTM International, 100 Barr Harbor Drive, PO Box C700, W. Conshohocken, PA 19428-2959; phone: (610) 832-9500; e-mail: service@astm.org; Internet site: www.astm.org.

D. **ANSI,** the American National Standards Institute, is also a not-for-profit, non-governmental organization.
1. ANSI does not develop standards, but it serves as the U.S. representative to international standard-setting organizations such as the International Accreditation Forum (IAF) and the International Organization for Standardization (ISO). It also accredits national organizations, such as ASTM, that develop standards.
2. Contact information: American National Standards Institute, 1819 L Street NW, Suite 600, Washington DC 20036; phone: (212) 642-4900; Internet site: www.ansi.org.

E. **USP,** The United States Pharmacopeial Convention, is another not-for-profit, non-governmental organization. USP publishes the *USP/NF,* commonly referred to simply as *USP.*
1. The *USP* was originally published every 10 years following its decennial convention; in 1970 the convention and book publication moved to a 5- year cycle, and currently *USP* is published annually. This is a book of standards, some of which are legally enforceable and some of which are advisory. The General Tests and Assays chapters of the *USP* (those with chapter numbers below ⟨1000⟩) are potentially legally enforceable; General Chapters (those with chapter numbers above ⟨1000⟩) are informational.
2. *USP* Chapter ⟨795⟩ "Pharmacy Compounding," which is in the category of potentially enforceable standards, has the following statement on standards for equipment: "Equipment should be of appropriate design and size for compounding and suitable for the intended purpose" (2). Although *USP* General Information Chapter ⟨1176⟩ "Prescription Balances and Volumetric Apparatus" is numbered in the advisory section, it would be legally enforceable if mentioned in a state or federal law.
3. Contact information: United States Pharmacopeial Convention, Inc., 12601 Twinbrook Parkway, Rockville, MD 20852; phone: (800) 822-8772; Internet site: www.usp.org.

F. With this information in mind, it is important to remember the following:
1. Standards, such as those in *Handbook 44,* ASTM E 617–97, or *USP,* that have been developed by the government or private agencies are there for use by the state and fed-

eral governments in regulating commerce and protecting public health and safety. Voluntary standards promulgated either by government agencies or not-for-profit organizations can become legally enforceable if these standards are written into federal laws or state statutes or administrative codes.

2. Although the practice of pharmacy is regulated primarily by state statutes and administered by state boards of pharmacy, the federal government does have an acknowledged role, principally through the Federal Food, Drug and Cosmetic Act and the Controlled Substances Act.

3. Although the potential for voluntary standards to be **legally enforceable** is dependent on individual state statutes and federal laws, these standards provide invaluable guidance to pharmacists in selecting and using weighing and measuring equipment and apparatus.

III. BALANCES AND WEIGHING

A. **Definitions:** In selecting a balance for purchase or for use in compounding, the pharmacist needs to be familiar with the following terms:

1. Capacity: The maximum weight, including containers and tares, that can be placed on a balance pan.

2. Sensitivity (also referred to as Sensitivity Requirement or Sensitivity Reciprocal): The smallest weight that gives a perceptible change in the indicating element (e.g., one subdivision deflection of the indicator pointer on the index plate of a double-pan balance; one number change on the digital display of an electronic single-pan balance).

3. Readability: The smallest weight increment that can be read on the dial, weighbeam, or digital display of a balance. The term is used mostly in specification descriptions for electronic balances. For these, it is the smallest increment on the digital display (e.g., 0.001 g). The readability on double-pan balances is determined by the value of the hash-mark increments on the graduated dial (e.g., each mark stands for 0.01 g). Many double-pan prescription balances have two scales on the same dial, one in the metric (0.01 g) system and one in the apothecary (0.2 gr) system. **Great care must be exercised when using these dials to ensure that the intended scale is being read.**

4. Precision: The reproducibility of the weighing measurement as expressed by a standard deviation. This term is used primarily in specifications on electronic balances.

5. Accuracy: The closeness of the displayed weight, as measured by the balance, to the true weight, as known by the use of a calibration weight or weights. This value is given in some electronic balance descriptions in lieu of a precision specification.

B. Prescription Balances

1. A prescription balance is described in the *USP* General Information Chapter ⟨1176⟩ Prescription Balances and Volumetric Apparatus as:

> "a scale or balance adapted to weighing medicinal and other substances required in prescriptions or in other pharmaceutical compounding. It is constructed so as to support its full capacity without developing undue stresses, and its adjustment is not altered by repeated weighings of capacity load" (3).

Chapter ⟨1176⟩ goes on to describe, in detail, the attributes of a Class A prescription balance, also known as a double-pan torsion balance.

2. Class A Prescription Balance

   a. These balances are now designated Class III by the National Institute for Standards and Technology (NIST).

   b. Sensitivity: They meet or exceed a sensitivity requirement of 6 mg with no load and with a load of 10 g on each pan.

   c. Capacity: The 4th edition of *Handbook 44* gave the assumed capacity of a Class A balance to be 15.5 g (the approximate weight of half an apothecary ounce) unless a larger capacity was stated in the manufacturer's specifications for that par-

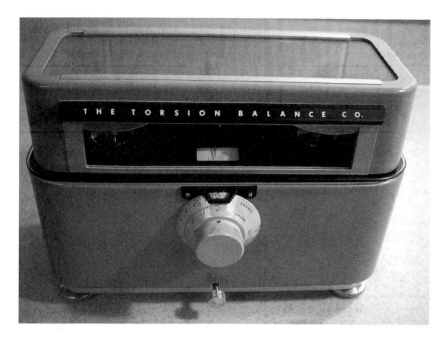

Double-pan torsion balance

ticular balance. While many balance brands have capacities exceeding 15.5 g, such as 60 or 120 g, it is usually impractical to weigh amounts greater than 15 to 30 g on a double-pan balance because heavier weights cause excessive wear on the balance internal parts, and because the volume occupied by larger weights of most powders and dry ingredients is difficult to contain on weighing papers, boats, or dishes without spilling.

3. Electronic single-pan balances

    a. Although the *USP* specifies that a Class A Prescription Balance be used for all weighing operations required in prescription compounding, a note at the beginning of Chapter ⟨1176⟩ states that other balances may be used provided they give equivalent or better accuracy.

    b. Sensitivity and features: Electronic, single-pan balances with internal weights, digital display features, and readability and precision of 1 mg are available at rel-

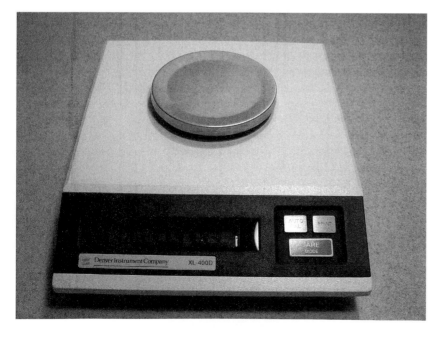

Electronic balance

atively reasonable costs. Some brands have other useful features, such as "parts counting."

   c. Capacity: Although capacities vary with the brand and model, balances with capacities of 100 to 210 g are commonly available for balances with readability and precision of 1 mg.

   d. Most pharmacists who have used these balances find them easier to use and more accurate than a traditional double-pan torsion balance. Although appropriately selected electronic balances meet or exceed the requirements for prescription balances as stated in the *USP*, the pharmacist should consult with his or her state board of pharmacy to determine if a given balance meets the applicable state statutes or codes for pharmacy equipment before purchasing an electronic balance.

4. Minimum Weighable Quantity (MWQ): The MWQ must be determined for any balance being used for compounding.

   a. A maximum 5% error is the generally accepted standard for weighing operations used in compounding (3).

   b. To avoid errors of 5% or more on a Class III (A) balance with a measured sensitivity requirement of 6 mg, do not weigh less than 120 mg of any drug or chemical; for example, 5% × 120 mg = 6 mg.

   c. A smaller MWQ may be used on a more sensitive balance. For example, a balance with a sensitivity requirement of 5 mg would have a MWQ of 100 mg because 5% × 100 mg = 5 mg. If an amount of drug or chemical is needed that is less than the MWQ that was determined for that balance, an aliquot method of measurement may be used. Methods of calculating aliquot amounts are presented in Chapter 9, Aliquots Calculation.

5. Balance testing

   a. *USP* general guidelines

      (1) Chapter ⟨1176⟩ states, "All balances should be calibrated and tested frequently using appropriate test weights, both singly and in combination" (3).

      (2) Chapter ⟨795⟩ Pharmacy Compounding states, "Equipment and accessories used in compounding should be inspected, maintained, and cleaned at appropriate intervals to ensure the accuracy and reliability of their performance" (2).

   b. Frequency of testing: As can be seen from the above statements, the frequency of balance testing is not explicitly stated and is therefore subject to interpretation and professional judgment. For balances with limited use, annual or semiannual testing may be adequate. For balances with moderate use, monthly checks are preferred, and those balances used extensively should be tested even more frequently.

   c. Records of testing: A balance-testing record should be maintained by the pharmacy; the record should include the date, the type of testing and calibration procedures performed, the results, and the name or initials of the person who performed the procedures. A sample testing record sheet for a Class III torsion balance is shown in Figure 13.1.

   d. Repair and reconditioning of balances: For balances that need to be repaired or reconditioned, contact the service department of the balance manufacturer. There are also companies that have the equipment and expertise to test, calibrate, recondition, and repair torsion and electronic balances. One such company is Pharmaceutical Balance Systems (phone: 262-691-3693; e-mail: info@pharmacybalances.com); information is available at their Internet site at www.torsionbalance.com, accessed December 2002.

   e. Testing procedures for electronic balances

      (1) Testing and calibration procedures for electronic balances are given in the use and maintenance manual provided by the balance manufacturer.

      (2) The usual procedure involves the use of special test calibration weights, which may be provided with the balance or purchased separately. Usually ANSI/ASTM Class 1 (NBS Class S) weights are required.

■ **Figure 13.1** Balance Testing for a Torsion Balance

Date_____

Balance Brand and Model Number_____

Test Weight Brand and Class_____

Pharmacist/Technician_____

Before proceeding with the balance tests, do the following:

1. Position the balance on flat, level surface away from drafts and air currents.
2. Check that the weighbeam rider or dial-in weights are at zero.
3. Using balance leveling feet, bring balance into equilibrium with the indicator at the zero position on index plate. Check this before each of the following tests.

Test	Results	Pass/Fail
Sensitivity Requirement		
1. Place a 6-mg weight on one of the empty balance pans. Release the balance pans.How many divisions is the indicator deflected on the index plate? To pass, the indicator must deflect 1 or more divisions.		
2. Place a 10-g weight in the center of each pan and place the 6-mg weight on one of the empty pans. How many divisions is the indicator deflected on the index plate? To pass, indicator must deflect 1 or more divisions		
Arm Ratio Test		
1. Place a 30-g weight in the center of each balance pan. Release the balance pans. Is the indicator deflected on the index plate? If no deflection, pass. If indicator deflected, perform 2.		
2. Place a 20-mg weight on the balance pan for the lighter side. Is the indicator back to the rest point or farther? If yes, pass; if no, fail.		
Shift Test		
1. Place a 10-g weight in the center of the left pan. Place a second 10-g weight on the right pan and successively move that weight toward the right, left, front, and back of the pan. In each case, is the indicator deflected? If no, pass. If indicator deflected, perform 2.		
2. If indicator deflected with any of the above shifts, add a 10-mg weight to the balance pan of the lighter side. Is the indicator back to the rest point or farther? If yes, pass; if no, fail.		
3. Place a 10-g weight in the center of the right pan. Place another 10-g weight on the left pan and successively move that weight toward the right, left, front, and back of the pan. If each case, is the indicator deflected? If no, pass. If indicator deflected, perform 4.		
4. If indicator deflected with any of the above shifts, add a 10-mg weight to the balance pan of the lighter side. Is the indicator back to the rest point or farther? If yes, pass; if no, fail.		
5. Move the 10-g weights to all different positions on both balance pans, e.g., both left, both right, one left and one right, both back, both front, one back and one front, etc. Is the indicator deflected on the index plate? If no, pass. If indicator deflected, perform 6.		
6. If indicator deflected with any of the above shifts, add a 10-mg weight to the balance pan of the lighter side. Is the indicator back to the rest point or farther? If yes, pass; if no, fail.		
Rider and Graduated Beam Tests		
1. Place a 500-mg weight on the left balance pan. Move the rider or the dial-in weight to the 500-mg position. Is the indicator deflected on the index plate? If no, pass. If the indicator is deflected, perform 2.		
2. If the indicator is deflected, place a 6-mg weight on the balance pan for the lighter side. Is the indicator back to the rest point or farther? If yes, pass; if no, fail		
3. Place a 1-g weight on the left balance pan. Move the rider or the dial-in weight to the 1-g position. Is the indicator deflected on the index plate? If no, pass. If the indicator is deflected, perform 4.		
4. If the indicator is deflected, place a 6-mg weight on the balance pan for the lighter side. Is the indicator back to the rest point or farther? If yes, pass; if no, fail.		

This balance passes the above performance tests.   Signed:_____

f. Testing procedures for Class III (A) Balances

(1) Test weights: ANSI/ASTM Class 4 (NBS Class P) or better weights are recommended for testing Class III prescription balances. This weight set should be reserved for testing the balance and for checking weights that are routinely used for compounding. Dial-in weights on double-pan torsion balances may not be used to calibrate the balance because an internal mechanism does not constitute a valid standard.

(2) The *USP* Chapter ⟨1176⟩ specifies the following tests to be performed on Class III (A) prescription balances. As stated above, a sample testing procedure with the details of these tests is shown in Figure 13.1.

(a) Sensitivity Requirement

(b) Arm Ratio Test

(c) Shift Tests

(d) Rider and Graduated Beam Tests

(3) The test for Sensitivity Requirement deserves some additional comment. The *USP* gives the following instructions regarding this test: "Level the balance, determine the rest point, and place a 6-mg weight on one of the empty pans. Repeat the operation with a 10-g weight in the center of each pan. The rest point is shifted not less than one division on the index plate each time the 6-mg weight is added" (3). Unfortunately, many weight sets available to pharmacies do not contain the 6-mg weight required for this test; the smallest weight in a set may be a 10-mg weight. A modified sensitivity requirement test may still be performed using other weights of comparable size, provided a linear relationship is established for the range of measurement. The procedure is as follows:

(a) Put weighing papers or weighing dishes on each balance pan.

(b) Bring the balance into equilibrium using the leveling feet at the front of the balance.

(c) Place one 10-mg weight on the right-hand balance pan.

(d) Release the pan arrest and read the number of divisions the balance indicator is deflected on the index plate: _____

(e) Repeat steps (c) and (d) using a 20-mg weight. How many units is the balance indicator shifted on the index plate now? _____

A linear relationship exists if the number found in (e) is two times that in (d); that is, double the weight gives double the deflections.

If a linear relationship exists, the sensitivity requirement can be calculated as shown below. For this example, a 10-mg weight was found to give 1.5 deflections, and a 20-mg weight gave 3 deflections (a linear relationship was established).

$$\frac{10 \ mg \ weight}{1.5 \ deflections} = \frac{x \ mg \ weight}{1 \ deflections} \quad x = 6.7 \ mg \ weight$$

In this example, the balance does not meet the Class III balance requirement. Remember, for a Class III balance, the sensitivity requirement must be 6 mg or less. In this case, a weight greater than 6 mg (6.7 mg) was needed to give one deflection.

C. Weights

1. Weights are to be stored in a rigid, compartmentalized box and should be handled with special forceps or tweezers to prevent contamination (3).

2. Metric and apothecary weights

a. Metric weights are the preferred weights to use in compounding.

b. While the *USP* no longer recognizes the apothecary system, it does allow either metric or apothecary weights to be used in compounding (3), and the 2002 edition of *Handbook 44* contains published tolerances for apothecary weights (1).

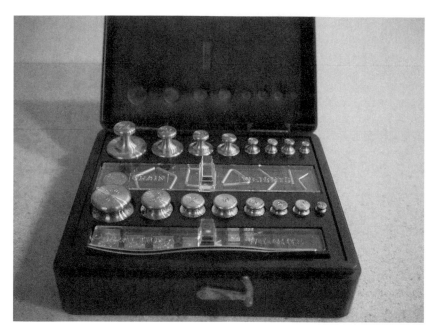

Weight set

    c. Some weight sets contain both metric and apothecary weights in the same box. These sets should be used with extreme caution because it is easy to select a weight from the wrong system. This is especially true when people who are not familiar with both systems use these weights.

3. All weights must have cylindric construction, and coin-type weights should not be used (3).

4. The *USP* recommends the use of Class P (ANSI/ASTM Class 4) or better weights for prescription compounding, but states that Class Q weights may be used because they do have tolerances within the limits of accuracy for Class III prescription balances (3). When purchasing a weight set for use in compounding, the pharmacist should require information from the vendor on the class of the weight set, because catalog descriptions such as "precision metric weight set" and "accurate weights" do not give sufficient information.

5. The situation with classes of weights is a bit confusing since the designations have recently been changed. The letter designations, such as P and Q, no longer specify weight classes but rather design limitations of weights, such as range of density of materials, surface area, surface finish, corrosion resistance, and hardness. Number designations 0 through 7 are now used to specify weight classes in the U.S., and the international standard, International Recommendation R111, from Organisation Internationale de Metrologie Legale (OIML) use classes E1, E2, F1, F2, M1, M2, and M3. The specifications for the various weight classes are shown in Table 13.1 (4).

    a. The following information, which is quoted from chapter ⟨41⟩ "Weights and Balances" of the *USP* is helpful in making conversions between the older letter classes and the newer U.S. number classes.

        Class 1 weights are designated as high-precision standards for calibration. They may be used for weighing accurately quantities below 20 mg. (For weights of 10 g or less, the requirements of class 1 are met by *USP XXI* class M.)

        Class 2 weights are used as working standards for calibration, built-in weights for analytical balances, and laboratory weights for routine analytical work. (The requirements of class 2 are met by *USP XXI* class S.)

        Class 3 and class 4 weights are used with moderate-precision laboratory balances. (Class 3 requirements are met by *USP XXI* class S-1; class 4 requirements are met by *USP XXI* class P.) (5)

TABLE 13.1 Metric Weight Tolerances

| Size | International Organization R111 | | | | ANSI/ASTM E 617 | | | | | | NBS Circular 547 Section 1 | | | | | NIST 105-1 |
	F1	F2	M1	M2*	Class 1**	Class 2**	Class 3	Class 4	Class 5	Class 6	M**	S	S-1	P	Q	F
100 g	0.5	1.5	5	15	0.25	0.50	1.0	2.0	9	10	0.50	0.25	1.0	2.0	9.0	20
50 g	0.30	1.0	3.0	10	0.12	0.25	0.6	1.2	5.6	7	0.25	0.12	0.60	1.2	5.6	10
30 g					0.074	0.15	0.45	0.90	4.0	5	0.15	0.074	0.45	0.90	4.0	6.0
20 g	0.25	0.8	2.5	8	0.074	0.10	0.35	0.70	3.0	3	0.10	0.074	0.35	0.70	3.0	4.0
10 g	0.20	0.6	2.0	6	0.05	0.074	0.25	0.50	2.0	2	0.050	0.074	0.25	0.50	2.0	2.0
5 g	0.15	0.5	1.5	5	0.034	0.054	0.18	0.36	1.3	2	0.034	0.054	0.18	0.36	1.3	1.5
3 g					0.034	0.054	0.15	0.30	0.95	2	0.034	0.054	0.15	0.30	0.95	1.3
2 g	0.12	0.4	1.2	4	0.034	0.054	0.13	0.26	0.75	2	0.034	0.054	0.13	0.26	0.75	1.1
1 g	0.10	0.3	1.0	3	0.034	0.054	0.10	0.20	0.50	2	0.034	0.054	0.10	0.20	0.50	0.9
500 mg	0.08	0.25	0.8	2.5	0.010	0.025	0.080	0.16	0.38	1	0.010	0.025	0.080	0.16	0.38	0.72
300 mg				2.0	0.010	0.025	0.070	0.14	0.30	1	0.010	0.025	0.070	0.14	0.30	0.61
200 mg	0.06	0.20	0.6	1.5	0.010	0.025	0.060	0.12	0.26	1	0.010	0.025	0.060	0.12	0.26	0.54
100 mg	0.05	0.15	0.5		0.010	0.025	0.050	0.10	0.20	1	0.010	0.025	0.050	0.10	0.20	0.43
50 mg	0.04	0.12	0.4		0.010	0.014	0.042	0.085	0.16		0.010	0.014	0.042	0.085	0.16	0.35
30 mg					0.010	0.014	0.038	0.075	0.14		0.010	0.014	0.038	0.075	0.14	0.30
20 mg	0.03	0.10	0.3		0.010	0.014	0.035	0.070	0.12		0.010	0.014	0.035	0.070	0.12	0.26
10 mg	0.025	0.08	0.25		0.010	0.014	0.030	0.060	0.10		0.010	0.014	0.030	0.060	0.10	0.21
5 mg	0.020	0.06	0.20		0.010	0.014	0.028	0.055	0.080		0.010	0.014	0.028	0.055	0.080	0.17
2 mg	0.020	0.06	0.20		0.010	0.014	0.025	0.050	0.060		0.010	0.014	0.025	0.050	0.060	0.12
1 mg	0.020	0.06	0.20		0.010	0.014	0.025	0.050	0.050		0.010	0.014	0.025	0.050	0.050	0.10

Note: All tolerances for these class and ranges are in milligrams. *Maintenance Tolerances **Individual
Information for this table was taken from *Troemner Mass Standards Handbook* (4). Additional classes and weight sizes can be obtained from the accrediting association or the *Troemner Mass Standards Handbook*.

b. More complete information on the new U.S. classes can be found in ASTM Standard E617, "Standard Specifications for Laboratory Weights and Precision Mass Standards." The document with the standard as of the year 2002 is E617-97 (the number 97 refers to the year of the most recent revision). Copies of ASTM Standard E 617 are available for purchase from ASTM through its web site or by using the contact information for ASTM given at the beginning of this chapter.

c. Sometimes there is confusion over the standards for weights given in *USP* chapter ⟨1176⟩ and chapter ⟨41⟩. Chapter ⟨1176⟩ was written specifically for prescription compounding. The standards for weights given in chapter ⟨41⟩ of the *USP* were written for "accurate weighing" in *USP* assays and not for general prescription compounding by pharmacists. The recommendation that a weight class be chosen so that the tolerance of the weights does not exceed 0.1% of the amount weighed as given in chapter ⟨41⟩ is not a requirement for weighings done in prescription compounding.

D. Weighing papers and dishes

1. When weighing drugs or chemicals, these substances are never placed directly on the balance pan; a disposable weighing paper, boat, or dish is placed on the balance pan, and the drug or chemical is placed on the paper or in the boat or dish. A fresh weighing paper or dish is used for each drug or chemical weighed. There are several reasons for using these devices: 1) they protect the balance pan from harmful or corrosive chemicals, 2) they prevent cross-contamination of drugs and chemicals, and 3) they eliminate the necessity of washing the balance pan between weighing different drugs or chemicals.

2. Weighing paper

a. Glassine papers are preferred for weighing. They have a smooth, shiny surface that does not absorb materials placed on them, and drugs and chemicals are easily slipped off for complete transfers. Glassine papers come in various sizes, from 3" × 3" to 6" × 6".

b. Some pharmacists use powder papers as weighing papers because they prefer the rectangular shape or sizes available. These papers are available in vegetable

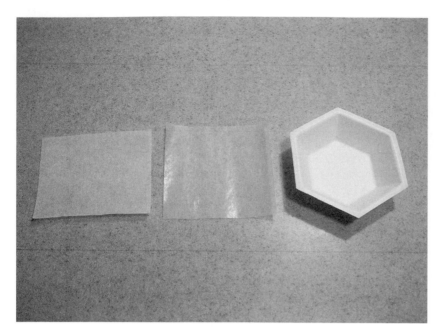

Weighing papers and dishes

parchment paper and come in various sizes. They are acceptable for most purposes, but they are more absorbent than glassine and should not be used for weighing thick liquids such as Coal Tar and Ichthammol.

c. Weighing papers should be creased to create a depression or "boat," which helps to contain the substance being weighed and prevents spilling on the balance pans or balance platform. This depression can be formed in many ways: pinching each of the four corners of the paper; folding the paper in quarters and then opening the sheet; making ¼" to ½" lengthwise folds along each side, to name a few.

3. Weighing dishes

a. Weighing dishes are available in a variety of sizes, shapes, and materials. Most vendors of compounding supplies have dishes made of aluminum and polystyrene plastic. They come in capacity sizes ranging from approximately 5 to 250 mL and are shaped as round pans, rectangles, boats, canoes, and hexagons.

b. Although these are very handy and they more securely contain substances being weighed, they are also more expensive than weighing papers. They have the added advantage of being useful for weighing liquids because they have rigid sides that will contain a liquid being weighed.

E. Recommended Weighing Procedures
Note: The following section gives general information and procedures for weighing both on a torsion and on an electronic digital balance. Abbreviated stepwise procedures are given in Figures 13.2 and 13.3. (The weighing procedure when using a torsion balance is also demonstrated on the CD that accompanies this book.) Figures 25.1 and 25.2 in Chapter 25 have specific weighing procedures for compounding capsules.

1. Weighing on a Torsion Balance

a. Position the balance on a flat, level surface in an area that is away, as much as is possible, from drafts or air currents.

b. Check to be sure that the weighbeam rider or the dial-in weights are at the zero position.

c. Using the leveling feet at the front of the balance, bring the balance into equilibrium. Equilibrium is reached when the index pointer, called the balance indicator, either comes to rest at the center on the index plate, or travels an equal number of divisions to the right and left of the center. If air currents in the room affect the movement of the balance pans, the balance lid should be closed. This is also true when determining balance during the weighing procedure.

■ **Figure 13.2** Procedure for Weighing on a Torsion Balance

1. Position the balance on a flat, level surface in an area that is away from drafts or air currents

2. Check to be sure that the weighbeam rider or the dial-in weights are at the zero position.

3. Using the leveling feet at the front of the balance, bring the balance into equilibrium. If air currents in the room affect the movement of the balance pans, the balance lid should be closed. This is also true when determining balance during the weighing procedure.

4. Place a weighing paper or dish on each balance pan. These should be positioned on the balance pans so that they do not interfere with the free movement of the pans.

5. With the weighing papers or dishes in place, repeat the process of using the leveling feet to bring the balance pans into equilibrium.

6. During the entire weighing procedure, keep the balance pans arrested when adding anything to the balance pans.

7. Add the appropriate external and dial weights to the balance. Handle external weights with tweezers or forceps. **External weights are added to the right-hand balance pan.** This is important because the dial-in weights are added to that side.

8. Using a spatula, add **material to be weighed** to the weighing paper or dish **on the left-hand balance pan.**

9. Release the arresting mechanisms and observe the balance pointer to determine if you have transferred the desired amount of material, or if too much or too little material was added.

10. If the pans are not in balance, arrest the pans before adding or removing material. Repeat steps 8. and 9. until the index pointer indicates that equilibrium has been reached. As you approach the required weight of material, you may release the balance arrest as you slowly and carefully add very small amounts of material until the exact weight is reached.

11. Arrest the balance pans and remove the weights, both external and dial-in. As you do this, recheck the weights to be sure you have selected the desired weights. Return the external weights to their appropriate compartments in the weight box.

12. If any powder or liquid was inadvertently spilled on the balance pan or platform, clean the balance.

■ **FIGURE 13-3** PROCEDURE FOR WEIGHING ON AN ELECTRONIC BALANCE

1. Position the balance on a flat, level surface in an area that is away from drafts or air currents.

2. Turn the balance on and press the tare button; the digital display should show 0.000 g. If air currents in the room are affecting the balance (the numbers on the digital display will drift up and down), the balance lid should be closed or an air current shield should be put in place. This is also true when determining balance during the weighing procedure.

3. Place a weighing paper or dish on the balance pan. If a weighing paper is being used, it should be positioned so that it does not interfere with the balance lid if it needs to be closed during the weighing procedure.

4. Press the tare button again to tare out the weight of the weighing paper or dish; the digital display should show 0.000 g.

5. Using a spatula, add material to be weighed to the weighing paper or dish on the balance pan until the desired weight appears on the digital display.

6. If any powder or liquid was inadvertently spilled on the balance pan or platform, clean the balance.

d. Place a weighing paper or dish on each balance pan. These should be positioned on the balance pans so that they do not interfere with the free movement of the pans.

e. With the weighing papers or dishes in place, repeat the process of using the leveling feet to bring the balance pans into equilibrium. This is necessary because there may be minor differences in the weights of weighing papers or dishes even with the same type and size.

f. During the entire weighing procedure, keep the balance pans arrested when adding anything to the balance pans. This protects the delicate parts of the balance mechanism. Some newer torsion balances allow for the dial weights to be adjusted without arresting the balance pans. Notice below that the arresting procedure is not necessary with electronic balances. This is one of the reasons weighing can be accomplished more efficiently with electronic balances. With an electronic balance, material is added until the display indicates that the target weight has been reached.

g. Add the appropriate external and dial weights to the balance. Handle external weights with tweezers or forceps, never with your fingers. External weights are added to the right-hand balance pan. This is important because the dial-in weights are added to that side. If you were to use a combination of external and dial weights for a given weight, putting the external weights on the wrong side would result in a weight that is the difference of the two rather than the desired sum of the two. If you have not done weighing recently and have forgotten which is the proper side for the external weights, dial in some weight and observe which balance pan goes down; that is the side for the weights.

h. Using a spatula, add material to be weighed to the weighing paper or dish on the left-hand balance pan. When using a spatula for this purpose, you may find it helpful to hold the spatula between your thumb and middle finger so that the index finger is free to tap the blade of the spatula. This is a good way to tap off small, controlled amounts of drug from the spatula blade.

i. Release the arresting mechanism and observe the balance indicator to determine if you have transferred the desired amount of material, or if too much or too little material was added.

j. If the pans are not in balance, arrest the pans before adding or removing material. Repeat steps h and i until the position of the balance indicator on the index plate shows that equilibrium has been reached. As you approach the required weight of material, you may release the balance arrest as you slowly and carefully add very small amounts of material until the exact weight is reached.

k. Arrest the balance pans and remove the weights, both external and dial-in. As you do this, recheck the weights to be sure you have selected the desired weights. Return the external weights to their appropriate compartments in the weight box.

l. If any powder or liquid was inadvertently spilled on the balance pan or platform, clean the balance.

2. Weighing on an electronic digital balance

Refer to the operator's manual for weighing instructions specific to that balance. Some balances have several modes for different weighing systems and dual-capacity weighing ranges; be sure the balance is in the proper mode for weighing in the metric system and in the appropriate range for the weighing being done. The following steps give general procedures for most top-loading digital balances. A brief stepwise version is given in Figure 13.3.

a. Position the balance on a flat, level surface in an area that is away, as much as is possible, from drafts or air currents.

b. Turn the balance on and press the tare button; the digital display should show 0.000 g. If air currents in the room are affecting the balance (the numbers on the digital display will drift up and down), the balance lid should be closed. This is also true when determining balance during the weighing procedure. For balances that do not have attached lids, air current shields can be purchased or improvised.

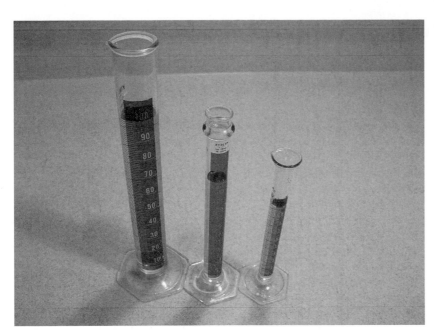

Cylindrical graduates

c. Place a weighing paper or dish on the balance pan. If a weighing paper is being used, it should be positioned so that it does not interfere with the balance lid if it needs to be closed during the weighing procedure.

d. Press the tare button again to tare out the weight of the weighing paper or dish; the digital display should show 0.000 g.

e. Using a spatula, add material to be weighed to the weighing paper or dish on the balance pan. When using a spatula for this purpose, you may find it helpful to hold the spatula between your thumb and middle finger so that the index finger is free to tap the blade of the spatula. This is a good way to tap off small, controlled amounts of drug from the spatula blade. As you approach the required weight of material, carefully add very small amounts of material until the exact weight is reached. If you overshoot the target weight, simply remove any excess powder or material with the spatula.

f. If any powder or liquid was inadvertently spilled on the balance pan or platform, clean the balance.

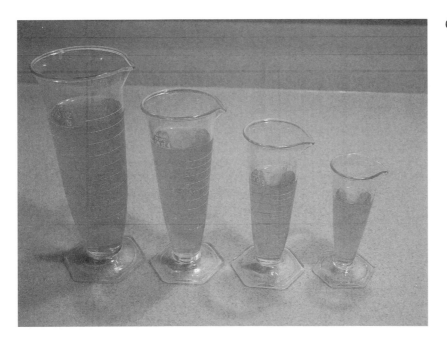

Conical graduates

IV. VOLUMETRIC APPARATUS AND MEASURING

A. Definitions

1. Capacity: The designated volume, at the maximum graduation, which the vessel will contain (labeled as "TC", meaning "to contain") or deliver (labeled as "TD," meaning "to deliver") at the temperature indicated on the vessel. Generally, graduates, pipettes, and burettes are calibrated TD, whereas volumetric flasks are calibrated TC.

2. Cylindrical graduate: A measuring vessel that is a right circular cylinder (that is, with sides parallel to each other and perpendicular to the base).

3. Conical graduate: A measuring vessel whose cross-section is circular but whose sides flare outward from its base. The circumference of the vessel is larger at the top graduation than at the lowest graduation marking.

B. Descriptions and standards for volumetric graduates

1. "Testing Glass Volumetric Apparatus," NBS Circular 602

   The *USP* lists pipets, burets, and cylinders that are graduated either in the metric or apothecary system as pharmaceutical devices used for measuring volumes of liquids. It states that these devices meet standards set down in NTIS COM-73-10504 (3). This document, also known as NBS Circular 602, "Testing Glass Volumetric Apparatus," was issued by NBS in 1959. It is now out of print, but the NIST Internet site states that the document can be obtained at a depository library for government publications, which can be located through a local library, or a copy may be requested through Interlibrary Loan.

   The standards set by this document, which apply to **cylindrical graduates** (the measuring devices most commonly used by pharmacists), are quoted below. Exact quotes are used here so there is no misunderstanding of the standards given in this document, which is now somewhat difficult to obtain. This information should be helpful to you in making informed decisions on the purchase of graduated cylinders. Many brands of graduated cylinders, which are available and marketed to pharmacists, do not meet these particular standards; however, it should be remembered that in most cases conformity with these standards is voluntary unless specifically mandated by state law. Consult the pharmacy codes and statutes for your state to find out what is required in the state where you practice.

   a. Material

   "The material should be of best-quality glass, transparent and free from striae, surface irregularities, and other defects which may distort the appearance of the liquid surface or the portion of the graduation line seen through the glass" (6).

   b. Design

   (1) "The cross section must be circular and the shape must permit complete emptying and draining and thorough cleaning" (6).

   (2) "Two scales are not permitted on the same piece of apparatus. For example, apparatus should not be graduated in both fluid ounces and milliliters" (6).

   (3) "The relation of the height to the diameter must be such that the graduation marks are not less than 1 mm apart, and also that the graduated height is at least five times the inside diameter" (6).

   c. Graduation lines

   (1) "Graduation lines shall be fine, clean, permanent, continuous, and of uniform width, perpendicular to the axis and parallel to the base of the apparatus. Line width should not exceed 0.3 mm for subdivided apparatus and 0.4 mm for single-line apparatus.

   All graduations must extend at least halfway around; and on subdivided apparatus at least every 10th mark, and on undivided apparatus, all marks must extend completely around the circumference. Subdivided apparatus must be provided with a sufficient number of lines of suitable length to facilitate reading.

The clear space between two adjacent marks must be not less than 1 mm wide. The spacing of marks on subdivided apparatus must show no apparent irregularities, and sufficient divisions must be numbered to readily indicate the intended capacity of any interval" (6).

   (2) "Subdivision lines shall be omitted between the base and the first numbered line. This will eliminate readings near the base which are difficult and not always accurate. The numbers indicating the capacity of the graduate at its different points should be placed immediately above the marks to which they refer" (6).

d. Basis of graduation

"Cylinders may be graduated either to contain or to deliver, but a scale numbered both up and down the length of the graduate is not permitted, as it is obvious that the same graduate cannot be correct both to contain and to deliver" (6).

e. Inscriptions

"Every instrument must bear in permanent legible characters the capacity, the temperature at which it is to be used, the method of use—that is, whether to contain or to deliver . . ." (6)

f. In summary, to comply with NTIS COM-73-10504 and *USP* standards, graduated cylinders for use in compounding should have the following characteristics:

   (1) Made of good-quality glass

   (2) Graduation marks that are clear and distinct (see specifications above)

   (3) Graduation marks in only one scale, either milliliters or ounces, but not both

   (4) Graduated either "to contain" or "to deliver"; in other words, cannot have a numbered scale both running up and also running down the side of the cylinder

   (5) No subdivision lines between the base and the first numbered graduation line
   Note: NBS Circular 602 has no stated requirement for the initial interval for cylindrical graduates as there is for cylindrical and conical graduates in *Handbook 44* (see below).

   (6) A permanent inscription with the capacity, the temperature at which the graduate is to be used, and whether it is calibrated TC (to contain) or TD (to deliver)

2. *Handbook 44*

The *USP* also lists conical graduates as acceptable measuring devices for prescription compounding and requires these to meet the standards described in *Handbook 44*, 4th Edition (3). As described at the beginning of this chapter, *Handbook 44* has been issued each year since 1949 (obviously it is currently well past the 4th edition). The section on graduates in *Handbook 44* applies to both cylindrical and conical graduates (1). The 2002 edition of *Handbook 44* has the following pertinent specifications for **cylindrical and conical graduates:**

a. Material

"A graduate shall be made of good-quality, thoroughly annealed, clear, transparent glass, free from bubbles and streaks that might affect the accuracy of measurement. The glass shall be uniform in thickness and shall not be excessively thick" (1).

b. Shape

"A graduate of a capacity of more than 15 mL (4 fluid drams) may be of either the cylindrical or circular conical type. A graduate of a capacity of 15 mL (4 fluid drams) or less shall be of the single-scale cylindrical type" (1).

c. Dimensional proportions

   (1) Conical

   "The inside measurement from the bottom of a circular conical graduate to the capacity graduation shall be not less than two times the inside diameter at the capacity graduation. The inside measurement from the bottom of the graduate to the point representing one-fourth of the capacity shall be not less than the inside diameter at that point" (1).

(2) Cylindrical

"The inside measurement from the bottom of a cylindrical graduate to the capacity graduation shall be not less than five times the inside diameter at the capacity graduation" (1).

d. Initial interval

"A graduate shall have an initial interval that is not subdivided, equal to not less than one-fifth and not more than one-fourth of the capacity of the graduate" (1).

e. Graduation designs

(1) General

"Graduations shall be perpendicular to the vertical axis of the graduate and parallel to each other. Graduations shall be continuous, of uniform thickness not greater than 0.4 mm (0.015 in), clearly visible, permanent, and indelible under normal conditions of use" (1).

(2) Single-scale graduates

"[T]he main graduations shall completely encircle the graduate and subordinate graduations shall extend at least one-half the distance around the graduate" (1).

(3) Double-scale graduates

"[T]here shall be a clear space between the ends of the main graduations on the two scales" (1).

f. Basis of graduation and inscription

"A graduate shall be graduated "to deliver" when the temperature of the graduate is 20°C (68°F), and shall be marked accordingly in a permanent and conspicuous manner" (1).

g. Capacities, graduation ranges and intervals, and number of graduations for the various sizes are given in a table of values in *Handbook 44*. See that document for details.

h. In summary, to comply with *USP* standards, conical graduates for use in compounding should have the characteristics given below. In states where statutes require compliance with *Handbook 44*, all graduates used in compounding should have these characteristics:

(1) Made of good-quality glass

(2) Graduation marks that are clear and distinct (see specifications above)

(3) Conical graduates must have a capacity of at least 15 mL (4 fluid drams)

(4) An initial graduation marking that is not less than one-fifth or more than one-fourth of the graduate capacity (e.g., for a 4-ounce [120 mL] conical graduate, the first graduation mark cannot be less than 24 mL or more than 30 mL [1 fluid ounce]).

(5) Note: There is no prohibition against a dual scale (milliliters and ounces) in *Handbook 44*, which is probably one reason why most conical graduates are available with graduation markings in both the metric and apothecary systems.

C. Descriptions and standards for medicine droppers

Standards are described for medicine droppers in the *USP*, both in the general chapter ⟨1176⟩ and in chapter ⟨1101⟩ Medicine Dropper.

1. Non-graduated medicine droppers: According to the *USP*, "an acceptable ungraduated medicine dropper has a delivery end 3 mm in external diameter and delivers 20 drops of water, weighing 1 g at a temperature of 15°. A tolerance of ±10% of the delivery specification is reasonable" (3).

a. Notice that the calibration is given in terms of water. Other liquids have different surface tensions and viscosities, which give different drop volumes. Therefore, if a dropper is to be used for measuring a liquid, it should be calibrated with the liquid to be measured. This is done by holding the dropper vertically and delivering a given number of drops into a small graduated cylinder and accurately measuring the volume.

      b. Because of the general availability and greater accuracy offered by syringes and pipets, non-graduated medicine droppers now have limited usefulness as measuring devices for compounding.

    2. Graduated medicine droppers: These have more stringent requirements. They must meet the specifications in section ⟨1101⟩ Medicine Dropper, which states: "The dropper, when held vertically, delivers water in drops each of which weighs between 45 mg and 55 mg" (7).

    3. Calibrated medicine droppers for administering doses of liquid drug products are available in both glass and plastic.

D. Descriptions of other volumetric apparatus

The following devices are not listed in the *USP* or *Handbook 44* as volumetric devices, but they are routinely used by pharmacists for measuring volumes when compounding prescriptions. Each has limitations, which should be considered.

    1. Syringes

      a. Plastic disposable syringes are available in sizes ranging from 0.5 mL to 60 mL.

      b. Small syringes of 1- and 3-mL capacities are useful for accurately measuring volumes less than the 2 mL minimum recommended for a 10-mL graduated cylinder.

      c. Syringes of the appropriate size are also preferred over graduated cylinders for measuring viscous liquids such as Glycerin or Mineral Oil, since these liquids drain slowly and incompletely from graduated cylinders.

      d. Special oral syringes are available and are recommended for giving more accurate measurement of doses than is possible with household measuring spoons. **If standard syringes are used for oral dosing, the tip cap, if present, should be removed before dispensing.** Fatalities have been reported when tip caps are inadvertently squirted in the throat of a patient when an oral liquid was administered.

    2. Graduated beakers

      a. Beakers are used in the pharmacy as vessels for compounding solutions and for many other purposes. They are commonly available in sizes ranging from 50 to 1,000 mL. Larger-capacity beakers are available from some suppliers.

      b. Most glass beakers have painted graduation marks. Usually these markings do not give precise volume measurements and are not meant to be used for accurate measuring. Unless these beakers are calibrated and marked using water measured in

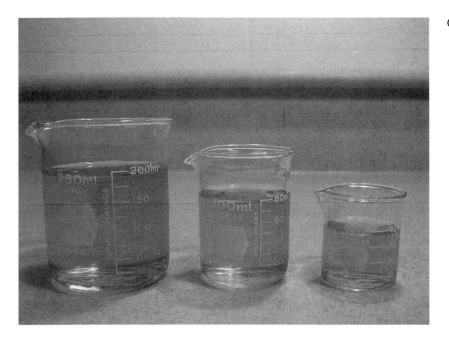

Graduated beakers

a graduated cylinder, they should not be used when accurate measuring is required, such as when "q.s.'ing" a preparation to a desired volume.

3. Graduated prescription bottles

    a. Amber plastic prescription bottles, commonly called prescription ovals, are used for dispensing liquid drug products and preparations. They are commonly available in 2, 3, 4, 6, 8, and 16 ounces (which correspond to metric capacities of 60, 90, 120, 180, 240, and 480 mL). They have graduation marks embossed in the plastic that run up the side of the bottle.

    b. Like graduated beakers, the volume markings on graduated prescription bottles are approximate.

        (1) The capacity markings are sufficiently accurate for measuring and dispensing a manufactured liquid product where the strength of the product is not dependent on the accuracy of the capacity markings.

        (2) Although graduated prescription bottles are not intended for the accurate measuring needed in compounding, in recent years the quality of some brands of prescription ovals has improved to the point where the graduation markings are quite accurate and well within the usual standard of ±5%. Pharmacists often prefer to q.s. liquid preparations in the final prescription bottles, especially when compounding thick liquid preparations, because there is no loss of material in transferring from a measuring cylinder. If prescription ovals are being used in this manner, the calibration markings on the bottles should be checked. This is done by accurately measuring water, or other compatible mobile liquid, in a graduated cylinder and using that to check the graduation and capacities markings on the bottles.

E. Selection and Use of Volumetric Apparatus

    1. For maximum accuracy in measuring, select a graduate or other volumetric device with a capacity equal to or slightly larger than the volume to be measured. For graduates, the smaller the volume to be measured as a percentage of the graduate capacity, the larger the potential percentage error from a given deviation in reading the meniscus. **The general rule is to measure volumes no less than 20% of the capacity of the graduate.**

    2. Cylindrical graduates are preferred for measurement over conical graduates. Because of the constant diameter of a cylindrical graduate, a given deviation in reading (e.g., ±1 mm) gives a constant error in a measured volume throughout the entire length of the graduate. This is not true for conical graduates, where the diameter continually increases from the base to the top graduation mark. Therefore, an error in reading the meniscus of ±1 mm can cause a volume error of 0.5 mL at any point on a 100-mL cylindrical graduate, but this same ±1-mm deviation can cause a much greater volume error (~1.8 mL) at the 100-mL mark of a 4-ounce conical graduate. According to the *USP*, conical graduates having a capacity of less than 25 mL should not be used in prescription compounding (3).

    3. When reading the volume of liquid in a graduate, the graduation mark, the meniscus of the liquid, and the line of sight should all be in alignment. This minimizes errors caused by the parallax effect.

    4. The following should be noted:

NBS Circular 602 sets standards for burets, flasks, pipettes, and cylindrical graduates of precision grade. Although *Handbook 44* addresses both cylindrical and conical graduates, the *USP* applies this document as a standard only to conical graduates. This means, as noted above, that by *USP* standard, the requirement for initial interval found in *Handbook 44* applies only to conical graduates, while the prohibition against a double scale in NBS Circular 602 applies only to cylindrical graduates.

This distinction is voided if a state statute or administrative code requires that pharmacies have equipment that conforms to only one of the standards. For example, if a state statute requires graduates that conform to NBS Circular 602, conical graduates would not meet the legal requirements for that state. If a statute requires conformity with the standards of *Handbook 44*, both cylindrical and conical graduates would be acceptable, but both types would be required to meet the initial interval standard of *Handbook 44*. This standard may be difficult to meet because manufacturers generally make cylindrical graduates that conform to NBS Circular 602, which does not have this requirement.

V. SUMMARY

Standards for weighing and measuring equipment change from time to time, and new and improved devices are becoming more generally available. This is part of the reason for updates to pharmacy practices acts being written in a more generic way. For example, instead of specifying a particular class of balance or weights or the number, size, and type of measuring device, a revised practice act may state that the pharmacist use equipment of appropriate size and design for the intended purpose; it leaves the selection of the equipment to the professional judgment of the pharmacist. Pharmacists should be knowledgeable about these issues and new standards for measuring devices so they can make informed decisions about the equipment they use in their practice and in making recommendations for updates to state pharmacy practice standards.

References

1. NIST Handbook 44, 2002 Edition, Specifications, Tolerances, and Other Technical Requirements for Weighing and Measuring Devices. National Institute of Standards and Technology. http://ts.nist.gov/ts/htdocs/230/235/h442002.htm, accessed November 2002.
2. The 2002 United States Pharmacopeia 25/National Formulary 20. Rockville, MD: The United States Pharmacopeial Convention, Inc., 2001; 2054.
3. The 2002 United States Pharmacopeia 25/National Formulary 20. Rockville, MD: The United States Pharmacopeial Convention, Inc., 2001; 2227–2228.
4. Troemner Mass Standards Handbook. Philadelphia, PA: Troemner, Inc., 2000; 6–7.
5. The 2002 United States Pharmacopeia 25/National Formulary 20. Rockville, MD: The United States Pharmacopeial Convention, Inc., 2001; 1869.
6. Hughes JC. Testing Glass Volumetric Apparatus. National Bureau of Standards Circular 602, The National Technical Information Service, Springfield, VA 22151, 1959; 1–4.
7. The 2002 United States Pharmacopeia 25/National Formulary 20. Rockville, MD: The United States Pharmacopeial Convention, Inc., 2001; 2205.

PART 4

PHARMACEUTICAL NECESSITIES

CHAPTER 14

Pharmaceutical Solvents

I. GENERAL INFORMATION

A. Water is the most commonly used and most desirable solvent-vehicle for liquid drug products and preparations for all uses.

B. Other solvents-vehicles frequently used as ingredients in drug products and compounded preparations include Alcohol, Isopropyl Alcohol, Glycerin, Propylene Glycol, and Polyethylene Glycol 400.

C. Some other solvents are used pharmaceutically in processing drug products, for assays and tests, or for making specialty products and preparations such as Flexible Collodion. Examples include acetone, ether, and chloroform.

D. Oils used as pharmaceutical solvents-vehicles include a variety of vegetable oils and mineral oil. Examples include Corn Oil, Cottonseed Oil, and Almond Oil. Some special vegetable and essential oils are used primarily as flavors and scents. The *National Formulary* section of the *USP–NF* has monographs for various oils of this type, such as Anise Oil, Lemon Oil, and Rose Oil. These are discussed in Chapter 20, Colors, Flavors, Sweeteners, and Scents.

E. The *USP–NF* lists official articles classified as solvents and vehicles in a table, USP and NF Excipients, Listed by Categories. These are given in Table 14.1. Notice that some articles are listed in both categories and some, such as Sterile Water for Inhalation and Dehydrated Alcohol, are not listed at all. The following chapter describes those articles most frequently encountered in pharmacy compounding and practice.

F. In reading and interpreting the current chapter, note that this text employs the usual convention of using upper-case first letters for words designating official *USP–NF* articles (e.g., Alcohol, Purified Water, etc.) and lower-case first letters for words designating the chemical substances (e.g., ethyl alcohol, water, etc.).

II. WATER

A. General information
   1. When water is used in making official *USP* preparations, it must meet the criteria specified in the *USP* for the type of preparation being made. For example, the water used for making parenteral products must meet the requirements for injections found in Chapter ⟨1⟩ Injections of the *USP*.

TABLE 14.1 USP and NF Excipients Categorized as Solvents and Vehicles (4)

Solvent	Vehicle
Acetone	FLAVORED AND/OR SWEETENED
Alcohol	Aromatic Elixir
Alcohol, Diluted	Benzaldehyde Elixir, Compound
Amylene Hydrate	Peppermint Water
Benzyl Benzoate	Sorbitol Solution
Butyl Alcohol	Syrup
Corn Oil	OLEAGINOUS
Cottonseed Oil	Alkyl (C 12–15) Benzoate
Diethylene Glycol Monoethyl Ether	Almond Oil
Ethyl Acetate	Corn Oil
Glycerin	Cottonseed Oil
Hexylene Glycol	Ethyl Oleate
Isopropyl Alcohol	Isopropyl Myristate
Methyl Alcohol	Isopropyl Palmitate
Methylene Chloride	Mineral Oil
Methyl Isobutyl Ketone	Mineral Oil, Light
Mineral Oil	Octyldodecanol
Peanut Oil	Olive Oil
Polyethylene Glycol	Peanut Oil
Propylene Glycol	Safflower Oil
Sesame Oil	Sesame Oil
Water for Injection, Sterile	Soybean Oil
Water for Irrigation, Sterile	Squalene
Water, Purified	STERILE
	Sodium Chloride Injection, Bacteriostatic
	Water for Injection, Bacteriostatic

2. The basic starting ingredient for all *USP* water items is potable (drinking) water as defined in the General Notices of the *USP*: "Potable water meeting the requirements for drinking water as set forth in the regulations of the federal Environmental Protection Agency may be used in the preparation of official substances" (1). This means that drinking water may be used in the manufacturing and preparation of USP drug substances, including water articles. Drinking or tap water does not, however, meet the standards as an ingredient in dosage forms. Water for making dosage forms must be one of the official *USP* monograph water articles as described below.

B. *USP–NF* water articles

1. Purified Water USP (2,3)
   H_2O MW = 18.02
   a. Preparation
      (1) Made from water complying with the U.S. Environmental Protection Agency (EPA) National Primary Drinking Water Regulations or comparable regulations of the European Union or Japan
      (2) Processed by distillation, ion-exchange treatment, reverse osmosis, or other suitable method
      (3) No added substances (such as preservatives)
   b. Description: Clear, colorless, odorless liquid
   c. Standards
      (1) Meets USP requirements for Total organic carbon ⟨643⟩ and Water conductivity ⟨645⟩.
      (2) Bacterial endotoxins (pyrogens): no standard
      (3) Bacteriologic purity: complies with EPA regulations for drinking water
   d. Packaging and storage: When packaged, use tight containers.
   e. Labeling: When packaged, label method of preparation.

    f. Uses

      (1) It is used as a solvent-vehicle for the preparation of pharmaceutical dosage forms for internal or external use.

      (2) It is not for use when sterility is required unless it meets the requirements under *USP* Sterility Tests ⟨71⟩ or is first sterilized by filtration or autoclaving. It must then be protected from microbial contamination.

      (3) It is not for use in making parenteral products unless it can be assured that it meets the requirements for sterility and bacterial endotoxins for parenteral administration.

2. Sterile Purified Water USP (2,3)

  a. Preparation

    (1) Made from Purified Water that has been sterilized and suitably packaged

    (2) No added substances (such as preservatives)

  b. Description: Clear, colorless, odorless liquid

  c. Standards

    (1) Meets USP requirements for Total organic carbon ⟨642⟩ and Water conductivity ⟨645⟩.

    (2) Bacterial endotoxins (pyrogens): no standard

    (3) Bacteriologic purity: Meets requirements in Chapter ⟨71⟩ for Sterility

    (4) pH: between 5.0 and 7.0

    (5) Other standards as given in the *USP* for Ammonia, Calcium, Chloride, Sulfate, and Oxidizable substances

  d. Packaging and storage: suitable tight containers

  e. Labeling: Label with method of preparation and that this is not for parenteral use.

  f. Uses

    (1) It is used as a solvent-vehicle for the preparation of pharmaceutical dosage forms for internal or external use.

    (2) It is not for parenteral administration.

3. Water for Injection USP (2,3)

  a. Preparation

    (1) Purified by distillation or reverse osmosis

    (2) No added substances (such as preservatives)

  b. Description: Clear, colorless, odorless liquid

  c. Standards

    (1) Bacterial endotoxins (pyrogens): not more than 0.25 USP Endotoxin Units per mL

    (2) All requirements for Purified Water

  d. Uses: Water for Injection is a starting material for making parenteral products. It must be processed further either before use or during product preparation. The *USP* monograph has the following note on its use:

    "NOTE—Water for Injection is intended for use as a solvent for the preparation of parenteral solutions. Where used for the preparation of parenteral solutions subject to final sterilization, use suitable means to minimize microbial growth, or first render the Water for Injection sterile and thereafter protect it from microbial contamination. For parenteral solutions that are prepared under aseptic conditions and are not sterilized by appropriate filtration or in the final container, first render the Water for Injection sterile and thereafter, protect it from microbial contamination" (2).

4. Sterile Water for Injection USP (2,3)

  a. Preparation

    (1) Made from Water for Injection that is sterilized and suitably packaged

    (2) No added substances (such as preservatives)

  b. Description: Clear, colorless, odorless liquid

  c. Standards

    (1) All requirements given for Sterile Purified Water

    (2) Particulate matter: Meets requirements in Chapter ⟨788⟩.

        (3) Bacterial endotoxins (pyrogens): Not more than 0.25 USP Endotoxin Units per mL

        (4) Bacteriologic purity: Meets requirements given for Sterile Purified Water (Chapter ⟨71⟩ for Sterility)

  d. Packaging and storage: Single-dose glass or plastic containers not larger than 1 liter. Glass containers of Type I or Type II glass are preferred.

  e. Labeling: Label to indicate that no preservative or other substance has been added. Also label that it is not suitable for intravascular injection unless it is first made approximately isotonic by the addition of a suitable solute.

  f. Uses

        (1) Base vehicle for large-volume parenteral fluids

        (2) Solvent for drugs intended for parenteral use

5. Sterile Water for Inhalation USP (2,3)

  a. Preparation

        (1) Made using Water for Injection that is sterilized and suitably packaged

        (2) No added substances, except that antimicrobial agents may be added when the water is to be used in humidifiers or other devices in which it may become contaminated

  b. Description: Clear, colorless solution

  c. Standards

        (1) All requirements given for Sterile Purified Water except pH

        (2) Bacterial endotoxins (pyrogens): Not more than 0.5 USP Endotoxin Units per mL

        (3) Bacteriologic purity: Meets USP sterility requirements

        (4) pH: 4.5 to 7.5

  d. Packaging and storage: Glass or plastic containers; Type I and II glass preferred for glass containers

  e. Labeling: Label that it is for inhalation therapy only and not for parenteral use.

  f. Uses

        (1) In humidifiers to add moisture to the environment

        (2) As a solvent for drugs to be administered by inhalation

        (3) The following is a note on use in the *USP* monograph:
NOTE—"Do not use Sterile Water for Inhalation for parenteral administration or for other sterile compendial dosage forms" (2).

6. Sterile Water for Irrigation USP (2,3)

  a. Preparation

        (1) Made from Water for Injection that is sterilized and suitably packaged

        (2) No added substances (such as preservatives)

  b. Description: Clear, colorless, odorless liquid

  c. Standards

        (1) All requirements given for Sterile Purified Water

        (2) Bacterial endotoxins (pyrogens): Meets the endotoxin test under Water for Injection

        (3) Bacteriologic purity: Meets requirements given for Sterile Purified Water

  d. Packaging and storage: Single-dose glass or plastic containers. Glass containers of Type I or Type II glass are preferred. Containers may have volumes in excess of 1 liter and may be designed with a closure to facilitate easy, rapid emptying.

  e. Labeling: Label to indicate that no preservative or other substance has been added. Also, the labels "For irrigation only" and "Not for injection" must be conspicuous.

  f. Uses

        (1) Irrigation fluid

        (2) Solvent for drugs to be administered by irrigation, usually for local effect

7. Bacteriostatic Water for Injection USP (2,3)
   a. Preparation
      (1) Made from Sterile Water for Injection that has been sterilized and suitably packaged
      (2) Added substances: one or more suitable antimicrobial agents are added
   b. Description: Clear, colorless liquid, odorless, or possibly having the odor of the added antimicrobial agent(s)
   c. Standards
      (1) Particulate matter: Meets requirements for Sterile Water for Injection
      (2) Bacterial endotoxins (pyrogens): Not more than 0.5 USP Endotoxin Units per mL
      (3) Bacteriologic purity: Meets USP sterility requirements
      (4) pH: 4.5 to 7.0
      (5) Meets the requirements of Chapter ⟨51⟩ Antimicrobial Preservatives—Effectiveness and label claim for content of the antimicrobial agent(s)
      (6) Meets all requirements for Sterile Purified Water except pH, Ammonia, Chloride, and Oxidizable substances
   d. Packaging and storage: Single-dose or multiple-dose glass or plastic containers not larger than 30 mL. Glass containers of Type I or Type II glass are preferred.
   e. Labeling: Label with name and quantity of preservative(s). Also label in boldface capital letters with contrasting color (preferably red): **NOT FOR USE IN NEWBORNS.**
   f. Uses
      (1) As a solvent for drugs to be given parenterally when a preserved solution is desired and when the antimicrobial agent(s) do not cause compatibility problems with the chosen drug or drugs
      (2) Is not to be used when large volumes are needed for parenteral administration. If large volumes are needed (greater than 30 mL), Sterile Water for Injection should be used. Even with moderate volumes (over 5 mL), Sterile Water for Injection is preferred.

III. ALCOHOLS

A. General information
   1. In organic chemistry, alcohols have the general formula R-OH, where R represents a general hydrocarbon group. In pharmacy, when the term "alcohol" is used, it has a more restricted meaning. In the General Notices section of the *USP*, it states:
      "Alcohol—All statements of percentages of alcohol, such as under the heading *Alcohol content*, refer to percentage, by volume of C_2H_5OH at 15.56°. Where reference is made to C_2H_5OH, the chemical entity possessing absolute (100 percent) strength is intended.

      Alcohol—Where 'alcohol' is called for in formulas, tests, and assays, the monograph article *Alcohol* is to be used" (1).

      Therefore, when a prescription order or pharmaceutical formula calls for alcohol, the monograph product Alcohol USP is to be used. Another alcohol such as isopropyl alcohol should not be used when the term "alcohol," without modifier, is written.
   2. If a prescription order calls for a specific alcohol, such as isopropyl alcohol, that specified alcohol must be used. Different alcohols may not be substituted in prescription or medications orders without the consent of the prescriber, anymore than, for example, may Aspirin be substituted for Acetaminophen. Alcohols vary greatly in their relative toxicities; a single carbon atom separates the pharmaceutically useful ethyl alcohol from the toxic methyl alcohol. Be sure to use only alcohols that are approved for the intended purpose, either external or internal use, or as a solvent for processing.

3. Calculations involving content and labeling of alcohol have been the subject of some confusion. Explanations and multiple examples can be found in Chapter 7, Quantity and Concentration Expressions and Calculations.

B. *USP–NF alcohol (R-OH) articles*

    1. Ethyl Alcohol (Ethanol)

          CH_3CH_2OH C_2H_6O MW = 46.07

      a. Alcohol USP (2,3)

          (1) Content: Not less than 92.3% and not more than 93.8%, by weight (w/w), corresponding to not less than 94.9% and not more than 96.0%, by volume (v/v), of C_2H_5OH

          (2) Description: Clear, colorless, mobile, volatile liquid; flammable; boils at 78°; has a characteristic odor.

          (3) Specific gravity: between 0.812 and 0.816

          (4) Labeling: "The content of alcohol in a liquid preparation shall be stated on the label as a percentage (v/v) of C_2H_5OH" (1).

          (5) Solubility: Miscible with water, isopropyl alcohol, glycerin, acetone, propylene glycol, polyethylene glycol 400, ether, and chloroform. Will mix with castor oil, but not other fixed oils and not with mineral oil.

          (6) It is used as a solvent-vehicle for the preparation of pharmaceutical dosage forms for internal or external use. It is an effective antiseptic-disinfectant, being germicidal in concentrations above 60%. Its usual concentration as an antiseptic-disinfectant is 70%.

          (7) Packaging and storage: Tight containers, remote from fire

      b. Dehydrated Alcohol USP (2,3)

          (1) Content: Not less than 99.2%, by weight (w/w), corresponding to not less than 99.5%, by volume (v/v), of C_2H_5OH

          (2) Description: Clear, colorless, mobile, volatile liquid; flammable; boils at 78°; has a characteristic odor

          (3) Specific gravity: not more than 0.7964

          (4) Use this preparation when "dehydrated" or "absolute" alcohol is written in a formula (1).

          (5) Packaging and storage: Tight containers, remote from fire

      c. Dehydrated Alcohol Injection USP (2,3)

          (1) The injection is dehydrated alcohol that is suitable for parenteral use.

          (2) Description: Clear, colorless, mobile, volatile liquid; flammable; boils at 78°; has a characteristic odor

          (3) Specific gravity: not more than 0.8035

          (4) It meets the requirements for Dehydrated Alcohol plus the requirements for parenteral products found in Chapter ⟨1⟩ Injections of the General Tests and Assays chapters of the *USP*. These include specifications for sterility, pyrogenicity, particulate matter, and other contaminants.

          (5) Packaging and storage: Single-dose containers with Type I glass preferred. Container headspace may have inert gas.

      d. Diluted Alcohol NF (2,3)

          (1) Content: A mixture of Alcohol and water with not less than 41.0% and not more than 42.0%, by weight (w/w), corresponding to not less than 48.4% and not more than 49.5%, by volume (v/v), of C_2H_5OH

          (2) Description: Clear, colorless, mobile liquid with a characteristic odor

          (3) Specific gravity: between 0.935 and 0.937

          (4) Made by mixing equal volumes of Alcohol USP and Purified Water. Mixing 500 mL of each gives 970 mL of Diluted Alcohol.

          (5) Packaging and storage: Tight containers, remote from fire

    e. Rubbing Alcohol USP (2,3)

        (1) Alcohol content: 68.5% to 71.5% by volume of dehydrated alcohol

        (2) Other content: It is made in accordance with the specifications of Formula 23-H (U.S. Treasury Department, Bureau of Alcohol, Tobacco, and Firearms): 8 parts by volume of acetone, 1.5 parts by volume of methyl isobutyl ketone, and 100 parts by volume of ethyl alcohol. In addition to containing water, ethyl alcohol, and denaturants, Rubbing Alcohol may also contain stabilizers, perfumes, or dyes that are FDA-approved for use in drugs. In each 100 mL it has not less than 355 mg sucrose octaacetate or not less than 1.4 mg of denatonium benzoate.

        (3) Description: Like Alcohol, except it may be colored because of addition of dye. Odor depends on presence of other additives such as perfumes.

        (4) Specific gravity: between 0.869 and 0.877

        (5) Rubbing Alcohol is for external use only. It may be used as a solvent-vehicle for drugs that are being formulated into topical products. It is an effective antiseptic-disinfectant.

        (6) Labeling: Label that it is flammable.

        (7) Packaging and storage: Tight containers, remote from fire

2. Isopropyl alcohol (2-Propanol)

    $CH_3CHOHCH_3$ C_3H_8O MW = 60.10

    a. Isopropyl Alcohol USP (2,3)

        (1) Content: Not less than 99.0% of C_3H_8O

        (2) Description: Transparent, colorless, mobile, volatile, flammable liquid with a characteristic odor

        (3) Specific gravity: between 0.783 and 0.787

        (4) Solubility: Miscible with water, alcohol, glycerin, propylene glycol, polyethylene glycol 400, acetone, ether, and chloroform. It is immiscible with fixed oils and mineral oil.

        (5) Isopropyl Alcohol is for external use only. It may be used as a solvent-vehicle for drugs that are being formulated into topical products. In concentrations $\geq$ 70% it is an effective disinfectant. It is somewhat superior to ethyl alcohol as an antiseptic.

        (6) Packaging and storage: Tight containers, remote from heat

    b. Isopropyl Rubbing Alcohol USP (2,3)

        (1) Content: Not less than 68.0% and not more than 72.0% by volume (v/v) of isopropyl alcohol, the remainder consisting of water, with or without stabilizers, perfume oils, and color additives that are certified by the FDA for use in drugs

        (2) Description: Like Isopropyl Alcohol, except it may be colored because of addition of dye. Odor depends on the presence of other additives such as perfumes.

        (3) Specific gravity: between 0.872 and 0.883

        (4) Isopropyl Rubbing Alcohol is for external use only. It may be used as a solvent-vehicle for drugs that are being formulated into topical products. It is an effective antiseptic-disinfectant.

        (5) Packaging and storage: Tight containers, remote from heat

    c. Azeotropic Isopropyl Alcohol USP (2,3)

        (1) Content: Not less than 91.0% and not more than 93.0% of isopropyl alcohol, by volume (v/v), the remainder consisting of water

        (2) Description: Like Isopropyl Alcohol

        (3) Specific gravity: between 0.815 and 0.810

        (4) Packaging and storage: Tight containers, remote from heat

IV. GLYCOLS

A. General information

1. Glycols are simply dihydroxy alcohols. Because of their chemical structure, they have more than one site for hydrogen bonding and therefore, relative to their molecular weights, they have higher water solubility and higher boiling points (are less volatile) than a comparable single hydroxy alcohol. For example, ethyl alcohol boils at 78°C, while the structurally comparable dihydroxy ethylene glycol has a boiling point of 197°C. Ethylene glycol owes its usefulness as an antifreeze to its unique glycol properties of low freezing point, high boiling point, and high water solubility. Similarly, polyethylene glycols have high water solubility even though they are high-molecular-weight organic compounds.

2. As with alcohols, glycols vary greatly in their relative toxicities, and a single carbon atom separates the pharmaceutically useful and nontoxic propylene glycol from the very toxic ethylene glycol. Be sure to use only glycols approved for the intended purpose, either external or internal use.

B. *USP–NF glycol articles*

1. Glycerin USP (Glycerol) (2,3)

   $C_3H_8O_3$ MW = 92.01

   Glycerin

   $$HOCH_2 \long!!!! CH \long!!!! CH_2OH$$
   with OH on the central CH

   a. Content: Not less than 99.0% and not more than 101.0% of $C_3H_8O_3$
   b. Description: Clear, colorless, viscous liquid. Practically odorless, hygroscopic, neutral pH.
   c. Specific gravity: not less than 1.249
   d. Solubility: Miscible with water, ethyl alcohol, isopropyl alcohol, propylene glycol, and polyethylene glycol 400; is soluble to the degree of 1 g/15 mL in acetone; insoluble in chloroform, ether, fixed oils, mineral oil, and volatile oils
   e. It is used as a solvent-vehicle for the preparation of pharmaceutical dosage forms for internal or external use. It has humectant and preservative properties.
   f. Packaging and storage: Tight containers

2. Glycerin Oral Solution USP (2,3)
   a. Content: Not less than 95.0% and not more than 105.0% of $C_3H_8O_3$
   b. Description: Like Glycerin USP except pH between 5.5 and 7.5
   c. Solubility: Like Glycerin USP
   d. It is used as a solvent-vehicle for the preparation of pharmaceutical oral dosage forms.
   e. Packaging and storage: Tight containers

3. Glycerin Ophthalmic Solution USP (2,3)
   a. Content: Not less than 98.5% of $C_3H_8O_3$. It may contain one or more suitable antimicrobial preservatives.
   b. Description: Like Glycerin Oral Solution USP except it is sterile
   c. Solubility: Like Glycerin USP
   d. For ophthalmic use
   e. Packaging and storage: Tight containers of glass or plastic with volume not greater than 15 mL and protected from light. The container or carton is sealed and tamper-proof so that sterility is ensured at opening.

4. Propylene Glycol USP (2,3)

$C_3H_8O_2$ MW = 76.09

Propylene Glycol

$$CH_3 \underset{}{\overset{\overset{\displaystyle OH}{|}}{CH}} CH_2OH$$

 a. Content: Not less than 99.5% of $C_3H_8O_2$
 b. Description: Clear, colorless, viscous liquid. Practically odorless, hygroscopic.
 c. Specific gravity: between 1.035 and 1.037
 d. Solubility: Miscible with water, ethyl and isopropyl alcohol, acetone, glycerin, polyethylene glycol 400, chloroform, and ether; dissolves many volatile oils, but is immiscible with fixed oils and mineral oil
 e. It is used as a solvent-vehicle for the preparation of pharmaceutical dosage forms for internal or external use. It is also useful as a humectant and preservative.

5. Polyethylene Glycol NF (2,3)
 a. Polyethylene Glycol, also known as PEG, is an addition polymer of ethylene oxide and water. It has the formula: $H(OCH_2CH_2)_nOH$ where n represents the number of oxyethylene groups.
 b. PEG is labeled with a number indicating the average nominal molecular weight of the Polyethylene Glycol. The numbers range from 200 to 8000; polyethylene glycols 200, 300, 400, and 600 are liquids at room temperature and the higher molecular polymers are waxy solids. (See Chapter 23, Table 23.1.)
 c. Polyethylene Glycol 400 is the most common liquid PEG used as a solvent-vehicle in making pharmaceutical dosage forms for both internal and external use. It is a clear, colorless, slightly hygroscopic, viscous liquid with a slight odor. It congeals at 6°C and has a specific gravity at 25° of 1.12.
 d. Solubility: All PEGs are soluble in water and many are organic solvents. PEG 400 is miscible with water, ethyl and isopropyl alcohol, acetone, glycerin, and propylene glycol. It is immiscible with fixed oils and mineral oil.
 e. Recommended packaging: Tight containers

V. KETONES

A. General information
 1. There are only two official solvent-vehicles in the ketone group, Acetone and Methyl Isobutyl Ketone. Methyl ethyl ketone is not an official substance, but it is described in the reagent section of the *USP* because it is used as a solvent for assays, tests, and processing.
 2. Official ketones have limited usefulness because of their volatility, flammability, and toxicity. They do have some unique solvent properties that make them useful.

B. Acetone NF (2,3)

CH_3COCH_3 C_3H_6O MW = 58.08

 1. Description: Transparent, colorless, mobile, volatile liquid that boils at 56.5°C. Has a distinctive odor. A 1 in 2 solution with water has neutral pH.
    CAUTION—*Acetone is very flammable. Do not use where it may be ignited.*
 2. Specific gravity: 0.788 (not >0.789)
 3. Solubility: Miscible with water, alcohol, ether, chloroform, and most oils
 4. Packaging and storage: Use tight containers and store remote from fire.

VI. OILS

A. General information
  1. The following are solvent-vehicle oils official in the *USP-NF*.
  2. As stated in the introduction to this chapter, some special vegetable and essential oils are used primarily as flavors and scents. The *National Formulary* section of the *USP–NF* has monographs for various oils of this type such as Anise Oil, Lemon Oil, and Rose Oil. These are discussed in Chapter 20, Colors, Flavors, Sweeteners, and Scents.

B. *USP–NF* oils
  1. Almond Oil NF (2,3)
      a. Description: Clear, pale straw-colored or colorless, oily liquid. Clear at −10°C, congeals at −20°C.
      b. Specific gravity: 0.910 to 0.915
      c. Solubility: Insoluble in water, slightly soluble in alcohol, miscible with mineral oil, other fixed oils, ether, chloroform, and solvent hexane
  2. Castor Oil USP (2,3)
      a. Description: Pale, yellowish or a nearly colorless, transparent, viscid liquid. Has a faint, mild odor.
      b. Specific gravity: 0.957 to 0.961
      c. Solubility: Insoluble in water and mineral oil, soluble in alcohol, miscible with dehydrated alcohol, other fixed oils, glacial acetic acid, chloroform, and ether
  3. Corn Oil NF (2,3)
      a. Description: Clear, light yellow, oily liquid with a faint characteristic odor
      b. Specific gravity: 0.914 to 0.921
      c. Solubility: Insoluble in water, slightly soluble in alcohol, miscible with mineral oil, other fixed oils, ether, chloroform, and solvent hexane
  4. Cottonseed Oil NF (2,3)
      a. Description: Pale yellow, oily liquid. Odorless or nearly so. Particles of fat may separate beginning at 10°C, solidifies at 0° to –5°C.
      b. Specific gravity: 0.915 to 0.921
      c. Solubility: Insoluble in water, slightly soluble in alcohol, miscible with mineral oil, other fixed oils, ether, chloroform, and solvent hexane
  5. Mineral Oil USP (2,3)
      a. Description: Colorless, transparent, oily liquid. Odorless at room temperature.
      b. Specific gravity: 0.845 to 0.905
      c. Solubility: Insoluble in water and in alcohol, soluble in volatile oils. Miscible with most fixed oils but not with Castor Oil.
  6. Light Mineral Oil NF (2,3)
      a. Description: Colorless, transparent, oily liquid. Odorless at room temperature.
      b. Specific gravity: 0.818 to 0.880
      c. Solubility: Insoluble in water and in alcohol, soluble in volatile oils. Miscible with most fixed oils but not with Castor Oil.
  7. Olive Oil NF (2,3)
      a. Description: Pale yellow, or light greenish-yellow oily liquid. Has a characteristic odor.
      b. Specific gravity: 0.910 to 0.915
      c. Solubility: Insoluble in water, slightly soluble in alcohol, miscible with mineral oil, other fixed oils, ether, and chloroform
  8. Peanut Oil NF (2,3)
      a. Description: Colorless or pale yellow oily liquid. May have a nutty odor.
      b. Specific gravity: 0.912 to 0.920
      c. Solubility: Insoluble in water, very slightly soluble in alcohol, miscible with mineral oil, other fixed oils, ether, and chloroform

9. Safflower Oil USP (2,3)
   a. Description: Light yellow oil. Becomes thick and rancid on prolonged exposure to air.
   b. Specific gravity: 0.921
   c. Solubility: Insoluble in water, slightly soluble in alcohol, miscible with other fixed oils, ether, and chloroform
10. Sesame Oil NF (2,3)
   a. Description: Pale yellow, oily liquid. Practically odorless.
   b. Specific gravity: 0.916 to 0.921
   c. Solubility: Insoluble in water, slightly soluble in alcohol, miscible with mineral oil, other fixed oils, ether, chloroform, and solvent hexane
11. Soybean Oil USP (2,3)
   a. Description: Clear, pale yellow oily liquid with a characteristic odor
   b. Specific gravity: 0.916 to 0.922
   c. Solubility: Insoluble in water, slightly soluble in alcohol, miscible with mineral oil, other fixed oils, ether, and chloroform

References

1. The 2002 United States Pharmacopeia 25/National Formulary 20. Rockville, MD: The United States Pharmacopeial Convention, Inc., 2001; 5.
2. The 2002 United States Pharmacopeia 25/National Formulary 20. Rockville, MD: The United States Pharmacopeial Convention, Inc., 2001: Official Monographs.
3. USP DI Vol. III, 22d ed. Englewood, CO: MICROMEDEX, Inc. 2002: Chemistry and Compendial Requirements.
4. The 2002 United States Pharmacopeia 25/National Formulary 20. Rockville, MD: The United States Pharmacopeial Convention, Inc., 2001; 2497–2499.

CHAPTER 15

Preservatives

I. DEFINITION

"Antimicrobial preservatives are substances added to nonsterile dosage forms to protect them from microbiological growth or from microorganisms that are introduced inadvertently during or subsequent to the manufacturing process. In the case of sterile articles packaged in multiple-dose containers, antimicrobial preservatives are added to inhibit the growth of microorganisms that may be introduced from repeatedly withdrawing individual doses.

Antimicrobial agents should not be used as a substitute for good manufacturing practices or solely to reduce the viable microbial population of a nonsterile product or to control the presterilization bioburden of multidose formulations during manufacturing." (1)—*USP*

II. USES

A. Preservatives should be added to extemporaneously compounded preparations when there is a possibility of microbial contamination and growth, either at the time of preparations or during use by the patient or caregiver.

B. In *USP* Chapter ⟨1151⟩ Pharmaceutical Dosage Forms, antimicrobial agents are explicitly mentioned and required for most dosage forms containing water and for one nonaqueous system, ophthalmic ointments (2):

1. Emulsions (including semisolid or ointment-type emulsions): "All emulsions require an antimicrobial agent because the aqueous phase is favorable to the growth of microorganisms."

2. Suspensions: "Suspensions intended for any route of administration should contain suitable antimicrobial agents to protect against bacteria, yeast, and mold contamination."

3. Oral solutions: "Antimicrobial agents to prevent the growth of bacteria, yeasts, and molds are generally also present."

4. Ophthalmic solutions: "Each solution must contain a suitable substance or mixture of substances to prevent the growth of, or to destroy, microorganisms accidentally introduced when the container is opened during use. Where intended for use in surgical procedures, ophthalmic solutions, although they must be sterile, should not contain antibacterial agents, since they may be irritating to the ocular tissues."

5. Ophthalmic ointments: "Ophthalmic ointments must contain a suitable substance or mixture of substances to prevent growth of, or to destroy, microorganisms accidentally introduced when the container is opened during use, unless otherwise directed in the individual monograph, or unless the formula itself is bacteriostatic."

C. The requirements for antimicrobial agents in parenteral products are treated in *USP* Chapter ⟨1⟩, Injections:

"A suitable substance or mixture of substances to prevent the growth of microorganisms must be added to preparations intended for injection that are packaged in multiple-dose containers, regardless of the method of sterilization employed, unless one of the following conditions prevails: (1) there are different directions in the individual monograph; (2) the substance contains a radionuclide with a physical half-life of less than 24 hours; (3) the active ingredients are themselves antimicrobial. Such substances are used in concentrations that will prevent the growth of or kill microorganisms in the preparations for injection" (3).

III. WHEN IS IT NOT NECESSARY TO ADD A PRESERVATIVE?

A. The preparation will be used immediately. This assumes that the preparation is made using appropriate techniques that avoid contamination while it is being made and administered.

B. No water is present. Generally, microorganisms require water for growth, so products that contain no water, such as tablets, powders, and hydrocarbon ointments, are not media for growth. Exceptions to this rule include ophthalmic ointments and nonaqueous injections when the *USP* specifically requires an antimicrobial agent.

C. The pH of the medium is either < 3 or > 9.
   Note: Although the above pH range for inhibition of growth holds true for most microorganisms, certain resistant molds have been shown to grow in media with pH below 3 (4).

D. Ingredient(s) that have antimicrobial properties are already present in the formulation.

IV. WHEN ARE PRESERVATIVES CONTRAINDICATED?

A. Neonates

B. Ophthalmic solutions intended for use in eyes during eye surgery, with non-intact corneas, or for intraocular injection

C. Parenteral products with volumes greater than 30 mL

V. ALTERNATIVE STRATEGIES WHEN PRESERVATIVES ARE NEEDED, BUT ARE CONTRAINDICATED

A. Prepare a single dose and use immediately.

B. Prepare a limited quantity that will be used within a short time period, store under refrigeration, and label with a short expiration period.

VI. PROPERTIES OF THE IDEAL PRESERVATIVE

A. Effective at a low, nontoxic concentration against a wide variety of organisms

B. Chemically stable under normal conditions of use, over a wide pH and temperature range

C. Soluble at the required concentration

D. Compatible with a wide variety of drugs and auxiliary agents

E. Free from objectionable odor, taste, color, or stinging

F. Nontoxic and nonsensitizing both internally and externally at the required concentration

G. Reasonable cost

H. Unreactive (does not adsorb, penetrate, or interact) with containers or closures

VII. ANTIMICROBIAL PRESERVATIVES LISTED IN THE *USP 25-NF 20*

A. Table 15.1 gives the articles listed as antimicrobial preservatives in the *USP 25-NF 20* (5). Some chemicals, although not listed by the *USP* as preservatives, have antimicrobial properties and may be useful as preservatives in formulated preparations.

B. The preservatives used most commonly in extemporaneous compounding are described below.
  1. To facilitate selection of an antimicrobial preservative when formulating a preparation, the agents are organized by suitability for route of administration (for example, oral, topical, and ophthalmic).
  2. The descriptions and solubilities presented here give a composite of information from the Chemistry and Compendial Requirements section of the *USP DI Vol. III* (6), *The Merck Index* (7), the *Handbook of Pharmaceutical Excipients* (8), and other references as cited. For additional information on each agent, consult the *Handbook of Pharmaceutical Excipients*.

VIII. PRESERVATIVES FOR ORAL DOSAGE FORMS

A. Alcohols and Glycols
  1. Ethyl Alcohol CH_3CH_2OH MW = 46.07
    a. Official products of ethyl alcohol that are suitable for oral use:
      (1) Alcohol USP
      (2) Dehydrated Alcohol USP
      (3) Dehydrated Alcohol Injection USP
      (4) Diluted Alcohol NF

TABLE 15.1   Antimicrobial Preservatives Listed in the *USP25-NF20* (5)

Benzalkonium Chloride	Chlorobutanol	Phenol	Propylparaben Sodium
Benzalkonium Chloride Solution	Chlorocresol	Phenylethyl Alcohol	Sodium Benzoate
Benzethonium Chloride	Cresol	Phenylmercuric	Sodium Dehydroacetate
Benzoic Acid	Dehydroacetic Acid	AcetatePhenylmercuric Nitrate	Sodium Propionate
Benzyl Alcohol	Ethylparaben	Potassium Benzoate	Sorbic Acid
Butylparaben	Methylparaben	Potassium Sorbate	Thimerosal
Cetylpyridium Chloride	Methylparaben Sodium	Propylparaben	Thymol

> **Note:** Rubbing Alcohol USP is a product containing ethyl alcohol, but it may **not** be used orally. It contains denaturants that are toxic orally.

b. Description and Solubility: See Chapter 14, Pharmaceutical Solvents.

c. Effective Concentration

(1) Effective concentration depends on the pH of the solution and the amount of "free water."

> Note: "Free water" is the water in a preparation that is not bound by interaction with other molecules. Originally the term was used to represent the amount of water in a preparation that is not tied up by interaction with sucrose in the ratio of 85 g of sucrose to 45 mL of water. This 85:45 ratio of sucrose to water is called the USP Syrup Equivalent because it is the proportion of these ingredients in the formula for Syrup NF (Simple Syrup), which is a saturated, self-preserving solution. Obviously, other dissolved molecules can also reduce the activity of water. For example, a salt, such as potassium chloride, or a highly hydrated polymer, such as methylcellulose, also binds water in an aqueous solution, but the degree of these interactions has not been documented. It is important to realize that these interactions do occur, and when these ingredients are in a liquid preparation, they do effectively reduce the "free water" in that product.

(2) The alcohol concentration should be 15% (Acid)—17.5% (Neutral or mildly alkaline) of the free water (9).

(3) Although the 15–17.5% range seems high, the percentage actually needed for most preparations is far less because these percentages apply only to the "free water." Consider the following example:

Mineral Oil Emulsion USP (10)

Mineral Oil	500 mL
Acacia	125 g
Syrup	100 mL
Vanillin	40 mg
Alcohol	60 mL
Purified Water, a sufficient quantity to make	1,000 mL

If you add the approximate volumes of all the ingredients (in the case of the solids, acacia and vanillin, you have to estimate the powder volume) and subtract this quantity from 1,000 mL, you get the approximate "free water" volume: 1,000 mL − (500 + 100 + 60 + ~40 [powder volume estimate]) = 300 mL. This is the amount of water that must be preserved with alcohol. The quantity of ethyl alcohol in this prescription is: 95% × 60 mL = 57 mL. This quantity represents only 5.7% of the total product, but it is 19% of the "free water" (19% × 300 mL = 57 mL).

(4) One commonly seen guideline of alcohol content for preservation of liquid formulations is 5–10% alcohol. In using this figure, one should be aware of its origins: it comes from a rough estimate of the free water available in the "average" product. Therefore, if you have a prescription order that contains a large proportion of "free water," you should add extra alcohol for adequate preservation.

2. Propylene Glycol

$C_3H_8O_2$ MW = 76.09

Propylene Glycol

$$CH_3 - \underset{\underset{OH}{|}}{CH} - CH_2OH$$

a. Official product: Propylene Glycol USP

b. Description and Solubility: See Chapter 14, Pharmaceutical Solvents.

c. Effective Concentration

(1) In most situations, Propylene Glycol is effective at a concentration of 10% w/v, although inhibition of growth of certain molds requires up to 30% w/v (11,12).

(2) Propylene Glycol potentiates several other preservatives. A 2% to 5% concentration of Propylene Glycol, while ineffective as a sole preservative, potentiated the effect of a methyl and propyl paraben combination, especially at their minimal effective concentration. The various combinations tested were found to be effective against bacteria, molds, and yeast but were ineffective against bacterial spores until they entered the vegetative stage (13). This effect on paraben efficacy is especially useful because the concentration at which the parabens exert their antimicrobial effect is so close to their solubility. Although parabens are particularly useful for preserving vulnerable syrups that have a neutral pH, because of their poor water solubility, it is often difficult to dissolve a sufficient concentration of parabens to achieve adequate preservation. In this study, both a 2% and a 5% concentration of Propylene Glycol allowed the minimum inhibitory concentration of Methylparaben to be reduced from 0.18% to 0.1% when combined with 0.02% Propylparaben (13).

3. Glycerin

$C_3H_8O_3$ MW = 92.01

Glycerin

$$HOCH_2 - \overset{\overset{\displaystyle OH}{|}}{CH} - CH_2OH$$

a. Official product: Glycerin USP

b. Description and Solubility: See Chapter 14, Pharmaceutical Solvents.

c. Effective Concentration

(1) Although Glycerin preserves at concentrations $\geq$ 50%, at lower concentrations it may actually act as a nutrient for some microorganisms. This is because Glycerin's activity as an antimicrobial agent depends solely on an osmotic effect rather than any innate toxicity to microorganisms (12).

(2) While glycerin is not often used as a sole preservative, it is frequently used with Alcohol to reduce the volume of alcohol necessary to preserve a preparation.

4. Benzyl Alcohol

C_7H_8O MW = 108.14

Benzyl alcohol

a. Official product: Benzyl Alcohol NF

b. Description: Colorless liquid; faint, aromatic odor; sharp, burning taste; neutral pH; flammable

c. Solubility: 1 g/30 mL water; freely soluble in 50% alcohol; miscible with alcohol and fixed and volatile oils

d. Effective Concentration: Bacteriocidal at 1–2% (14)

e. Benzyl Alcohol is listed here because it is approved for oral products; however, it is not typically used in these preparations because of its sharp, burning taste. It is used frequently in manufactured parenteral products, in which it is especially useful because of its local anesthetic properties. It may be used in topical preparations and, in fact, has been used therapeutically as a local anesthetic to relieve itching when mixed with equal parts of alcohol and water (15). Although listed as an approved preservative for ophthalmic products (16), it is not commonly found in ophthalmic preparations.

   f. Benzyl Alcohol is most effective at pH less than 5 and has minimal activity at pH 8 and above. It is incompatible with methylcellulose and its activity is reduced by nonionic surfactants such as polysorbate 80 (8).

B. Organic Acids

  1. Benzoic Acid/Sodium Benzoate/Potassium Benzoate

    a. Official products include:

      (1) Benzoic Acid USP

        $C_7H_6O_2$ MW = 122.12

Benzoic Acid

      (2) Sodium Benzoate NF

      (3) Potassium Benzoate NF

    b. Descriptions

      (1) Benzoic Acid: White crystals, scales, or needles; slight aromatic odor; volatile at warm temperatures; pK_a = 4.19; pH of a saturated solution = 2.8

      (2) Sodium Benzoate: White granular or crystalline powder; practically odorless; slightly hygroscopic but stable in air. Has an unpleasant sweet and salty taste. Sodium Benzoate is the most commonly used salt of benzoic acid.

      (3) Potassium Benzoate: White granular or crystalline powder; practically odorless; stable in air

    c. Solubilities

      (1) Benzoic Acid: 1 g/300 mL of water (0.33%), or 3 mL of alcohol; soluble in fixed oils

      (2) Sodium Benzoate: 1 g/2 mL of water, or 75 mL of alcohol.

      (3) Potassium Benzoate: soluble in water and alcohol

    d. Effective concentration

      (1) Benzoic Acid is the active preservative form, and its effective concentration is 0.1–0.3% (17).

      (2) Because its effective concentration is so close to its solubility, Benzoic Acid is often dissolved as the sodium salt (Sodium Benzoate), which is very water-soluble. The amount present as the active form is then dependent on the pH of the solution. This amount can be estimated using the Henderson–Hasselbalch equation.

      (3) Benzoic Acid/Sodium Benzoate is ineffective in solutions with a pH above 5. This means that in deciding the effectiveness of this preservative, you must know the pH of the liquid you wish to preserve. Most fruit-flavored and cola fountain syrups have pH's around 3 and are effectively preserved with Benzoic Acid/Sodium Benzoate. Depending on method of preparation, Syrup NF has a pH of 5 to 6.5, so it may or may not be adequately protected. Methylcellulose 1% gel has a pH of approximately 6 and Sodium Carboxymethylcellulose 1% gel has a pH of about 7, so these would probably not be preserved. The monographs of some official liquid preparations give pH ranges for these liquids. The pH of manufactured liquid drug products is often given in the product package insert. An alternative easy way to determine the approximate pH of a liquid product is to use pH paper or a pH meter.

      (4) Its effectiveness may be reduced by nonionic surfactants such as polysorbate 80.

(5) Benzoic Acid/Sodium Benzoate is widely used as a preservative, especially in foods. It has most of the properties of an ideal preservative. Its biggest drawback is the pH dependence of its effectiveness.

2. Sorbic Acid/Potassium Sorbate

   a. Official products include:

      (1) Sorbic Acid NF

         $C_6H_8O_2$ MW = 112.13

Sorbic Acid

      (2) Potassium Sorbate NF

   b. Descriptions

      (1) Sorbic Acid: White crystalline powder; pK_a 4.76

      (2) Potassium Sorbate: White crystals or powder

   c. Solubilities

      (1) Sorbic Acid: listed in *Remington: The Science and Practice of Pharmacy* as 1 g/1,000 mL of water (0.1%); *The Merck Index* gives a water solubility of 0.25% (1 g/400 mL) at 30° and 3.8% (1 g/26 mL) at 100°. The solubility in alcohol is 1 g/10 mL and in propylene glycol, 1 g/19 mL.

      (2) Potassium Sorbate: very soluble in water, 1 g/4.5 mL, and moderately soluble in alcohol, 1 g/35 mL

   d. Effective Concentration

      (1) Sorbic Acid is the active form, with an effective concentration of 0.05–0.2% (17).

      (2) Sorbic acid has properties and problems that are similar to those of Benzoic Acid. Like Benzoic Acid, Sorbic Acid has an effective concentration that is very close to its solubility. Because of this, the salt form, Potassium Sorbate, which is very soluble in water, is often used. As with Benzoic Acid, the amount that is present in the active acid form is dependent on the pH of the solution. Because Sorbic Acid has a slightly higher pK_a than Benzoic Acid, it has a higher ratio of active to inactive form at the pH levels common to oral products. It reportedly has little antimicrobial activity above pH 6 (18).

      (3) Sorbic Acid is widely used as a preservative in foods. It is one of the least toxic preservatives, with a reported oral LD_{50} in rats of 7.36 g/kg (7). While it has low toxicity orally, irritation of the skin in topical products has been reported.

C. Esters of p-Hydroxybenzoic Acid (Parabens)

   1. Official products of parabens include:

      a. Methylparaben NF

         $C_8H_8O_3$ MW = 152.15

Methylparaben

      b. Methylparaben Sodium NF

    c. Propylparaben NF

       $C_{10}H_{12}O_3$ MW = 180.20

Propylparaben

    d. Propylparaben Sodium NF

2. Descriptions
   a. Methylparaben: Small, colorless crystals, or white, crystalline powder; practically odorless; slight burning taste
   b. Methylparaben Sodium: White, hygroscopic powder
   c. Propylparaben: Small, colorless crystals, or white powder
   d. Propylparaben Sodium: White, odorless, hygroscopic powder
3. Solubilities
   a. Methylparaben: 1 g/400 mL of water (0.25%), or 3 mL of alcohol. It is soluble in glycerin (1 g/60 mL) and propylene glycol (1 g/5 mL). Insoluble in mineral oil; solubility in fixed oils varies.
   b. Propylparaben: 1 g/2,500 mL of water (0.04%), or 1.5 mL of alcohol
   c. The sodium salts are more soluble, but they are formed only at a relatively high pH (~9), and at this pH the molecule is fairly unstable because of hydrolysis of the ester group.
4. Effective concentration
   a. Methylparaben: 0.05–0.25% (Lower part of range is effective only when used in combination with another preservative such as Propylparaben, Benzyl Alcohol, or Propylene Glycol.)

   Methylparaben has a water solubility that is identical to its effective concentration. Because it is a rather hydrophobic powder, it is somewhat difficult to dissolve in aqueous solutions. If the product will tolerate a small amount of alcohol or propylene glycol, the powder can first be dissolved in a minimal amount of Alcohol or Propylene Glycol. Methylparaben has many properties of an ideal preservative, including activity over a wide pH range. Its major problem is its poor water solubility. Its effectiveness is enhanced by 2-5% Propylene Glycol (13).

   b. Propylparaben: 0.02–0.04% (Most effective when used in combination with another preservative such as Methylparaben. A concentration of 0.035% is the maximum acceptable concentration for parenteral products.)

   Propylparaben would be a great preservative if it were more water-soluble. It is rarely used by itself because it is impossible to get enough dissolved for sufficient preservative action. It is most often used in combination with Methylparaben. Combinations of paraben esters have a synergistic effect. A combination of 0.18% of Methylparaben to 0.02% Propylparaben is common and has been approved for use as a preservative for certain parenteral products. Like Methylparaben, Propylparaben is hydrophobic and is difficult to dissolve in water. Furthermore, Propylparaben is used in such a small amount that for the small quantities used in extemporaneous formulation, an aliquot is required. If the product will tolerate a small amount of alcohol or propylene glycol, the powder can first be dissolved in a minimal amount of Alcohol or Propylene Glycol. One possible stock solution has the following formula:

Methylparaben	9 g
Propylparaben	1 g
Propylene Glycol q.s. ad	100 mL

Two milliliters of this stock solution in each 100 mL or 100 g of preparation will provide 0.18% Methylparaben, 0.02% Propylparaben, and approximately 2% Propylene Glycol.

5. Parabens are approved for use in oral, topical, ophthalmic, and parenteral products. They can be sensitizing when used externally or on mucous membranes, and can cause allergic reactions. These have not been reported when these agents are taken orally or used parenterally.

IX. PRESERVATIVES FOR TOPICAL PRODUCTS (EXCEPT OPHTHALMIC PRODUCTS)

A. Alcohols and Glycols
1. Ethyl alcohol: See description above and in Chapter 14, Pharmaceutical Solvents. One official product of ethyl alcohol that is not suitable for oral use, but may be used topically, is Rubbing Alcohol USP. It is described in Chapter 14.
2. Isopropyl Alcohol $CH_3CHOHCH_3$
   C_3H_8O MW = 60.10
   a. Although Isopropyl Alcohol may not be used internally because of its toxicity, it is safe for external use and is an effective preservative for topical products.
   b. Official Products, Descriptions, and Solubility: See Chapter 14, Pharmaceutical Solvents.
   c. Effective concentration: Same as ethyl alcohol
3. Propylene Glycol: See description above.
4. Glycerin: See description above.
5. Benzyl Alcohol: See description above.

B. Organic Acids
1. Benzoic Acid: See description above.
2. Sorbic Acid: See description above.

C. Esters of p-Hydroxybenzoic Acid (Parabens): See description above.

D. Organic Mercurial Derivatives
1. Official products
   a. Phenylmercuric Acetate NF
      $C_8H_8HgO_2$ MW = 336.74

      Phenylmercuric Acetate

   b. Phenylmercuric Nitrate NF

      Phenylmercuric Nitrate

Phenylmercuric Nitrate is a mixture of phenylmercuric nitrate and phenylmercuric hydroxide (10).

    c.   Thimerosal USP

         $C_9H_9HgNaO_2S$ MW = 404.81

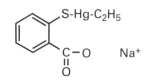

Thimerosal

    d.   Thimerosal Topical Solution USP

    e.   Thimerosal Tincture USP

2. Descriptions

    a.   Phenylmercuric Acetate NF: White crystalline powder; odorless; pH of a saturated solution = 4

    b.   Phenylmercuric Nitrate NF: White crystalline powder with mild aromatic odor. Affected by light. Saturated solutions are acid to litmus.

    c.   Thimerosal USP: Light cream-colored, crystalline powder with a slight odor. Affected by light. pH of a 1% solution = 6.7.

    d.   Thimerosal Topical Solution USP: Clear liquid. Sensitive to some metals. Affected by light. pH: 9.6–10.2.

    e.   Thimerosal Tincture USP: Transparent, mobile liquid with the odor of acetone and alcohol. Sensitive to some metals. Affected by light. Alcohol content: 45.0–55.0%.

3. Solubilities

    a.   Phenylmercuric Acetate (PMA): listed in *Remington's Pharmaceutical Sciences,* 18th ed., as 1 g/180 mL water, 225 mL alcohol; *The Merck Index* gives 1 g/600 mL water, soluble in alcohol and acetone.

    b.   Phenylmercuric Nitrate (PMN): listed in *Remington's Pharmaceutical Sciences,* 18th ed., as 1 g/600 mL water, slightly soluble in alcohol or glycerin; *The Merck Index* gives 1 g/1,250 mL water, slightly soluble in alcohol, moderately soluble in glycerin. Soluble in propylene glycol.

         Note: The *Handbook of Pharmaceutical Excipients* states for both compounds that the compendial values and laboratory values on solubility vary considerably. This can be seen in the values above.

    c.   Because PMN and PMA are used in very dilute concentrations, stock solutions are useful. Convenient concentrations of aqueous stock solutions are 1:2,000 and 1:10,000.

    d.   Thimerosal: 1 g/1 mL water, 8 mL (*Merck*) or 12 mL (*Remington*) alcohol

4. Effective concentrations

    a.   Phenylmercuric Acetate and Nitrate: May be used for topical products in a range of 0.002–0.01%. The usual concentration for ophthalmic solutions is 0.002–0.004%, with 0.004% the maximum allowed for eye products (19).

         Used primarily to preserve parenterals and eye and nasal products. All mercurial compounds can be sensitizing.

    b.   Thimerosal: 0.001–0.02%. The maximum acceptable concentration for ophthalmic products is 0.01% (19); the maximum for parenteral products is 0.04%.

5. Incompatibilities

    a.   Phenylmercuric acetate and nitrate precipitate with halides and anionic emulsifying agents, suspending agents, and drugs such as penicillin and fluorescein. They also are incompatible with tragacanth, starch, talc, silicates, sodium metabisulfite, aluminum and other metals, ammonia and its salts, amino acids, sulfur compounds, rubber, and some plastics. Disodium edetate and sodium thiosulfate may cause inactivation of PMN or PMA. Activity may be lost because of sorption onto polyethylene surfaces of containers, closures, or droppers (8,20).

    b.   Thimerosal is a sodium salt that precipitates in acidic solutions. It also is incompatible with aluminum and other metals, silver nitrate, sodium chloride solutions, lecithin, phenylmercuric compounds, large cations such as quaternary ammonium compounds, thioglycolate, and proteins. Sodium metabisulfite and the EDTA compounds can reduce its antimicrobial effectiveness. In solution it may sorb to some plastics and rubber closures (8,20).

E. Salts of Quaternary Ammonium Bases
Note: Although the quaternary ammonium preservatives may be used in oral dosage forms, they are listed here because they are used primarily in topical and ophthalmic drug products and preparations.
  1. Official products
    a. Benzalkonium Chloride NF

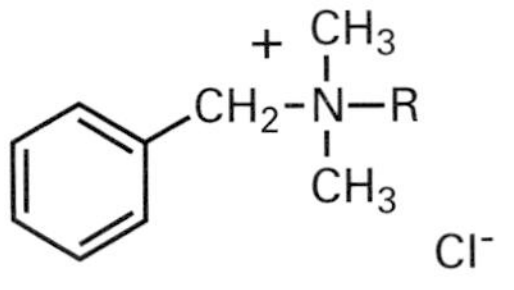

$$R = C_8H_{17} \text{ to } C_{18}H_{37} \quad \text{(Mixture)}$$
Benzalkonium chloride

Benzalkonium Chloride is a mixture of alkyl-benzyldimethylammonium chlorides with the general formula $[C_6H_5CH_2N(CH_3)_2R]Cl$, in which R represents a mixture of alkyls, including groups beginning with $n\text{-}C_8H_{17}$ and extending through higher homologs, with $n\text{-}C_{12}H_{25}$, $n\text{-}C_{14}H_{29}$, and $n\text{-}C_{16}H_{33}$ providing the majority of R groups (10).

    b. Benzalkonium Chloride Solution NF
Benzalkonium Chloride Solution contains benzalkonium chloride in solution. The solution may also contain a suitable coloring agent and may contain not more than 10% alcohol. This solution should not be mixed with ordinary soaps or with anionic detergents since they may decrease or destroy its bacteriostatic activity (10).

    c. Benzethonium Chloride USP
      $C_3H_8O_2$ MW = 76.09

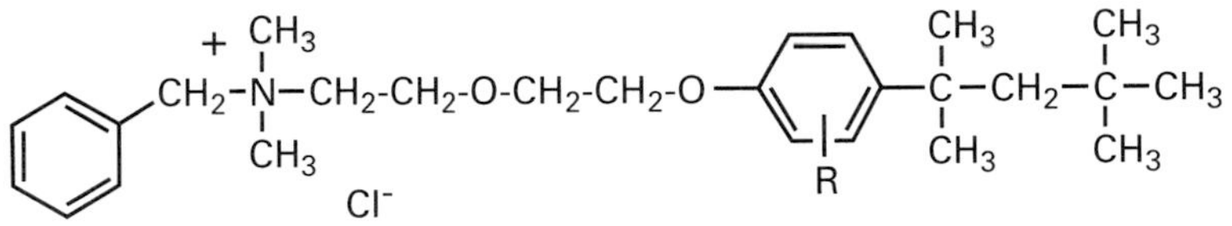

Benzethonium chloride   R = H

    d. Benzethonium Chloride Topical Solution USP
Benzethonium Chloride Topical Solution is an aqueous solution of the chemical (10).

    e. Benzethonium Chloride Tincture USP has the formula shown here (10):

Benzethonium Chloride	2 g
Alcohol	685 mL
Acetone	100 mL
Purified Water, a sufficient quantity to make	1,000 mL

    f. Cetylpyridium Chloride USP
      $C_{21}H_{38}ClN \cdot H_2O$ MW = 358.00

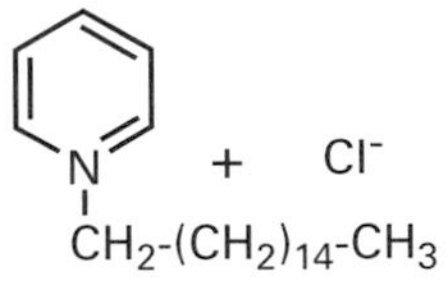

Cetylpyridium chloride

    g. Cetylpyridinium Chloride Topical Solution USP
Cetylpyridinium Chloride Topical Solution is an aqueous solution of the chemical (10).

  2. Descriptions

    a. Benzalkonium Chloride (BAC): White or yellowish-white amorphous powder, thick gel or gel-like pieces; hygroscopic; mild odor with a very bitter taste. Slightly alkaline (pH = 5–8 for a 10% w/v solution). Solutions foam when shaken.

    b. Benzethonium Chloride: White crystals; mild odor with a bitter taste. The pH of a 1% solution = 4.8–5.5.

    c. Cetylpyridinium Chloride: White powder; mild odor with a bitter taste

  3. Solubilities

    a. Benzalkonium Chloride: very soluble in water, alcohol, and acetone

    b. Benzethonium Chloride: 1 g/mL of water, alcohol, or acetone

    c. Cetylpyridinium Chloride: very soluble in water and alcohol

  4. Effective concentrations

    a. Benzalkonium Chloride: 0.004–0.02% (21). The usual concentration for preservation is 0.01%, with 0.013% the maximum allowed for ophthalmics (19). The preservative action of Benzalkonium Chloride is somewhat unpredictable at the 0.01% concentration used for ophthalmic solutions. Its bacteriocidal properties are improved by the addition of 0.1% Edetate (EDTA). It can be irritating to the eye and its solutions may be sensitizing. Benzalkonium chloride is available as 1:750, 10%, 17%, and 50% w/v aqueous solutions and as a 1:750 tincture.

    b. Benzethonium Chloride: 0.01–0.02% (21). The usual preservative concentration and the maximum allowed for ophthalmics is 0.01% (19). Benzethonium Chloride is available as the powder.

    c. Cetylpyridinium Chloride: 0.01–0.02% (21). Cetylpyridinium Chloride is available as the powder.

  5. Incompatibilities: The salts of quaternary ammonium bases have many incompatibilities. For example, *Martindale: The Extra Pharmacopeia* lists the following incompatibilities for Benzalkonium Chloride: soaps, anionic drugs and detergents, nonionic surfactants in high concentrations, citrates, iodides, nitrates, permanganates, salicylates, silver salts, tartrates, fluorescein sodium, hydrogen peroxide, kaolin, lanolin, some sulfonamides, some components of commercial rubber mixes, and boric acid 5% (but not less than or equal to 2%) (20). The *Handbook of Pharmaceutical Excipients* also lists zinc oxide and zinc sulfate (8). Cetylpyridinium Chloride, but not Benzalkonium Chloride, is reported to be inactivated by methylcellulose (22).

X. PRESERVATIVES FOR OPHTHALMIC PRODUCTS

A. All ophthalmic products must be sterile. Preparations in multi-dose containers must contain a suitable preservative to prevent the growth of microorganisms that may be introduced inadvertently into the product during use.

B. Preservatives commonly used in commercial ophthalmic products are given in Table 15.2 (16). Chlorobutanol, which is not used for oral or topical preparations, is described below. Preservatives that are frequently used in extemporaneous compounding of ophthalmic

TABLE 15.2 Preservatives Commonly Used in Ophthalmic Products (16)

Benzalkonium Chloride	Disodium ETDA	Propylparaben
Benzethonium Chloride	Methylparaben	Sodium Benzoate
Cetylpyridium Chloride	Phenylethyl Alcohol	Sodium Propionate
Chlorhexidine	Phenylmercuric Acetate	Sorbic acid
Chlorobutanol	Phenylmercuric Nitrate	Thimerosal

preparations, but that are also used in oral and topical preparations, have been described previously.

C. Chlorobutanol

$C_4H_7Cl_3O$(anhydrous)   MW = 177.46
                    and/or(hemihydrate)   186.46

$$CH_3-\underset{\underset{OH}{|}}{\overset{\overset{CH_3}{|}}{C}}-CCl_3$$

Chlorobutanol

1. Official product: Chlorobutanol NF
2. Description: Colorless to white crystals with a camphor-like odor and taste
3. Solubility: 1 g/125 mL, water although it is somewhat difficult to dissolve. Also, 1 g/0.6 mL alcohol and 10 mL glycerin. It is freely soluble in volatile oils.
4. Effective concentration: 0.5% (19)

5. Incompatibilities
   a. Is incompatible with silver nitrate and the sodium salts of sulfonamides
   b. Hydrolyzes to hydrochloric acid in solutions with pH's at or above neutrality; should be used in solutions buffered at 5.0–5.5
   c. Activity may be lost because of sorption onto polyethylene or rubber surfaces of ophthalmic containers or droppers.
   d. Is inactivated by the macromolecules polysorbate 80 and polyvinylpyrrolidone, but not by methylcellulose (22). Also interacts with carboxymethylcellulose, with resulting reduced antimicrobial activity (8).
6. Chlorobutanol is used for ophthalmic and parenteral products. It is not used for oral preparations because of its camphor-like odor and taste. Its use as an ophthalmic preservative is limited because of its instability except at acid pH and because it acts slowly in killing organisms.

References

1. The 2002 United States Pharmacopeia 25/National Formulary 20. Rockville, MD: The United States Pharmacopeial Convention, Inc., 2001; 1869.
2. The 2002 United States Pharmacopeia 25/National Formulary 20. Rockville, MD: The United States Pharmacopeial Convention, Inc., 2001; 2213-2225.
3. The 2002 United States Pharmacopeia 25/National Formulary 20. Rockville, MD: The United States Pharmacopeial Convention, Inc., 2001; 1834.
4. Barr M, Tice LF. The preservation of aqueous sorbitol solutions. JAPhA Sci Ed 1957; 46: 221–223.
5. The 2002 United States Pharmacopeia 25/National Formulary 20. Rockville, MD: The United States Pharmacopeial Convention, Inc., 2001; 2496.
6. USP DI Vol. III, 22d ed. Englewood, CO: MICROMEDEX, Inc., 2002: Chemistry and Compendial Requirements.
7. Budavari S, ed. The Merck Index, 11th ed. Rahway, NJ: Merck & Co., Inc., 1989.
8. Kibbe AH. Handbook of Pharmaceutical Excipients, 3d ed. Washington DC: American Pharmaceutical Association and Pharmaceutical Press, 2000.
9. Gabel LF. The relative action of preservatives in pharmaceutical preparations. JAPhA 1921; 10: 767–768.
10. The 2002 United States Pharmacopeia 25/National Formulary 20. Rockville, MD: The United States Pharmacopeial Convention, Inc., 2001: Official Monographs.
11. Rae J. The preservative properties of ethylene and propylene glycol. Pharm J 1938; 140: 517.
12. Barr M, Tice LF. A study of the inhibitory concentrations of glycerin-sorbitol and propylene glycol-sorbitol combinations on the growth of microorganisms. JAPhA Sci Ed 1957; 46: 217–218.
13. Prickett PS, Murray HL, Mercer NH. Potentiation of preservatives (parabens) in pharmaceutical formulations by low concentrations of propylene glycol. J Pharm Sci 1961; 50: 316-320.

14. Leszczynska-Bakal H, Smmazynski T. Preservation of pharmaceutical preparations by chemical compounds with antibacterial activity. Paper presented at Symposium on Preservatives used in Cosmetics, Bointe Pollena, May 30, 1974.

15. Hoover JE, ed. Remington's Pharmaceutical Sciences, 14th ed. Easton, PA: Mack Publishing Co., 1970; 1066.

16. Handbook of Nonprescription Drugs, 10th ed. American Pharmaceutical Association, Washington DC, 1993; 357.

17. Entrekin DN. Relation of pH to preservative effectiveness I acid media. J Pharm Sci 1961; 50: 743–746.

18. Eklund T. The antimicrobial effect of dissociated and undissociated sorbic acid at different pH levels. J Appl Bacteriol 1983; 54: 383–389.

19. FDA Advisory Review Panel on OTC Ophthalmic Drug Products. Final Report, December 1979.

20. Reynolds JEF, ed. Martindale: The extra pharmacopoeia, 30th ed. London: The Pharmaceutical Press, 1993; 785.

21. Allen LV. Preservatives and compounding. US Pharmacist 1994; 19: 84.

22. King RE. Dispensing of Medication, 9th ed. Easton, PA: Mack Publishing Co., 1984; 148.

CHAPTER 16

Antioxidants

I. DEFINITIONS

A. **Oxidation/reduction** (redox) reactions involve the transfer of one or more oxygen or hydrogen atoms or the transfer of electrons (1). Writing an electron-transfer in equation form, where e^- represents an electron and n the number of electrons:

$$\text{reduced form} \rightleftharpoons \text{oxidized form} + ne^-$$

Table 16.1 shows examples of the various types of oxidation.

B. **Auto-oxidations** are oxidations that occur spontaneously under normal conditions of preparation, packaging, and storage.

C. A **free radical** is a chemical species that has an unshared electron in its outer shell. (Oxygen [O_2] has an electronic configuration with two unshared electrons in its outer shell.)

D. **Antioxidants** are substances that prevent or inhibit oxidation. They are added to dosage forms to protect components of the dosage form that are subject to chemical degradation by oxidation.

E. **Chelating agents** are organic compounds that can form complexes with metal ions, and in so doing inactivate the catalytic activity of the metal ions in the oxidation process.

II. USES

A. Antioxidants and/or chelating agents may be added to manufactured pharmaceutical products and to extemporaneously compounded preparations when the product or preparation contains an ingredient or ingredients, either an active ingredient or a dosage form component, that is subject to chemical degradation by oxidation.

B. For compounded preparations, the decision by the pharmacist whether or not to add an antioxidant or chelating agent is made by taking into consideration the susceptibility of the ingredient(s) to degradation, the dosage form, the targeted site of drug delivery (e.g., topical, oral, ophthalmic, parenteral, etc.), the packaging for the preparation, the anticipated conditions of storage and use of the preparation, and the beyond-use time period desired or needed.

TABLE 16.1 Examples of Oxidation Types

Examples of Oxidation Types

Process	Reduced form	Oxidized form
Electron-transfer	Fe^{+2}	Fe^{+3}
	H_2	$2 H^+$
	$2 I^-$	I_2
	H_2O_2	$O_2 + 2H^+$
Addition of oxygen (or loss of hydrogen)	CH_4	CH_3OH
	CH_3OH	$H_2C{=}O$
	$H_2C{=}O$	$HCOOH$
	$HCOOH$	CO_2
Loss of hydrogen	RCH_2CH_2R	$RCH{=}CHR + H_2$
	$2 RSH$	$RSSR + H_2$

III. MECHANISM FOR AUTOXIDATION OF PHARMACEUTICAL COMPOUNDS

To appreciate how antioxidants and chelating agents function in preventing or retarding oxidation, it is helpful to have a basic understanding of the oxidation process. Oxidation is complex, and the following is just a brief outline of this process. For an excellent review on the subject of oxidation in pharmaceutical products and preparations, see the chapter on oxidation and photolysis in *Chemical Stability of Pharmaceuticals* (2).

A. Oxidation Reactions

Auto-oxidation of pharmaceutical ingredients occurs by a series of free radical chain reactions, including initiation, propagation, and termination.

1. Initiation

$$\text{Initiator} \rightarrow R\cdot + H\cdot$$

Note: This reaction may be catalyzed by heat, light, and metal ions.

2. Propagation

$$R\cdot + O_2 \rightarrow RO_2\cdot \text{(peroxy radical)}$$

$$RO_2\cdot + RH \rightarrow ROOH + R\cdot$$

3. Termination

$$RO_2\cdot + RO_2\cdot \rightarrow \text{stable products}$$

$$RO_2\cdot + R\cdot \rightarrow \text{stable products}$$

$$R\cdot + R\cdot \rightarrow \text{stable products}$$

B. To prevent or inhibit oxidation, the stabilizing compound must prevent or interfere with initiation or propagation, or it must participate in a termination step.

1. Chelating agents inhibit oxidation by complexing metal ions that act as catalysts for some oxidation reactions.

a. Metal ions, such as Fe^{+3}, Cu^{+2}, Co^{+3}, Ni^{+2}, and Mn^{+2}, can act as initiators of oxidation because they each have an unshared electron in their outer shell.

b. Drug products and preparations may easily be contaminated by trace amounts of metals because these contaminants may be present in minute amounts, even in high-quality compounding ingredients and on the surfaces of compounding equipment and packaging materials.

c. Chelating agents, such as ethylenediaminetetraacetic acid (also known as EDTA or Edetic Acid), Citric Acid, and Tartaric Acid, act by binding the metal ions through complexation. Their binding capacity is pH-dependent because it depends on the degree of ionization of these organic acids; they are most effective when fully ionized so they lose their ability to complex at low pH.

2. Antioxidants may function by one of the following mechanisms:

   a. Some are compounds that are easily oxidized; they have lower oxidation potentials than the drugs they are intended to protect and are preferentially oxidized. These agents act as so-called oxygen scavengers. Examples include the sulfites, Ascorbic Acid, Monothioglycerol, and Sodium Formaldehyde Sulfoxylate.

   b. Some antioxidants act as chain terminators. They provide a readily available hydrogen atom or an electron and, in the process, are converted to free radicals that are not sufficiently reactive to sustain the chain reaction. Their free radicals either are intrinsically stable or they will combine with other radicals in a termination step. All of the oil system antioxidants listed below act as chain terminators. The water-soluble antioxidant Monothioglycerol may also act as a chain terminator.

   c. Some antioxidants are reducing agents; they reduce a drug or component that has been oxidized. Ascorbic Acid and Sodium Thiosulfate may act as reducing agents.

C. Environmental factors that affect oxidation, such as temperature, light, and pH, are discussed in Chapter 34.

IV. PROPERTIES OF THE IDEAL ANTIOXIDANT/CHELATING AGENT

A. Effective at a low, nontoxic concentration

B. Stable and effective under normal conditions of use, over a wide pH and temperature range

C. Soluble at the required concentration

D. Compatible with a wide variety of drugs and auxiliary agents

E. Free from objectionable odor, taste, or stinging

F. Colorless in both the original and oxidized form

G. Nontoxic and nonsensitizing both internally and externally at the required concentration

H. Reasonable cost

I. Unreactive (does not adsorb, penetrate, or interact) with containers or closures

V. ANTIOXIDANTS LISTED IN THE *USP 25-NF 20*

Table 16.2 gives the chemicals listed as antioxidants in the *USP 25-NF 20* (3). This table has divided the antioxidants into two categories: those commonly used for aqueous systems and those most commonly used for oil systems (4).

TABLE 16.2   Antioxidants Listed in the *USP25-NF20* (3)

Antioxidants for Aqueous Systems	Antioxidants for Oil Systems
Ascorbic Acid	Ascorbyl Palmitate
Hypophosphorous Acid	Butylated Hydroxyanisole
Monothioglycerol	Butylated Hydroxytoluene
Potassium Metabisulfite	Propyl Gallate
Sodium Metabisulfite	Tocopherol
Sodium Thiosulfate	Tocopherols Excipient
Sodium Formaldehyde Sulfoxylate	
Sulfur Dioxide	

VI.   CHELATING AGENTS LISTED IN THE *USP 25-NF 20*

A.   Edetate Calcium Disodium, Edetate Disodium, and Edetic Acid (EDTA) are the three compounds listed by the *USP/NF* as chelating agents (3).

B.   Although not listed as chelating agents, Citric Acid USP and Tartaric Acid NF are official compounds that may act as chelating agents.

VII.   ANTIOXIDANTS FOR AQUEOUS SYSTEMS

The descriptions and solubilities presented here give a composite of information from the *Handbook of Pharmaceutical Excipients* (5), the Chemistry and Compendial Requirements section of the *USP DI Vol. III* (6), and *The Merck Index* (7). For additional information on each agent, consult the *Handbook of Pharmaceutical Excipients*.

A.   Ascorbic Acid USP

Ascorbic Acid

1. Description: White or slightly yellow crystals or powder; odorless. Gradually darkens on exposure to light. Reasonably stable in dry state, but oxidizes in solution. Solutions have a sour, acid taste, with a pH of 2 to 3. $pK_{a1} = 4.17$, $pK_{a2} = 11.57$.
2. Solubilities: 1 g/3 mL water, 30 mL alcohol, 20 mL propylene glycol, 100 mL glycerin; practically insoluble in vegetable oils
3. Effective concentration: 0.05–3.0% (8)

B.   Sodium Bisulfite ($NaHSO_3$) and Metabisulfite ($Na_2S_2O_5$)
   1. Description
      a. Sodium Bisulfite: White or yellowish white crystals or powder with the odor of sulfur dioxide; disagreeable taste. Unstable in air, losing some SO_2 and gradually oxidizing to the sulfate. Aqueous solutions are acid to litmus.
      b. Sodium Metabisulfite NF: Colorless crystals or white powder with a sulfurous odor; acid and saline taste. Slowly oxidizes to sulfate on exposure to air and moisture. Aqueous solutions are acid to litmus with pH of 5% solution = 3.5 − 5.0. The metabisulfite is less hygroscopic and more stable than the bisulfite.
   2. Solubilities
      a. Sodium Bisulfite: 1 g/4 mL water, 70 mL alcohol
      b. Sodium Metabisulfite NF: 1 g/2 mL water; soluble in glycerin; slightly soluble in alcohol
   3. Effective concentrations
      a. Sodium Bisulfite: 0.1% (9)
      b. Sodium Metabisulfite NF: 0.02–1.0% (8)
   4. Sulfite warnings: Sulfites are known to cause allergic-type reactions in certain susceptible individuals. Although the number of affected individuals is small, in 1986, a section (§201.22) was added to the Food, Drug and Cosmetic Act to require a warning on all prescription drug products that contain sulfite. The warning statement is: "Contains (*insert the name of the sulfite, e.g., sodium metabisulfite*), a sulfite that may cause allergic-type reactions including anaphylactic symptoms and life-threatening or less severe asthmatic episodes in certain susceptible people. The overall prevalence of

sulfite sensitivity in the general population is unknown and probably low. Sulfite sensitivity is seen more frequently in asthmatic than in nonasthmatic people" (10). Although this warning is not required on prescription labels, it is prudent to discuss with a patient the addition of a sulfite to any compounded preparation. It also is wise to include on the prescription label the name and quantity of any sulfite added to a drug preparation.

C. Sodium Thiosulfate USP $Na_2S_2O_3 \cdot 5H_2O$
1. Description: Large colorless crystals or coarse crystalline powder. It effloresces in dry air at temperatures above 33° and slightly deliquesces in moist air. Aqueous solutions are neutral or slightly alkaline (pH 6.5–8).
2. Solubility: 1 g/0.5 mL water; insoluble in alcohol
3. Effective concentration: 0.05%

D. Sodium Formaldehyde Sulfoxylate NF $HOCH_2SOONa$
1. Description: White crystals or hard white masses with an odor of garlic. Aqueous solutions practically neutral.
2. Solubility: Freely soluble in water; slightly soluble in alcohol
3. Effective concentration: 0.005–0.5% (8)

VIII. ANTIOXIDANTS FOR OIL SYSTEMS

The descriptions and solubilities presented here give a composite of information from the *Handbook of Pharmaceutical Excipients* (5), the Chemistry and Compendial Requirements section of the *USP DI Vol. III* (6), and *The Merck Index* (7). For additional information on each agent, consult the *Handbook of Pharmaceutical Excipients*.

A. Ascorbyl Palmitate NF

Ascorbyl Palmitate

1. Description: White to yellowish-white powder with a characteristic odor
2. Solubility: Very slightly soluble in water and in vegetable oils; 1 g in 9.3 mL alcohol
3. Effective concentration: 0.01–0.2% (8)

B. Butylated Hydroxyanisole (BHA) and Butylated Hydroxytoluene (BHT)

Butylated Hydroxyanisole

Butylated Hydroxytoluene

1. Descriptions
    a. Butylated Hydroxyanisole NF (BHA): White or slightly yellow powder or waxy solid with a faint odor
    b. Butylated Hydroxytoluene NF (BHT): White or pale yellow crystalline solid with a faint odor
2. Solubilities
    a. Butylated Hydroxyanisole NF (BHA): Insoluble in water; freely soluble in alcohol (95%) and propylene glycol; soluble in 50% or higher alcohol, isopropyl alcohol, fats, and oils
    b. Butylated Hydroxytoluene NF (BHT): Insoluble in water, glycerin, and propylene glycol; soluble in alcohol, isopropyl alcohol, and acetone. It is more soluble in vegetable oils and fats than is BHA.
3. Effective concentrations
    a. Butylated Hydroxyanisole NF (BHA): 0.005–0.01% (4)
    b. Butylated Hydroxytoluene NF (BHT): 0.01% (4)

C.   Propyl Gallate NF

Propyl Gallate

1. Description: White, crystalline powder with a very slight odor. pH of a 0.1% solution = 5.9. Has some antimicrobial activity in addition to its antioxidant properties. Unstable at high temperatures.
2. Solubility: Slightly soluble in water (1 g/1,000 mL at 20°); freely soluble in alcohol (1 g/3 mL at 20°); 1 g/2.5 mL propylene glycol; solubility in fixed and mineral oils varies with the oil
3. Effective concentration: 0.005–0.15% (4)

D.   α-Tocopherol (Vitamin E USP)

α-Tocopherol

Vitamin E

1. Description: Clear, yellow, or greenish-yellow viscous oil. Practically odorless. Unstable to light and air, so store in airtight container under inert gas, protected from light.
2. Solubility: Insoluble in water; soluble in alcohol; miscible with acetone and vegetable oils
3. Effective concentration: 0.01–0.1% (4)

IX. CHELATING AGENTS

The descriptions and solubilities presented here give a composite of information from the *Handbook of Pharmaceutical Excipients* (5), the Chemistry and Compendial Requirements section of the *USP DI Vol. III* (6), and *The Merck Index* (7). For additional information on each agent, consult the *Handbook of Pharmaceutical Excipients*.

A. Edetic Acid NF

Edetic Acid

1. Description: White, crystalline powder. The pH of a 0.2% solution is 2.2 with the four pK_a values = 2.00, 2.67, 6.26, and 10.26. Has some reported independent antimicrobial activity and has synergistic effect with some antimicrobial agents, such as Benzalkonium Chloride and parabens.
2. Solubility: Very slightly soluble in water (1 g/2,000 mL given in *The Merck Index*; 1 g/500 mL given in *Handbook of Pharmaceutical Excipients*)
3. Effective concentration: 0.1% (8)

B. Disodium Edetate USP

Disodium Edetate

1. Description: White, crystalline powder, slightly acid taste. pH of solutions reported as 4.3–4.7 and as 5.3. The disodium salt of edetate is reported to reduce the antimicrobial activity of the mercurial antimicrobial agents phenylmercuric nitrate and thimerosal.
2. Solubility: Soluble in water (1 g/11 mL); slightly soluble in alcohol
3. Effective concentration: 0.1% (4)

C. Calcium Disodium Edetate
1. Description: White crystalline granules or powder; odorless; tasteless; slightly hygroscopic but stable in air. pH of solutions reported as approximately 7 and as 4–5. The

synergistic effect on antimicrobial activity is reported to be lost in the presence of calcium ions.

2. Solubility: Soluble in water (1 g/2 mL), very slightly soluble in alcohol
3. Because the calcium in Calcium Disodium Edetate is preferentially exchanged for lead and other toxic heavy metals, Calcium Disodium Edetate is used primarily as a therapeutic agent for lead poisoning and for removing other heavy metals from the circulation while not removing calcium from the circulation, cells, and bones. It is available as Edetate Calcium Disodium Injection, Calcium Disodium Versenate®, which is 200 mg/mL (20%).
4. Effective concentration: 0.1%

D. Citric Acid USP

$$CH_2COOH$$
$$HO-\!\!\!\!-COOH$$
$$CH_2COOH$$

Citric acid

1. Description: Colorless or translucent crystals or white, granular or crystalline powder. Is available as both the monohydrate and anhydrous solid, and these powders will take up water or effloresce depending on the form and the relative humidity. The pH of a 1% solution is 2.2 with the three pK_a values = 3.13, 4.76, and 6.40.
2. Solubility: 1 g/mL in water and alcohol
3. Effective concentration: 0.3–2.0% (5)
4. Citric Acid is used primarily to adjust pH and as a buffering agent, but it used as an antioxidant synergistically with other agents because of its chelating properties.

E. Tartaric Acid USP

$$COOH$$
$$H-\!\!\!\!-OH$$
$$HO-\!\!\!\!-H$$
$$COOH$$

Compound 3
(+) Tartaric acid
(R,R)

1. Description: Colorless or translucent crystals or white crystalline powder; odorless; tart; stable in air. The pH of a 1.5% solution is 2.2 with its two pK_a values = 2.93 and 4.23.
2. Solubility: 1 g/0.75 mL water and 2.5 mL alcohol; soluble in glycerin
3. Effective concentration: varies
4. Tartaric Acid is used primarily to adjust pH and as a buffering agent, but it is used as an antioxidant synergistically with other agents because of its chelating properties.

References

1. Connors KA, Amidon GL, Stella VJ. Chemical stability of pharmaceuticals, 2nd ed. New York: John Wiley & Sons, 1986; 83.
2. Connors KA, Amidon GL, Stella VJ. Chemical stability of pharmaceuticals, 2nd ed. New York: John Wiley & Sons, 1986; 82–114.
3. The 2002 United States Pharmacopeia 25/National Formulary 20. Rockville, MD: The United States Pharmacopeial Convention, Inc., 2001; 2496.
4. Lachman L. Antioxidants and chelating agents as stabilizers in liquid dosage forms. Drug & Cosm Ind' Jan-Feb 1968.

5. Kibbe AH. Handbook of Pharmaceutical Excipients, 3d ed. Washington DC: American Pharmaceutical Association and Pharmaceutical Press, 2000.

6. USP DI Vol. III, 22d ed. Englewood, CO: MICROMEDEX, Inc. 2002: Chemistry and Compendial Requirements.

7. Budavari S, ed. The Merck Index, 11th ed. Rahway, NJ: Merck & Co., Inc., 1989.

8. Swarbrick J, Boylan JC, eds. Encyclopedia of pharmaceutical technology, Vol. 1. New York: Marcel Dekker Inc., 1988; 441.

9. FDA Advisory Review Panel on OTC Ophthalmic Drug Products. Final Report, Dec. 1979.

10. 21 CFR § 201.22 (b)

CHAPTER 17

Buffers And pH Adjusting Agents

I. DEFINITIONS

A. An **acid** may be defined as:
1. A substance that, when dissolved in water, yields hydrogen ions, H^+ (**Arrhenius theory**)
2. A species that yields protons, H^+ (**Bronsted-Lowry theory**)
3. An electron pair acceptor (Lewis theory)

B. A **base** may be defined as:
1. A substance that, when dissolved in water, gives hydroxide ions, OH^- (Arrhenius theory)
2. A species that can accept a proton (Bronsted-Lowry theory)
3. An electron pair donor (Lewis theory)
   In pharmaceutical systems, we usually are dealing with solutions that contain water; therefore, the Arrhenius and Bronsted-Lowry definitions are most suitable for our purposes.

C. A **buffer** is a compound or a mixture of compounds that, when present in a solution, resists changes in the pH of the solution when small quantities of acid or base are added to the solution.

D. **Buffer capacity** is a measure of the resistance to change in the pH of a solution when acids or bases are added to the solution.

E. Many useful equations have been derived to deal with the subject of acid-base chemistry. A list of those equations most useful in pharmaceutical systems is given in Table 17.1. Example calculations using these equations are also given.

II. USES

Buffers or agents to adjust the pH of solutions may be added to manufactured pharmaceutical products or to extemporaneously compounded preparations for any of the following reasons:

A. For preparations that are intended to be applied to the sensitive membranes of the eye or nasal passages or that may be injected into muscles, blood vessels, organs, tissue, or lesions, it is desirable to adjust the pH of the preparation to a level that is close to the physiologic pH of the tissue. This is done to minimize tissue damage and pain or discomfort experienced by the patient.

B. The absorption, and therefore the therapeutic effectiveness, of certain drugs may be improved when they are present either in an ionized or nonionized state. This state may be manipulated and maintained by adjusting the pH of the medium.

C. The chemical stability of many drugs in solution may be improved by maintaining the pH of the solution in a particular range.

D. The aqueous solubility of many organic drugs depends on the degree to which these weak electrolytes are present in ionic form. This, in turn, may depend on the pH of the solution.

III. BUFFER CAPACITY

A. Buffer capacity, β, is defined by the formula:

$$\beta = \frac{\Delta B}{\Delta pH}$$

where ΔB is the gram equivalents per liter of strong acid or strong base added to the buffer solution

ΔpH is the resulting pH change

The larger β is, the greater the buffer capacity of the system (that is, its ability to resist a pH change).

B. While buffer capacity can be determined for a system by using the above formula, it is not often calculated in compounding situations. Because of the limited beyond-use datings needed for compounded drug preparations, exact buffer capacities are not required. (For a detailed treatment of the subject of buffer capacity, refer to a book on physical pharmacy [1].)

C. Even though we rarely calculate buffer capacity, it is helpful to understand the concept in principle and to understand the circumstances under which buffer capacity is maximized.
1. Solutions of strong acids like HCl will resist a change in pH at or below pH 3. In fact, the standard buffer solution identified by the *USP* for the pH range 1.2–2.2 is a 0.2 M solution of HCl to which KCl has been added as a neutral salt for proper electrolyte concentration (2).
2. Similarly, strong bases like NaOH give good buffer capacity at pH 11 or above.
3. The most common buffer systems consist of a combination of a weak acid and its salt (i.e., its conjugate base) or a weak base and its salt (i.e., its conjugate acid).
   a. The Henderson-Hasselbalch equation, also known as the buffer equation, relates the pH of a solution, which contains an acid-base conjugate pair, to their dissociation constant and the concentrations of the species in the solution. This equation and sample problems are shown in Table 17.1.
   b. Acid-base conjugate pairs have their greatest buffer capacity when the pH of the solution is equal to their pK_a, and buffer capacity of an acid-base pair is effective in the range $pH = pK_a \pm 1$.
4. Buffer capacity is related to the concentration of the buffer; the greater the concentration of the buffer, the greater the resistance to a change in pH.
5. High buffer capacity is sometimes undesirable. For example, when a drug is most stable at a pH that differs considerably from the physiologic pH at the site of administration, a compromise must be found. One possible solution is to use a buffer that maintains the pH at the desirable level for stability but has a relatively low buffer capacity, so that upon administration, the body's natural buffering systems will rapidly alter the pH of the solution to a more comfortable level.

TABLE 17.1 Equations Useful in Acid-Base and Buffer Calculations

General Equations

$$pH = -\log[H_3O^+]$$
$$pOH = -\log[OH^-]$$
$$pH + pOH = pK_w = 14$$
$$pK_a = -\log K_a$$
$$pK_b = -\log K_b$$
$$pK_a + pK_b = pK_w = 14$$

K_a is the dissociation constant for a weak acid.

For: $HA + H_2O \rightleftharpoons H_3O^+ + A^-$

$$K_a = \frac{[H_3O^+][A^-]}{[HA]}$$

K_b is the dissociation constant for a weak base

For: $B + H_2O \rightleftharpoons BH^+ + OH^-$

$$K_b = \frac{[BH^+][OH^-]}{[B]}$$

Generally K values for all drugs, both acids and bases, are now reported as K_as.

Specific Equations	Examples
For a strong acid: $pH = -\log[C_a] = -\log[H^+]$	0.1 N HCl $pH = -\log[C_a] = -\log[0.1] = 1$
For a strong base: $pOH = -\log[OH^-] = -\log[C_b]$ or $pH = pK_w + \log[C_b]$	0.1 N NaOH $pH = pK_w + \log[C_b] = 14 + \log[0.1]$ $= 14 - 1 = 13$
For a weak acid: $pH = \frac{1}{2}pK_a - \frac{1}{2}\log[C_a]$	0.1 N Acetic Acid (HOAc);$pK_a = 4.76$ $pH = \frac{1}{2}(4.76) - \frac{1}{2}\log[0.1]$ $= 2.38 - (-0.5) = 2.88$
For a weak base: $pOH = \frac{1}{2}pK_b - \frac{1}{2}\log[C_b]$ or $pH = \frac{1}{2}pK_w + \frac{1}{2}pK_a + \frac{1}{2}\log[C_b]$	0.1 N Sodium Acetate (the conjugate base of Acetic Acid) $pH = 7 + 2.38 + \frac{1}{2}\log[0.1] = 8.88$
For a diprotic (H_2A) acid: Solution with only the acid $pH = \frac{1}{2}pK_{a1} - \frac{1}{2}\log[C_a]$ Notice that this is the same equation as for a weak acid. See the note at the bottom of this table.	0.1 M H_2CO_3; $pK_{a1} = 6.37$; $pK_{a2} = 10.33$ $pH = \frac{1}{2}(6.37) - \frac{1}{2}\log[0.1]$ $= 3.185 - (-0.5) = 3.685$
For a diprotic (H_2A) acid: Solution with only the ampholyte, HA^- $pH = \frac{1}{2}pK_{a1} + \frac{1}{2}pK_{a2}$ See the note at the bottom of this table.	0.1 M $NaHCO_3$ $pH = \frac{1}{2}(6.37) + \frac{1}{2}(10.33)$ $= 3.185 + 5.165 = 8.35$
For a diprotic (H_2A) acid: Solution with only the diacidic base, A^{-2} $pH = \frac{1}{2}pK_w + \frac{1}{2}pK_{a2} + \frac{1}{2}\log[C_b]$ See the note at the bottom of this table.	0.1 M Na_2CO_3 $pH = \frac{1}{2}(14) + \frac{1}{2}(10.33) + \frac{1}{2}\log(0.1)$ $= 7 + 5.165 + (-0.5) = 11.67$
For conjugate acid-base pairs: $pH = pK_a + \log\frac{[conjugate\ base]}{[conjugate\ acid]}$ For acids this is often written: $pH = pK_a + \log\frac{[salt]}{[acid]}$ For bases this is often written: $pH = pK_a + \log\frac{[base]}{[salt]}$ These are all equivalent forms of the Henderson-Hasselbalch equation.	Ex. #1: 0.1 M HOAc and 0.1 M NaOAc $pH = 4.76 + \log\frac{[0.1]}{[0.1]} = 4.76 + \log 1$ $= 4.76 + 0 = 4.76$ Ex. # 2 0.1 M HOAc and 0.2 M NaOAc $pH = 4.76 + \log\frac{[0.2]}{[0.1]} = 4.76 + 0.30$ $= 5.06$ Ex. # 3 0.1 NH_4OH (ammonia) and 0.1 M NH_4Cl $pK_b = 4.76\ pK_a$ (for conjugate acid) $= 9.24$ $pH = 9.24 + \log\frac{[0.1]}{[0.1]} = 9.24$ Ex. #4 0.1 NH_4OH and 0.2 M NH_4Cl $pH = 9.24 + \log\frac{[0.1]}{[0.2]} = 9.24 - 0.30$ $= 8.94$

Note: You may recall from previous coursework that the equations presented in this table are simplified versions of more complex (and more accurate) equations. They are based on assumptions that do not hold in all cases. (For example, $pK_w = 14$ only at 25°C.) They do give the sort of approximations that are helpful in the practical situations encountered in compounding. For a detailed treatment of this subject, the reader may wish to review chapters on ionic equilibria and buffered and isotonic solutions in a book on physical pharmacy (1) or an equivalent text.

IV. SELECTING A BUFFER SYSTEM OR A COMPOUND TO ADJUST pH

A. First, consider the route of administration for the dosage form.

1. Ingredients to buffer or adjust pH must be nontoxic for the intended route of administration. This is an important factor to consider. For example, Tables 17.2 through 17.6 (3–8) give the formulas for some buffer systems that were developed primarily for ophthalmic solutions. They contain Boric Acid or Sodium Borate, common ingredients for ophthalmic solutions. These would not be satisfactory for systemic drug preparations because borate is toxic systemically.

2. For oral liquid preparations, buffer compounds should not have a disagreeable odor or taste.

3. Agents used for parenteral preparations must be in sterile form or must be rendered sterile.

4. Agents for any route of administration should be nonirritating at the needed concentration.

B. Consider the easiest systems first.

1. If a formula merely calls for the adjustment of pH to a given level, usually a dilute solution (0.1–0.2 N) of HCl or NaOH may be used. Be aware of possible compatibility considerations with the chloride ion in HCl. For example, if a drug is available as a salt with an uncommon anion, such as mesylate, the chloride may cause precipitation because the hydrochloride salt of that drug is less soluble.

2. Sodium Bicarbonate Injection is often used to raise the pH of some parenteral preparations.

TABLE 17.2–17.6   Ophthalmic Buffer Solutions

TABLE 17.2   Boric Acid Solution pH = 5

Boric Acid, crystals	19 g
Purified Water, q.s.	1000 mL

TABLE 17.3   Gifford Ophthalmic Buffer (3)

Acid Stock Solution		Alkaline Stock Solution	
Boric Acid	12.4 g		
Potassium Chloride	7.4 g	Sodium Carbonate Monohydrate	24.8 g
Purified Water, q.s.	1000 mL	Purified Water, q.s.	1000 mL
mL of Boric Acid Solution		mL of Sodium Carbonate Solution	pH
30		0.05	6.0
30		0.1	6.2
30		0.2	6.6
30		0.3	6.8
30		0.5	6.9
30		0.6	7.0
30		1.0	7.2
30		1.5	7.4
30		2.0	7.6
30		3.0	7.8
30		4.0	8.0
30		8.0	8.5

TABLE 17.4 Palitzsch Ophthalmic Buffer (4)

Acid Stock Solution		Alkaline Stock Solution	
Boric Acid	12.404 g	Sodium Borate Decahydrate	19.108 g
Purified Water, q.s.	1000 mL	Purified Water, q.s.	1000 mL

mL of 0.2 M Boric Acid Solution	mL of 0.05 M Sodium Borate Solution	pH
97	3	6.8
94	6	7.1
90	10	7.4
85	15	7.6
80	20	7.8
75	25	7.9
70	30	8.1
65	35	8.2
55	45	8.4
45	55	8.6
40	60	8.7
30	70	8.8
20	80	9.0
10	90	9.1

TABLE 17.5 Sodium Acetate-Boric Acid Stock Solution (5)

Acid Stock Solution pH 7.6		Acid Stock Solution pH about 5	
Sodium Acetate Trihydrate, NF	20 g	Boric Acid, Crystals	19 g
Purified Water, q.s.	1000 mL	Purified Water, q.s.	1000 mL

mL of Sodium Acetate Solution	mL of Boric Acid Solution	pH of Resulting Solution
–	100	5
5	95	5.7
10	90	6.05
20	80	6.3
30	70	6.5
40	60	6.65
50	50	6.75
60	40	6.85
70	30	6.95
80	20	7.1
90	10	7.25
95	5	7.4
100	…	7.6

3. For oral or topical liquids, consider using a preformulated vehicle. Many of the available flavored syrups and liquid vehicles contain buffers or ingredients that function as buffers. See Chapter 21, Vehicles for Liquid Preparations, for descriptions and specifications.

4. For an easily made buffer in the low- to mid-pH range (3.6–5.6), the Acetate Buffer given in Table 17.7 is useful (9). It may be used for systemic, topical, or ophthalmic drug preparations. If isotonicity is needed (see Tables 17.7 and 17.8), the appropriate quantities of Sodium Chloride are also given; if any of the preparation ingredients are incompatible with halides, Sodium Nitrate or Dextrose, in equal osmolar quantities (see Chapter 10), can be substituted for the Sodium Chloride.

5. If a **concentrated** buffer is desired in the low- to mid-pH range (2.5–6.5), the Citrate Buffer in Table 17.9 can be used. When combined in the ratios given, the resulting

TABLE 17.6 Atkins and Pantin Ophthalmic Buffer (6)

Acid Stock Solution		Alkaline Stock Solution	
Boric Acid	12.405 g		
Sodium Chloride	7.50 g	Sodium Carbonate, Anhydrous	21.2 g
Purified Water, q.s.	1000 mL	Purified Water, q.s.	1000 mL

mL of 0.2 M Boric Acid Solution	mL of 0.2 M Sodium Carbonate Solution	pH
93.8	6.2	7.6
91.7	8.3	7.8
88.8	11.2	8.0
85.0	15.0	8.2
80.7	19.3	8.4
75.7	24.3	8.6
69.5	30.5	8.8
63.0	37.0	9.0
56.4	43.6	9.2
49.7	50.3	9.4
42.9	57.1	9.6
36.0	64.0	9.8
29.1	70.9	10.0
22.1	77.9	10.2
15.4	84.6	10.4
9.8	90.2	10.6
5.7	94.3	10.8
3.5	96.5	11.0

Note: The footnotes given for the ophthalmic buffer solutions given in Tables 17.2–17.7 reference the original published journal articles. A review of these solutions is given in *Remington's Pharmaceutical Sciences*, 14th ed. (7)

solution has a molarity of 0.33 M. This buffer can be diluted 10-fold and still have adequate buffer capacity.

6. For preparations to be buffered between pH 6 and 8, Sorenson's Phosphate Buffer is a useful system. It can be used for systemic, topical, or ophthalmic preparations. Its formula is shown in Table 17.8. It has a relatively high buffer capacity. If an isotonic solution is needed, Sodium Chloride in the amounts given in the table can be added; if any of the product ingredients are incompatible with halides, Sodium Nitrate or Dextrose, in equal osmolar quantities (see Chapter 10), can be substituted for the Sodium Chloride.

TABLE 17.7–17.8 Isotonic Multi-Purpose Buffer Solutions

TABLE 17.7 Modified Walpole Acetate Buffer (9)

pH	Acetic Acid 99% mL/100 mL	Sodium Acetate Anhydrous g/100 mL	Sodium Chloride to make isotonic g/100 mL
3.6	1.11	0.123	0.28
3.8	1.06	0.197	0.28
4.0	0.98	0.295	0.27
4.2	0.88	0.435	0.26
4.4	0.76	0.607	0.24
4.6	0.61	0.804	0.22
4.8	0.48	0.984	0.21
5.0	0.35	1.156	0.19
5.2	0.25	1.296	0.18
5.4	0.17	1.402	0.17
5.6	0.11	1.484	0.16

This buffer is suitable for internal, external, or ophthalmic use.

TABLE 17.8   Sorensen's Modified Phosphate Buffer (8)

Acid Stock Solution, M/15 Sodium Biphosphate		Alkaline Stock Solution, M/15 Sodium Phosphate	
*Sodium Biphosphate, Anhydrous	8.006 g	Sodium Phosphate, Anhydrous	9.473 g
Purified Water, q.s.	1000 mL	Purified Water, q.s.	1000 mL
mL of M/15 Sodium Biphosphate Solution mL)	mL of M/15 Sodium Phosphate Solution	pH	Sodium Chloride Required for Isotonicity (Gm/100
90	10	5.9	0.52
80	20	6.2	0.51
70	30	6.5	0.50
60	40	6.6	0.49
50	50	6.8	0.48
40	60	7.0	0.46
30	70	7.2	0.45
20	80	7.4	0.44
10	90	7.7	0.43
5	95	8.0	0.42

*Sodium biphosphate, monohydrated 9.208 Gm may be used.
This buffer is suitable for internal, external, or ophthalmic use.

7. For ophthalmic solutions that require buffering in the mid-acid range (~5), Boric Acid 1.9% is easy to make and has an appropriately low buffer capacity for this situation.

C. If a customized buffer solution must be made, follow these steps:
   1. Select a compound or combination of compounds that can give you a pH in the range you desire.
      a. As discussed above, this may be a strong acid, a strong base, or a conjugate pair. If using a conjugate pair, the pK_a of the conjugate acid should be within one pH unit of the desired pH.

TABLE 17.9   Concentrated Multi-Purpose Buffer Solution

TABLE 17.9   Citrate Buffer

Acid Stock Solution, M/3 Citric Acid		Alkaline Stock Solution, M/3 Sodium Citrate	
*Citric Acid Monohyrate	70 g	Sodium Citrate Dihydrate	98 g
Purified Water, q.s.	1000 mL	Purified Water, q.s.	1000 mL
*Citric Acid Anhydrous 64 g may be substituted			
mL of M/3 Citric Acid Solution		mL of M/3 Sodium Citrate Solution	pH
92		8	2.5
82		18	3.0
68		32	3.5
58		42	4.0
44		56	4.5
28		72	5.0
14		86	5.5
6		94	6.0
2		98	6.5

Both compounds combined yield a concentration of 0.33 M.
This buffer is suitable for internal, external, or ophthalmic use.

b. For possible conjugate pairs, you may want to consult the table in the appendix section of the CD that accompanies this book. This table gives the pK_as of a large number of drugs and reference compounds.

c. Be sure that your choice is chemically stable, is sufficiently soluble, is compatible with the other ingredients in the formulation, is free from odor and color, and is nonsensitizing and nontoxic by the route of administration being used.

d. Examples of some possible choices are:

pH Range	Buffer
pH 1–3	HCl
pH 2.5–6.5	Citrate Buffer
pH 3.6–5.6	Acetate Buffer
pH 6–8	Sorenson's Phosphate Buffer
pH 8–9	Sodium Bicarbonate
pH 9–11	Sodium Bicarbonate/Sodium Carbonate
pH 11–13	NaOH

2. Calculate the concentration of each compound needed.

a. You may use the appropriate equation from Table 17.1 (remembering that these equations can only give approximations), or one of the buffer formulas from Tables 17.2–17.9.

b. If an acid-base conjugate pair is selected, recall that the Henderson-Hasselbalch equation gives you just the ratio of concentrations. From the calculated ratio, select the specific concentrations for the ingredients based on the fact that adequate buffer capacity can be had with final concentrations of 0.05 to 0.5 M (1).

3. After the solution is made, use pH paper or a pH meter to measure the pH of the solution and make adjustments as needed.

V. ACIDIFYING, ALKALIZING, AND BUFFERING AGENTS

Table 17.10 shows compounds that are official articles in the *USP25-NF20* and that are categorized by *USP-NF* as excipients used as acidifying, alkalizing and buffering agents (10).

TABLE 17.10 *USP-NF* Articles Categorized as Acidifying, Alkalizing, or Buffering Agents (10)

Acidifying Agents	Alkalizing Agents	Buffering Agents
Acetic Acid	Strong Ammonia	Acetic Acid
Glacial Acetic Acid	Solution	Ammonium Carbonate
Citric Acid	Ammonium Carbonate	Ammonium Phosphate
Fumaric Acid	Diethanolamine	Boric Acid
Hydrochloric Acid	Potassium Hydroxide	Citric Acid
Diluted Hydrochloric Acid	Sodium Bicarbonate	Lactic Acid
Malic Acid	Sodium Borate	Phosphoric Acid
Nitric Acid	Sodium Carbonate	Potassium Citrate
Phosphoric Acid	Sodium Hydroxide	Potassium Metaphosphate
Diluted Phosphoric Acid	Trolamine	Monobasic Potassium
Propionic Acid		Phosphate
Sulfuric Acid		Sodium Acetate
Tartaric Acid		Sodium Citrate
		Sodium Lactate Solution
		Dibasic Sodium Phosphate
		Monobasic Sodium Phosphate

References

1. Martin A, Bustamante P. Physical pharmacy, 4th ed. Philadelphia: Lea & Febiger, 1993; 143–185.
2. The 2002 United States Pharmacopeia 25/National Formulary 20. Rockville, MD: The United States Pharmacopeial Convention, Inc., 2001; 2340.
3. Gifford SR. Reaction of buffer solution and of ophthalmic drugs. Arch Ophthalmol 1935; 13: 78.
4. Palitzsch S. Use of borax and boric acid solutions in the colorimetric measurement of the hydrogen ion concentration of sea water. Biochem Z 1915; 70: 333.
5. Neuwald F, et al. Galenical and pharmacological research on the composition of aqueous ophthalmic pharmaceuticals. I. Stability of some compounds used as ophthalmic pharmaceuticals, II. A generally useful buffer. Pharm Ztg Ver Apotheker-Ztg 1957; 102: 40, 51–52 and 1958; 103: 12.
6. Atkins WR, Pantin GF. Buffer mixture for the alkaline range of hydrogen-ion concentration determinations. Biochem J 1926; 20: 102.
7. Deardorff DL. Ophthalmic Solutions. In: Hoover JE, ed. Remington's pharmaceutical sciences, 14th ed. Easton, PA: Mack Publishing Co., 1970; 1553–1555.
8. Sörensen SL. Enzyme studies. II. The measurement and importance or the hydrogen ion concentration in enzyme reactions. Biochem Z 1909; 21: 131 and 22: 352.
9. Schumacher GE. Buffer formulations. Am J Hosp Pharm 1966; 23: 629.
10. The 2002 United States Pharmacopeia 25/National Formulary 20. Rockville, MD: The United States Pharmacopeial Convention, Inc., 2001; 2496.

CHAPTER 18

Viscosity-inducing Agents

I. DEFINITIONS

A. **Viscosity** is a measure of the resistance to flow of a system under an applied stress. The more viscous a liquid, the greater the applied force required to make it flow at a particular rate. This is expressed mathematically by Newton's Law of Flow (1):

$$\frac{F}{A} = \eta \frac{dv}{dr}$$

where F/A is shearing stress, the force per unit area required to bring about flow
dv/dr is the rate of shear
η is the coefficient of viscosity, usually referred to as just viscosity

B. The traditional unit of viscosity is the **poise,** which is defined as the shearing force in dynes required to produce a velocity of 1 cm/sec between two parallel planes of a liquid each 1 cm^2 in area and separated by a distance of 1 cm.

C. The unit of viscosity commonly used in pharmacy is the **centipoise** (cp, plural cps), which is equal to 0.01 poise.

D. In the more recently adopted International System of Units (SI), the basic unit of viscosity is **Pascal sec** (Pa s) or Newton/m^2–sec^{-1}, which equals 10 poise. The SI unit of viscosity commonly used to report viscosities of pharmaceutical liquids is the **milliPascal sec** (mPa s), which conveniently is numerically equal to the viscosity value in centipoise. The various units of viscosity can be illustrated with the viscosity of water, which is approximately 1 cps at 20°C.

1 cps = 0.01 poise = 0.001 Pa s = 1 mPa s

The SI System's mPa s viscosity units are now used for reporting viscosity values in books such as the *Handbook of Pharmaceutical Excipients.*

E. While "thick" liquids are generally more viscous than "thin" liquids, there is not a direct relationship between perceived "thickness" and viscosity. The viscosity values for some common substances are given in Table 18.1; these give some feeling for relative centipoise (or mPa s) values.

F. **Viscosity-inducing agents** are molecules that interact with water molecules to form a structured system that interrupts the flow of the molecules past one another. They are hydrophilic colloids that are classified either as soluble macromolecules or particulate association colloids (2).

TABLE 18.1	Absolute Viscosity of Some Newtonian Liquids at 20°C (1)
Liquid	**Viscosity (cps)**
Castor Oil	1000
Chloroform	0.563
Ethyl Alcohol	1.19
Glycerin 93%	400
Olive Oil	100
Water	1.0087

Reprinted with Permission from Martin A, Bustamante P. Physical Pharmacy, 4th ed. Philadelphia: Lea & Febiger, 1993:455. Copyright Williams & Wilkins Co.,Baltimore

1. The soluble macromolecules are linear or branched-chain polymers that dissolve molecularly in water. They are classified as colloidal dispersions because the individual molecules are in the colloidal particle size range, exceeding 50–100 Å. They are further classified into one of three groups: natural polymers, semisynthetic cellulose derivatives, and synthetic polymers.

2. The particulate association colloids are water-insoluble particles that hydrate strongly. They include inorganic silicates, colloidal silicon dioxide, and microcrystalline cellulose.

G.   Newtonian and Non-Newtonian Flow (1)

1. Pure liquids and dilute solutions (like those in Table 18.1) exhibit **Newtonian flow**, which means that their viscosity, η, is characterized by a single value. The relationship between shearing stress (F'/A) and rate of shear (dv/dr) is linear: a plot of shearing stress versus rate of shear gives a straight line; the slope of the line, η, is constant and the line passes through the origin (Fig. 18.1A).

2. Many pharmaceutical systems exhibit non-Newtonian flow patterns. The viscosity of these systems is not constant; rather, it depends on the shearing stress or force applied. Liquid and solid heterogeneous dispersions, such as suspensions, emulsions, colloidal dispersions, and ointments and creams, are non-Newtonian systems. These are further classified into three different groups, based on their flow characteristics: plastic, pseudoplastic, and dilatant. It is helpful for pharmacists who compound drug preparations to have some understanding of these systems. A brief description follows; for a more detailed treatment, refer to a book on physical pharmacy (1) or the chapter on rheology in *Remington The Science and Practice of Pharmacy* (3).

   a. **Pseudoplastic systems** are sometimes called "shear thinning systems" because their viscosity decreases with increasing shear stress. In this case, a plot of shearing stress versus rate of shear initially starts at the origin and appears Newtonian, but the slope begins to decrease, giving a curved line (Fig. 18.1B). Pharmaceutical systems that exhibit pseudoplastic behavior are the colloidal dispersions of the natural gums, such as acacia and tragacanth, and the synthetic and semisynthetic hydrophilic polymers, such as methylcellulose and carboxymethylcellulose.

   b. **Plastic systems** exhibit Newtonian flow patterns, but only after a certain shearing stress, called the yield value, is reached. In this case the plot of shearing stress versus rate of shear does not go through the origin. In other words, a plastic system exhibits infinite viscosity (the slope, $\eta = \infty$) and does not flow at all until the yield value is reached; once flow is established, the system behaves like a Newtonian system (Fig. 18.1C). Plastic flow is a desirable property in disperse systems in which the force of gravity on small particles is not enough to overcome the yield value; that is, suspension particles do not settle and emulsion droplets do not cream but, under the larger stresses of shaking, pouring, rubbing, or syringing, the system flows. Plastic flow is produced by structured systems of flocculated particles in concentrated suspensions or emulsions.

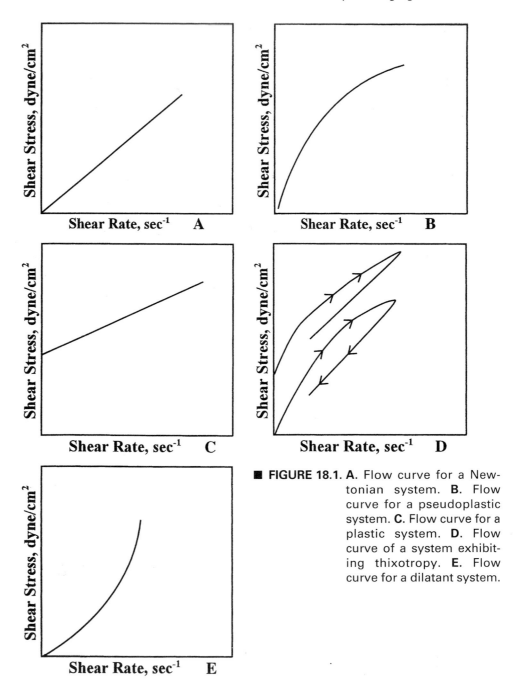

FIGURE 18.1. A. Flow curve for a Newtonian system. **B.** Flow curve for a pseudoplastic system. **C.** Flow curve for a plastic system. **D.** Flow curve of a system exhibiting thixotropy. **E.** Flow curve for a dilatant system.

c. **Thixotropy** is a property of many plastic and pseudoplastic systems in which the consistency lost when shear is applied (e.g., shaking) takes some finite amount of time for recovery (Fig. 18.1D). This is a desirable property of liquid pharmaceutical dispersions: the dispersion becomes fluid when the product is shaken; the product remains fluid long enough for a dose to be poured or a topical product to be applied; the system then regains its consistency rapidly enough on standing so that the suspended particles do not settle. Catsup is a nonpharmaceutical example of a thixotropic system. Bentonite Magma, consisting of flocculated colloidal clay particles, and several of the structured liquids marketed as suspending vehicles for compounding, are examples of pharmaceutical thixotropic systems.

d. **Dilatant systems** act oppositely of pseudoplastic systems. They are called shear-thickening systems because their viscosity increases with increasing shear stress (Fig. 18.1E). Suspensions that have high concentrations of deflocculated particles may exhibit dilatant behavior. One common example of a dilatant system is a starch-in-water slurry. This system flows when left at rest, but firms up when pressure is applied. Dilatant systems may cause problems with high-speed mixing equipment used in formulation; these materials may solidify under conditions of high shear and damage the equipment. Dilatancy must also be avoided in injectable suspensions because the high shear stress that results when pushing a liquid through a small needle bore may cause the syringe to lock—not a pleasant experience for the patient.

II. THE ROLE OF VISCOSITY IN FORMULATION

Increased viscosity can offer both advantages and disadvantages with respect to formulating liquid and semisolid preparations. Understanding the meaning of viscosity and the various types of flow behavior is useful to the pharmacist in selecting appropriate formulation ingredients.

A. For topical products, appropriate viscosity is essential in achieving desirable smoothness and consistency so that the product will be easy to apply, will remain in contact with the affected area, and will feel good to the patient.

B. Palatability of oral liquid products is often enhanced by formulating the product with appropriate viscosity. This provides what is sometimes referred to as desirable "mouth feel." Viscous vehicles also may improve the perceived flavor of oral liquids by reducing the contact of bad-tasting drugs with the taste buds on the tongue.

C. High viscosity is a disadvantage when dissolving drugs to make solutions because diffusion, and therefore rate of dissolution, decreases as viscosity increases. This is why pharmacists do not dissolve drugs directly in viscous vehicles, but rather first dissolve them in a minimum quantity of water or other low-viscosity solvent and then combine the resulting solution with the desired viscous vehicle.

D. If increased viscosity is the only formulation goal, a high-viscosity liquid, such as glycerin, or a concentrated aqueous solution of a soluble micromolecule, such as sucrose or sorbitol, may be used.

E. If a structured system is needed to retard the settling or creaming rate of the particles or oil droplets in disperse systems, the selection and addition of a viscosity-inducing agent that gives pseudoplastic, plastic, or thixotropic flow is required.

III. SUSPENDING AND/OR VISCOSITY INDUCING AGENTS LISTED IN *USP 25-NF 20*

A. Table 18.2 gives the articles listed as suspending and/or viscosity-inducing agents in the *USP 25-NF 20* (4). This is not a complete list of all agents used in this way; some compounds, although not on this list, are used for these purposes in manufactured products and compounded preparations.

B. The agents used most commonly as suspending or viscosity-increasing agents in extemporaneous compounding are described in the section below. For each agent, the text gives the information needed for selection and use of a suitable compound: a description of each compound, including the pH of its dispersions, its solubility, incompatibilities, suggestions for preparing and preserving its dispersions, possible uses for the compound, and some advantages and disadvantages in its use.

TABLE 18.2 USP and NF Excipients Categorized as Suspending and/or Viscosity-increasing Agents (4)

Acacia	Gelatin
Agar	Guar Gum
Alginic Acid	Hydroxyethyl Cellulose
Aluminum Monostearate	Hydroxypropyl Cellulose
Attapulgite, Activated	Hydroxypropyl Methylcellulose
Attapulgite, Colloidal Activated	Magnesium Aluminum Silicate
Bentonite	Methylcellulose
Bentonite, Purified	Pectin
Bentonite Magma	Polyethylene Oxide
Carbomer 910, 934, 934P, 940, 941, and 1342	Polyvinyl Alcohol
	Povidone
Carboxymethylcellulose Calcium	Propylene Glycol Alginate
Carboxymethylcellulose Sodium	Silicon Dioxide
Carboxymethylcellulose Sodium 12	Silicon Dioxide, Colloidal
Carrageenan	Sodium Alginate
Cellulose, Microcystalline and Carboxymethylcellulose Sodium	Tragacanth
	Xanthan Gum
Dextrin	

IV. VISCOSITY-INDUCING AGENTS

The descriptions and solubilities presented here give a composite of information from *Remington: The Science and Practice of Pharmacy* (5), the *Handbook of Pharmaceutical Excipients* (6), *The Merck Index* (7), official monographs in the *USP-NF* (8), the Chemistry and Compendial Requirements section of the *USP DI Vol. III* (9), and other references as cited. Additional information on each agent, including references to original research journal articles, can be found in the *Handbook of Pharmaceutical Excipients*.

A. Semi-synthetic Cellulose Derivatives
    1. Methylcellulose USP

$R = CH_3$ or H

    a. Description
        (1) Methylcellulose is a polymer formed by the methylation of cellulose to form methyl ether linkages. The degree of methylation is regulated to yield polymers with a controlled number of sites for hydrogen bonding. This, together with polymer chain length, determines the degree to which the polymer increases the viscosity of its water solutions or gels. These solutions or gels exhibit pseudoplastic flow characteristics.
        (2) Methylcellulose is white, fibrous powder or granules. The pH of a 1% dispersion is 5.5 to 8.0.
        (3) Methylcellulose is available in various viscosity grades: 15, 25, 100, 400, 1,500, and 4,000 cps are the most commonly available grades. The grade number refers to the viscosity of a 2% aqueous solution at 20°C.
    b. Solubility: Methylcellulose is insoluble or practically insoluble in acetone, alcohols, glycols, hot water, and saturated salt solutions, but it is soluble in glacial acetic acid. It swells in water and produces a clear to opalescent, viscous colloidal solution that is neutral to litmus.

c. Incompatibilities

(1) Methylcellulose is stable to alkalies and dilute acids but coagulates from solution with high concentrations of salts of mineral acids, with moderate to high concentrations of salts of polybasic acids, and with phenols and tannins. This is reported to be prevented by the addition of alcohol or glycol diacetate (5).

(2) It is also incompatible with aminacrine hydrochloride, Chlorocresol, mercuric chloride, Silver Nitrate, Cetylpyridium Chloride (but not Benzalkonium Chloride), *p*-hydroxybenzoic acid, *p*-aminobenzoic acid, and the parabens (6). Benzyl Alcohol is also stated to be incompatible with Methylcellulose.

d. Preparation of dispersions

While the hydrogen bonding sites make possible the formation of clear viscous gels of Methylcellulose, they are also responsible for the difficulty with which its solutions are made. If you were to add water at room temperature to Methylcellulose powder, a clumpy mess would result. This is because water forms hydrogen bonds rapidly with the Methylcellulose on the outside of the powder bed, forming a very viscous layer and preventing water penetration to the rest of the powder. Hydration of the powder and clear gel formation would eventually occur, but this takes a long time. Listed below are three methods for successful dispersion of Methylcellulose in water:

(1) Heat to boiling a portion (approximately one third) of the total water needed for the dispersion. Add the Methylcellulose powder and stir to completely wet the powder. Add the remaining water as cold water or ice chips and stir. This method is useful when you need to make a relatively clear solution quickly.

(2) Heat to boiling the total amount of water needed for the solution. Disperse the Methylcellulose in the water. Put the cloudy dispersion in a refrigerator and gently stir or agitate frequently until a clear viscous solution results. This method is not useful when you need the solution immediately because it takes a minimum of 4 hours to convert the nonviscous, cloudy dispersion to a clear, viscous gel.

(3) Place the Methylcellulose powder in a glass mortar and wet the powder completely with a minimum amount of Alcohol or Glycerin; then with trituration gradually add cold water to the final desired volume. This method is useful when boiling water is not readily available; however, the gels that result may not be crystal clear. Furthermore, there may be cases when you want to avoid Alcohol or Glycerin in a formulation. This method is particularly handy when the formulation contains an alcohol or glycol as an ingredient and the end product is a suspension or emulsion in which clarity is not essential.

e. Preservation of aqueous dispersions

(1) Although pure solutions or gels of Methylcellulose do not support bacterial or mold growth as readily as comparable preparations of the natural polymers (e.g., acacia and tragacanth), preservatives are recommended for Methylcellulose solutions because they are liable to microbial spoilage.

(2) Because the pH of Methylcellulose solutions is between 5.5 and 8.0, the organic acid preservatives Benzoic Acid/Sodium Benzoate and Sorbic Acid/Potassium Sorbate would not be effective unless the pH of the solution is adjusted to a level of 5.0 or below.

(3) As stated above, Methylcellulose is incompatible with the parabens, Benzyl Alcohol, and Cetylpyridium Chloride. For Methylcellulose solutions with pH above 5.0, this leaves the following possibilities for preservatives: Alcohol, Propylene Glycol, and Benzalkonium or Benzethonium Chloride.

f. Uses

(1) Methylcellulose is used extensively by the pharmaceutical industry in both oral and topical products. It is used both in solid dosage forms and in emulsions, suspensions, and solutions.

(2) These polymers are also used therapeutically as bulk laxatives, diet aids, and in artificial tears products.

(3) In compounding, Methylcellulose is useful for making sugar-free vehicles to use in formulating oral solutions and suspensions. It can also be used as a viscosity-inducing agent for topical liquid and gel preparations when a film is acceptable.

(4) A 1% gel of Methylcellulose 1,500 cps dispersed in Purified Water or Water for Irrigation gives a liquid vehicle that is useful for many purposes. Although there are published formulas like this that are preserved with 0.2% Sodium Benzoate, the pH of Methylcellulose solutions is not favorable to preservation with this agent.

(5) A 5% gel of Methylcellulose 1,500 cps dispersed in Purified Water or Water for Irrigation gives a soft semisolid gel that can be used for topical or vaginal preparations.

g. Advantages of Methylcellulose

(1) It produces aesthetically pleasing, clear, colorless, odorless gels.

(2) Its gels have a neutral pH and are stable over a wide pH range, approximately 3 to 12.

(3) It is a nonelectrolyte with no ionizable groups, so it is compatible with many other ingredients and drugs; it is not reactive with quaternary nitrogen compounds (such as Benzalkonium Chloride), weak acids, or the salts of weak bases.

(4) It is relatively unaffected by moderate concentrations of univalent ions.

(5) Although not soluble in alcohol or most other organic solvents, its solutions tolerate relatively high alcohol concentrations.

(6) It is not a sugar, so it is useful when a sugar-free vehicle is needed.

(7) It is effective as a viscosity-inducing agent at low concentrations, so vehicles made with Methylcellulose are not hypertonic. If necessary, its solutions can be made isotonic by adding compatible solutes.

(8) Methylcellulose solutions and gels are less susceptible to bacterial and mold growth than are the natural polymer dispersions.

h. Disadvantages

(1) Flavoring and sweetening are required for palatability when the solutions are used as vehicles for oral drug preparations.

(2) Because Methylcellulose depends on hydrogen bonding for its solubility in water, drugs or chemicals that strongly associate with water can dehydrate Methylcellulose molecules and cause their separation from solution. Compatibility problems occur with high concentrations of univalent ions and moderate concentrations of polyvalent ions. Methylcellulose is also dehydrated by phenolic substances, including Phenol and Resorcinol.

(3) Methylcellulose is not soluble in alcohol or most other organic solvents, although its aqueous solutions do tolerate fairly high concentrations of alcohol.

(4) The solutions support bacterial or mold growth, especially when nutrients such as organic drugs, sweeteners, or flavors are added.

(5) The solutions are somewhat difficult to prepare.

2. Carboxymethylcellulose Sodium USP (Sodium CMC)

   a. Description

     (1) Sodium CMC is structurally similar to methylcellulose except that the methyl groups are replaced with —$CH_2COO^-Na^+$ moieties. Although Sodium CMC has properties similar to Methylcellulose, there are some differences, due mainly to the ionic centers in Sodium CMC molecules.

     (2) It is a white to cream-colored powder or granules. The powder is hygroscopic, and in conditions of high humidity it can absorb large amounts of water. It has a pK_a of 4.3, and a 1% w/v aqueous solution has a pH of approximately 7.5.

(3) Sodium CMC comes in three basic viscosity grades: low, medium, and high. These are sometimes designated LF (1% aqueous solution = 25–50 cps), MF (1% aqueous solution = 400–800 cps), and HF (1% aqueous solution = 1,500–3,000 cps).

(4) Table 18.3 gives the percent concentrations in water of various viscosity-inducing agents needed to give a viscosity of 800 cps. Notice that a 1.7% Methylcellulose 1,500 cps solution gives approximately the same viscosity as a 1.9% solution of medium-viscosity Sodium CMC. Based on this observation, you can conclude that Methylcellulose 1,500 cps is approximately equal to medium-viscosity Sodium CMC in its ability to induce viscosity. Table 18.3 gives useful information when it is necessary to substitute one viscosity-increasing agent for another in a formulation.

b. Solubility: Sodium CMC is insoluble or practically insoluble in acetone, alcohol, glycols, and most other organic solvents. Its solubility in water varies with the degree of substitution on the polymer. It disperses in both hot and cold water to form clear, colloidal solutions.

c. Incompatibilities
(1) Because Sodium CMC molecules interact with water using both hydrogen bonding and ion-dipole interactions, they are less susceptible to dehydration than Methylcellulose, but are subject to the normal incompatibilities of its weak electrolyte group.

(2) Because it is the salt of a weak carboxylic acid, it is more sensitive to pH than Methylcellulose. Although its solutions will tolerate a fairly wide pH range (2–10), they are most stable in the range of pH 5 to 10 and exhibit maximum viscosity at pH 7 to 9 (6).

(3) Its solutions tolerate a fairly high concentration of alcohol or glycols.

(4) Sodium CMC, as a large anionic molecule, has potential incompatibilities with quaternary nitrogen compounds such as Benzethonium and Benzalkonium Chloride, and with acids and the salts of some weak bases.

(5) It is also incompatible with soluble iron salts and some other metals such as aluminum, mercury, and zinc (6).

d. Preparation of dispersions
(1) *Remington*'s statement that it is easily dispersed in water to form colloidal solutions is somewhat of an overstatement: When water is added to the powder or granules, clumps of partially hydrated powder result; fortunately, the powder hydrates fully and disperses to form a clear solution in 1 to 2 hours.

(2) Although Sodium CMC gels are made more easily than are Methylcellulose solutions, CMC powder clumps initially when either hot or cold water is

TABLE 18.3   Comparative Viscosities of Various Suspending Agents (17)

Suspending Agent	% Concentration to give 800 cps
Acacia	35 (for 600 cps)
Tragacanth	2.8
Methylcellulose 100 cps	3.5
Methylcellulose 400 cps	2.4
Methylcellulose 1500 cps	1.7
Carboxymethylcellulose, low	4.1
Carboxymethylcellulose, medium	1.9
Carboxymethylcellulose, high	0.7
Bentonite	6.3
Veegum	6.0

Reprinted with permission from Gerding PW, Sperandio GJ. JAPhA Prac Ed 1954;15:356.

added. As stated above, these solutions clear in 1 to 2 hours irrespective of the temperature of the water added.

- **(3)** Carboxymethylcellulose Sodium Paste USP is a thick semisolid with a concentration of 16.5% Sodium CMC in water (8).
- **(4)** Gels of Sodium CMC can be made from sols by the addition of controlled amounts of polyvalent cations, such as aluminum. If too much electrolyte is added or if it is added too rapidly, precipitation of the polymer results (10).

- **e.** Preservation of aqueous dispersions
  - **(1)** It is recommended that aqueous solutions of Sodium CMC be preserved if stored for an extended period of time (6).
  - **(2)** Selection of a preservative for Sodium CMC solutions poses a dilemma. The pH of its solutions is too high for effective use of the organic acids, and Sodium CMC is incompatible with the quaternary ammonium preservatives. Methylparaben by itself does not preserve these solutions adequately, but the combination with Propylparaben in Propylene Glycol, which is described in Chapter 15 can be used. Alcohol and/or Propylene Glycol are possibilities, depending on the circumstances.

- **f.** Uses

  Its uses are similar to those of Methylcellulose.

- **g.** Advantages of Sodium Carboxymethylcellulose
  - **(1)** Because of its ionic centers, it interacts with water through ion-dipole interactions and is therefore less easily dehydrated than is Methylcellulose, which depends solely on hydrogen bonding with water. As a result Sodium CMC gels are less affected by high concentrations of electrolytes. Sample Prescription 26.2 in Chapter 26, Solutions, illustrates this effect. As stated previously, controlled amounts of polyvalent cations cause gelation of CMC solutions.
  - **(2)** Although it is not soluble in alcohol or most other organic solvents, its solutions tolerate high alcohol concentrations.
  - **(3)** It is more stable than Methylcellulose to phenolic-type compounds.

- **h.** Disadvantages
  - **(1)** Because of its ionic centers, which are salts forms of weak carboxylic acids, it has the potential for interactions and incompatibilities characteristic of these groups.
  - **(2)** Its gels have a pH of approximately 7.5; therefore, preservatives such as Benzoic Acid/Na Benzoate and Sorbic Acid/K Sorbate, which require a pH of 5 or below for activity, are not effective in solutions of Sodium CMC.

3. Hydroxypropyl Methylcellulose USP
- **a.** Description
  - **(1)** Hydroxypropyl Methylcellulose is a propylene glycol ether of methylcellulose. It is official in the *USP* with varying degrees of substitution, which confer several levels of viscosity induction.
  - **(2)** It is a white or slightly off-white, fibrous or granular powder. It is odorless and tasteless.
  - **(3)** Its solutions have a pH similar to that of Methylcellulose, with a 1% solution having a pH range of 5.5 to 8.0.
- **b.** Solubility: It swells in water to produce a clear or opalescent, viscous colloidal dispersion. Upon heating it is converted from a sol to a gel. This can be reversed with cooling. It is practically insoluble in alcohol, but soluble in mixtures of water and alcohol or water and isopropyl alcohol as long as the alcohol content does not exceed 50%.
- **c.** Incompatibilities
  - **(1)** Like Methylcellulose, Hydroxypropyl Methylcellulose does not have any ionic groups, so it does not have incompatibilities associated with these groups.
  - **(2)** It solutions are most stable between pH 3 and 11 (6).

d. Preparation of liquid dispersions

Solutions of Hydroxypropyl Methylcellulose are prepared in a similar manner to those of Methylcellulose.

(1) One method is to add the Hydroxypropyl Methylcellulose powder to hot water (80 to 90°C) with agitation to ensure complete wetting of the powder; cold water or ice chips are then added to form a clear, gel-like solution (6,11).

(2) An alternative method may be used when the formulation contains alcohol or glycol as an ingredient. With this method, the Hydroxypropyl Methylcellulose is added to the organic solvent in a ratio of 5 to 8 parts of solvent to 1 part of the powder. Cold water is then used to q.s. the preparation to desired volume (6).

(3) A manufactured gel vehicle of Hydroxypropyl Methylcellulose is Liqua-Gel®. In addition to Purified Water and the polymer, Liqua-Gel® contains Propylene Glycol and Glycerin plus preservatives and pH-adjusting and buffering agents. It is described in Chapter 21, Vehicles for Liquid Preparations.

e. Preservation of aqueous dispersions

(1) As with Methylcellulose, the pH of Hydroxypropyl Methylcellulose solutions is between 5.5 and 8.0, so the organic acid preservative Benzoic Acid/Sodium Benzoate would not be effective unless the pH of the solution is adjusted to a level of 5.0 or below. Sorbic Acid/Potassium Sorbate would also be ineffective unless the pH is 6.0 or below.

(2) Manufactured ophthalmic solutions are preserved with Benzalkonium Chloride, so this would be a good choice as a preservative. Alcohol and Propylene Glycol are also possible preservatives, depending on the dosage form and route of administration.

(3) Although the following incompatibilities have only been documented with Methylcellulose, because of its structural similarity with Hydroxypropyl Methylcellulose, the following preservatives should be avoided: parabens, Benzyl Alcohol, and Cetylpyridium Chloride.

4. Hydroxypropyl Cellulose NF

a. Description

(1) Hydroxypropyl Cellulose, also known as Klucel®, is a partially substituted poly(hydroxypropyl) ether of cellulose. It is official in the *NF*, which states that it contains not more than 80.5% of hydroxypropyl groups. It may contain not more than 0.6% of silica or other anticaking agent (8).

(2) It is an off-white powder, odorless and tasteless.

(3) Its solutions have a pH similar to that of Methylcellulose, with a 1% solution having a pH range of 5.0 to 8.5.

b. Solubility: It is freely soluble in water below 38° but is insoluble in hot water and precipitates as flocs between 40° and 45°; it is soluble in many polar solvents like short-chain alcohols (alcohol, isopropyl alcohol, etc.) and glycols such as propylene glycol, but is insoluble in glycerin. It is also insoluble in aliphatic hydrocarbons such as oils and aromatic hydrocarbons. For a thorough description of the solubility characteristics of this interesting compound, refer to the *Handbook of Pharmaceutical Excipients* (6).

c. Incompatibilities

(1) Like Methylcellulose, Hydroxypropyl Cellulose does not have any ionic groups, so it does not have incompatibilities associated with these groups.

(2) It is incompatible with Methylparaben and Propylparaben (6).

(3) Solutions of Hydroxypropyl Cellulose are stable at pH 6 to 8; at low pH it is subject to acid hydrolysis and at high pH it may undergo oxidative degradation (6).

(4) As with Methylcellulose, Hydroxypropyl Cellulose can be dehydrated by moderate to high concentrations of electrolytes. For a rather complete table of compatibility with inorganic salts at a range of concentrations, see the Hydroxypropyl Cellulose monograph in the *Handbook of Pharmaceutical Excipients* (6).

d. Preparation of liquid dispersions

Preparing colloidal dispersions of Hydroxypropyl Cellulose requires some patience.

(1) The powder is sprinkled, in portions, upon Purified Water or a hydroalcoholic solution; a water or water-alcohol mixture is required for gel formation because a gel may not form if only alcohol is used (12).

(2) Allow each portion to become thoroughly wetted without stirring. (Do not stir or agitate the preparation until **all** the powder is thoroughly wetted.)

(3) The preparation is then agitated (stirred or shaken), and it is allowed to stand with occasional agitation for 24 hours. It may be placed in a refrigerator.

(4) If needed, Purified Water is added to bring the preparation to the desired final volume, and the preparation is agitated to obtain a uniform, clear dispersion.

e. Preservation of aqueous dispersions

(1) Because of its high degree of substitution, Hydroxypropyl Cellulose is relatively resistant to growth of bacteria and molds. When in aqueous solution a preservative is recommended when prolonged storage is required (6).

(2) Alcohol, Isopropyl Alcohol, or Propylene Glycol would be acceptable preservatives, depending on the use of the preparation (e.g., Isopropyl Alcohol is not for internal use).

f. Uses

The substitution of hydroxypropyl groups reduces the water solubility of this compound but promotes its solubility in alcohols and glycols. This makes it a useful viscosity-inducing agent for elixirs and topical alcoholic gels. Sample Prescription 30.7 in Chapter 30 illustrates the use of Hydroxypropyl Cellulose for making a gel preparation.

B. Natural Polymers

1. Acacia NF

a. Description

(1) Also known as Gum Arabic, Acacia is a natural gum harvested from the stems and branches of various species of the Acacia tree. As a natural product, it is a mixture of components, the main constituents being calcium, magnesium, and potassium salts of arabic acid, a polysaccharide. As such, Acacia contains large anions and its solutions are acid to litmus. The pH of a 5% w/v solution is 4.5 to 5.0.

(2) Acacia is available as flakes, spheroidal tears, granules, or powder. It is ivory or yellowish-white in color. It has a bland taste and is odorless.

b. Solubility: Acacia forms light-beige colloidal dispersions in twice its weight of water. It is soluble in glycerin (1 g/20 mL), propylene glycol (1g/20 mL), and water (1 g/2.7 mL). It is practically insoluble in alcohol.

c. Incompatibilities

(1) Acacia is similar to Sodium CMC in that it interacts with water using both hydrogen bonding and ion-dipole interactions. This makes it less susceptible to dehydration than Methylcellulose, but, like Sodium CMC, it is subject to the normal incompatibilities of its weak electrolyte groups.

(2) Acacia powder contains peroxidase, which acts as an oxidizing agent for drugs or other ingredients that are susceptible to oxidation. Examples of labile drugs include phenolic and catechol compounds, tannins, and alkaloids such as atropine, morphine, cocaine, physostigmine, and related compounds. The peroxidase can be destroyed by heating acacia solutions at 100°C for a few minutes (5).

(3) It is precipitated from solution by heavy metals and borax. The borax precipitation can be prevented by the addition of glycerin (5).

(4) It is incompatible with large cations, such as quaternary ammonium compounds.

(5) It contains the polyvalent ions calcium and magnesium and has incompatibilities associated with these ions.

(6) A more complete list of incompatibilities can be found in an older edition of *Remington's Pharmaceutical Sciences* or *Martindale The Extra Pharmacopoeia.*

d. Preparation of liquid dispersions

(1) Although Acacia is almost completely soluble in twice its weight of water, like MC and CMC it tends to clump up when mixed directly with water. This clumping can be prevented by first wetting the acacia powder with glycerin or by first diluting the acacia powder with other powdered ingredient(s) present in the formulation. This latter method is used in preparing Acacia Syrup, which is described in Chapter 21, Vehicles for Liquid Preparations.

(2) Acacia Mucilage, which was formerly official in the *National Formulary,* is a solution of 35% w/v acacia in water with 0.2% benzoic acid as a preservative.

(3) Acacia Syrup was an official formulation until *NF XVII*. It has recently been readmitted with the First Supplement to *NF 20*. As stated above, its formula and method of preparation are described in Chapter 21, Vehicles for Liquid Preparations.

e. Preservation of aqueous dispersions

(1) Because Acacia is a natural product, its raw material could contain microbial contamination. The *NF* monograph for Acacia states that it must meet the requirements of the tests for absence of *Salmonella* (8). Appropriate precautions should be taken with the purchase of Acacia and with making aqueous preparations, including the use of preservatives, conservative beyond-use dates, and, when possible, refrigeration.

(2) With the pH of its solutions in the 4.5 to 5.0 range, aqueous liquid preparations of Acacia are ideal for using the organic acid preservatives, Benzoic Acid/Sodium Benzoate and Sorbic Acid/Potassium Sorbate. Alcohol and Propylene Glycol may also be used.

(3) Because Acacia is incompatible with large cations, the quaternary ammonium preservatives Benzalkonium Chloride, Benzethonium Chloride, and Cetylpyridium Chloride should not be used.

f. Uses

(1) Acacia Syrup was at one time a very commonly used vehicle for extemporaneous compounding of oral solutions and suspensions. It has in recent years been largely replaced by gels of the semi-synthetic gums, such as Methylcellulose and Sodium Carboxymethylcellulose and by specialty manufactured vehicles such as Ora Sweet®, Ora Plus®, and Suspendol®.

(2) Acacia powder is unique in that it forms stable oil-in-water emulsions using simple compounding equipment such as a mortar and pestle.

g. Advantages of Acacia

(1) It is stable over a wide pH range of 2 to 10.

(2) Although it is not soluble in alcohol, its solutions tolerate alcohol concentrations up to 35% (5).

(3) Its mucilages contain no sucrose, so they are useful when a sugar-free vehicle is needed (Acacia does contain polysaccharides). Note that Acacia Syrup contains a large amount of sucrose, so this preparation may not be used when a sugar-free vehicle is required.

h. Disadvantages

(1) Flavoring and sweetening are required for palatability (Acacia Syrup is flavored and sweetened; Acacia solutions are often mixed with flavored syrups such as Syrup NF, or artificially flavored cherry or orange syrup).

(2) Acacia has numerous compatibility problems, as described above.

(3) Unless preserved with an antimicrobial agent, Acacia solutions and emulsions are excellent media for bacterial or mold growth. Usually refrigeration is also recommended. Fortunately Acacia is compatible with several preservatives, as described above.

(4) Like the semi-synthetic cellulose polymers, Acacia dispersions are somewhat difficult to prepare.

(5) Acacia solutions are not as aesthetically appealing as the solutions made with synthetic and semi-synthetic polymers; they do not have that colorless, crystal-clear appearance.

2. Tragacanth NF

a. Description

(1) Like acacia, tragacanth is a natural gum. It comes from various species of the plant *Astragalus*.

(2) Tragacanth contains bassorin, which is a complex mixture of methoxylated acids that absorb water to form a gel. It also contains tragacanthin, which is a polysaccharide of glucuronic acid and arabinose. This fraction forms a colloidal solution when mixed with water. The pH of a 1% w/v aqueous dispersion is 5 to 6.

b. Solubility: Although Tragacanth is practically insoluble in water, alcohol, and other organic solvents, it swells in 10 times its weight of either hot or cold water to give beige-colored colloidal dispersions, which are sols or semi-gels depending on the concentration and conditions.

c. Incompatibilities

(1) Tragacanth contains anionic species that have the same types of incompatibilities as Sodium CMC and Acacia.

(2) It is compatible with moderate to relatively high salt concentrations (6).

(3) It has some reported compatibility problems with various preservatives, and some of these are pH-dependent. For example, at pH 7, it reportedly reduces the antimicrobial effectiveness of Methylparaben and Chlorobutanol, but it does not have this adverse effect at pH 5 and below. As expected, it reduces the effectiveness of the quaternary ammonium compound Benzalkonium Chloride and also has some effect on Phenylmercuric Acetate and Phenol (6).

d. Preparation of liquid dispersions

(1) Pure Tragacanth dispersions are very difficult to make. The following description from the 20th edition of *Remington* illustrates this point:

"Introduced into water, Tragacanth absorbs a certain proportion of that liquid, swells very much, and forms a soft adhesive paste, but does not dissolve. If agitated with an excess of water, this paste forms a uniform mixture; but in the course of one or two days the greater part separates, and is deposited, leaving a portion dissolved in the supernatant fluid. The finest mucilage is obtained from the whole gum or *flake* tragacanth. Several days should be allowed for obtaining a uniform mucilage of the maximum strength" (5).

(2) When other ingredients are permitted in a formulation, the preparation of liquid dispersions of Tragacanth is easier.

(a) The Tragacanth powder can be wetted first with Glycerin or Propylene Glycol using trituration in a mortar. An aqueous solution may then be added gradually with trituration until a smooth, thick liquid or gel is obtained.

(b) If the formulation contains powdered ingredients such as sucrose, the dry Tragacanth should be mixed with the powder first, and then the liquid ingredients added with trituration.

(3) Tragacanth mucilage was last official in *National Formulary XII*. This preparation is an aqueous solution that contains Benzoic Acid 0.2% and Glycerin 18% in addition to Tragacanth 6% (5).

e. Preservation of aqueous dispersions

(1) Because Tragacanth is a natural product, its raw material could contain bacterial contamination, and reports of contamination have been published (6). The *NF* monograph for Tragacanth states that it must meet the requirements of the tests for absence of *Salmonella* and *Escherichia coli* (8). Appropriate precautions should be taken with the purchase of Tragacanth and with making aqueous preparations of this natural product, including the use of preservatives, conservative beyond-use dates, and, when possible, refrigeration.

(2) With the normal pH of its solutions in the 5 to 6 range, aqueous liquid preparations of Tragacanth may be preserved by the organic acid preservative Sorbic Acid/Potassium Sorbate. If the pH is controlled at pH 5 or below, Benzoic Acid/Sodium Benzoate or Methylparaben may be used. Alcohol and Propylene Glycol are also possible preservatives.

(3) Because Tragacanth is incompatible with large cations, the quaternary ammonium preservatives Benzalkonium Chloride, Benzethonium Chloride, and Cetylpyridium Chloride may not be used.

f. Uses

(1) Tragacanth is rarely used by itself but is useful as an auxiliary emulsifier and viscosity-increasing agent.

(2) Gels of Tragacanth can be made by adding Glycerin or Propylene Glycol. These elements decrease the solubility of the tragacanth and produce a semisolid gel. Ephedrine Sulfate Jelly NF XII contains 1% Ephedrine sulfate, 1% Tragacanth, and 15% Glycerin in Purified Water. The formula and method of preparation are given in Table 22.2 in Chapter 22, Ointment Bases.

g. Advantages of Tragacanth

(1) As can be observed from Table 18.3, Tragacanth is a better viscosity-inducing agent than Acacia.

h. Disadvantages

(1) Tragacanth dispersions are very difficult to make.

(2) Tragacanth contains anionic species that have the same types of incompatibilities as Sodium CMC and Acacia.

(3) As with Acacia, solutions of Tragacanth are prone to mold and microbial growth.

(4) In most cases Tragacanth solutions and gels require the use of additional viscosity-inducing agents or flavored syrups for quality preparations.

(5) Because they lack that colorless, crystal-clear appearance of the synthetic and semi-synthetic polymers, Tragacanth solutions are not as aesthetically appealing.

3. Xanthan Gum NF

a. Description

(1) Xanthan gum is a high-molecular-weight polysaccharide gum that is made by fermentation of a carbohydrate, then purified by recovery with isopropyl alcohol. It contains three different monosaccharides: glucose, mannose, and glucuronic acid as the sodium, potassium, or calcium salt.

(2) It is a cream-colored fine powder; it is tasteless and has a slight odor. The pH of a 1% solution is in the range 6 to 8.

b. Solubility: It is soluble in hot and cold water to give viscous dispersions. Information on its solubility in alcohol is conflicting. *Remington* states that 1 g dissolves in 3 mL of alcohol and *Dispensing of Medication* says that it is freely soluble in alcohol; however, the *Handbook of Pharmaceutical Excipients* says that it is practically insoluble in alcohol.

c. Incompatibilities

(1) Solutions of Xanthan Gum are compatible with nearly all univalent and divalent cations, with polyols, alcohol, chelating agents, and with most preservatives (11).

(2) Aqueous solutions are stable over a wide pH range reported as 1 to 10 (11) or 3 to 12 (6), and over a temperature range of 10 to 60°C (6).

(3) Because of the anionic nature of the glucuronic acid groups, Xanthan Gum shows incompatibilities that are similar to Sodium CMC and Acacia: it is incompatible with large cationic drugs, surfactants, polymers, and preservatives.

(4) Solutions of Xanthan Gum are stable to the addition of up to 60% of water-miscible solvents such as acetone, alcohol, and isopropyl alcohol (6).

(5) Xanthan Gum has reported incompatibility with Sodium CMC and some drugs such as Amitriptyline, Tamoxifen, Verapamil, and Aluminum Hydroxide Gel (6). For additional information on compatibility and stability, refer to the Xanthan Gum monograph in the *Handbook of Pharmaceutical Excipients*.

   d. Preparation of liquid dispersions

(1) If a pure dispersion in water is needed, place the water in a beaker and, using a high-speed stirrer (such as a magnetic stirring device), stir the water to form a vortex. Slowly sprinkle the Xanthan Gum onto the water to obtain a uniform dispersion. Dispersion may be aided by the use of moderate heat (45°C or less).

(2) When other ingredients are permitted in the formulation, the preparation of a liquid dispersion of Xanthan Gum can be made by first wetting the powder with Glycerin or Propylene Glycol using trituration in a mortar. An aqueous solution may then be added gradually with trituration until a smooth, thick liquid or gel is obtained.

   e. Preservation of aqueous dispersions

(1) Because Xanthan Gum is made by a fermentation process, microbiological contamination would be possible. The *NF* monograph for Xanthan Gum states that it must meet the requirements of the tests for absence of *Salmonella* and *Escherichia coli* (8). Appropriate precautions should be taken with the purchase of Xanthan Gum and with making aqueous preparations, including the use of preservatives.

(2) With the normal pH of its solutions in the 6 to 8 range, aqueous liquid preparations of Xanthan Gum may be preserved with a combination of Methylparaben and Propylparaben. If the pH is controlled at 5 or below, Benzoic Acid/Sodium Benzoate or Sorbic Acid/Potassium Sorbate may be used. Alcohol and Propylene Glycol are also possible preservatives.

(3) Because Xanthan Gum is incompatible with large cations, the quaternary ammonium preservatives Benzalkonium Chloride, Benzethonium Chloride, and Cetylpyridium Chloride may not be used.

   f. Uses

(1) Xanthan gum is used as a suspending and emulsifying agent in concentrations of 0.2% to 0.5%. At concentrations of 1% and above it gives viscous, soft-gel solutions (10).

(2) There are several official liquid vehicle preparations of Xanthan Gum in the *NF 20*, including Xanthan Gum Solution, Suspension Structured Vehicle, and Sugar-Free Suspension Structured Vehicle. Two additional official vehicles containing Xanthan Gum have been proposed, Oral Suspension Vehicle and Oral Liquid Vehicle Sugar-Free. Furthermore, there are several manufactured liquid vehicles that contain Xanthan Gum, including Ora Plus®, Ora-Sweet SF®, and Suspendol-S®. All of these are discussed in Chapter 21, Vehicles for Liquid Preparations.

4. Sodium Alginate NF

   a. Description

(1) Sodium Alginate is a polysaccharide product extracted from brown seaweeds using dilute alkali. It consists mainly of the sodium salt of Alginic Acid, which is a polyuronic acid (10).

    (2) It is a yellowish-white coarse or fine powder; practically odorless and tasteless. The pH of a 1% w/v solution is 7.2.

  b. Solubility

    (1) It is slowly soluble in water, forming viscous colloidal solutions that may be converted into a gel by the addition of divalent cations, particularly calcium, or by the reduction of pH (10).

    (2) It is insoluble in alcohol and in hydroalcoholic solutions that contain greater than 30% alcohol. It is also insoluble in aqueous solutions when the pH is below 3. This is because of the conversion of its carboxylate ions to un-ionized carboxylic acids groups.

  c. Incompatibilities

    (1) Sodium Alginate solutions are most stable between pH 4 and 10 (6). As stated above, below pH 3, the free acid precipitates.

    (2) Sodium Alginate is reported to be incompatible with acridine derivatives, crystal violet, Phenylmercuric Acetate and Nitrate, and heavy metals. Alcohol concentrations of greater than 5% are also reported to be incompatible (6).

    (3) As stated above, the addition of calcium salts and other divalent cations causes gelation; depending on the situation, this can be considered either a desired outcome or an incompatibility. Other electrolytes also affect the viscosity of Sodium Alginate solutions, with low concentrations causing an increase in viscosity and high concentrations a precipitation of the polymer. For example, a Sodium Chloride concentration of 4% or greater causes precipitation of Sodium Alginate from solution (6).

  d. Preparation of liquid dispersions

    (1) Preparation of Sodium Alginate solutions is similar to that for Xanthan Gum. If a pure dispersion in water is needed, place the water in a beaker and, using a high-speed stirrer (such as a magnetic stirring device), stir the water to form a vortex. Slowly sprinkle the Sodium Alginate onto the water to obtain a uniform dispersion. Dispersion may be aided by the use of moderate heat (45°C or less).

    (2) When other ingredients are permitted in the formulation, the preparation of a liquid dispersion of Sodium Alginate can be made by first wetting the powder with Glycerin or Propylene Glycol using trituration in a mortar. An aqueous solution may then be added gradually with trituration until a smooth, thick liquid or gel is obtained.

  e. Preservation of aqueous dispersions

    (1) Because Sodium Alginate is extracted from seaweed, microbiological contamination is possible. The *NF* monograph for Sodium Alginate states that the total bacterial count may not exceed 200 per g, and tests for *Salmonella* and *Escherichia coli* must be negative (8). Appropriate precautions should be taken with the purchase of Sodium Alginate and with making aqueous preparations, including the use of preservatives, conservative beyond-use dates, and, when possible, refrigeration.

    (2) With the normal pH of its solutions at 7.2, aqueous liquid preparations of Sodium Alginate may be preserved with a combination of Methylparaben and Propylparaben or, for external use preparations, either 0.1% chlorocresol or 0.1% chloroxylenol (6). If the pH of the preparation is controlled at pH 5 or below, Benzoic Acid/Sodium Benzoate or Sorbic Acid/Potassium Sorbate may be used. Alcohol has limited usefulness because, as stated above, Sodium Alginate is incompatible with alcohol content of 5% or greater.

    (3) Because Sodium Alginate is the salt of a polycarboxylic acid compound, it is probably incompatible with large cations like the quaternary ammonium preservatives Benzalkonium Chloride, Benzethonium Chloride, and Cetylpyridium Chloride. These should not be used as preservatives.

f. Uses

(1) Sodium Alginate is used as a suspending agent in concentrations of 1% to 5% and as a stabilizer for emulsions at 1% to 3%. At concentrations of 5% to 10% it gives creams and pastes (6). It is used in the food and pharmaceutical industries for multiple purposes.

5. Carrageenan NF

a. Description

(1) Carrageenan is a hydrocolloid extracted from red seaweeds using water or dilute alkali. It consists mainly of potassium, sodium, calcium, magnesium, and ammonium sulfate esters of galactose and 3,6-anhydrogalactose copolymers (8). There are three types of carrageenan, kappa and iota, which are gelling polymers, and lambda, which is a nongelling polymer (6).

(2) It is a yellowish-brown to white coarse or fine powder; it is odorless and tasteless.

b. Solubility

(1) All three types hydrate rapidly in cold water, but only lambda-carrageenan (all salts) and sodium carrageenan (all types) dissolve completely at 20°. Aqueous solutions of the gelling types, kappa-carrageenan and iota-carrageenan, must be heated to 80° for dissolution when potassium and calcium ions are present.

(2) Carrageenan mixtures are generally insoluble in organic solvents and in oils.

c. Incompatibilities

(1) Carrageenan solutions are most stable at pH 9. In acid solution it reportedly depolymerizes (7).

(2) It reacts with cationic compounds (6). It precipitates proteins if the pH of the solution is below the isoelectric point for the protein (7).

d. Preparation of liquid dispersions

(1) The *NF* monograph states that not more than 30 mL of water is required to dissolve 1 g at 80°C (8).

(2) When other ingredients are permitted in the formulation, the preparation of a liquid dispersion of Carrageenan can be made by first wetting the powder with Glycerin or Propylene Glycol using trituration in a mortar. An aqueous solution may then be added gradually with trituration until a smooth, thick liquid or gel is obtained.

e. Preservation of aqueous dispersions

(1) Because Carrageenan is extracted from seaweed, microbiological contamination is possible. The *NF* monograph for Carrageenan states that the total bacterial count may not exceed 200 per g, and tests for *Salmonella* and *Escherichia coli* must be negative (8).

(2) With the normal pH of its solutions in the basic range, Carrageenan may be preserved with a combination of Methylparaben and Propylparaben. If the pH of the preparation is controlled at pH 5 or below, Benzoic Acid/Sodium Benzoate or Sorbic Acid/Potassium Sorbate may be used.

(3) As stated above, Carrageenan reacts with cations and therefore it is probably incompatible with the quaternary ammonium preservatives Benzalkonium Chloride, Benzethonium Chloride, and Cetylpyridium Chloride. These would not be good choices as preservatives.

f. Uses

(1) Carrageenan is used as a suspending agent, as a viscosity-inducing agent, and as an excipient in tablet, capsule, and suppository formulations. It is used in the food and pharmaceutical industries for multiple purposes.

(2) Carrageenan is an ingredient in a vehicle proposed for addition to *NF 20*, Oral Suspension Vehicle. The formula is given in Chapter 21, Vehicles for Liquid Preparations.

C. Synthetic Polymers
  1. Carbomer NF
    a. Description
      (1) Also known as Carbopol®, Carbomer is a high-molecular-weight copolymer of acrylic acid. As can be seen in Table 18.2, various types and grades are official in the *NF*. Several of these are available from vendors of compounding drugs and chemicals. The "P" suffix identifies a highly purified product that is suitable for oral use. The *NF* monographs for carbomers without a "P" specify that these compounds be labeled to indicate that they are not for internal use (8).
      (2) Carbomers are white, fluffy powders furnished as the free acid. They are hygroscopic and have a slight characteristic odor. The pH of a 1% aqueous dispersion is 2.5 to 3.0.
      (3) Carbomers 934 and 940 are two readily available carbomers.
        (a) In Carbomer 934, the acrylic acid is cross-linked with allyl ethers of sucrose. It forms clear gels with water. The viscosity of a neutralized 0.5% aqueous dispersion of Carbomer 934 is between 30,500 and 39,400 cps (8).
        (b) In Carbomer 940, the acrylic acid is cross-linked with allyl ethers of pentaerythritol. It forms similar clear gels with hydroalcoholic systems. The viscosity of a neutralized 0.5% aqueous dispersion of Carbomer 940 is between 40,000 and 60,000 cps (8).
    b. Solubility: Carbomers are soluble in water. After dispersion in aqueous media, the acid groups of these polymers are neutralized with an alkali hydroxide or amine base to give very-high-viscosity gelled systems. After neutralization they are soluble in alcohol and glycerin.
    c. Incompatibilities
      (1) Carbomers are incompatible with phenol and resorcinol, cationic polymers, strong acids, and high concentrations of electrolytes (6).
      (2) The viscosity of Carbomer gels may be decreased by the addition of electrolytes (10). Some grades are more tolerant to ion content than others.
      (3) As indicated below in the section on preparation, the viscosity and quality of a carbomer dispersion are dependent on the pH of the solution. The viscosity of the system is greatly reduced if the pH is adjusted above 12 or below 3 (6).
      (4) Carbomer dispersions are photosensitive and should be protected from light (13). Stability to light is reportedly improved by the addition of benzophenone with 0.05 to 0.1% Edetic Acid (EDTA) (6,13).
    d. Preparation of liquid dispersions
      (1) Liquid dispersions of carbomers are made by carefully dusting the powder onto the desired liquid vehicle with vigorous stirring or using a high-speed mixer. When the dispersion is in this fluid form, other ingredients can easily be added and dispersed. The preparation is then allowed to stand until entrapped air bubbles can escape.
      (2) The dispersions are gelled by adding an inorganic base, such as sodium, potassium or ammonium hydroxide, borax, or sodium carbonate or bicarbonate. An amount of base approximately equivalent to 0.4 grams of sodium hydroxide is needed to neutralize 1 gram of Carbomer (6,13). Organic amine bases such as triethanolamine may also be used (7,13,14). The formulas and methods of preparation of several Carbomer gels are given in Table 22.2 in Chapter 22, Ointment Bases.
      (3) The final pH of the preparation is an important factor in gel viscosity and quality. Some sources recommend that it be adjusted to neutrality (10), while others state that a range of 6 to 11 is satisfactory (6,13).
      (4) The viscosity of these systems can be increased by the addition of polyols, such as propylene glycol and glycerin, because they hydrogen-bond with the polymer (10).

e. Preservation of aqueous dispersions

(1) Aqueous dispersions of Carbomer are susceptible to microbial growth and should be preserved. Recommended preservatives include 0.1% chlorocresol, 0.18% Methylparaben with 0.02% Propylparaben, or 0.1% Thimerosal (6).

(2) Benzalkonium Chloride and Sodium Benzoate at a concentration of 0.1% or greater give cloudy dispersions with reduced viscosity (6).

f. Uses

(1) Although Carbomer 934P is approved for oral use, Carbomers are used most frequently in topical products.

(2) Carbomers may be used as emulsifying agents (0.1% to 0.5% concentration), suspending agents (0.5% to 1% concentration), and gelling agents (0.5% to 2% concentration) (6).

2. Poloxamer NF

a. Description

(1) Also know as Pluronic®, Poloxamer is a block copolymer of ethylene oxide and propylene oxide. It is available in several types; the properties of a particular type depend on the average molecular weight of the type and on the relative proportions of polyoxyethylene and polyoxypropylene present in the copolymer.

(2) The physical state of the polymer type is designated by a letter attached to the name, "L" for liquid, "P" for paste, and "F" for flake. The *NF* lists five poloxamers in the Poloxamer monograph: four that are solids, 188 (commercial grade F-68), 237 (commercial grade F-87), 338 (commercial grade F-108), and 407 (commercial grade F-127), and one liquid, 124 (commercial grade L-44) (6,8).

(3) The type of Poloxamer most often seen in formulas for compounded preparations is Poloxamer 407, brand name Pluronic® F-127. This compound is a white, practically odorless, tasteless solid with an average molecular weight of 9,840 to 14,600. It melts at 56°C. The pH of a 2.5% solution is 5.0 to 7.4 (6,8,15).

(4) Poloxamers have the unique property of forming micelles at low concentrations and clear, thermoreversible gels at concentrations at or above 20%. Thermoreversibility means that they are liquids at cool (e.g., refrigerated) temperatures but are gels when warmed to body temperature (15).

b. Solubility: Solubility varies with the type and grade; Poloxamer 407 is freely soluble in water, alcohol, and isopropyl alcohol (6,15).

c. Incompatibilities

(1) Although poloxamers are relatively stable solids, they are subject to oxidation. The official monograph states that they may contain a suitable antioxidant, but the product must be labeled with the name and quantity of the antioxidant added (8).

(2) Aqueous solutions of poloxamers are also quite stable and are reported to tolerate the presence of acids, alkalis, and metal ions (6).

(3) Inorganic salts can cause compatibility problems with Poloxamer gels if the concentration of the salt in solution is too high. It is important to be aware of this property because formulas for Poloxamer gels often contain buffer solutions; if the concentration of the buffer is too high, the desired gel will not form. The critical molal concentrations of the salts vary with the salt but are in the range of 0.1 to 0.3 molal (16).

(4) Poloxamer 188 is reported to be incompatible with phenols and parabens at some concentrations (6).

d. Preparation

(1) Poloxamer gels are not difficult to make, but they do take time. They can be prepared by adding the granules or flakes to water and stirring to dissolve. At the 20% concentration, a "snowball" is often the result, so stirring to dissolve is not possible. Amazingly, when this preparation is placed in a refrigerator for several hours or overnight, a clear, viscous liquid solution results. A sample formula and procedure for making a Poloxamer gel is given in Table 22.2 in Chapter 22, Ointment Bases.

    (2) Prepared Poloxamer 20% gels, which are buffered and preserved, may be purchased from pharmaceutical vendors. A typical formulation includes a citrate/phosphate buffer with Sorbic Acid and Methyl- and Propylparaben as preservatives.

    (3) Often Poloxamer gels are combined with a lecithin-isopropyl palmitate solution, which acts as an emollient, emulsifier, and penetration enhancer. This solution may be prepared by adding 10 g of soya lecithin to 10 g of isopropyl palmitate and allowing the mixture to set overnight. Typically 20 grams of the lecithin-isopropyl palmitate solution is included for each 100 mL of finished Poloxamer gel. The prepared lecithin-isopropyl palmitate solution is also available from several pharmaceutical vendors. The manufactured solution comes already preserved, but if the solution is made in the pharmacy, a preservative must be added. Sample Prescription 30.8 in Chapter 30 illustrates the use of this poloxamer-lecithin organogel in a compounded preparation.

  e. Preservation of aqueous dispersions

    (1) Poloxamer aqueous solutions are subject to microbial growth and must be preserved.

    (2). Depending on the pH of the solution, the organic acid preservatives Benzoic Acid/Sodium Benzoate or Sorbic Acid/Potassium Sorbate may or may not be effective. Some formulas include citrate and/or phosphate buffers, or other pH-adjusting agents to control the pH at 5 or below, and then use Sorbic Acid or Potassium Sorbate as the preservative.

    (3) Because Poloxamer is soluble in either alcohol or isopropyl alcohol, these may also be considered, depending on the concentration and use (Isopropyl Alcohol may not be used for internal use preparations). Propylene Glycol is also a possible preservative, as are the parabens.

  f. Uses

    (1) Depending on the type, Poloxamer polymers have a wide variety of uses in pharmaceutical products. They are used as emulsifiers, suspending agents, solubilizing agents, wetting agents, and binders or coating ingredients in tablets (6).

    (2) For compounding, Poloxamers are used most often as viscosity-inducing agents for topical gels. In recent years, they have been used in making extemporaneous transdermal systems.

3. Polyvinyl alcohol and povidone or polyvinylpyrrolidone are two other examples of synthetic polymers used as viscosity-inducing agents. They are available from vendors of compounding products and supplies. For information on these agents, consult the *Handbook of Pharmaceutical Excipients*.

D. Particulate Association Colloids

  1. Bentonite NF

    a. Description

      (1) Bentonite is a natural clay product that consists mainly of colloidal, hydrated aluminum silicate ($Al_2O_3 \cdot 4SiO_2 \cdot H_2O$). It may also contain calcium, magnesium, and iron. The *NF 20* lists two solid Bentonite articles, Bentonite and Purified Bentonite, and the aqueous suspension Bentonite Magma. Purified Bentonite is Bentonite that has been processed to remove grit and non-swellable ore components (8). Veegum® is a silicate with similar properties; it is the purified product of magnesium aluminum silicate.

(2) Bentonite has the disadvantage of having a rather unappealing, gray appearance and an "earthy" taste. Veegum® is white or cream-colored and odorless and has a somewhat better appearance.

(3) Both are anionic, and their dispersions have pH's in the range of 9 to 10.5.

b. Solubility: Bentonite is insoluble in water, but instead absorbs water and swells to approximately 12 times its original volume to form suspensions or gels. It is practically insoluble in alcohol, isopropyl alcohol, glycerin, and fixed oils.

c. Incompatibilities

(1) Although Bentonite is insoluble in water-miscible solvents, its aqueous suspensions will tolerate these in fairly high concentrations: 30% alcohol, isopropyl alcohol, propylene glycol, or polyethylene glycol, and 50% glycerin (6).

(2) The ability of Bentonite to absorb water is decreased by acids and acid salts, which cause its suspensions and gels to break down. In contrast, small amounts of alkaline compounds such as magnesium oxide will enhance its gelling properties. It is most stable at pH 7 and above (5).

(3) Bentonite particles are anionic, and either flocculation or breakdown of the suspension is possible with the addition of electrolytes or positively charged suspensions; the outcome depends on the concentrations (6).

d. Preparation of dispersions

(1) Bentonite Magma NF is a 5% w/w suspension of Bentonite in water. Its formula and method of preparation are given in the *NF* (8):

Bentonite	50 g
Purified Water, a sufficient quantity to make	1,000 g

Sprinkle the Bentonite, in portions, upon 800 g of hot Purified Water, allowing each portion to become thoroughly wetted without stirring. Allow it to stand with occasional stirring for 24 hours. Stir until a uniform magma is obtained, add Purified Water to make 1,000 g, and mix.

Making Bentonite Magma is a very finicky process, so follow these instructions to the letter. The *NF* also gives a method using a high-speed blender, but this method is not as reliable and can be very messy.

(2) When Bentonite is included as an ingredient in an aqueous formulation, it should be first triturated with a nonaqueous liquid such as Glycerin or with the formulation powdered ingredients before adding the water or aqueous portion (6).

(3) Bentonite Magma has a tendency to get thicker and more gel-like with aging; this factor should be considered in determining quantities to prepare for stock suspensions and when setting beyond-use dates on formulated preparations.

e. Preservation of aqueous dispersions

(1) The monographs of all three *NF* articles, Bentonite, Purified Bentonite, and Bentonite Magma, contain microbial limits that state that these articles must meet the test for absence of *Escherichia coli*.

(2) Bentonite and Veegum® both absorb cationic preservatives, therefore probably reducing their effectiveness. Nonionic and anionic preservatives are reported to be unaffected by the clay itself (6), but since Bentonite and Veegum® lose their viscosity below pH 6, preservatives, such as the organic acids, that are only effective below pH 5 or 6 would not be useful in aqueous preparations of Bentonite or Veegum®. Possible effective preservatives include the parabens, Alcohol, Isopropyl Alcohol (for external use products), and Propylene Glycol.

(3) The official Bentonite Magma does not contain a preservative.

f. Uses

(1) Bentonite and Veegum® are approved for both oral and topical use. In suspensions they offer the advantage of producing plastic, thixotropic systems, so they are very good at suspending solid ingredients. They are most useful in preparations that have sufficient quantities of opaque solids because these powders mask their somewhat unappealing appearance. An example of this is Calamine Lotion USP, which contains Calamine and Zinc Oxide and uses Bentonite Magma as the suspending medium.

(2) Bentonite and Veegum® can be made in concentrations ranging from 2% to 10%: the 2% concentration gives a rather thin lotion, the 5% magma has a nice thixotropic structure that is easily pourable when shaken, the 7% suspension is just pourable, and the 10% concentration produces a semisolid preparation.

2. Colloidal Silicon Dioxide NF and Silicon Dioxide NF

  a. Description

    (1) Colloidal Silicon Dioxide, also known as colloidal silica or Cab-O-Sil®, is SiO_2. It is a submicroscopic silica prepared by high-temperature vapor hydrolysis of a silicon compound.

    (2) Colloidal Silicon Dioxide is distinguished in the *NF* from plain Silicon Dioxide. Silicon Dioxide NF, SiO_2xH_2O, is obtained by precipitating dissolved silica in a solution of sodium silicate. The *NF* further distinguishes two types of plain Silicon Dioxide, depending on the method of preparation, and instructs that the type be appropriately labeled. One type, silica gel, is prepared by adding a mineral acid to the sodium silicate solution; the second type, precipitated silica, is very fine particles produced by destabilization of a sodium silicate solution.

    (3) Colloidal Silicon Dioxide is a light, white, very fine (approximately 15 nm) powder; it is odorless, tasteless, hygroscopic, and nongritty. The pH of 4% dispersions is in the range 3.5 to 4.4.

  b. Solubility: Both regular and Colloidal Silicon Dioxide are insoluble in water and practically insoluble in organic solvents and acids except hydrofluoric acid, but are soluble in hot solutions of alkali hydroxides. Colloidal Silicon Dioxide forms colloidal dispersions with water.

  c. Incompatibilities

    (1) Both forms are quite inert and do not have significant compatibility problems.

    (2) Colloidal Silicon Dioxide is an effective viscosity-inducing agent when in aqueous dispersions at pH of 7.5 and below. Above pH 7.5, the viscosity-inducing property decreases up to pH 10.7, when the compound dissolves to form soluble silicates (6).

  d. Method of preparation of liquid dispersions

  Although insoluble in water, Silicon Dioxide and Colloidal Silicon Dioxide are easily wet by water. Colloidal Silicon Dioxide forms aqueous dispersions at pH 7.5 and below.

  e. Preservation of aqueous dispersions

    (1) Aqueous dispersions of Colloidal Silicon Dioxide have a pH in the acid range (3.5 to 4.4), where the organic acid preservatives are effective.

    (2) Because silicon dioxide is unreactive, most other preservatives should be effective antimicrobial agents in its aqueous dispersions.

  f. Uses

    (1) The silica gel type of Silicon Dioxide is used in compounding as a filtering aid and as a suspending agent. It is a suspending ingredient in several official compounded suppositories (e.g., Morphine Sulfate Suppositories USP and Progesterone Vaginal Suppositories USP).

    (2) Colloidal Silicon Dioxide is widely used in the pharmaceutical industry as a glidant in tablets and capsules and as a suspending and thickening agent in emulsions, suspensions, suppositories, and aerosols. It confers structure and thixotropy on suspensions, gels, and semi-solid systems (6).

3. Microcrystalline Cellulose NF and Microcrystalline Cellulose and Carboxymethyl-cellulose Sodium NF
   a. Description
      (1) Microcrystalline Cellulose, also known as Avicel®, is cellulose that has been partially depolymerized by treatment with mineral acids, and the resulting material is purified (8). Although it is a derivative of cellulose, it is classified as a particulate association colloid because it does not dissolve molecularly in water.
      (2) Microcrystalline Cellulose is also available combined with the semi-synthetic cellulose derivative Carboxymethylcellulose Sodium in an official *NF* product that is a colloid-forming mixture (8).
      (3) Microcrystalline Cellulose is a fine, white, free-flowing, crystalline powder that is odorless and tasteless. It is available in a variety of grades with varying particle sizes and moisture contents, which confer different properties and uses.
      (4) The combination product Microcrystalline Cellulose and Carboxymethylcellulose Sodium is a whitish powder that is tasteless and odorless. Particle size varies from fine to coarse. The pH of its dispersions is in the range of 6 to 8. The Carboxymethylcellulose Sodium (Sodium CMC) portion makes up between 8.3% and 18.8%, depending on the grade.
   b. Solubility
      (1) Microcrystalline Cellulose is insoluble in water, dilute acids, and most organic solvents. It is slightly soluble in dilute alkali (e.g., 5% NaOH).
      (2) The combination product is also insoluble in organic solvents and dilute acids, but the powder will swell in water and gives a white, opaque dispersion or gel with nice structure for suspending solid particles.
   c. Incompatibilities: Microcrystalline Cellulose is a very stable compound, but it is incompatible with strong oxidizing agents (6). The combination product has the incompatibilities of Sodium CMC (see that description above under Carboxymethylcellulose Sodium).
   d. Preparation of liquid dispersions
      (1) Microcrystalline Cellulose is generally not used by itself as a viscosity-increasing agent for liquid preparations.
      (2) The combination product is used to produce dispersions or gels with nice structure for suspending solid particles. The method of preparing a liquid dispersion of this combination is essentially the same as for Sodium CMC.
   e. Preservation of aqueous dispersions
      (1) When in solid state, the Microcrystalline Cellulose does not require a preservative.
      (2) As stated above, for liquid dispersions the combination product of Microcrystalline Cellulose with Sodium CMC (or a similar combination) is used. In this case, the acceptable preservatives are limited to those useful for dispersions of the soluble polymer, such as for Sodium CMC (see that section above).
   f. Uses
      (1) Microcrystalline Cellulose is a useful ingredient in making tablets and capsules; it is used as a binder, diluent, lubricant, and disintegrant (6).
      (2) Because it has good flow properties, Microcrystalline Cellulose is useful as a diluent in compounding capsules using small-scale "capsule machines." For this purpose it has the advantage over soluble polymers in that it does not hydrate rapidly to form viscous gels surrounding the capsule powder when it comes into contact with the aqueous solutions in the stomach. Such viscous layers can retard the release of active ingredient from the capsule material.
      (3) The combination product Microcrystalline Cellulose and Carboxymethylcellulose Sodium produces thixotropic dispersions that are useful as suspending vehicles (6).

References

1. Martin A, Bustamante P. Physical pharmacy, 4th ed. Philadelphia: Lea & Febiger, 1993; 453–460.
2. Schott H. Colloidal dispersions. In: Gennaro AR, ed. Remington: The science and practice of pharmacy, 20th ed. Philadelphia: Lippincott Williams and Wilkins, 2000; 307-308.
3. Schott H. Rheology. In: Gennaro AR, ed. Remington: The science and practice of pharmacy, 20th ed. Philadelphia: Lippincott Williams and Wilkins, 2000; 335-355.
4. The 2002 United States Pharmacopeia 25/National Formulary 20. Rockville, MD: The United States Pharmacopeial Convention, Inc., 2001; 2496.
5. Reilly Jr WJ. Pharmaceutical necessities. In: Gennaro AR, ed. Remington: The science and practice of pharmacy, 20th ed. Philadelphia: Lippincott Williams and Wilkins, 2000; 1030–1034, 1042, 1046-1047.
6. Kibbe AH. Handbook of pharmaceutical excipients, 3rd ed. Washington DC: American Pharmaceutical Association and Pharmaceutical Press, 2000.
7. Budavari S, ed. The Merck Index, 11th ed. Rahway, NJ: Merck & Co., Inc., 1989.
8. The 2002 United States Pharmacopeia 25/National Formulary 20. Rockville, MD: The United States Pharmacopeial Convention, Inc., 2001: Official Monographs.
9. USP DI Vol. III, 22d ed. Englewood, CO: MICROMEDEX, Inc., 2002: Chemistry and Compendial Requirements.
10. Lieberman HA, Rieger MM, Banker GS, eds. Pharmaceutical dosage forms: Disperse systems volume 2, 2nd ed. New York: Marcel Dekker, Inc., 1996; 407–409.
11. Lieberman HA, Rieger MM, Banker GS, ed. Pharmaceutical dosage forms: Disperse systems volume 2, 2nd ed. New York: Marcel Dekker, Inc., 1996; 204–205.
12. Allen LV, ed. Piroxicam 0.5% in an alcoholic gel. IJPC 1997; 1:181.
13. Allen LV, ed. Featured excipient carbopols (carbomers). IJPC 1997; 1:265–266.
14. Siegel FP, Ecanow B. Dermatologicals. In: King RE, ed. Dispensing of medications, 9th ed. Easton, PA: Mack Publishing Co., 1984; 80.
15. Allen LV, ed. Featured excipient: poloxamer. IJPC 1997; 1:190–191.
16. Pandit NK, Kisaka J. Loss of gelation ability of Pluronic® F127 in the presence of some salts. Int J Pharmaceut 1996; 145:129–136.
17. Gerding PW, Sperandio GJ. Factors affecting the choice of suspending agents in pharmaceuticals. JAPhA Prac Ed 1954;15:356–359.

CHAPTER 19

Surfactants and Emulsifying Agents

I. DEFINITIONS

A. **Surface-active agents**, also called **surfactants**, are molecules or ions that are adsorbed at interfaces (1).

1. The molecular structure of these substances is composed of two parts: a hydrophilic (water-loving) portion that orients itself toward water or other relatively polar liquids or solids, and a hydrophobic (water-hating) or lipophilic (oil-loving) part that orients itself toward oil or other nonpolar solids, liquids, or gas (e.g., air).

2. Surfactants orient themselves at interfaces so as to reduce the interfacial free energy produced by the presence of the interface (2). They lower the surface tension between a liquid and a gas (e.g., air) or the interfacial tension between two liquids.

3. Surfactants can function as wetting agents, detergents, foaming agents, dispersing agents, solubilizers, and emulsifying agents.

   Note: A detailed discussion of interfacial phenomena is beyond the scope of this text. For more information on this subject refer to a book on physical pharmacy (1), or the chapter on interfacial phenomena in *Remington: The Science and Practice of Pharmacy* (2).

B. An **emulsifying agent** is a compound that concentrates at the interface of two immiscible phases, usually an oil and water. It lowers the interfacial free energy, reduces the interfacial tension between the phases, and forms a film or barrier around the droplets of the immiscible, discontinuous phase as they are formed and prevents the coalescence of the droplets.

A discussion of the emulsification process and of liquid emulsions can be found in Chapter 29, Liquid Emulsions. Semisolid emulsions, creams and ointments, are described in Chapters 22, Ointment Bases, and 30, Ointments, Creams, Gels, and Pastes.

II. DESIRABLE PROPERTIES OF EMULSIFYING AGENTS (3)

A. Molecular Structure

1. Although emulsifying agents must contain both hydrophilic and lipophilic parts, neither portion may be too strongly dominant. If the hydrophilic part of the molecule is completely dominant, the substance does not concentrate at the water-oil interface; it remains dissolved in the water phase. By the same token, if the lipophilic portion is

too strong, the substance remains dissolved in the oil. A good emulsifier should have a reasonable balance between its hydrophilic and lipophilic groups.

2. As a general rule, emulsifying agents in which the hydrophilic groups are relatively dominant produce oil-in-water (o/w) emulsions; those in which the lipophilic groups are strongest favor the production of water-in-oil (w/o) emulsions, and those with nearly equal balance may give either type, depending on the circumstances. The examples below illustrate.

   a. In the soap sodium stearate, the hydrophilic group —COO^-Na^+ is somewhat dominant over the lipophilic hydrocarbon chain $C_{17}H_{35}$—. As a result, sodium stearate is soluble in water and insoluble in oil. It does possess sufficient balance between the groups so that it concentrates at the oil-water interface and it produces oil-in-water emulsions.

   b. In contrast, calcium stearate contains two long hydrocarbon chains, rather than one, so that the lipophilic groups dominate. Calcium stearate is insoluble in water and soluble in oil and promotes the formation of water-in-oil emulsions.

   c. In both cases, the ionic portion is required. If a substance such as an acid is added to an emulsion stabilized by one of these emulsifiers, the equilibrium for the reaction $R\text{-}COO^- \rightleftharpoons R\text{-}COOH$ shifts to the right. The un-ionized form now predominates; the required hydrophilic-lipophilic balance is destroyed and the emulsifier leaves the water-oil interface and dissolves in the oil.

B. The emulsifier must produce a stable film at the interface.

1. Some surface-active agents are capable of producing emulsions, but the emulsions separate on standing or storage because the surfactant is incapable of producing stable, strong barriers to prevent the coalescence of the dispersed droplets.

2. Agents such as these may be useful if combined with a second substance that acts as a stabilizer. The surfactant is then referred to as the primary emulsifying agent and the stabilizer as the secondary or auxiliary emulsifier. An example of such a system is the use of the primary emulsifier Sodium Lauryl Sulfate with the auxiliary emulsifier Stearyl Alcohol in Hydrophilic Ointment USP.

C. The emulsifying agent should be stable to chemical degradation.

D. The emulsifying agent should be reasonably inert and should not interact chemically with any of the other ingredients in the formulation.

E. If the emulsifier is liable to microbiological attack, adequate precautions must be taken.

1. In the emulsion section of *USP* Chapter ⟨1151⟩ Pharmaceutical Dosage Forms, it states that all emulsions require the addition of a suitable preservative because the water phase is vulnerable to the growth of microorganisms.

2. Other possible precautions when emulsifiers favor the growth of microorganisms include the use of refrigeration and short beyond-use datings.

F. The substance should be nontoxic and nonirritating to skin or mucous membranes.

G. Depending on its use, it should be relatively odorless, tasteless, and colorless.

H. It should have a reasonable cost.

III. CLASSIFICATION AND CHARACTERISTICS OF SURFACTANTS AND EMULSIFYING AGENTS

A. *Water-soluble polymers:* The water-soluble or hydrophilic polymers may be grouped either by their origin or based on their electrical charge (4).

1. Based on their origin, there are three classes of water-soluble polymers: natural polymers, derivatives of cellulose, and synthetic hydrophilic polymers.

    a. The natural polymers include polysaccharides, such as Acacia, agar, Pectin, Sodium Alginate, Xanthan Gum, and Tragacanth, and polypeptides, such as casein and Gelatin.

    b. The cellulose derivatives are semi-synthetic products, made by chemical modification of cellulose to yield soluble polymers. Examples include Methylcellulose, Sodium Carboxymethylcellulose, and Hydroxyethyl and Hydroxypropyl Cellulose.

    c. The synthetic water-soluble polymers include vinyl polymers such as Polyvinyl Alcohol and Povidone (polyvinylpyrrolidone), Carbomer, which is a copolymer of acrylic acid, and Polyethylene Glycols.

  2. Based on electrical charge, the hydrophilic polymers are either uncharged or anionic; cationic polymers are uncommon.

    a. Examples of the nonionic or uncharged polymers include Methylcellulose and Ethylcellulose, Hydroxyethyl and Hydroxypropyl Cellulose, Pyroxylin, Polyethylene Oxide, Polyvinyl Alcohol, and Povidone (polyvinylpyrrolidone),

    b. Examples of anionic polymers include Acacia, Alginic Acid, Pectin, Tragacanth, Xanthan Gum, and Carbomer at a pH favoring the ionic form of the acid group, and Sodium Alginate, and Sodium Carboxymethylcellulose.

  3. Water-soluble polymers have the following characteristics in common:

    a. They favor o/w emulsions.

    b. They have the advantage of being viscosity-building agents in addition to having surface activity.

    c. With the exception of some of the natural gums, most of the water-soluble polymers are used as auxiliary emulsifying agents.

  4. Other properties of the water-soluble polymers depend on the particular chemical structure of the polymer. These agents are discussed in detail in Chapter 18, Viscosity-inducing Agents. Information is given on their individual properties, solubilities, incompatibilities, formulation methods, and uses.

B. *Anionic Soaps and Detergents*

  1. Soft soaps

    a. These are salts of fatty acids in which the positive ion is univalent, such as Na^+, K^+, and NH_4^+. The most common fatty acids are stearic (C-18), oleic (C-18Δ9cis), palmitic (C-16), and lauric (C-12).

    b. Often the emulsifier is formed at the time of emulsification by adding an alkali base (e.g., NaOH, KOH, NH_4OH, sodium borate) or an organic amine base (e.g., triethanolamine) to a fixed oil that contains a sufficient amount of fatty acid.

      (1) Soaps with an organic amine as the cation are more balanced and less hydrophilic and form more stable emulsions than the alkali soap emulsifiers (5).

      (2) Emulsions made with alkali soap emulsifying agents sometimes require the addition of auxiliary emulsifiers for stable emulsions.

    c. Soft soaps are water-soluble and/or water-dispersible.

    d. They usually form o/w emulsions.

      (1) The classical vanishing creams and other water-washable creams of this type are o/w emulsions that use soft soap emulsifiers.

      (2) Two exceptions are Rose Water Ointment and Cold Cream. These are w/o emulsions formed when a solution of Sodium Borate (borax) is added to melted White and Cetyl Esters Waxes, which contain sufficient fatty acids for the formation of a soap emulsifier.

    e. Soft soaps give emulsions with a pH in the basic range.

      (1) The alkali soap emulsions have a pH in the range of 8–10 (6) and are most stable above pH 10 (5).

      (2) The organic bases give soaps that have a lower neutrality point (about pH 8), with the pH of the emulsions nearer to neutrality and more stable to changes in pH (5).

   f. Soap emulsifiers are weak electrolytes (salts of a carboxylic acid [R-COO⁻], a weak acid) and require this ionic center for their surface activity. This means that any drug or other ingredient that neutralizes that ionic center will destroy an emulsion stabilized by these emulsifiers. Problematic ingredients include drugs or additives that are acids or that produce an acid pH (e.g., phenol, salicylic acid) because lowering the pH shifts the equilibrium in favor of the weakly dissociated, oil-soluble R-COOH form.

   g. Soft soaps are incompatible with multivalent cations (Mg^{++}, Ca^{++}) because these replace the univalent ion, forming the multiple hydrocarbon chain soap of the multivalent ion. This shifts the hydrophilic-lipophilic balance of the molecule in favor of the lipophilic type. This new emulsifier favors the opposite type of emulsion (w/o) and may cause the emulsion to "crack" or coalesce.

   h. Soaps are also incompatible with high concentrations of electrolytes and with high-molecular-weight cations (6) such as the preservatives Benzalkonium Chloride and Benzethonium Chloride. The anionic portion of the soap binds these preservatives and renders them inactive.

   i. Soft soaps are unsuitable emulsifiers for internal-use emulsions because of their soapy taste and laxative action (5).

2. Hard soaps

   a. These are salts of fatty acids in which the positive ion is divalent or trivalent (Ca^{+2}, Mg^{+2}, Zn^{+2}, Al^{+3}). The most common hard soap is calcium oleate. This is formed by reacting calcium hydroxide in Calcium Hydroxide Topical Solution (also known as Lime Water) with oleic acid found in Olive Oil and certain other fixed oils.

   b. Hard soaps are oil-soluble and water-insoluble.

   c. They form w/o emulsions.

   d. Like soft soaps, these are salts of a carboxylic acid (R-COO⁻), a weak acid, which gives the weakly dissociated R-COOH form upon addition of drugs or other ingredients that are acids or that produce an acid pH. Hard soaps are particularly sensitive to acid ingredients (5).

   e. The R-COO⁻ groups of hard soaps may interact with and bind high-molecular-weight cations like Benzalkonium Chloride.

   f. Hard soaps are unsuitable for internal-use emulsions.

3. Detergents

   a. These are salts of alkyl sulfates, sulfonates, phosphates, and sulfosuccinates. Two examples of detergents from this group that are commonly used in pharmaceuticals are Sodium Lauryl Sulfate and dioctyl sodium sulfosuccinate (Docusate Sodium).

   b. Detergents are very hydrophilic and are soluble in water.

   c. They always form o/w emulsions.

   d. As strong electrolytes, they are more stable to acids, such as phenolic compounds and salicylic acid, and are not sensitive to high concentrations of electrolytes.

   e. Because their ionic centers strongly repel each other, detergents do not form firm, intact barriers. These surfactants are most often used in conjunction with secondary non-ionic emulsifiers such as Cetyl or Stearyl Alcohol.

   f. Like soaps, detergents are unsuitable for internal use emulsions because of their soapy taste and laxative action.

C. *Cationic surfactants*

   1. The cationic surfactants are quaternary ammonium compounds such as Benzalkonium Chloride, Benzethonium Chloride, and Cetylpyridinium Chloride.

   2. They are very hydrophilic and are very soluble in water.

   3. Cationic surfactants do not make good emulsifiers but are useful as antimicrobial agents. Their properties and uses as antimicrobial agents are discussed in Chapter 15, Preservatives.

D. *Finely divided solids*

1. These are usually finely divided hydrophilic inorganic solids. When these solids are in a very fine state of subdivision, they tend not to be easily wetted by liquids, and they orient at interfaces, forming a barrier to coalescence. The most common examples of this type include the colloidal clays, Bentonite and Veegum,® and metallic hydroxides, such as Magnesium Oxide and Zinc Oxide.

2. Large quantities of finely divided solids, which are in a product formulation for therapeutic purposes, may function as emulsifiers if an appropriate order of mixing is used. An example is the emulsification of 25% Mineral Oil with 75% magnesia magma (Haley's M-O®).

3. The finely divided solids are not usually used by themselves but are useful as auxiliary emulsifiers. An exception is the Magnesia Magma-Mineral Oil emulsion mentioned above. Here, the finely divided Magnesium Oxide of magnesia magma serves as the sole emulsifier agent for the Mineral Oil (6).

4. Hydrophilic solids favor o/w emulsions and are used most often as auxiliary emulsifier for this emulsion type. There are, however, examples of hydrophilic solids present in w/o formulations. An example is the presence of the hydrophilic solids Calamine and Zinc Oxide in Calamine Liniment, a w/o emulsion that has calcium oleate as the primary emulsifying agent.

5. Finely divided hydrophobic solids favor the formation of w/o emulsions. If a large quantity of a hydrophobic solid is added to a system with the primary emulsifier favoring an o/w emulsion, the final emulsion type is difficult to predict. An example is the formulation of an oral o/w emulsion of the water-insoluble hydrophobic drug, sulfadiazine, with a non-ionic emulsifying system that favors an o/w emulsion. Depending on the exact conditions, the result may be either a w/o or an o/w emulsion. Because o/w emulsions are preferred for oral products, the formation of a w/o emulsion in this case may create a compounding problem.

E. *Natural non-ionic surfactants*

1. These include fatty acid alcohols, such as Stearyl Alcohol and Cetyl Alcohol, wool fat or wool wax and its derivatives, wool alcohols and Cholesterol, and derivatives of other natural waxes, such as spermaceti and Cetyl Esters Wax (synthetic spermaceti). These are available as fractions of the natural products or their synthetic versions.

2. Some of the natural waxes, such as wool wax, Lanolin USP (wool fat), hydrous lanolin (hydrous wool fat) and its synthetic version Hydrophilic Petrolatum USP, are complex mixtures of oils, waxes, and emulsifiers. The purified emulsifying agents in Hydrophilic Petrolatum are the non-ionic emulsifiers Stearyl Alcohol and Cholesterol. Lanolin and hydrous lanolin contain mixtures of similar natural emulsifiers. All are capable of absorbing water to form w/o emulsions. These are discussed in more detail in Chapter 22, Ointment Bases.

3. Although the purified fractions and their synthetic counterparts may be used to produce w/o emulsions, they are also commonly used as auxiliary emulsifiers to stabilize o/w emulsions when a powerful o/w emulsifying agent, such as a detergent, is present as the primary emulsifier. An example of such a system is the o/w cream Hydrophilic Ointment USP. In this product, Sodium Lauryl Sulfate is the primary emulsifier, with Stearyl Alcohol as the auxiliary emulsifying agent.

F. *Synthetic non-ionic surfactants*

1. These are complex esters and ester-ethers, derived from polyols, alkylene oxides, fatty acids, and fatty alcohols. The hydrophilic portion of these molecules consists of free hydroxyl and oxyethylene groups. The lipophilic part has long-chain hydrocarbons of fatty acids and fatty alcohols. Although they are given a chemical designation based on the primary component, these are actually complex mixtures of closely related derivatives. For example, Sorbitan Monooleate, also known as Span 80, is a mixture, but the primary component is sorbitan monooleate. Polysorbate 80 (Tween 80) is polyoxyethylene 20 sorbitan monooleate; the 20 indicates that there are approximately 20

moles of ethylene oxide for each mole of sorbitol and sorbitol anhydride. Commonly used non-ionic surfactants include various Spans, Tweens, Arlacels, and Myrjs.

2. Non-ionic surfactants have the following characteristics in common.

   a. They are neutral compounds that are stable over a wide pH range.

   b. They are relatively insensitive to the presence of high concentrations of electrolytes.

   c. They are heat stable.

   d. Because these compounds do not possess significant innate ability as viscosity-inducing agents, depending on the water–oil phase ratio and the melting point of the oil phase, emulsions made with these agents may require auxiliary viscosity-inducing agents or a viscous vehicle for the external phase.

   e. Non-ionic surfactants are mixed in various proportions to give either w/o or o/w emulsions. The appropriate amounts of individual emulsifiers needed to form a specific emulsion type can be determined using a mathematic system called the HLB system. This system assigns numeric values to fats and oils and to emulsifiers based on the relative amounts of hydrophilic and lipophilic portions present in these molecules. Examples of the calculation and use of the HLB system can be found in Chapter 29, Liquid Emulsions.

References

1. Martin A, Bustamante P. Physical pharmacy, 4th ed. Philadelphia: Lea & Febiger, 1993; 370.
2. Bummer PM. Interfacial phenomena. In: Gennaro AR, ed. Remington: The science and practice of pharmacy, 20th ed. Philadelphia: Lippincott Williams and Wilkins, 2000; 282–283.
3. Spalton LM. Pharmaceutical emulsions and emulsifying agents. Brooklyn, NY: Chemical Publishing, Inc., 1950; 4–6.
4. Schott H. Colloidal dispersions. In: Gennaro AR, ed. Remington: The science and practice of pharmacy, 20th ed. Philadelphia: Lippincott Williams and Wilkins, 2000; 307–308.
5. Spalton LM. Pharmaceutical emulsions and emulsifying agents. Brooklyn, NY: Chemical Publishing, Inc., 1950; 8–10.
6. Ecanow B. Liquid medications. In: King RE, ed. Dispensing of medications, 9th ed. Easton, PA: Mack Publishing Co., 1984; 112–113.

CHAPTER 20

Colors, Flavors, Sweeteners, and Scents

I. COLORS

A. Colors are substances added to drug products solely for the purpose of imparting color.
1. They must be nontoxic and inactive pharmacologically.
2. They may not be added to injectable or ophthalmic preparations (1).
3. They must follow FDA regulations concerning the use of colors (1).
4. They should not be employed to disguise poor product quality.

B. Colors are added to improve patient acceptance of a product.
1. The color added to an oral product is usually selected to coincide with or complement the flavor given to the preparation. For example, cherry-flavored preparations are usually colored red, orange-flavored preparations are colored orange, mint-flavored preparations may be green or white, and so on.
2. Flesh-toned colors may be added to topical preparations so that the preparation blends with the color of the skin and is less visible.

C. The colors used in pharmaceutical products are either natural colors or synthetic dyes.
1. Natural colors that are used in drug products fall into two classes: mineral pigments and plant pigments.
   a. Examples of mineral pigments include Red Ferric Oxide, Titanium Oxide, and carbon black. Red Ferric Oxide is the red component that, when added to white Zinc Oxide powder, gives the pink-colored powder Calamine. Titanium Oxide is a white pigment that is often added to oral or topical preparations and cosmetics. It is also used in tablet coatings and in capsule shells to render them opaque.
   b. Plant pigments include colors such as indigo, saffron, and beta-carotene.
2. Synthetic dyes
   a. As their name indicates, synthetic dyes are chemically synthesized. The first dyes of this sort were synthesized from aniline; because aniline was extracted from coal tar, this whole class of colors is often referred to either as aniline dyes or coal tar dyes.
   b. Synthetic dyes owe their colors to the presence of certain unsaturated groups called chromophores. Often conjugation of unsaturated systems is a requirement for color. The color of the dye or its intensity can be altered by the presence of other groups called auxochromes (2).

    c. Dyes used in foods, drugs, and cosmetics must be certified by the FDA for such use.

      (1) FD&C dyes may be used in foods, drugs, and cosmetics.

      (2) D&C dyes are certified for use in drugs and cosmetics.

      (3) External D&C dyes are restricted for use in externally applied drugs and cosmetics.

      (4) It is important to keep abreast of the current legal status of dyes used in drug products because changes do occur. For example, Amaranth, formerly certified FD&C Red #2, was at one time used extensively in processed food products and was the most frequently used dye in compounding pharmaceutical preparations. In 1976 it was banned from use in foods, drugs, and cosmetics.

    d. Dyes may be affected by changes in pH, and most are labile to either oxidation or reduction reactions. These changes may affect the dye's solubility, may change its color or hue, or may destroy its color all together. Table 20.1 lists several water-soluble FD&C certified dyes that are currently available from vendors of compounding drugs and chemicals. The table shows factors that affect the stability of each of these dyes (3). This information is helpful in selecting a particular dye for a product being prepared.

3. Recommended dye concentrations for drug preparation

    a. Appropriate concentrations of dye can best be determined by trial. The general guidelines below may be helpful.

    b. Liquids

      (1) The concentration of dye needed to impart a satisfactory color to a liquid drug preparation is so small that it is usually most convenient to make a stock solution of the dye and use a dropper or 1-mL syringe to measure the desired quantity.

      (2) Color may develop with a concentration of 0.001% to 0.0005%; a tint may result with a concentration as low as 0.0001% (2).

      (3) Rather than purchasing powdered dyes, some pharmacists find it more convenient to buy food coloring from the grocery store. These colors are FD&C-approved and may be used for drug preparations. Their stability in the preparation, however, cannot be predicted unless the exact dye is specified on the label. Some labels do give this information. For example, a bottle of green food color was labeled: water, propylene glycol, FD&C Blue #1, FD&C Yellow #5, 0.1% Propylparaben as a preservative.

TABLE 20.1 Stability of Some FD&C Certified Dyes to Various Factors Which May Influence Their Color Stability in Pharmaceutical Preparations (3)

FD&C Certified dyes	Acid	Alkali	Light	Reducing Agents	Oxidizing Agents	pH value[a]
FD&C Blue # 1 (Brilliant Blue)	Moderate	Moderate	Good	Good	Poor	4.9–5.6
FD&C Blue # 2 (Indigo Carmine)	Good	Moderate	Poor	Moderate	Poor	8.5
FD&C Green # 3 (Fast Green FCF)	Good	Poor	Good	Good	Poor	4.2–5.8
FD&C Red # 3 (Erythrosine)	Poor	Good	Fair	Moderate	Fair	7.7
FD&C Yellow # 5 (Tartrazine)	Good	Good	Good	Poor	Fair	6.8
FD&C Yellow # 6 (Sunset Yellow FCF)	Good	Good	Good	Poor	Fair	6.6
FD&C Red # 40	Good	Good	Good	Poor	Fair	7.3

[a]pH values of 1% aqueous solutions (or suspensions).

    c. Powders

      (1) A concentration of approximately 0.1% would give a pastel color to white powders (2). The dye should be incorporated using geometric dilution and trituration.

II. FLAVORS AND SWEETENERS

A. Although intuitively we all know what flavor is, this characteristic is difficult to adequately define and quantify in precise terms. This is because flavor embodies a group of sensations including taste, smell, touch, sight, and sometimes even sound.

B. Even a single sensation such as taste is difficult to describe: although the four primary tastes are sweet, sour, salty, and bitter, even a combination of these taste types could never be expected to describe the taste of a ripe strawberry or a frosty glass of root beer.

C. Flavors and sweeteners are added to oral dosage forms to improve patient acceptance of the preparation. Selecting a desirable flavor for a compounded drug preparation is important because patient compliance with a medication regimen may depend on the flavor of the drug preparation. This is especially true with children.

    1. Flavors may be added to improve the palatability of a bland preparation or to mask the unpleasant taste of an active ingredient. Bitter is the most objectionable taste to patients and is unfortunately the most common taste for drugs.

    2. As with coloring, determining the type and amount of flavor and sweetener is best done by trial.

    3. When possible, selection of flavoring for a drug preparation should be done in consultation with the patient.

      a. Flavor preference is somewhat age-related. Children tend to prefer sweet, fruity, and bubblegum-type flavors, whereas adults often favor flavors like chocolate, coffee, licorice, maple, or butterscotch.

      b. Flavors are also a matter of personal preference; for example, some patients love the taste of chocolate, while others dislike it. Although a certain flavor may do the best job of masking a particular drug taste, it is not useful if the intended patient dislikes that flavor.

      c. Be aware that some patients associate bitter taste with drug potency and effectiveness.

      d. Always check with patients for possible allergy to specific flavors.

D. It is useful to recognize that there are some correlations between certain chemical types and the four primary tastes.

    1. Sour taste is the result of H^+ ions and is proportional to the hydrogen ion concentration and the compound's lipid solubility (2). Therefore, obviously acids and phenols would generally exhibit sour tastes, but tannins, alum, and lactones are also reported to have this characteristic (2).

    2. Salty tastes are associated with inorganic or low-molecular-weight ionic compounds, such as sodium chloride (thus the name "salt"), ammonium chloride, potassium gluconate, and sodium salicylate.

    3. When one of the ions in a salt is a high-molecular-weight compound, such as Diphenhydramine HCl, the taste is usually bitter. Free bases and amides such as Caffeine, Amphetamine, and Codeine are also bitter.

    4. Sweetness is most often associated with the low-molecular-weight polyhydroxy compounds, such as sucrose, sorbitol, and mannitol, but various other groups may give intensely sweet compounds. Imides such as saccharin and amino acid combinations such as those in aspartame are very sweet; these structure–activity relationships are unpredictable, and in fact both of these compounds, widely used as sweeteners, were discovered by accident.

    5. Unsaturation in organic compounds may give sharp, burning tastes (2).

E. Methods of Improving the Palatability of Oral Preparations (2,4)

1. Blending

   a. Blended flavors often give improved taste. For example, Compound Orange Spirit, which is illustrated below, is a blend that has been found to give a pleasant flavor.

   b. Try to select a flavor that either blends with or is associated with the drug taste or type. Further improvement may be achieved by then adding a sweetener or blending in another complementary flavor.

      (1) A sour drug tastes best when flavored with a citrus or fruity flavor plus an added sweetener.

      (2) Antacids are most often associated with mint flavor, so this would be a good choice for this type of preparation. The flavor will be improved further by adding a sweetener.

      (3). Bitter taste can often be improved by adding a salty, sweet, or sour flavor.

2. Masking or overshadowing

   a. To cover up the taste of the drug, add a flavor and/or sweetener that has an intense, long-lasting taste. Peppermint, wintergreen (methyl salicylate), and licorice (glycyrrhiza) are examples of compounds of this type.

   b. Up to a point, increasing the concentration of a flavor or sweetener increases the intensity of its flavor.

3. Physical

   a. Because solubility is a requirement for taste, a bad-tasting drug can be rendered tasteless by using an insoluble form of the drug or by precipitating the drug from solution by altering the pH or the solvent system of the drug preparation.

   b. Oils can be emulsified; for example, Castor Oil Emulsion is much more palatable than liquid Castor Oil.

   c. A viscous vehicle can be used to reduce the contact of the drug with the taste buds on the tongue.

4. Chemical

   Chemical methods are used most frequently in drug-product manufacturing. In this case, the drug may be complexed, a pro-drug can be made, and so on.

5. Physiological

   a. The addition of an extremely small quantity of an anesthetizing agent can be used. Examples include Menthol, Peppermint Oil, and sodium phenolate.

   b. Effervescence can be added to the preparation or the patient can be instructed to take the medication with a carbonated beverage. Carbon dioxide anesthetizes the taste buds.

   c. The preparation can be stored in the refrigerator. Cold both reduces the intensity of disagreeable tastes and anesthetizes the taste buds.

F. Sweeteners

1. Table 20.2 gives the articles listed as sweetening agents in the *USP 25-NF 20* (5). Although this list is representative of the most commonly used agents, it is not a complete list of all agents used as sweeteners in foods and in drug products and preparations. The *Handbook of Pharmaceutical Excipients* lists and describes a number of other compounds used by manufacturers and pharmacists. Some very nice natural sweeteners, such as stevia powder, are available from some pharmaceutical vendors and health food stores.

2. Desirable properties of sweeteners include: colorless, odorless, soluble in water at the concentration needed for sweetness, pleasant taste with no bitter aftertaste, chemically stable at normal temperatures of use and storage, stable over a broad pH range, non-carcinogenic, and nontoxic.

3. Polyhydroxy compounds

   Note: The solubilities and descriptions given below are abstracted from *Remington: The Science and Practice of Pharmacy* (6) and *The Merck Index* (7).

TABLE 20.2 USP and NF Excipients Categorized as Flavors and Perfumes and Sweetening Agents (5)

Flavors and Perfumes	Sweetening Agents
Anethole	Aspartame
Benzaldehyde	Dextrates
Ethyl Vanillin	Dextrose
Menthol	Dextrose Excipient
Methyl Salicylate	Fructose
Monosodium Glutamate	Mannitol
Peppermint	Saccharin
Peppermint Oil	Saccharin Calcium
Peppermint Spirit	Saccharin Sodium
Rose	Sorbitol
Stronger Rose Water	Sorbitol Solution
Thymol	Sucralose
Vanillin	Sucrose
	Sugar, Compressible
	Sugar, Confectioner's
	Syrup

  a. Sucrose NF

    (1) Description: Colorless or white crystals or powder; odorless, sweet taste, neutral to litmus

    (2) Solubility: 1 g/0.5 mL water, 170 mL alcohol, less than 0.2 mL boiling water

    (3) Available as pure crystals or powder, as Syrup NF (described in Chapter 21, Vehicles for Liquid Preparations), and as Confectioner's Sugar NF, which is 96% sucrose mixed with corn starch in a fine, white powder.

  b. Sorbitol NF

    (1) Description: White powder, granules, or flakes; hygroscopic; odorless; neutral to litmus

    (2) Solubility: 1 g/0.45 mL water; slightly soluble in alcohol

    (3) Sweetness: approximately 0.5–0.7 times as sweet as sucrose (8)

    (4) Available as powder or as the 70% Sorbitol Solution USP (described in Chapter 21, Vehicles for Liquid Preparations)

    (5) When vigorously mixed with liquid Polyethylene Glycol (e.g., PEG 300 or 400), a waxy, water-soluble gel with a melting point of 35–40°C may result (9).

  c. Mannitol USP

    (1) Description: White, crystalline powder or granules; odorless; neutral to litmus

    (2) Solubility: 1 g/5.5 mL water, 83 mL alcohol, 18 mL glycerin

    (3) Sweetness: approximately 0.7 times as sweet as sucrose; very smooth "mouth feel" (8)

    (4) For nonsterile products and preparations, Mannitol is available as powder and as granules. It is also available as a sterile injection in concentrations ranging from 5% to 25%, which are used parenterally for the treatment of oliguria, and to treat elevated intracranial and intraocular pressures. Incompatibilities of these solutions can be found in a current edition of *The Handbook of Injectable Drugs.*

    (5) Mannitol is an isomer of Sorbitol, and whereas Sorbitol is hygroscopic, Mannitol does not sorb water even at high relative humidity (9).

4. Saccharin compounds

  a. Saccharin NF

    (1) Description: White, odorless crystals or powder; solutions acid to litmus (pH = 2.0)

    (2) Solubility: 1 g/290 mL water, 31 mL alcohol, 25 mL boiling water, 50 mL glycerin

    (3) Sweetness: approximately 500 times as sweet as sucrose in dilute solution, with sweetness detectable at 1:100,000 concentration (7); 60 mg is equivalent in sweetening power to 30 g of sucrose (6)

    (4) Available as powder, Saccharin is used in a concentration of 0.02–0.5% (9).

  b. Saccharin Sodium USP (also known as soluble saccharin)

    (1) Description: White, odorless crystals or powder; the dihydrate effloresces; pH of a 10% solution is reported to be 6.6 (9)

    (2) Solubility: 1 g/1.5 mL water, 50 mL alcohol, 3.5 mL propylene glycol

    (3) Sweetness: approximately 300–500 times as sweet as sucrose in dilute solution (7,8). Bitter aftertaste noticeable at moderate to high concentration.

    (4) Available as powder and as soluble tablets, 15, 30, and 60 mg. An official USP article, Saccharin Sodium Oral Solution, has a pH range of 3.0–5.0.

    (5) Sodium Saccharin has the advantage of high water solubility. In oral solutions and syrups, it is used in a concentration range of 0.04% to 0.6%. It works synergistically with other sweeteners such as aspartame and cyclamates (9).

  c. Saccharin Calcium USP

    (1) Description: White, odorless crystals or powder

    (2) Solubility: 1 g/2.6 mL water, 4.7 mL alcohol

    (3) Sweetness: approximately 300 times as sweet as sucrose in dilute solution (6)

    (4) Available as powder

    (5) Calcium Saccharin has the advantage of good solubility in both water and alcohol, so it is easy to use in both syrups and elixirs.

  d. Since 1974, when studies were released by the Canadian Health Protection Branch linking saccharin to induction of bladder tumors in rats, there has been controversy about the safety of saccharin. Manufactured products or processed foods that contain saccharin must bear a warning about the possible carcinogenicity of this compound. It is generally thought that in moderate amounts, saccharin is safe for consumption. The Joint Food and Agriculture Organization/World Health Organization (FAO/WHO) Expert Committee on Food Additives recommends 2.5 mg/kg as an acceptable daily intake for saccharin or one of its salts (8).

  5. Aspartame NF

  a. Aspartame is a combination of two amino acids, L-aspartic acid and L-phenylalanine in its methyl ester form. Both amino acids are found in regular protein foods. Neither is sweet by itself (8).

  b. Description: White, odorless powder. The manufactured product Equal® contains dextrose and maltodextrin as diluents for improved flow properties. The pH of a 0.8% solution is 4.5 to 6.0 (9).

  c. Solubility: Slightly soluble in water, 1 g/100 mL, with increased solubility in acidic solutions (8). Slightly soluble in alcohol (9). Diluents or other excipients in commercial products may have more limited water solubility.

  d. Sweetness: Aspartame is approximately 180 times as sweet as sucrose (8). It works synergistically with other sweeteners such as saccharin (9).

  e. Aspartame is not stable to heat (e.g., heat sterilization, baking in an oven).

  f. Because Aspartame contains phenylalanine, it should not be used by phenylketonurics (people with an inherited inability to metabolize phenylalanine).

G. Flavors

  1. Table 20.2 gives the articles listed as flavors and perfumes in the *USP 25-NF 20* (5).

  a. Although this list is representative of some commonly used agents, it is not a very complete list of flavors used in foods and in drug products and preparations. Furthermore, approximately 16 monographs for flavoring agents that were formerly official in the *USP* or *NF* have been readmitted with the First Supplement to the *NF 20*. These are listed in Table 20.3.

TABLE 20.3 Flavoring Agents Added to *NF 20* in First Supplement (10)

Anise Oil	Clove Oil
Caraway	Fennel Oil
Caraway Oil	Lemon Oil
Cardamom Oil	Licorice Fluidextract
Cardamom Seed	Orange Oil
Compound Cardamom Tincture	Sweet Orange Peel Tincture
Cherry Juice	Vanilla
Chocolate	Vanilla Tincture

   b. *Remington: The Science and Practice of Pharmacy* has a more complete list of flavoring agents and has monograph descriptions for a number of compounds used by manufacturers and pharmacists.

2. A wide variety of flavor concentrates are available from numerous sources.

   a. Vendors of compounding drugs and chemicals are a good source of flavors. Catalogs from some of these companies have long lists of available flavor concentrates; some companies even offer special flavors, such as beef, liver, and fish, that are intended for compounding for animals. Some of the concentrates indicate that they can be used at concentrations of 0.2–0.5%.

   b. Food stores, including grocery stores and stores that specialize in supplies for baking and candy making, are another source of flavors.

   c. Some pharmaceutical suppliers also specialize in marketing flavors and scents for compounding. One such company is LorAnn Oil (1-800-248-1302).

3. Most flavors are available either as oils (e.g., Lemon Oil, Orange Oil) or as alcoholic concentrates. If an oil is to be added to an aqueous solution, it must be solubilized first by adding it to Alcohol, Glycerin, Propylene Glycol, or a similar solvent that is approved for oral use.

4. Often blended flavors give improved taste. Two examples of blended flavors are Compound Orange Spirit and Compound Cardamom Tincture. The formula given here for Compound Orange Spirit (6) illustrates this type of flavoring agent.

Orange Oil	200 mL
Lemon Oil	50 mL
Coriander Oil	20 mL
Anise Oil	5 mL
Alcohol, a sufficient quantity to make	1,000 mL

   Mix the oils with sufficient alcohol to make the product measure 1,000 mL.
   Alcohol Content: 65% to 75%

III. SCENTS

A. Scents may be added to topical preparations to improve their esthetic appeal.

B. As stated above, Table 20.2 gives the articles listed as flavors and perfumes in the *USP 25-NF 20* (5).

C. Two readily available scents are:

1. Methyl Salicylate NF, which is synthetic oil of wintergreen

2. Rose scent, which is available in a variety of forms

   a. The official forms are Rose Oil NF, which is a colorless or light yellow oil, and Stronger Rose Water, which is a saturated solution of Rose Oil in water. Stronger Rose Water can be diluted with an equal volume of Purified Water to make Rose Water.

    b. Vendors of compounding supplies may also have rose scent available as Artificial Rose Oil and/or Soluble Rose Fluid.

D. As stated previously, some pharmaceutical suppliers specialize in marketing flavors and scents for compounding.

References

1. The 2002 United States Pharmacopeia 25/National Formulary 20. Rockville, MD: The United States Pharmacopeial Convention, Inc., 2001; 6.
2. Reilly Jr WJ. Pharmaceutical necessities. Gennaro AR, ed. Remington: The science and practice of pharmacy, 20th ed. Philadelphia: Lippincott Williams and Wilkins, 2000; 1017–1018.
3. Booth RE, Dale JK. Compounding and dispensing information. In: King RE, ed. Dispensing of medications, 9th ed. Easton, PA: Mack Publishing Co., 1984; 397.
4. Roy GM. Taste masking in oral pharmaceuticals. Pharm Technol 1994; 18: 84–99.
5. The 2002 United States Pharmacopeia 25/National Formulary 20. Rockville, MD: The United States Pharmacopeial Convention, Inc., 2001; 2498.
6. Reilly Jr WJ. Pharmaceutical necessities. Gennaro AR, ed. Remington: The science and practice of pharmacy, 20th ed. Philadelphia: Lippincott Williams and Wilkins, 2000; 1020–1027.
7. Budavari S, ed. The Merck Index, 11th ed. Rathway, NJ: Merck & Co., Inc., 1989.
8. Murphy DH. A practical compendium on sweetening agents. Am Pharm 1983; 23:32–37.
9. Kibbe AH. Handbook of pharmaceutical excipients, 3d ed., Washington DC: American Pharmaceutical Association and Pharmaceutical Presss, 2000.
10. The 2002 United States Pharmacopeia 25/National Formulary 20, First Supplement. Rockville, MD: The United States Pharmacopeial Convention, Inc., 2002: Official Monographs.

CHAPTER 21

Vehicles for Liquid Preparations

I. INTRODUCTION

A. A vehicle for a liquid dosage form may be a pharmaceutical solvent, a solution, an emulsion, or a suspension.

B. The desired or required properties of the vehicle depend on the route of administration for the preparation and the type of solvent system needed or desired. The definitions and descriptions of pharmaceutical solvents are given in Chapter 14. The various types of liquid systems, such as syrup, elixir, spirit, suspension, and emulsion, are given in Chapters 26 through 29, which discuss each individual liquid dosage form type. The ingredients used in liquid vehicles are described in Chapters 14 through 20.

C. This chapter discusses the general properties of liquid vehicles for oral and topical products and gives examples and descriptions of potential vehicles. For ease of use, the information in this chapter is divided into two sections: vehicles for oral use and vehicles for topical use.

II. VEHICLES FOR ORAL LIQUID PREPARATIONS

A. Restrictions
   1. Neonates (birth to 1 month): Add only the essentials.
      a. Alcohol and preservatives should not be added. The organ and enzyme systems of these tiny infants are not fully mature and do not metabolize alcohol and preservatives efficiently (1-4).
      b. Because colors, flavors, and sweeteners are not needed, they also should be avoided.
      c. Hypertonic solutions should not be used—that is, no concentrated sugar syrups, 70% sorbitol, and so on. The gastrointestinal tracts of neonates are delicate; there are reports of injury to the GI tracts of neonates caused by administration of hypertonic solutions (5-7).
      d. A 1% Methylcellulose Gel that is preservative-free is a suitable liquid vehicle for this age group.
   2. Children: Use judgment based on the child's age; infants are obviously more sensitive than are 2- to 6-year-olds.
      a. Use little to no alcohol (1). In practical terms, this means use the minimum amount of alcohol that is necessary for solubility purposes if a solution is

needed. Do not use alcohol as a preservative when there are alternatives. Alcohol content can be minimized even for solubility purposes by the addition of a less toxic solvent such as Glycerin. For example, a recommended formula for Phenobarbital Elixir cuts down on the alcohol content by the addition of Glycerin.

b. Preservatives are not contraindicated, but, especially for infants, should be used only when necessary. In some cases you may substitute refrigeration and a short beyond-use date for the preservative. If this is done, be certain that the caregiver understands the importance of proper storage conditions and the hazards associated with administering a preparation that has passed its beyond-use date.

3. Adults: You may use anything that is approved for oral use. There are some restrictions based on particular patient type or disease state.

a. Diabetics: No sugar. Alcohol only if necessary, and never with oral antidiabetic agents, such as Chlorpropamide, which may give a disulfiram reaction.

b. Patients with NG tubes: No restrictions, but there is no need to add auxiliary agents such as flavors, sweeteners, or colors.

c. Patients who are alcoholics, or patients on a drug that gives a disulfiram reaction: No alcohol.

B. Pharmacist-prepared Liquid Vehicles

Many of the liquid vehicles described below may be customized and made with or without preservatives, alcohol, flavors, and sweeteners.

1. Sucrose-based vehicles

a. Syrup NF (Simple Syrup)

(1) This saturated solution of sucrose in water is highly hypertonic. It is an 85% w/v or 65% w/w solution of sucrose in water. Its specific gravity is 1.3.

(2) It has the following formula (8):

Sucrose	850 g
Purified Water, a sufficient quantity to make	1,000 mL

Method of preparation: It may be prepared by adding sucrose to boiling water or by percolation, as described in the NF monograph. If heat is used, care must be exercised to prevent caramelization of the Sucrose.

(3) If made correctly, Syrup is fully saturated and self-preserving. However, if it is diluted in any way, it will support mold or other microbial growth. Precautions, such as storage under refrigeration or addition of a preservative, must be taken when Syrup is diluted in compounding. Syrup has a pH in the range of 5 to 7.

(4) It is available from pharmaceutical vendors, in which case it is preserved, usually with Sodium Benzoate or Potassium Sorbate. It can be diluted to give liquid vehicles of various concentrations, and other ingredients, such as flavors, may be added.

b. Citric Acid Syrup

(1) This syrup, also known as Syrup of Lemon, was formerly official in the *USP*. It contains 1 g of Citric Acid dissolved in 1 mL of Purified Water, 1 mL of Lemon Tincture, and Syrup sufficient to make 100 mL of product (9).

(2) Citric Acid Syrup has an acid pH, which is useful for drugs that need an acid vehicle for stability or solubility purposes.

(3) Like Syrup NF, Citric Acid Syrup is a saturated sucrose solution that is hypertonic and self-preserving unless diluted. It may be preserved with Sodium Benzoate/Benzoic Acid or Potassium Sorbate/Sorbic Acid.

c. Acacia Syrup NF

(1) Acacia Syrup was formerly official in *NF XVI* and has been readmitted to *NF 20* with the First Supplement to *USP 25-NF 20*. It has the following formula (10):

Acacia, granular or powdered	100 g
Sodium Benzoate	1 g
Vanilla Tincture	5 mL
Sucrose	800 g
Purified Water, a sufficient quantity to make	1,000 mL

Method of preparation: Accurately weigh each solid ingredient. Mix the Acacia, Sodium Benzoate, and Sucrose; then add 425 mL of Purified Water, and mix well. Heat the mixture on a steam bath until dissolved. When cool, remove the scum, add Vanilla Tincture and sufficient Purified Water to make the product measure 1,000 mL, and strain, if necessary.

(2) Like Syrup NF, Acacia Syrup is a very hypertonic solution. Although flavored and sweetened, it is somewhat bland. It has a nice "mouth feel." It is more difficult to make than a simple sucrose-based syrup.

d. Oral Liquid Vehicle

(1) A sugar-base vehicle, called Oral Liquid Vehicle, has been proposed for introduction to the *National Formulary* (11). Its method of preparation would be similar to that for Syrup NF.

Oral Solution Vehicle	
Sucrose	80 g
Glycerin	5 g
Sorbitol	5 g
Sodium Phosphate, Dibasic	120 mg
Citric Acid, Monohydrate	200 mg
Potassium Sorbate	100 mg
Methylparaben	100 mg
Purified Water, a sufficient quantity to make 100 mL	

(2) It could be used in place of Syrup NF and has the advantage of containing preservatives. Its citrate/phosphate buffer confers a pH in the 4 to 5 range.

e. Sucrose–Xanthan Gum Structured Vehicle

(1) The formula below is for a sucrose-sweetened structured vehicle that is official in *NF 20*.

Suspension Structured Vehicle NF (8)	
Potassium Sorbate	0.15 g
Xanthan Gum	0.15 g
Citric Acid, Anhydrous	0.15 g
Sucrose	20 g
Purified Water, a sufficient quantity to make	100 mL

Method of preparation: Accurately weigh each solid ingredient. Transfer the Potassium Sorbate to a beaker and add 50 mL of Purified Water to dissolve the Potassium Sorbate. Using a magnetic stirring device or manually stirring, slowly sift the Xanthan Gum into the vortex while slowly stirring. Apply minimal heat and add the Citric Acid and the Sucrose and stir to mix. Add a sufficient quantity of Purified Water to obtain a final volume of 100 mL, and stir to thoroughly mix.

Labeling: Shake well before using.

Beyond-use date: 30 days from the day of compounding.

(2) This vehicle has the advantage of including a preservative–buffer system, and it contains Xanthan Gum, which confers some structure that makes it especially useful as a suspending vehicle. Its disadvantage is that it is more difficult to make than a simple sucrose-based vehicle.

f. Other sugar-based flavored syrups

(1) Several flavored syrups that were formerly official in the *USP* or *NF* have been readmitted to the *NF* through the First Supplement to *USP 25-NF 20*. These include Cherry Syrup, Chocolate Syrup, and Orange Syrup. Because these syrups contain natural flavors as ingredients, they are best when freshly made. For example, the Orange Syrup monograph warns that it should not be used if it has a terebinthine odor or taste (10). The ingredients for each of these syrups are given here; for details on their preparation, consult the *NF* monograph (10).

- **(a)** Cherry Syrup: Cherry Juice 475 mL, Sucrose 800 g, Alcohol 20 mL, Purified Water sufficient to make 1,000 mL
- **(b)** Chocolate Syrup (also called Cocoa Syrup): Chocolate 180 g, Sucrose 600 g, Liquid Glucose 180 g, Glycerin 50 mL, Sodium Chloride 2 g, Vanillin 0.2 g, Sodium Benzoate 1 g, Purified Water sufficient to make 1,000 mL
- **(c)** Orange Syrup: Sweet Orange Peel Tincture 50 mL, Citric Acid (anhydrous) 5 g, Talc 15 g, Sucrose 820 g, Purified Water sufficient to make 1,000 mL

(2) The First Supplement to *USP 25-NF 20* also contains monographs for Fennel Oil and Anise Oil, which are made by steam extraction, and for Licorice Fluidextract (also known as glycyrrhiza fluidextract), which is made by percolation and extraction of ground Licorice. These components have been used to make Glycyrrhiza Syrup (last official in *USP XVIII*), which contains Fennel Oil 0.05 mL, Anise Oil 0.5 mL, Licorice Fluidextract 250 mL, and sufficient Syrup to make 1,000 mL of preparation (9).

(3) These natural product syrups are time-consuming to make and are probably less tasty to most children than the manufactured artificially flavored syrups described in the next section. "Natural" syrups may be preferred by some patients.

g. Aromatic Elixir NF

(1) Aromatic Elixir is useful when a sweetened, flavored, hydroalcoholic vehicle is needed.

(2) This official elixir has the following formula (8):

Suitable essential oil(s)	
Syrup	375 mL
Talc	30 g
Alcohol, Purified Water, each a	
sufficient quantity, to make	1,000 mL

Method of preparation: Dissolve the oil(s) in 250 mL of Alcohol. Add the 375 mL of Syrup in portions with stirring. Add 250 mL of Purified Water with stirring. Mix the Talc with the liquid and filter through a filter that has been wetted with Diluted Alcohol, returning the filtrate until a clear liquid is obtained. Add sufficient Diluted Alcohol to make the liquid measure 1000 mL. Alcohol content: 21.0–23.0%

(3) This elixir, also known as Simple Elixir, was originally made using 1.2% Compound Orange Spirit as the essential oils flavor. The Compound Orange Spirit is made by mixing Orange, Lemon, Coriander, and Anise Oils in alcohol (the formula is given in Chapter 20, Colors, Flavors, Sweeteners, and Scents). A more recent Aromatic Elixir formula substitutes small quantities of Orange (2.4 mL), Lemon (0.6 mL), Coriander (0.24 mL), and Anise (0.06 mL) Oils for the Compound Orange Spirit (9).

h. Iso-Alcoholic Elixir

(1) Iso-Alcoholic Elixir, also known as Iso-Elixir, was formerly official in the *National Formulary*. It actually consists of two elixirs: Low-Alcoholic Elixir, which contains 8–10% alcohol, and High-Alcoholic Elixir, which contains 73–78% alcohol. These elixirs are mixed in established ratios to give vehicles of desired alcohol concentrations.

(2) The formulas for Low and High Alcoholic Elixirs and the Volume-Percent Alcohol table can be found in older editions of *Remington: The Science and*

Practice of Pharmacy. The 19th edition of *Remington* has the vehicle formulas but not the table with volume-percent alcohol ratios.

2. Sugar-free Sorbitol-based vehicles
   a. Sorbitol is the monosaccharide D-glucitol. It has a pleasant, non-artificial, sweet taste with about half the sweetness of sucrose. It is added as a sweetener to sugar-free products. It has the added advantage in liquid preparations of preventing sugar-crystallization or "cap lock."
   b. Sorbitol Solution USP
      (1) The official Sorbitol Solution USP is an aqueous solution containing in each 100 grams of solution, 70 grams of total solids consisting mostly of D-sorbitol with small amounts of mannitol and other isomer polyhydric alcohols. By USP specifications, it can contain no less than 64 g of D-sorbitol per 100 g of solution (8).
      (2) It is a clear, colorless, odorless liquid with the consistency of syrup. It has a sweet taste and is neutral to litmus. Its specific gravity is 1.285 (9).
      (3) Sorbitol Solution can be made from Sorbitol NF, which is a white powder with a water solubility of 1 g in 0.45 mL of water (9). The official 70% w/w solution is also available from pharmaceutical vendors. This can be diluted to give liquid vehicles of various concentrations. Other ingredients, such as flavors, may be added.
      (4) Saturated solutions are self-preserving, but lesser concentrations require the same precautions as sucrose syrups.
      (5) If large quantities are consumed, this syrup can have a laxative effect.
3. Oral liquid vehicles made with natural and synthetic polymers
   a. Various natural and synthetic polymers can be used by the pharmacist to make oral liquid vehicles that have a good consistency; if desired, they may be made sugar-free.
   b. The compounds commonly used are the semi-synthetic cellulose derivatives (such as Methylcellulose [MC], Sodium Carboxymethylcellulose [Sodium CMC], Hydroxypropyl Cellulose, and Hydroxypropyl Methylcellulose), the synthetic polymers (such as Carbomer), and the natural polymers (such as Acacia, Tragacanth, Xanthan Gum, and Sodium Alginate). Details about these compounds, including their properties, solubilities, incompatibilities, and methods for preparing and preserving their solutions, are given in Chapter 18, Viscosity-inducing Agents.
   c. Methylcellulose and Sodium Carboxymethylcellulose
      (1) MC and Sodium CMC can be purchased as pure powders from various vendors of compounding supplies. Solutions and gels of these agents can be made in a wide range of viscosities by selecting an appropriate grade and concentration. As indicated above, methods of preparing solutions of these agents and suitable preservatives are discussed in Chapter 18.
      (2) Solutions of MC and Sodium CMC are clear, odorless, and tasteless. A 1% solution of either Methylcellulose 1,500 cps or Sodium CMC medium viscosity (sometimes labeled 7MF) gives a nice, sugar-free, non-hypertonic liquid vehicle that is suitable for making oral liquid preparations for neonates or other patients requiring this type of vehicle. Such a solution may also be used for topical preparations.
      (3) If used for older children or adults, solutions of MC or Sodium CMC may be customized by adding flavors or sweeteners to improve palatability. Sample Prescription 26.2 in Chapter 26, Solutions, illustrates this technique.
      (4) Often these solutions are mixed with Syrup or a flavored syrup to give a vehicle that has nice viscosity and "mouth feel" but is not as sweet or as highly hypertonic as a saturated sucrose or sorbitol syrup.
      (5) Methylcellulose is also available as the over-the-counter bulk laxatives Citrucel® (orange flavored with sucrose for sweetening) and Citrucel® SF (orange flavored with aspartame for sweetening). A similar product, Unifiber®, which is cellulose with corn syrup solids and Xanthan Gum, is also available.

(a) These powders contain no preservatives and give vehicles of moderate osmolarity, so they are especially useful when preparing oral liquid products for infants and children.

(b) The sugar-free products make good suspending media when extemporaneous products are needed for patients who cannot tolerate sugar.

(c) A proportion of 1 g Citrucel® for each 30 mL of water gives a vehicle with nice consistency.

d. Acacia and Tragacanth

(1) The formula for Acacia Syrup NF, which is a flavored Acacia–Sucrose vehicle, is given above in the section on sugar-based liquid vehicles.

(2) Non-sweetened, non-flavored mucilages of Acacia and Tragacanth were formerly official preparations. The concentrations of the mucilages that were official are 35% for Acacia and 6% for Tragacanth. Each contained Benzoic Acid 0.2% as a preservative. If used for oral preparations, sweeteners and flavors should be added to improve palatability.

(3) Currently, mucilages of Acacia and Tragacanth are seldom used because they offer no real advantages over solutions of the synthetic polymers, and they have the disadvantage of being difficult to make and are especially good media for growth of molds and other microorganisms. Furthermore, they do not offer the esthetically pleasing clear, colorless solutions of the synthetic polymers.

e. Xanthan Gum solutions and structured vehicles

(1) The following are the formulas and directions for making two Xanthan Gum vehicles as given in *NF 20* (8). The first preparation is a non-flavored and non-sweetened vehicle that can be used for oral or topical preparations; the second is a sweetened sugar-free vehicle. A third Xanthan Gum vehicle is a sucrose-sweetened vehicle; it is described above with the sugar-based vehicles. All three give vehicles of good consistency and with some structure for suspending insoluble ingredients.

Xanthan Gum Solution NF (8)
Xanthan Gum
    for 0.1% Solution   100 mg
    for 1.0% Solution   1.0 g
Methylparaben   100 mg
Propylparaben   20 mg
Purified Water, a sufficient
         quantity to make   100 mL

Method of preparation: Propylparaben and Methylparaben have limited water solubility: Propylparaben 40 mg/100 mL of water and Methylparaben 250 mg/100 mL of water. For electronic balances with a minimum weighable quantity of 20 mg, weigh that quantity of Propylparaben and dissolve in 90 mL of Purified Water, using heat to about 50° and stirring. (For Class 3 balances with a minimum weighable quantity of 120 mg, multiply these quantities by 6 and take a 1/6 aliquot to give 90 mL with 20 mg of Propylparaben.) Weigh and add the 100 mg of Methylparaben with stirring to dissolve. (Again, if the balance has a minimum weighable quantity above 100 mg, an aliquot method may be needed.) Cool the solution and, using a blender or a magnetic stirring device or manually stirring, slowly sift the Xanthan Gum into the vortex, and continue to stir or blend for 2 minutes after the Xanthan Gum has been added. Add 10 mL of Purified Water, and blend or stir for 5 minutes. Allow to stand for 1 hour or longer for any foam to subside. Add Purified Water, if necessary, to make the final volume 100 mL and stir to obtain a uniform preparation.

Beyond-use date: 6 weeks from the day it was compounded

Sugar-Free Suspension Structured Vehicle NF (8)

Xanthan Gum	0.20 g
Saccharin Sodium	0.20 g
Potassium Sorbate	0.15 g
Citric Acid	0.10 g
Sorbitol	2.0 g
Mannitol	2.0 g
Glycerin	2.0 mL
Purified Water, a sufficient quantity to make	100 mL

Method of preparation: Accurately weigh and measure all ingredients. Place 30 mL of Purified Water in a beaker and heat to about 50°C. Using a magnetic stirring device or manually stirring, slowly sift the Xanthan Gum into the vortex and continue to stir to blend. Transfer the Saccharin Sodium, Potassium Sorbate, and Citric Acid to a separate beaker and dissolve these in 50 mL of Purified Water. Using moderate heat, incorporate the Sorbitol, Mannitol, and Glycerin into this mixture. Add the previously prepared Xanthan Gum dispersion to this mixture and stir to mix. Add a sufficient quantity of Purified Water to obtain a final volume of 100 mL, and mix thoroughly.
Labeling: Shake well before using.
Beyond-use date: 30 days from the day of compounding.

(2) Three additional vehicles have been proposed for introduction to the *National Formulary* (11). The first (Oral Solution Vehicle) is a sugar-based vehicle; it is described above with the sucrose-based vehicles. The second (Oral Suspension Vehicle) is a non-flavored and non-sweetened vehicle with some structure for suspending insoluble ingredients. Although intended for oral preparations, it contains no flavors or sweeteners, so it could be used for oral or topical preparations. The third is a sweetened sugar-free vehicle with some structure for suspending insoluble ingredients. The formulas for these vehicles are given here. Their methods of preparation would be similar to those outlined above. These vehicles give very nice preparations, but they contain multiple ingredients and are somewhat time-consuming to prepare; similar manufactured vehicles offer the same advantages.

Oral Suspension Vehicle	
Cellulose Microcrystalline	800 mg
Xanthan Gum	200 mg
Carrageenan	150 mg
Carboxymethylcellulose Sodium, High Viscosity	25 mg
Sodium Phosphate, Dibasic	120 mg
Citric Acid, Monohydrate	250 mg
Simethicone	0.1 mL
Potassium Sorbate	100 mg
Methylparaben	100 mg
Purified Water, a sufficient quantity to make	100 mL

Oral Solution Vehicle Sugar-Free	
Xanthan Gum	50 mg
Glycerin	10 mL
Sorbitol Solution	25 mL
Saccharin Sodium	100 mg
Citric Acid, Monohydrate	1.5 g
Sodium Citrate	2.0 g
Potassium Sorbate	100 mg
Methylparaben	100 mg
Purified Water, a sufficient quantity to make	100 mL

C. Manufactured Liquid Vehicles

    1. A wide variety of liquid vehicles for oral preparations are currently available.

        a. These products offer the obvious advantage of convenience.

        b. All of these vehicles contain preservatives, which is beneficial from the viewpoint of microbiological stability, but which may limit their usefulness in certain populations, such as neonates.

        c. For certain standard vehicles such as Syrup NF and Cherry Syrup, and some popular commercial vehicles such as Ora-Sweet®, Ora-Sweet SF®, and Ora-Plus®, stability studies for numerous drugs have been published. This is helpful to the pharmacist in assigning beyond-use dates.

    2. Sugar-based vehicles

        a. Syrup NF (Simple Syrup), artificially fruit-flavored syrups such as cherry and orange syrup, chocolate syrup, and cola syrup are available from vendors of pharmacy compounding supplies and from some food stores and candy and soda fountain supply wholesalers. These syrups have pH's in the acid range and usually contain either Sodium Benzoate or Potassium Sorbate as a preservative. Most of these vehicles are hypertonic.

        b. Ora-Sweet® is a citrus-berry-flavored vehicle especially made for compounding oral liquid preparations. It contains Sucrose, Glycerin, and Sorbitol to prevent "cap-lock," Methylparaben and Potassium Sorbate as preservatives, flavors, and Citric Acid and Sodium Phosphate as a buffer and antioxidant system. It has a pH of 4.2. Although the vehicle itself is hypertonic, with an osmolality of 3,240 mOsm/kg, it may be diluted up to 50% without losing its taste and texture properties (12,13).

        c. Aromatic Elixir NF is available from several vendors of compounding ingredients and supplies. Its formula is given in the previous section on pharmacist-prepared vehicles. Aromatic Elixir contains 21% to 23% alcohol and is useful when a hydro-alcoholic oral vehicle is needed.

    3. Sugar-free, artificially sweetened vehicles

        a. Sorbitol Solution USP is available as the 70% w/w solution from several vendors of compounding ingredients and supplies. Its formula and description are given in the previous section on pharmacist-prepared vehicles. This is a hypertonic solution.

        b. Ora-Sweet SF® is a citrus-berry-flavored, sugar-free, alcohol-free vehicle made for compounding oral liquid preparations when a specialized vehicle of this type is needed. It contains Xanthan Gum, Glycerin, and Sorbitol to give it body and texture, Sodium Saccharin for sweetness, Methyl- and Propylparaben and Potassium Sorbate as preservatives, Citric Acid and Sodium Citrate as a buffering and antioxidant system, and flavors. It has a pH of 4.2. Although the vehicle itself is hypertonic, with an osmolality of 2,150 mOsm/kg, it may be diluted up to 50% without losing its taste and texture properties (12,13).

    4. Non-sweetened vehicles

        a. These vehicles provide structured systems especially useful for suspending insoluble ingredients in liquid preparations. They may be used as vehicles for either oral or topical preparations but must be sweetened and/or flavored if a palatable preparation for oral use is needed.

        b. Ora-Plus® is a thixotropic vehicle containing Microcrystalline Cellulose, Sodium Carboxymethylcellulose, Xanthan Gum, and Carrageenan as suspending agents, as well as preservatives, buffers, and an antifoaming agent. It contains no sugar, sweeteners, flavors, or alcohol. It has a pH of 4.2 and a more nearly isotonic osmolality of 230 mOsm/kg. It may be diluted up to 50% without losing its suspending properties. It is marketed specifically for compounding oral suspensions (12,13).

        c. Suspendol-S® is marketed for compounding suspensions for vaginal and rectal use but may also be used for compounding oral suspensions. It is described below in the section on vehicles for topical administration.

III. VEHICLES FOR TOPICAL LIQUID PRODUCTS

A. Restrictions

There are not as many restrictions on vehicles for preparations intended for topical administration.

1. The pharmacist must be sure that the patient is not allergic to any of the ingredients in the preparation.
2. Ingredients that may be sensitizing or irritating should be avoided.
3. If the product is to be used on denuded areas, osmolarity should be considered.

B. Pharmacist-prepared Liquid Vehicles for Topical Administration

1. Various natural and synthetic polymers can be used by the pharmacist to make liquid vehicles for topical preparations. The natural gums, such as Acacia, Tragacanth, and Xanthan Gum, and the semi-synthetic cellulose derivatives, such as Methylcellulose and Sodium Carboxymethylcellulose, are described previously in this chapter and in Chapter 18, Viscosity-inducing Agents.
2. Synthetic polymers, such as Carbomer and Poloxamer, are described in Chapter 18, Viscosity-inducing Agents.
3. Hydrophilic particulate colloids, such as Bentonite, Veegum®, Colloidal Silicon Dioxide, and Microcrystalline Cellulose are described in Chapter 18, Viscosity-inducing Agents.

C. Manufactured Liquid Vehicles

1. Some liquid vehicles made specifically for compounding topical preparations are available from pharmaceutical suppliers. Several examples are given here to illustrate useful ingredients and formulations. This list is just a sampling; other products of this type can be found in the ointment and lotion base sections of drug information references such as *Drug Facts and Comparisons* or *The Handbook of Nonprescription Drugs*.

   a. Suspendol-S® is especially marketed for vaginal and rectal preparations, but it is also a general suspending vehicle. It contains an acrylic polymer resin, a silicone defoaming agent, Methylparaben, Polysorbate 80, and buffers for a pH of 5.5 (12).

   b. Liquaderm–A® is a hydroalcoholic solution that was formulated as a vehicle for topical preparations with active ingredients that require a high concentration of alcohol/glycol solvents for dissolution. It contains 68% Isopropyl Alcohol, 20% Propylene Glycol, 3% Glycerin, and the emulsifying–wetting agent laureth-4 (polyoxyethylene 4 lauryl ether). It has a pH of 5.5. It is sold in a special 2-ounce bottle with an applicator filter top (12,14).

   c. Liqua–Gel® is a water-soluble liquid lubricating gel with a viscosity of approximately 80,000 cps. It contains Purified Water, Propylene Glycol, Glycerin, Hydroxypropyl Methylcellulose, Sodium Phosphate, and Boric Acid as pH-adjusting agents, and Potassium Sorbate, diazolidinyl urea, Methylparaben, and Propylparaben as preservatives. It has a pH of approximately 5.0 (12). Other similar vehicles include K-Y Jelly® and Lubricating Jelly (15).

   d. E-Solve® Lotion contains 85% absolute alcohol, Propylene Glycol, lauramide-DEA, Hydroxypropyl Cellulose, Titanium Dioxide, Polysorbate 20, Polyvinylpyrrolidone, Polysorbate 80, Talc, and iron oxides (15).

   e. C-Solve® Lotion contains SD alcohol 40B, Glycerin, Polysorbate 20 and 80, Hydroxyethyl Cellulose, Polyvinylpyrrolidone, hydrolyzed animal protein, collagen, and imidazolidinyl urea (15).

   f. Vehicle/N® Solution contains 45% SD alcohol 40, laureth-4, Propylene Glycol, and 4% Isopropyl Alcohol and Vehicle/N Mild ® Solution contains 37.5% SD alcohol 40, laureth-4, and 5% Isopropyl Alcohol (15).

   g. Solvent–G® Liquid contains 55% SD alcohol 40B, laureth-4, Propylene Glycol, and Isopropyl Alcohol (15).

Note: The letter SD with alcohol stands for "specially denatured"; the numbers, such as 40 and 40B, signify the particular denaturants used. For more detailed information on this, consult the Code of Federal Regulations, Title 27, Volume 1, Part 1 to 199, which is available on the Internet at www.atf.treas.gov/regulations/27cfr21.htm or the journal article, Allen LV, Jr. Featured excipient: specially denatured alcohols. IJPC 2002; 5:380–383.

2. Many commercial topical liquids marketed for other purposes, such as cleansers, lubricants, and emollients, are suitable suspending media for topical products. Three examples are given here.

   a. Cetaphil® Lotion contains Cetyl Alcohol, Stearyl Alcohol, Sodium Lauryl Sulfate, Propylene Glycol, and parabens (15).

   b. Spectro-Jel® contains iodo-methylcellulose, carboxypolymethylene, Cetyl Alcohol, Sorbitan Monooleate, fumed silica, triethanolamine stearate, glycol polysiloxane, Propylene Glycol, Glycerin, and 5% Isopropyl Alcohol (15).

   c. Nutraderm® Lotion contains Mineral Oil, Sorbitan Stearate, Stearyl Alcohol, Sodium Lauryl Sulfate, Cetyl Alcohol, Carbomer-940, parabens, and Triethanolamine (15).

References

1. Committee on Drugs, American Academy of Pediatrics. Ethanol in liquid preparations intended for children. Pediatrics 1984; 73: 405–407.
2. Gershanik J, Boecler B, Ensley H, et al. The gasping syndrome and benzyl alcohol poisoning. N Engl J Med 1982; 307: 1384–1388.
3. Martin G, Finberg L. Propylene glycol: a potentially toxic vehicle in liquid dosage form. J Pediatr 1970; 77: 877–878.
4. Arulanantham K, Genel M. Central nervous system toxicity associated with ingestion of propylene glycol. J Pediatr 1978; 93: 515–516.
5. White KC, Harkavy KL. Hypertonic formulas resulting from added oral medications. Am J Dis Child 1982; 136: 931–933.
6. Charney EB, Bodurtha JN. Intractable diarrhea associated with the use of sorbitol. J Pediatr 1981; 98: 157–158.
7. Ernst JA, Williams JM, Glick M, et al. Osmolality of substances used in the intensive care nursery. Pediatrics 1983; 72: 347–352.
8. The 2002 United States Pharmacopeia 25/National Formulary 20. Rockville, MD: The United States Pharmacopeial Convention, Inc., 2001: Official Monographs.
9. Reilly Jr WJ. Pharmaceutical necessities. In: Gennaro AR, ed. Remington: The science and practice of pharmacy, 20th ed. Philadelphia: Lippincott Williams and Wilkins, 2000; 1020–1029.
10. The 2002 United States Pharmacopeia 25/National Formulary 20, First Supplement. Rockville, MD: The United States Pharmacopeial Convention, Inc., 2002: Official Monographs.
11. Pharmacopeial Forum, Vol. 28, No. 6. Rockville, MD: The United States Pharmacopeial Convention, Inc., 2003; 1998–2000.
12. Paddock Laboratories Product Information. Minneapolis, MN: Paddock Laboratories, Inc.
13. Personal correspondence with Paddock Laboratories Customer Service Department. Minneapolis, MN: Paddock Laboratories, Inc.
14. Paddock Laboratories. Material Safety Data Sheets. Minneapolis, MN: Paddock Laboratories, Inc.
15. Drug Facts and Comparisons 2002. St. Louis, MO: Facts and Comparisons, 2002.

CHAPTER 22

Ointment Bases

I. DEFINITIONS

A. **Ointments:** "Ointments are semisolid preparations intended for external application to the skin or mucous membranes (1)." —*USP*

B. According to the *USP*, there are four general classes of ointments bases (1):
1. Hydrocarbon
2. Absorption
3. Water-removable
4. Water-soluble

C. **Creams:** Although creams meet the general definition of an ointment, they have been given a separate class description in the *USP;* this description gives some historic perspective on the use of this term, and then states that the term *cream* is now reserved for ointment bases of the water-removable class.

> "Creams are semisolid dosage forms containing one or more drug substances dissolved or dispersed in a suitable base. The term has traditionally been applied to semisolids that possess a relatively fluid consistency formulated as either water-in-oil (e.g., *Cold Cream*) or oil-in-water (e.g., *Fluocinolone Acetonide Cream*) emulsions. However, more recently the term has been restricted to products consisting of oil-in-water emulsions or aqueous microcrystalline dispersions of long chain fatty acids or alcohols that are water washable and more cosmetically and aesthetically acceptable (1)." —*USP*

D. Although pastes and most gels also fit the official *USP* definition of an ointment, they are also classified separately in the *USP*.
1. "**Gels** (sometimes called Jellies) are semisolid systems consisting of either suspensions made up of small inorganic particles or large organic molecules interpenetrated by a liquid (1)." —*USP*
2. "**Pastes** are semisolid dosage forms that contain one or more drug substances intended for topical application. One class is made from a single phase aqueous gel (e.g., *Carboxymethylcellulose Sodium Paste*). The other class, the fatty pastes (e.g., *Zinc Oxide Paste*), consists of thick, stiff ointments that do not ordinarily flow at body temperature, and therefore serve as protective coatings over the areas to which they are applied (1)." —*USP*

E. Although the word "ointment" has the general meaning given above, the term is also used more specifically by pharmaceutical manufacturers as part of a drug product name to indicate that the drug is incorporated into a specific ointment base type, a hydrocarbon ointment base (e.g., Hydrocortisone Ointment). They use the word cream as part of a drug product name to indicate that the drug is incorporated into a water-removable ointment base (e.g., Hydrocortisone Cream). For the purpose of this chapter, the term "ointment" is used in its most general sense as a topical semisolid preparation, and information is given here that includes all four ointment classes as well as pastes and gels.

F. **Emollient:** An agent that softens the skin or soothes irritation in skin or mucous membrane

G. **Protective:** A substance that protects injured or exposed skin surfaces from harmful or annoying stimuli

H. **Occlusive:** A substance that promotes retention of water in the skin by forming a hydrophobic barrier that prevents moisture in the skin from evaporating

I. **Humectant:** A substance that causes water to be retained because of its hygroscopic properties

II. DESIRABLE PROPERTIES OF OINTMENT BASES

A. Chemically and physically stable under normal conditions of use and storage

B. Nonreactive and compatible with a wide variety of drugs and auxiliary agents

C. Free from objectionable odor

D. Nontoxic, nonsensitizing, and nonirritating

E. Aesthetically appealing, easy to apply, and nongreasy

F. Remains in contact with the skin until removal is desired, then is removed easily

III. CLASSIFICATION AND CHARACTERISTICS OF OINTMENT BASES

A. As stated previously, the *USP* recognizes four general classes of ointment bases to be used therapeutically or as vehicles for active ingredients.
1. Hydrocarbon or oleaginous bases
   a. See Table 22.1 for characteristics and examples of these bases; see Table 22.2 for some sample formulas.
   b. Advantages
      (1) Inexpensive
      (2) Nonreactive
      (3) Nonirritating
      (4) Good emollient, protective, and occlusive properties
      (5) Are not water-washable so they stay on the skin and keep incorporated medications in contact with the skin
   c. Disadvantages
      (1) Poor patient acceptance because of their greasy nature
      (2) Are not removed easily with washing when this is desired (**Note**: they may be removed with Mineral Oil)
      (3) Cannot absorb water and can absorb only limited amounts of alcoholic solutions, so most liquid ingredients are difficult to incorporate into hydrocarbon bases, and aqueous skin secretions do not readily dissipate. Possible strategies for dealing with this difficulty are discussed in Chapter 30, Ointments, Creams, Gels, and Pastes.

TABLE 22.1   Characteristics of Ointment Bases

Base Type	Characteristics	Examples
Hydrocarbon (Oleaginous)	-Insoluble in water -Not water-washable -Anhydrous -Will not absorb water -Emollient -Occlusive -Greasy	White Petrolatum White Ointment Vegetable shortening (e.g., Crisco®) Vaseline®
Anhydrous Absorption	-Insoluble in water -Not water-washable -Anhydrous -Can absorb water -Emollient -Occlusive -Greasy	Hydrophilic Petrolatum Lanolin Aquaphor® Aquabase® Polysorb®
Water-in-Oil Emulsion Absorption	-Insoluble in water -Not water-washable -Contains water -Can absorb water (limited) -Emollient -Occlusive -Greasy	Hydrous Lanolin Cold Cream Eucerin® Hydrocream® Rose Water Ointment
Water-Removable (Oil-in-Water Emulsion)	-Insoluble in water -Water washable -Contains water -Can absorb water -Non-occlusive -Non-greasy	Hydrophilic Ointment Vanishing Cream Dermabase® Velvachol®
Water-Soluble	-Water soluble -Water washable -May contain water -Can absorb water (limited) -Non-occlusive -Non-greasy -Lipid-free	Polyethylene Glycol Ointment

Gels— Single-phase systems	-Water soluble
	-Water washable
	-Contain water
	-May contain alcohol
	-Can absorb additional
	  water
	-Non-occlusive
	-Non-greasy
	-Lipid-free
		Methylcellulose Gel
		Sodium
		  Carboxymethyl-
		  cellulose Gel
		Hydroxypropyl
		  Methylcellulose Gel
		  (Liqua-Gel®)
		Hydroxypropyl
		  Cellulose Gel
		Carbomer Gel
		Poloxamer Gel

2. Absorption Bases
   a. See Table 22.1 for characteristics and examples of these bases; see Table 22.2 for some sample formulas.
   b. Absorption bases have two subgroups:
      (1) Anhydrous absorption bases
          These are hydrocarbon bases that contain an emulsifier or emulsifiers that form water-in-oil emulsions when water or an aqueous solution is added.

TABLE 22.2 Ointment Base Formulas

Hydrocarbon (Oleaginous) Bases

White Ointment USP (7)

White Wax	50 g
White Petrolatum	950 g
To make	100 g

Melt the White Wax in a suitable dish on a water bath, add the White Petrolatum, warm until liquefied, then discontinue the heating, and stir the mixture until it begins to congeal.

Other Names: Simple Ointment

Anhydrous Absorption Bases

Hydrophilic Petrolatum USP (7)

Cholesterol	30 g
Stearyl Alcohol	30 g
White Wax	80 g
White Petrolatum	860 g
To make	1000 g

Melt the Stearyl Alcohol and White Wax together on a water bath, then add the Cholesterol, and stir until completely dissolved. Add the White Petrolatum, and mix. Remove from the bath, and stir until the mixture congeals.

Polysorb®

Petrolatum
Wax
Sorbitan Sesquioleate

Aquaphor®

Petrolatum
Mineral Oil
Mineral Wax
Woolwax Alcohol

Aquabase®

Petrolatum
Mineral Oil
Mineral Wax
Woolwax Alcohol
Sorbitan Sesquioleate

These bases will absorb significant amounts of water.

Water-In-Oil Emulsion Absorption Bases

Cold Cream (7)

Cetyl Esters Wax	125 g
White Wax	120 g
Almond Oil	560 g
Sodium Borate	5 g
Stronger Rose Water	25 mL
Purified Water	165 mL
Rose Oil	200 µl
To make about	1000 g

Cut the Cetyl Esters Wax and the White Wax into small pieces and melt them on a water bath. Add the Almond Oil and continue heating until the temperature of the mixture reaches 70°. Dissolve the Sodium Borate in the Stronger Rose Water and Purified Water which has been warmed to 70°. Gradually, with stirring, add the warm water solution to the melted oil phase and stir rapidly and continuously until the mixture has congealed (about 45°). Stir in the Rose Oil.

Note: The formula for Cold Cream is the same as for Rose Water Ointment except Mineral Oil replaces the Almond Oil and 190 mL of Purified Water is used since no fragrance is added. Neither Cold Cream nor Rose Water Ointment will absorb significant amounts of water.

Hydrocream®

Petrolatum	Mineral Oil
Mineral Wax	Cholesterol
Woolwax Alcohol	Parabens
Imidazolidinyl urea	Water

Eucerin®

Petrolatum	Mineral Oil
Woolwax Alcohol	Preservative
Mineral Wax	Water

Although they each contain water, Eucerin and Hydrocream® will absorb a moderate amount of extra water.

(Continued)

TABLE 22.2   Continued

Water-Removable (Oil-In-Water Emulsion) Bases

Hydrophilic Ointment USP (7)

Methylparaben	0.25 g
Propylparaben	0.15 g
Sodium Lauryl Sulfate	10 g
Propylene Glycol	120 g
Stearyl Alcohol	250 g
White Petrolatum	250 g
Purified Water	370 g
To make about	1000 g

Melt the Stearyl Alcohol and the White Petrolatum on a water bath. Continue heating until the temperature of the mixture is about 75°. Add the other ingredients to the water and heat to 75°. Add the aqueous portion to the wax mixture with stirring. Stir continuously until the mixture has congealed.

Dermabase®

Parabens
Sodium Lauryl Sulfate
Propylene Glycol
Cetyl and Stearyl Alcohols
Mineral Oil
Isopalmitate
Imidazolidinyl urea
White Petrolatum
Water

Hydrophilic Ointment and its brand counterparts such as Dermbase® will absorb about 30% water without thinning.

Soft Water-washable Base (9)

Stearic Acid	7 g
Cetyl Alcohol	2 g
Glycerin	10 g
Mineral Oil (Heavy)	20 g
Triethanolamine	2 g
Purified Water to make about	100 g

Combine the Cetyl Alcohol, Stearic Acid, and the Mineral Oil and melt on a water bath. Continue heating until the temperature of the mixture is about 70°. Add the other ingredients to the water and heat to 70°. Add the aqueous portion to the wax mixture with stirring. Stir continuously until the mixture has congealed.

Vanishing Cream Base (9)

Stearic Acid	18 g
Light Mineral Oil	2 g
Lanolin	0.5 g
Arlacel 83	2 g
Potassium Hydroxide	0.2 g
Sorbitol Solution 70%	3.7 g
Purified Water to make about	100 g

Combine the Stearic Acid, the Lanolin, the Arlacel, and the Mineral Oil and melt on a water bath. Continue heating until the temperature of the mixture is about 70°. Add the other ingredients to the water and heat to 70°. Add the aqueous portion to the oil mixture with stirring. Stir continuously until the mixture has congealed.

Water-Soluble Base	Paste

Polyethylene Glycol Ointment NF (7)

Polyethylene Glycol 3350	400 g
Polyethylene Glycol 400	600 g
To make	1000 g

Combine the two ingredients and heat on a water bath until the mixture is about 65°. Remove and stir until congealed. If a firmer ointment is desired, 100 g of PEG 400 may be replaced with an equal weight of PEG 3350. To make an ointment that will absorb 6 to 25% of an aqueous solution, replace 50 g of PEG 3350 with an equal weight of Stearyl Alcohol.

Zinc Oxide Paste USP (7)

Zinc Oxide	250 g
Starch	250 g
White Petrolatum	500 g
To make	1000 g

Incorporate the Zinc Oxide and Starch in the White Petrolatum and levigate until a smooth paste is obtained.

(Continued)

TABLE 22.2	Continued

Gels

Carbomer 934 Aqueous Jelly (10)

Carbomer 934	2 g
Triethanolamine	1.65 mL
Parabens	0.2 g
Purified Water, to make	100 mL

Dissolve the parabens in 95 mL of warm water and allow to cool. Add the Carbomer in small amounts to the solution while stirring vigorously (or use a high speed stirrer) until a uniform dispersion is obtained. Allow to stand until entrapped air can escape. Add the triethanolamine dropwise, stirring carefully to avoid entrapping air. Add Purified Water to make 100 mL.

Carbomer 934 Hydroalcoholic Jelly

Carbomer 934	0.625 g
Alcohol USP	50 mL
10% NaOH	dropwise to pH 6–7
Purified Water	49 mL

Disperse the Carbomer 934 in the Purified Water slowly with continuous stirring until a uniform dispersion is obtained. Dropwise add the NaOH solution to form the gel and obtain a pH in the range of 6–7. Very gradually add the Alcohol in small amounts with constant stirring. If the Alcohol is added too quickly, the gel will fall apart. Also, this formula will not work with Carbomer 940.

Carbomer 940 Alcoholic Gel

Carbomer 940	0.5 g
Isopropyl Alcohol 70%	71 mL
Triethanolamine	0.67 g
Purified Water	28 mL

Slowly add the Carbomer 940 to the Isopropyl Alcohol with constant stirring. Add the Triethanolamine to the Purified Water, then add this solution to the Carbomer-IPA solution while stirring slowly. Mix thoroughly until the gel formed.

Poloxamer Gel

Poloxamer 407	20 g
Parabens	0.2 g
Purified Water, to make	100 mL

Dissolve the parabens in 95 mL of warm water and allow to cool. Add the Poloxamer to the solution (Do not be surprised if you get a "snowball"). Cover the container, put in the refrigerator, and allow to hydrate overnight. A clear gel will result. Add Purified Water to make 100 mL.

Note: A manufactured 20% Poloxamer Gel which is preserved with Sorbic Acid and parabens and buffered with a citrate-phosphate buffer is available. Often Poloxamer gels are combined with a lecithin-isopropyl palmitate solution which adds emollient, emulsifier, and penetration enhancement properties. The lecithin-palmitate solution may be purchased or may be prepared by adding 10 g of soya lecithin to 10 g of isopropyl palmitate and allowing the mixture to set overnight. Usually 20 grams of the lecithin-palmitate solution is added for each 100 mL of finished Poloxamer gel. The manufactured lecithin solution comes already preserved, but if the solution is made in the pharmacy, a preservative must be added. Sample Prescription 30.8 in Chapter 30 shows an example of a preparation of this type.

Ephedrine Sulfate Jelly NF XII (10)

Ephedrine Sulfate	10 g
Tragacanth	10 g
Methyl Salicylate	0.1 g
Eucalyptol	1.0 mL
Pine Needle Oil	0.1 mL
Glycerin	150 g
Purified Water	830 mL

Dissolve the ephedrine sulfate in the Purified Water and add the Glycerin, Tragacanth and the other ingredients. Mix well and store in a closed container for one week, stirring or agitating occasionally.

(2) Water-in-oil emulsions

These are absorption bases that contain water, the amount depending on the base.

c. Advantages

(1) Moderately good protective, occlusive, and emollient properties

(2) Do not wash off easily, so they hold incorporated medications in contact with the skin

(3) Can absorb liquids

(a) Anhydrous absorption bases can absorb significant amounts of water and moderate amounts of alcoholic solutions.

(b) Because they already contain water, emulsion absorption bases absorb variable amounts of water and/or alcohol.

(4) Some lanolin-types have compositions somewhat like the sebaceous secretions of the skin. These are thought to have superior emollient properties. *Martindale: The Extra Pharmacopoeia* states that wool fat preparations mixed with suitable vegetable oils or with petrolatum give emollient ointments that penetrate the skin and enhance absorption (2).

d. Disadvantages

(1) Some bases in this group have poor patient acceptance.

(a) The anhydrous absorption bases have a greasy nature similar to that of Hydrocarbon bases.

(b) Some lanolin-type bases are somewhat sticky and have a mildly unpleasant odor.

(2) Not easily removed with washing

(**Note:** As with Hydrocarbon bases, they may be removed with Mineral Oil)

(3) Those bases containing wool wax or wool wax alcohols may be sensitizing. Efforts have been made to remove offending principles, including detergents and natural free fatty alcohols. This is reported to reduce the incidence of hypersensitivity to almost zero (3).

(4) Those with soap-type emulsifiers (e.g., Cold Cream, Rose Water Ointment) can have the compatibility problems associated with this type of emulsifying agent. This is discussed in the section on soft soaps in Chapter 19, Surfactants and Emulsifying Agents.

(5) Those that contain water may have chemical stability problems with ingredients that are sensitive to hydrolysis.

(6) Those containing water are also subject to microbial growth, and the *USP* requires that these contain a preservative (1).

3. Water-removable Bases

a. See Table 22.1 for characteristics and examples of these bases; see Table 22.2 for some sample formulas.

b. These are oil-in-water emulsions, also known as creams.

In former times, the term "cream" was used for **either** oil-in-water (e.g., Vanishing Cream) **or** water-in-oil (e.g., Cold Cream) emulsion bases, and it usually was used for bases with a more fluid consistency. Now the term is reserved for water-removable oil-in-water emulsion bases or microcrystalline dispersions of long-chain fatty acids or alcohols in water.

c. Advantages

(1) Nongreasy and therefore aesthetically pleasing

(2) Can be removed from the skin by washing

(3) Can absorb some water or alcohol; if the amount of liquid added reaches a critical amount, the base will thin out to a lotion.

(4) Will allow the dissipation of fluids from injured skin

d. Disadvantages

(1) Less protective, less emollient, and less occlusive than Hydrocarbon or Absorption bases

    (2) Those with soap-type emulsifiers can have compatibility problems. As stated above, this is discussed in the section on soft soaps in Chapter 19, Surfactants and Emulsifying Agents.

    (3) Those that contain water may have chemical stability problems with ingredients that are sensitive to hydrolysis.

    (4) Those containing water are also subject to microbial growth, and the *USP* requires that these contain a preservative (1).

    (5) Because water is the external phase, these bases may "dry out" due to evaporation of the water. This can be minimized by storage in tight containers; humectants may be added to retard dehydration.

  4. Water-soluble Bases

    a. See Table 22.1 for characteristics and examples of these bases; see Table 22.2 for a sample formula.

    b. These are greaseless ointment bases that are water-soluble. Most are polyethylene glycol-type ointment bases, and Polyethylene Glycol Ointment USP is the only official preparation in this class (1).

    c. Advantages

      (1) Are soluble in water, so are easily removed by washing

      (2) Leave no oil residue

      (3) Can absorb some water or alcohol; as the amount of liquid added increases, the base begins to thin out and eventually dissolves. The water-absorbing potential of Polyethylene Glycol Ointment can be improved by adding Stearyl Alcohol; the formula for this is shown in Table 22.2.

    d. Disadvantages

      (1) Irritating, especially on denuded or abraded skin or mucous membranes

      (2) Little to no emollient properties

      (3) PEG-type bases may have compatibility problems with incorporated drugs that are subject to oxidation.

      (4) Those that contain water may have the compatibility and stability problems associated with water, and a preservative is required.

B. Pastes

  1. Fatty pastes

    a. Fatty pastes have similar properties to ointments, but they are usually thicker and seem less greasy and more absorptive than ointments. This is because they contain high concentrations of solid ingredients that absorb water and aqueous solutions.

    b. They are better at absorbing skin secretions, and they are less penetrating and stay in place on the skin better than ointments.

    c. The *USP* lists two official products of this type: Zinc Oxide Paste (See Table 22.2) and Zinc Oxide and Salicylic Acid Paste.

  2. There are several other official pastes, each with unique makeup: Carboxymethylcellulose Sodium Paste is a single-phase aqueous gel containing 16% to 17% Sodium CMC; Magnesium Hydroxide Paste is a thick aqueous suspension containing 29% to 33% w/w Magnesium Hydroxide; Triamcinolone Acetonide Dental Paste is 0.1% Triamcinolone Acetonide in a paste of Pectin, Gelatin, Sodium CMC, Polyethylene, Mineral Oil, Guar Gum, and Tragacanth.

C. Gels

  1. As indicated in the definitions given at the beginning of this chapter, gels are semisolids that may be either single-phase or two-phase systems. Gels may be used topically, may be introduced into body cavities (nasal, vaginal, etc.), or may be used internally (e.g., Aluminum Hydroxide Gel).

    a. Single-phase systems (See Tables 22.1 and 22.2)

      (1) The single-phase systems contain soluble macromolecules, which are linear or branched-chain polymers that dissolve molecularly in water. They are classified as colloidal dispersions because the individual molecules are in the colloidal particle size range, exceeding 50–100 Å.

(2) The polymers are classified into one of three groups: natural polymers (e.g., Tragacanth), semisynthetic cellulose derivatives (e.g., Methylcellulose), and synthetic polymers (e.g., Carbomer). These groups are discussed in detail in Chapter 18, Viscosity-inducing Agents.

(3) The continuous phase for these gels is usually aqueous, but alcohols, polyols, and oils may also be used.

b. Two-phase systems

(1) The two-phase systems consist of a concentrated network of particulate association colloids. These are water-insoluble particles that hydrate strongly. Examples include the official preparations Aluminum Hydroxide Gel and Bentonite Magma.

(2) These are thixotropic suspensions that are semisolids on standing but become fluid when agitated. The term "gel" is used when the dispersed particles are very small, and the term "magma" is used for gels with larger-sized particles.

(3) Several compounds that form association colloidal gels, including Bentonite, Microcrystalline Cellulose, and Colloidal Silicon Dioxide, are discussed in Chapter 18, Viscosity-inducing Agents.

IV. INGREDIENTS FOR OINTMENT BASES

A. The ingredients, formulas, methods of preparation, and/or descriptions of some ointment bases are given in Table 22.2.

B. Descriptions of ointment base ingredients, such as solvents, preservatives, and surfactants, which are contained in numerous types of dosage forms, can be found in the chapters covering those specific ingredient types.

C. Ingredients specific to ointment bases are described here; these include waxes, fatty alcohols, acids, and esters, and miscellaneous ointment bases and ingredients. The descriptions and solubilities presented here give a composite of information from *Remington: The Science and Practice of Pharmacy* (4,5), the *Handbook of Pharmaceutical Excipients* (6), official monographs in the *USP-NF* (7), and other references as cited. Additional information on each agent, including references to original research journal articles, can be found in the *Handbook of Pharmaceutical Excipients*.

1. Petrolatum USP and White Petrolatum USP

a. Description

(1) Petrolatum and White Petrolatum are mixtures of purified semisolid saturated hydrocarbons extracted from petroleum. White Petrolatum has undergone additional treatment so that it is nearly decolorized, and it is preferred for pharmaceutical preparations because it is reported to cause less hypersensitivity reactions. The *USP* monographs for both compounds state that they may contain suitable stabilizers.

(2) Petrolatum is a yellowish, translucent, soft unctuous mass. White Petrolatum is similar, but, as its name indicates, it is white. Both are tasteless and odorless and greasy to the touch. They have a melting point range of 38 to 60°C, and the specific gravity of the melt is 0.815 to 0.880.

b. Solubility: Practically insoluble in water, hot or cold alcohol, acetone, and glycerin; soluble in most volatile and fixed oils

c. Incompatibilities: The Petrolatums are quite stable, and there are few problems with incompatibilities. They do not mix with aqueous or hydroalcoholic solutions.

d. Uses

(1) White Petrolatum is a nice, all-purpose, soft ointment base. It is used both by itself and as a major component of combination ointment bases.

(2) If a stiffer base is desired, a portion of White Wax may be added (see the formula for White Ointment in Table 22.2).

    e. Other names
- **(1)** Petroleum: mineral jelly, petroleum jelly
- **(2)** White Petrolatum: white mineral jelly, white petroleum jelly, white soft paraffin, Vaseline®

2. Lanolin USP and Modified Lanolin USP

    a. Description

- **(1)** Lanolin and Modified Lanolin are the purified, fatty, wax-like substances obtained from the wool of sheep that has been cleaned, decolorized, and deodorized. Modified Lanolin has undergone additional treatment to reduce the contents of free lanolin alcohols and detergent and pesticide residues. This modified product is intended to reduce hypersensitivity reactions. The *USP* monographs for both compounds state that they contain not more than 0.25% water and they may contain not more than 0.02% of a suitable antioxidant.
- **(2)** Lanolin is a yellow, tenacious, unctuous mass with a slight characteristic odor. It melts between 38 and 44°C to give a clear or nearly clear yellow liquid. At 15°C it has a density of 0.932–0.945.
- **(3)** There is often confusion between Lanolin and hydrous lanolin. Hydrous lanolin, also known as Hydrous Wool Fat, contains 25% to 30% water. It is a yellowish-white ointment with a mild characteristic odor. Prior to *USP 23* hydrous lanolin was officially known as Lanolin, and the product now known as Lanolin was officially known as Anhydrous Lanolin. With *USP 23*, hydrous lanolin was deleted from the *USP* and the monograph for Anhydrous Lanolin was renamed Lanolin. You will still find references that use the older nomenclature.

    b. Solubility: Practically insoluble in water, but will take up twice its weight of water without separation; sparingly soluble in cold alcohol, but more soluble in boiling alcohol

    c. Incompatibilities: Lanolin is a natural product that may contain components that can act as oxidizing agents to sensitive ingredients.

    d. Uses

- **(1)** Lanolin may be used by itself, but it will also mix with vegetable oils or petrolatum to give an emollient base that is reported to penetrate the skin and give improved absorption of active ingredients (6).
- **(2)** As stated above, it will take up to twice its weight of water to form a water-in-oil emulsion.

    e. Other names: Wool fat, anhydrous lanolin, refined wool fat

3. Paraffin NF

    a. Description

- **(1)** Paraffin is a purified mixture of solid hydrocarbons from petroleum.
- **(2)** It is a colorless or white translucent solid; tasteless and odorless; slightly greasy to the touch. It has a congealing range of 47–65°C, depending on the grade, and the specific gravity of the melt is in the range 0.84 to 0.89.

    b. Solubility: Practically insoluble in water, alcohol, and acetone; freely soluble in volatile oils and most warm fixed oils

    c. Incompatibilities: Paraffin is a stable, nonreactive compound.

    d. Uses: a stiffening ingredient in ointment bases

    e. Other names: Paraffin wax, Hard Paraffin, Mineral Wax

4. White Wax NF

    a. Description

- **(1)** White Wax is the bleached, purified wax of honeybees. It consists mainly of esters of long-chain hydrocarbons, with myricyl palmitate the principal ester. It also contains free fatty acids and carbohydrates, with a small amount of free wax alcohols.
- **(2)** It is a yellowish-white translucent solid, nearly tasteless with a faint odor; melting point 62–65°; the specific gravity of the melted wax is approximately 0.95.

    b. Solubility: Insoluble in water and sparingly soluble in alcohol; soluble in fixed and volatile oils

    c. Incompatibilities: White wax is a fairly unreactive compound. The free fatty acids portion can react with bases such as sodium hydroxide to form soaps. This can be used to advantage in making an emulsion-type ointment base.

    d. Uses: a stiffening ingredient in ointment bases

    e. Other names: Bleached wax, White Beeswax

5. Cetyl Esters Wax NF

    a. Description

        (1) Cetyl Esters Wax is a mixture primarily of esters of saturated fatty alcohols and fatty acids (C_{14}–C_{18}). Cetyl Esters Wax is a synthetic substitute for the natural product spermaceti, which was formerly extracted from the head of sperm whales.

        (2) It is white to off-white translucent flakes with a faint odor and bland, mild taste; melting point 43–47°; when melted at 50°C, the specific gravity is 0.82 to 0.84

    b. Solubility: Insoluble in water; practically insoluble in cold alcohol but soluble in boiling alcohol; soluble in volatile and fixed oils; solubility in Mineral Oil is 14–22 mg/mL.

    c. Incompatibilities: Cetyl Esters Wax is quite stable and nonreactive; it is incompatible with strong acids or bases (6).

    d. Uses: a stiffening ingredient and emollient in ointment bases

    e. Other names: Synthetic Spermaceti

6. Cetyl Alcohol NF

    a. Description

        (1) Cetyl Alcohol is at least 90% cetyl alcohol, $CH_3(CH_2)_{14}CH_2OH$, with the remainder related alcohols, chiefly stearyl alcohol.

        (2) It is white, waxy flakes or granules with a faint odor and bland, mild taste; melting point 45–50°C, with specific gravity of the melt 0.908.

    b. Solubility: Insoluble in water but soluble in alcohol and in vegetable oils; when melted, it is miscible with fats, mineral oils, and paraffins.

    c. Incompatibilities: Cetyl Alcohol is quite stable and nonreactive; it is incompatible with strong oxidizing agents (6).

    d. Uses (6)

        (1) Cetyl Alcohol is used as a stiffening ingredient and emollient not only in ointment bases, but also in liquid emulsions and lotions, suppositories, and controlled-release solid dosage forms.

        (2) It is widely used in manufactured topical products because of its favorable properties for such formulations: emollient, water-absorptive, and emulsifying. It also gives these dosage forms a nice texture and consistency.

        (3) When applied to the skin, it is absorbed and retained in the epidermis. This accounts for its emollient, lubricating property. It leaves the skin feeling soft and smooth.

        (4) When added to oleaginous bases such as petrolatum, it increases their ability to absorb water. In fact, when 5% is added to petrolatum, the combination will absorb 40–50% of its weight in water.

        (5) It is used as an auxiliary emulsifier for both water-in-oil and oil-in-water emulsions. It is frequently used with detergent surfactants such as Sodium Lauryl Sulfate to form good barriers to coalescence.

7. Stearyl Alcohol NF

    a. Description

        (1) Content: At least 90% stearyl alcohol, $CH_3(CH_2)_{16}CH_2OH$, with the remainder related alcohols, chiefly cetyl alcohol

        (2) It is hard, white, waxy flakes or granules with a faint odor and bland, mild taste; melting point 55–60°C, with specific gravity of the melt 0.88–0.91.

    b. Solubility: Insoluble in water but soluble in alcohol, propylene glycol, and vegetable oils

    c. Incompatibilities: Stearyl Alcohol is quite stable and nonreactive; it is incompatible with strong oxidizing agents (6).

    d. Uses (6)

        (1) Stearyl Alcohol is used mainly as a stiffening ingredient, but it does have some emollient, water-absorptive, and emulsifying properties. It is used in ointment bases, liquid emulsions and lotions, suppositories, and controlled-release solid dosage forms.

        (2) As with Cetyl Alcohol, when added to oleaginous bases such as petrolatum, it increases their ability to absorb water.

        (3) In a concentration of 6% to 25%, it is used in Polyethylene Glycol Ointment to increase the water-absorbing ability of that water-soluble base (see the Polyethylene Glycol Ointment formula in Table 22.2).

8. Lanolin Alcohols NF

    a. Description

        (1) Lanolin Alcohols is a mixture of aliphatic alcohols, triterpenoid alcohols, and sterols that are obtained by the hydrolysis of Lanolin. It contains not less than 30% of cholesterol. It may contain an antioxidant.

        (2) It is a hard, waxy, amber solid; with a characteristic odor; melting point not below 56°C.

        (3) This product is a purified version of wool alcohols, which consist of a separated fraction containing cholesterol and other alcohols prepared by the saponification of grease from the wool of sheep (4).

    b. Solubility: Insoluble in water; slightly soluble in alcohol, soluble 1 part in 25 parts of boiling alcohol

    c. Incompatibilities: Incompatible with Coal Tar, Ichthammol, Phenol, and Resorcinol (6)

    d. Uses (6)

        (1) Lanolin Alcohol is used mainly as an auxiliary emulsifying agent in ointments and other topical preparations, but it does have some emollient and water-absorptive properties.

        (2) As with Cetyl and Stearyl Alcohol, when Lanolin Alcohols is added to oleaginous bases such as petrolatum, it increases their ability to absorb water; 5% Lanolin Alcohols added to petrolatum increases its ability to absorb water by three-fold.

    e. Other names: Wool Alcohols, Woolwax Alcohol

9. Cholesterol NF

        $C_{27}H_{46}O$ MW = 386.65

Cholesterol

    a. Description: White to light-yellow leaflets, needles, powder, or granules; almost odorless; melting point 147–150°; affected by light

    b. Solubility: Insoluble in water; 1 g/100 mL alcohol or 50 mL dehydrated alcohol (slowly); soluble in acetone, hot alcohol, and vegetable oils

    c. Incompatibilities: Cholesterol is a stable and nonreactive compound.

    d. Uses (6)

        (1) Cholesterol is used as an emulsifying agent in ointments and other topical preparations in concentrations of 0.3–5%.

        (2) It also has emollient and water-absorptive properties.

10. Glyceryl Monostearate NF

   a. Description

   (1) Glyceryl Monostearate is a mixture primarily of the mono-esters of glycerin with stearic acid, $CH_3(CH_2)_{16}COOH$, and palmitic acid, $CH_3(CH_2)_{14}COOH$. It may contain an antioxidant.

   (2) It is a whitish, waxlike solid with a slight, agreeable fatty odor and taste; does not melt below 55°C; specific gravity of the melt is 0.92; affected by light.

   b. Solubility: Insoluble in water; soluble in hot alcohol, acetone, mineral, or fixed oils

   c. Incompatibilities: The grades of Glyceryl Monostearate that are self-emulsifying (e.g., Arlacel 165®, Hodag CMS-D®, and others) are incompatible with acidic compounds.

   d. Uses (6)

   (1) Glyceryl Monostearate is used as a nonionic emulsifier for both oil-in-water and water-in-oil emulsions, both liquids and semisolids. It also has emollient properties and imparts texture and viscosity to topical preparations of various types.

   (2) It is also used in solid dosage forms for multiple purposes, including as a lubricant in tablet and capsule making and as a release modifier for controlled-release oral dosage forms, suppositories, and implants.

11. Stearic Acid NF

   a. Description

   (1) Stearic Acid NF is a mixture primarily of stearic acid, $CH_3(CH_2)_{16}COOH$, and palmitic acid, $CH_3(CH_2)_{14}COOH$. The content of stearic acid is not less than 40% and the content of both stearic and palmitic acids is not less than 90%. The *NF* also has a monograph for Purified Stearic Acid, in which the stearic acid content is not less than 90% and the combined acids content is not less than 96% of the total.

   (2) It is a hard, white to faintly yellowish, glossy, crystalline solid or powder with a slight odor and taste of tallow; it melts at approximately 55°, with the purified acid melting at 69–70°.

   (3) Both Stearic Acid and Purified Stearic Acid must be labeled for external use only unless it is made entirely from edible sources.

   b. Solubility: Practically insoluble in water; 1 g/20 mL alcohol, 25 mL acetone, soluble in propylene glycol

   c. Incompatibilities

   (1) As discussed below, Stearic Acid reacts with alkali and organic bases to form stearate soaps. In most cases this is an intended reaction, as with nascent soap emulsifying agents and with the in situ formation of sodium stearate in Glycerin Suppositories USP.

   (2) It also reacts with metal hydroxides to form water-insoluble stearates, and salts of zinc and calcium are reported to react with stearic acid in ointment bases to give lumpy preparations (6).

   d. Uses

   (1) Stearic Acid is widely used as an emulsifying and solubilizing agent in topical preparations. It is also used as a lubricant in tablet and capsule making.

   (2) Stearic Acid is the fatty acid part of a soap emulsifier used for water-removable o/w emulsion bases. The base part may be sodium or potassium hydroxide, sodium carbonate, or triethanolamine. When excess stearic acid is added, the unneutralized stearic acid is emulsified as part of the oil phase. This free stearic acid gives these creams a pearlescent luster; they are known as vanishing creams. Because of the inherent compatibility problems of soap emulsifiers, some newer vanishing cream formulations use nonionic surfactants, but stearic acid is still added for the desirable pearl luster.

12. Polyethylene Glycols (PEG) (7,8)

   a. Description

   (1) PEG has the general formula: $H—[OCH_2CH_2—]_nOH$.

   (2) Polyethylene glycols are available as various grades from 200 to 8000, where the assigned number indicates the average molecular weight, Those with numbers 200 through 600 are clear, viscous liquids; PEG 900 and 1000 are soft solids, and PEGs 1450 to 8000 are white, waxy solids or flakes. All are odorless and tasteless, and the pH of a 5% solution is in the range of 4.5 to 7.5. See Table 23.1 in Chapter 23 for more information on the densities and melting points of the individual grades.

b. Solubility: Although all are soluble in water and in many organic solvents, their solubilities depend on their molecular weight. See Table 23.1 in Chapter 23 for the solubility of individual grades in water. The liquid PEGs are soluble in acetone, alcohol, glycerin, and glycols; solid PEGs are soluble in acetone and alcohol, slightly soluble in aliphatic hydrocarbons, but insoluble in fats, fixed oils, and mineral oil.

c. Incompatibilities (6)

(1) Although these compounds are quite stable, Polyethylene Glycols may cause problems for compounds subject to oxidation because of the presence of residual peroxide impurities from the manufacturing process.

(2) Other reported incompatibilities include: reduced antibacterial activity of some antibiotics, including penicillin and bacitracin; reduced preservative effectiveness of the parabens due to binding with PEG; liquefaction of PEG bases with phenol, tannic acid, and salicylic acid (although the original USP formula for Benzoic and Salicylic Acid Ointment, also known as Whitfield's Ointment, used PEG Ointment as the base); discoloration of sulfanilamides; precipitation of sorbitol; and softening or other reactions with some plastics and some membrane filters.

d. Uses (6)

(1) Polyethylene Glycols are widely used in pharmaceutical products and preparations. They are used as ointment and suppository bases, as solvents, viscosity-increasing agents, plasticizers, and as lubricants in tablet and capsule making. They are approved for use in oral, topical, rectal, ophthalmic, and parenteral products.

(2) Their usefulness is limited by the fact that they may be irritating to delicate tissues, mucous membranes, and denuded skin. Although their water-solubility would seem to make them good vehicles to use on burned or denuded skin, they must be used with caution in these situations, both because of their irritating nature and because there have been reports of systemic toxicity due to absorption from these areas. There have also been reports of hypersensitivity reactions.

(3) The limitation for parenteral products is 30% v/v of PEG 300.

e. Other names: PEG, Carbowax®, Atpeg®, Hodag PEG®

References

1. The 2002 United States Pharmacopeia 25/National Formulary 20. Rockville, MD: The United States Pharmacopeial Convention, Inc., 2001; 2217–2220.
2. Reynolds JEF, ed. Martindale: The extra pharmacopoeia, ed. 30. London: The Pharmaceutical Press, 1993; 1111.
3. Clark EW, et al. Lanolin with reduced sensitizing potential. Contact Dermatitis 1977; 3: 69–74.
4. Swinyard EA, Lowenthal W. Pharmaceutical necessities. In: Gennaro AR, ed. Remington: The science and practice of pharmacy, 18th ed. Easton, PA: Mack Publishing Co., 1990; 1310–1312.
5. Reilly Jr WJ. Pharmaceutical necessities. In: Gennaro AR, ed. Remington: The science and practice of pharmacy, 20th ed. Philadelphia: Lippincott Williams and Wilkins, 2000; 1034–1037.
6. Kibbe AH. Handbook of pharmaceutical excipients, 3d ed. Washington DC: American Pharmaceutical Association and Pharmaceutical Press, 2000.
7. The 2002 United States Pharmacopeia 25/National Formulary 20. Rockville, MD: The United States Pharmacopeial Convention, Inc., 2001: Official Monographs.
8. Plaxco JM. Suppositories. In: King RE, ed. Dispensing of medications, 9th ed. Easton, PA: Mack Publishing Co., 1984; 93.
9. Ecanow B, Siegel FP. Dermatology. In: King RE, ed. Dispensing of medications, 9th ed. Easton, PA: Mack Publishing Co., 1984; 78–79.
10. Nairn JG. Solutions, emulsions, suspensions, and extracts. In: Gennaro AR, ed. Remington: The science and practice of pharmacy, 19th ed. Easton, PA: Mack Publishing Co., 1995; 1518.

CHAPTER 23

Suppository Bases

I. DEFINITIONS

A. **Suppositories:** "Suppositories are solid bodies of various weights and shapes, adapted for introduction into the rectal, vaginal, or urethral orifice of the human body. They usually melt, soften, or dissolve at body temperature. A suppository may act as a protectant or palliative to the local tissues at the point of introduction or as a carrier of therapeutic agents for systemic or local action" (1).—*USP*

B. According to the *USP*, there are five general classes of suppository bases:
  1. Cocoa Butter
  2. Cocoa Butter Substitutes
  3. Glycerinated Gelatin
  4. Polyethylene Glycol-Base
  5. Surfactant Base

II. DESIRABLE PROPERTIES OF SUPPOSITORY BASES

A. Chemically and physically stable under normal conditions of use and storage

B. Nonreactive and compatible with a wide variety of drugs and auxiliary agents

C. Free from objectionable odor

D. An aesthetically appealing appearance

E. Nontoxic, nonsensitizing, and nonirritating to sensitive tissues

F. Expansion–contraction characteristics such that it shrinks just enough on cooling so that it releases easily from suppository molds

G. Melts or dissolves in the intended body orifice to release the drug

H. Nonbinding of drugs

I. Mixes with or absorbs some water

J.   Viscosity low enough when melted to pour easily but high enough to suspend particles of solid drug

K.   Some wetting and/or emulsifying properties so that it will spread, disperse in, and release the active ingredient(s) at the administration site

III. CLASSIFICATION AND CHARACTERISTICS OF SUPPOSITORY BASES

The five general classes of suppository bases are described here. The descriptions and solubilities for bases or base ingredient are a composite of information from *Remington: The Science and Practice of Pharmacy* (2), the *Handbook of Pharmaceutical Excipients* (3), official monographs in the *USP-NF* (4), and other references as cited. Additional information on each agent, including references to original research journal articles, can be found in the *Handbook of Pharmaceutical Excipients*.

A.   Cocoa Butter NF
  1.   Description
     a.   Cocoa Butter is the fat from the seeds of *Theobroma cacao* (chocolate beans). It may be obtained either by expressing the oil from the seeds or by solvent extraction. Chemically it is a mixture of triglycerides of saturated and unsaturated fatty acids, primarily stearic, palmitic, oleic, lauric, and linoleic.
     b.   It is a mellow, yellowish solid with a mild odor and bland taste. It is a solid at room temperature but melts at body temperature with a melting point of 31–34°C. The specific gravity of the melt is 0.858–0.864. It is available as bars or grated.
     c.   Cocoa Butter does not contain emulsifiers so it does not absorb significant amounts of water. Tween 61, a tan, waxy, solid, nonionic surfactant, can be added (5–10%) to increase the water absorption properties of Cocoa Butter (5), although addition of nonionic surfactants reportedly gives suppositories with poor stability on storage (6).
  2.   Solubility: Insoluble in water, slightly soluble in alcohol, and soluble in boiling absolute alcohol
  3.   Incompatibilities: The most notable compatibility problem of Cocoa Butter is the lowering of its melting point with drugs such as Chloral Hydrate, Phenol, and Thymol. This can be overcome by the addition of 4–6% White Wax or 18–28% Cetyl Esters Wax, but determining the exact amount that will give an appropriate melting temperature can be difficult and time-consuming (7). A group of successful formulas for Chloral Hydrate suppositories, including some made with Cocoa Butter, has been published (8).
  4.   Advantages
     a.   Cocoa Butter is bland and nonirritating to sensitive membrane tissues. It is also an excellent emollient and is used alone or in topical skin products for this property.
     b.   Because Cocoa Butter has a variety of uses besides suppository making, it is readily available in many pharmacies. It is also one base that can be used for hand-molding suppositories—no special molds or equipment are needed. These two properties make this base useful when a custom suppository is needed on an emergency basis.
     c.   Cocoa Butter has a solidification temperature 12–13° below its melting point. This makes it easy to pour suppositories before the base solidifies (5).
     d.   Cocoa Butter is available in grated form. This eliminates one time-consuming aspect of compounding suppositories.
  5.   Disadvantages
     a.   Because of its relatively low melting point, Cocoa Butter and its suppositories must be stored either at controlled room temperature or in the refrigerator. It is recommended that storage temperature should not exceed 25°C.

b. Cocoa Butter has the further disadvantage of existing in several polymorphic forms that have even lower melting points, 18°, 24°, and 28–31°C (5). Cocoa Butter suppositories are therefore somewhat difficult to make by fusion.

   (1) Cocoa butter can very easily be overheated, and when it is, it may solidify as one of the lower-melting polymorphs. This means that the suppositories do not set up properly, and they may melt at room temperature, or the suppositories may liquefy when handled by the patient during insertion.

   (2) When melting Cocoa Butter, a warm water bath should be used and the temperature should be controlled closely. When melted, the base should have a slightly opalescent appearance. Once the molten Cocoa Butter has completely turned to a clear, straw-colored liquid, the desired melting point has been exceeded; all the stable β-crystals have been destroyed, and the suppositories will melt at a temperature below the desired 34–35°C. A sample procedure with appropriate temperatures for the warm water bath and the Cocoa Butter melt is given with Sample Prescription 31.1 in Chapter 31, Suppositories.

c. As with all fatty bases, Cocoa Butter suppositories may give poor and somewhat erratic release of some drugs. The release of a drug from a fatty suppository base, like Cocoa Butter, to the aqueous medium in the body cavity depends on the water/base partition coefficient of the drug. Because many organic drug molecules are water-insoluble and lipophilic unless present in an ionized salt form, this can be a problem.

   (1) For this reason, from a bioavailability point of view, water-soluble ionized (salt) forms of drugs (these have high water/base partition coefficients) should be used when possible with Cocoa Butter, particularly when a systemic effect is desired. For example, if a drug like Phenobarbital is being incorporated into a Cocoa Butter suppository base, the sodium salt of Phenobarbital is the preferred form of the drug to use.

   (2) For drugs, like Acetaminophen, that do not have a water-soluble form, Cocoa Butter and other fatty bases are not good choices for suppository bases (9).

B. Cocoa Butter Substitutes

   1. Description

   a. The *USP* has the following description of Cocoa Butter Substitutes:
   "Fat-type suppository bases can be produced from a variety of vegetable oils, such as coconut or palm kernel, which are modified by esterification, hydrogenation, and fractionation to obtain products of varying composition and melting temperatures (e.g., *Hydrogenated Vegetable Oil* and *Hard Fat*). These products can be so designed as to reduce rancidity. At the same time, desired characteristics such as narrow intervals between melting and solidification temperatures, and melting ranges to accommodate various formulation and climatic conditions, can be built in" (1).

   b. Chemically this type of base is composed primarily of mixtures of triglyceride esters of saturated fatty acids in the C-12 to C-18 range, with lesser amounts of mono- and diglycerides. Other possible additives include beeswax, lecithin, polysorbates, ethoxylated fatty alcohols, and ethoxylated partial fatty glycerides (3).

   c. Substitutes for Cocoa Butter were first developed in Europe during World War II because of the limited availability of natural Cocoa Butter. In recent years, suppliers of compounding materials in the U.S. have developed additional products of this type (6). While a number of commercial bases of this type have been described, Witepsol® and Fattibase® are the two most commonly available to compounding pharmacists. These are described below.

   d. Witepsol®

   (1) Witepsol® is a whitish, waxy, brittle solid that melts to a clear to yellowish liquid; it is nearly odorless and has a density of 0.95–0.98 at 20°C. It contains emulsifying agents and will absorb a small amount of water (3,6).

(2) Although the *Handbook of Pharmaceutical Excipients* lists 20 different grades of Witepsol®, the H15 grade is the most readily available to pharmacists. It has a melting point range of 33.5 to 35.5°C (3), which is quite close to its congealing range of 32–34°C (6).

(3) Although some pharmacists speak highly of Witepsol® bases, others report poor or uneven results. Although suppositories made with this base solidify rapidly and should contract to release easily from the mold, there are reports of problems with suppositories breaking into pieces when being removed from the suppository mold.

  e. Fattibase®

    (1) Fattibase® is an opaque, white, waxy solid; it is odorless and has a bland taste. Its specific gravity at 37°C is 0.89. It is a mixture of triglycerides from palm, palm kernel, and coconut oils together with self-emulsifying glyceryl monostearate and polyoxyl stearate, which serve as emulsifiers and suspending agents (10).

    (2) It has a melting point range of 32 to 36.5°C, but instructions from its manufacturer Paddock Labs state that the base should be heated slowly and evenly to 49–54°C before adding the active ingredients. The suppositories should be poured when the mixture is 43–49°C. The base should not be heated above 60°C, and the use of microwave ovens for heating the base is not recommended (10,11).

    (3) Fattibase® has found favor with many pharmacists who make suppositories with this type of base. It has the advantages of Cocoa Butter without the difficulties caused by the sensitive melting point range and polymorphism of Cocoa Butter. Its suppositories release well from molds; a light spraying with vegetable oil can be used if needed.

2. Solubility: Practically insoluble in water and slightly soluble in warm alcohol

3. Incompatibilities: The Cocoa Butter Substitutes may have some of the same temperature-lowering difficulties as seen with Cocoa Butter.

4. Advantages

  a. Fatty bases are favored because they are bland and nonirritating to sensitive membrane tissues.

  b. Some synthetic versions of Cocoa Butter, such as Fattibase®, are much easier to work with than Cocoa Butter. Unlike Cocoa Butter, they do not exist in polymorphic forms.

5. Disadvantages

  a. Because of their relatively low melting points, these bases and their suppositories must be stored either at controlled room temperature or in the refrigerator.

  b. As discussed above under Cocoa Butter, all fatty bases give poor and somewhat erratic release of water-insoluble drugs. For this reason, water-soluble ionized (salt) forms of drugs should be used when possible with fatty bases, particularly when a systemic effect is desired. For drugs that do not have water-soluble forms, fatty bases are not good choices as suppository bases.

  C. Glycerinated Gelatin Bases

    1. Description: This base consists of 70 parts of glycerin, 20 parts of gelatin, and 10 parts of water (1). The method of preparation is like that for glycerinated gummy gel base, which is described in Table 25.3 in Chapter 25.

    2. These bases are used infrequently because they are more difficult to make and offer few advantages.

    3. The base material has a soft, rubbery consistency (rather like the candy gummy worms), which makes them suitable for vaginal administration but not firm enough for rectal use.

    4. They do not melt, but dissolve slowly in the mucous secretions of the vagina; they have been recommended for sustained release of local antimicrobial agents (5). Glycerinated gelatin suppositories should be moistened before insertion.

5. Glycerinated gelatin suppositories are hygroscopic, so they must be dispensed in tight containers.

6. They are reported to support mold or bacterial growth, so they should be stored in the refrigerator and should contain a preservative (e.g., methylparaben 0.18%, propylparaben 0.02%) (6).

D. Polyethylene Glycol Bases

1. Description: Polyethylene glycol (PEG) suppository bases are composed of blends of various molecular-weight polyethylene glycol polymers. Polyethylene Glycol is described in Chapter 22, and properties of some PEG polymers that are used often for pharmaceutical applications are given in Table 23.1. Formulas for some PEG suppository bases are given in Table 23.2.

2. Some commercial polyethylene glycol suppository bases also contain additional components, such as surfactants. One widely used base is Polybase®; it contains a mixture of polyethylene glycols plus the emulsifier polysorbate 80. Polybase® is a white solid with an average molecular weight of 3,440 and a specific gravity of 1.177 at 24°C (10).

3. PEG suppository bases are formulated so they do not melt at body temperature, but rather dissolve in body fluids. Their suppositories should be moistened with water before insertion.

4. Advantages
   a. PEG suppositories are easily made by fusion.
   b. When formulated with an appropriate PEG blend, they dissolve in body cavity fluids and release the active ingredient(s), both hydrophilic and hydrophobic drugs. Provided there are sufficient aqueous secretions in the body cavity, they provide more reliable release of drug from the dosage form than do fatty bases.
   c. Because their melting points are easily controlled by appropriate blending, these bases and their suppositories do not require carefully monitored storage temperatures.

5. Disadvantages
   a. They are irritating to body cavity tissues, so they have less patient acceptance than do fatty base suppositories.
   b. They are incompatible with a long list of drugs, especially those prone to oxidation. Specific examples are given in the description of Polyethylene Glycol in Chapter 22.
   c. They interact with polystyrene, the plastic often used for prescription vials, so they should not be dispensed in these containers, unless the suppositories are first wrapped with foil or placed in individual polyethylene bags.

TABLE 23.1   Physical Properties of Polyethylene Glycols (12)

Grade (Ave. MW)	MW Range	Physical Form	Density at 20°C* or 60° C**	Melting Range °C	Solubility in Water Wt % 20°C	pH of 5% Solution
300	285–315	liquid	1.1250*	−15 to −8°	Complete	4.5 to 7.5
400	380–420	liquid	1.1254*	4 to 8°	Complete	4.5 to 7.5
600	570–630	liquid	1.1257*	20 to 25°	Complete	4.5 to 7.5
1000	950–1050	soft solid	1.0926**	37 to 40°	80	4.5 to 7.5
1450	1300–1600	soft solid or flake	1.0919**	43 to 46°	72	4.5 to 7.5
3350	3000–3700	flake or powder	1.0926**	54 to 58°	67	4.5 to 7.5
4600	4400–4800	flake or powder	1.0926**	57 to 61°	65	4.5 to 7.5
8000	7000–9000	flake or powder	1.0845**	60 to 63°	63	4.5 to 7.5

TABLE 23.2	Polyethylene Glycol (PEG) Bases (6)	

Base 1

PEG	8000	50%
PEG	1540	30%
PEG	400	20%

A good general purpose water soluble suppository base

Base 2

PEG	3350	60%
PEG	1000	30%
PEG	400	10%

A good general purpose base which is slightly softer and dissolves more readily

Base 3

PEG	8000	30%
PEG	1540	70%

This base has a higher melting point which is usually sufficient to compensate for the melting point lowering of drugs such as chloral hydrate

Base 4

PEG	8000	40%
PEG	400	60%

Base 5

PEG	8000	20%
PEG	400	80%

These bases have been used for progesterone suppositories. Personal communication to the author from practitioners report Base 5 to be superior for this purpose.

Base 6

PEG	8000	60%
PEG	1540	25%
Cetyl Alcohol		5%
Water		10%

This base can be used for water-soluble drugs

Bases 1, 2, 3, 4, and 6 are found in Reference 6: Plaxco JM. Suppositories. In: King RE, ed. Dispensing of medications, 9th ed. Easton, PA: Mack Publishing Co., 1984:93–94.

E. Surfactant or Water-dispersible Bases

   1. Several nonionic surfactants, such as polyoxyethylene sorbitan fatty acid esters and the polyoxyethylene stearates, are used alone or in combination with other suppository vehicle materials to make suppository bases (1).

   2. Bases of this type are not used as frequently for compounding because they are more complicated to formulate.

   3. If formulated correctly, these bases have desirable melting points and consistencies. Because they contain surfactants, there are readily dispersed in body cavity fluids.

   4. One blend that could be easily made in the pharmacy contains 60% Tween 61 and 40% Tween 60 (5). Both of these compounds are solids at room temperature. They are available through vendors of compounding drugs and chemicals.

F. Release of drug from suppository bases is unpredictable. In practice, because bioavailability studies are usually impracticable, it is important to monitor the effectiveness of the drug delivery system by frequent monitoring of therapeutic results.

References

1. The 2002 United States Pharmacopeia 25/National Formulary 20. Rockville, MD: The United States Pharmacopeial Convention, Inc., 2001; 2222.

2. Reilly Jr WJ. Pharmaceutical necessities. In: Gennaro AR, ed. Remington: The science and practice of pharmacy, 20th ed. Philadelphia, PA: Lippincott Williams and Wilkins, 2000; 1043.

3. Kibbe AH. Handbook of pharmaceutical excipients, 3d ed. Washington DC: American Pharmaceutical Association and Pharmaceutical Press, 2000.

4. The 2002 United States Pharmacopeia 25/National Formulary 20. Rockville, MD: The United States Pharmacopeial Convention, Inc., 2001: Official Monographs.

5. Coben LJ, Lieberman HA. Suppositories. In: Lieberman HA, Lachman L, Kanig J, eds. The theory and practice of industrial pharmacy, 3d ed. Philadelphia: Lea & Febiger, 1986; 564–588.

6. Plaxco JM. Suppositories. In: King RE, ed. Dispensing of medication, 9th ed. Easton, PA: Mack Publishing Co., 1984; 93–94.

7. King JC. Suppositories. In: Martin EW, ed. Dispensing of medication, 7th ed. Easton, PA: Mack Publishing Co., 1971; 849.

8. Schumacher GF. Chloral hydrate suppositories. Am J Hosp Pharm 1966; 23: 110.

9. Feldman S. Bioavailability of acetaminophen suppositories. In: Schumacher GE, ed. Biopharmaceutics and pharmacokinetics. Am J Hosp Pharm 1975; 32: 1173–1174.

10. Fattibase® Product Data Sheet, Paddock Laboratories, Minneapolis, MN.

11. Personal correspondence with Paddock Laboratories Customer Service Department. Minneapolis, MN: Paddock Laboratories, Inc.

12. Carbowax® Product Data Sheets, Union Carbide Chemicals and Plastics Company, Danbury, CT.

PART 5

DOSAGE FORMS AND THEIR PREPARATION

CHAPTER 24

Powders

I. DEFINITIONS

A. **Powders:** "Powders are intimate mixtures of dry, finely divided drugs and/or chemicals that may be intended for internal (Oral Powders) or external (Topical Powders) use" (1).—*USP*

B. **Efflorescent Powders:** These are drugs or chemicals that contain water of hydration that may be released when the powders are manipulated or are stored under conditions of low relative humidity (see Chapter 34 for more information).

C. **Hygroscopic Powders:** These are solid drugs or chemicals that absorb moisture from the air (see Chapter 34 for more information).

D. **Deliquescent Powders:** These are hygroscopic powders that may absorb sufficient moisture from the air to dissolve and form a solution (see Chapter 34 for more information).

E. **Pharmaceutical Eutectic Mixture:** This is a mixture of two or more substances that may liquefy when intimately mixed at room temperature (see Chapter 34 for more information).

II. USES

A. Topical bulk powders, often referred to as dusting powders, are applied to the skin for local effect.

B. Bulk powders for internal use offer a convenient method of dispensing nonpotent, powdered drugs that have doses that require moderate to large volumes of powder. Examples include antacids, bulk laxatives, and antidiarrheal medications. Bulk powders for internal use are dispensed in wide-mouth containers, and the dose is measured volumetrically by the patient or caregiver at the time of administration using a household measuring device, such as a measuring spoon or cup. Because of this imprecise method of measuring the dose, this dosage form is not used for drugs that require precise and accurate dosing.

C. Powders for internal use may also be encapsulated into hard-shell capsules or compressed into tablets. Although formulating powders into tablets and capsules is done principally by pharmaceutical manufacturers, capsules can easily be made extemporaneously by the pharmacist. Because the quantity of drug formulated into tablets and capsules can be measured accurately, these systems are ideal for potent drugs. For patients who cannot swallow tablets or capsules, divided powders or liquid dosage forms are two alternatives.

D. Powders may be dispensed as divided powders, also known as chartulae. In this case, the pharmacist weighs each dose of powder separately and places it in a small individual packet or polyethylene bag. The patient or caregiver empties the contents of the packet into a liquid vehicle or, if the drug is to be taken by mouth, may mix it with soft food, such as pudding or applesauce. This dosage form is useful when a solid dosage form is desired but the medication is not manufactured in the required dose, or it is supplied as capsules or tablets but the patient cannot swallow these dosage forms.

E. Because most drugs are solids, powders are used as primary ingredients for most other drug delivery systems.

III. ADVANTAGES OF SOLID DOSAGE FORMS OVER LIQUIDS

A. Drugs and chemicals are most stable as dry solids.

B. Because they are dry and compact, tablets, capsules, and divided powders are packaged, transported, administered, and stored more easily than are liquids.

C. Undesirable taste is more noticeable when substances are in solution than when in solid form. Objectionable taste can be concealed completely by enclosing the solid drug in capsules or coated tablets.

D. Accurate dosing is easier to achieve with dosage forms furnished as individual units, such as tablets, capsules, and divided powders.

E. Controlled release is much easier to achieve with solid dosage forms than with liquids.

IV. DESIRED PROPERTIES OF POWDERS

A. When intended for topical application, powders should be finely divided and have uniform particle size so as to be smooth to the touch and nonirritating to the skin. They should be free-flowing and should spread easily on the surface of the skin.

B. Powders for internal use should also be finely divided with uniform particle size because the rate of dissolution and therefore often the bioavailability of the drug depend on the particle size of the drug. Dissolution rate is expressed mathematically by the Noyes-Whitney equation:

$$\frac{dC}{dt} = K S(C_s - C)$$

where: dC/dt = change in concentration with change in time (or rate of dissolution)
K = the dissolution rate constant
S = surface area of the solid
C_s = solubility of the solid
C = concentration of the drug in solution at time = t

C. Because the surface area of a given amount of solid increases as the particle size is decreased for a given weight of solid, the smaller the particle size, the larger the surface area and the faster the rate of dissolution.

D. It is especially important for the particle size of bulk powders to be uniform because particles of different sizes tend to stratify on standing or when a powder is being transported. Stratification can result in inaccurate dosing.

E. Even when powder is being used as an ingredient for another dosage form, particle size is important because it affects the rate of dissolution, rate of settling (in suspensions), degree of comfort (in topical products), and bioavailability.

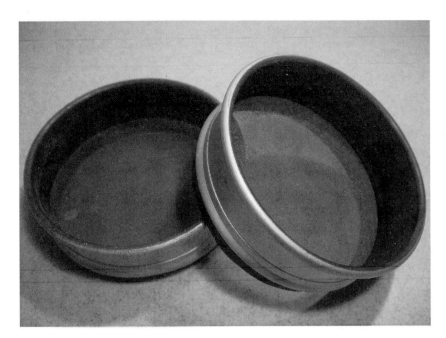

Mesh sieves

F. Particle size for most pharmaceutical powders is determined by sieving, and the descriptive terms used to classify powders have meaning in terms of percent of the powder sample that will pass through a sieve of a given fineness.

    1. Sieve properties are specified in the American Society for Testing and Materials (ASTM) Specification E11, U.S. Standard Sieve Series. Table 24.1 shows the sieve size openings for sieves used to measured particle size for powders of interest in pharmaceuticals. The table column "Sieve U.S. No." gives what is commonly referred to as mesh size, a number that comes from the number of openings per linear inch of the sieve mesh. The larger the mesh number, the smaller the particles must be to pass through that sieve.

    2. Powders almost never have a completely uniform particle size, but rather they have a size distribution. Therefore, even when using sieves to measure particle size, the results are reported as the percent of the sample that passes through a given sieve size

TABLE 24.1   Sizes of Standard Sieves

Sieve Size	Sieve U.S. No.
4.00 mm	5
2.00 mm	10
1.40 mm	14
1.00 mm	18
850 μm	20
710 μm	25
600 μm	30
500 μm	35
425 μm	40
355 μm	45
300 μm	50
250 μm	60
212 μm	70
180 μm	80
150 μm	100
125 μm	120
106 μm	140
90 μm	170
75 μm	200
63 mm	230

TABLE 24.2 Classification of Powders by Fineness (3)

Classification of Powder	d_{50} Sieve Opening (μm)
Very Course	> 1000
Coarse	355–1000
Moderately Fine	180–355
Fine	125–180
Very Fine	90–125

plus an upper and lower size boundary, or specifications will state that all the powder must pass through a sieve of a given mesh size. For example, the USP compounding monograph for Ketoconazole Oral Suspension states, "If Tablets are used, finely powder the Tablets such that they pass through a 40-mesh or 45-mesh sieve" (2).

3. Descriptive terms, such as fine or coarse, are used to describe powder fineness. The classification used by the USP for this purpose is given in Table 24.2, where the designation d_{50} means "the smallest sieve opening through which 50% or more of the material passes" (3).

4. Small sieves with mesh sizes useful for compounding are available from some vendors of compounding supplies.

V. PRINCIPLES OF COMPOUNDING FOR POWDERS

A. General Principles

1. In nearly all compounding situations, solids need to be in a fine state of subdivision. Unless the solid can be purchased as a fine powder, particle size reduction by the pharmacist is required.

2. The chemical composition and the processing of solids determine their degree of subdivision and physical properties. The properties of a given solid must be understood and considered to properly handle and manipulate the material when fabricating it into a solid dosage form or when incorporating it into another drug delivery system.

   a. Solids purchased as fine powders may need no further manipulation.

   b. Some drugs have fine particles, but these may have agglomerated on storage and may need to be broken down into the primary particles originally processed by the manufacturer.

   c. Some drugs and chemicals are available as crystals that can easily be crushed into fine powder using a standard compounding technique, such as trituration, described below.

   d. Some materials are not easy to pulverize. They may be waxy substances or hard crystals that do not crush into fine powder with simple trituration. If a fine state of subdivision is needed, these drugs may require special techniques, such as pulverization by intervention.

   e. Some solids have unique properties, such as deliquescence or intense color, that require special handling.

   f. Some solid drugs and chemicals are cytotoxic or hazardous substances; these too require special precautions and handling.

3. When two or more solids are being combined into one mixture, homogeneous blending of the powders is needed.

B. Particle Size Reduction

1. The process of particle size reduction is called **comminution.** The pharmaceutical industry has elaborate equipment and processes with which to produce finely divided powders with precisely controlled particle size. Although the equipment and methods available in the pharmacy are not nearly as efficient, they are adequate for the processing done by pharmacists in extemporaneous compounding.

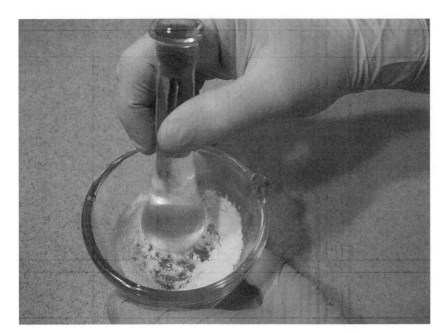

Trituration in a glass mortar

2. Methods of comminution available to the pharmacist

    a. **Trituration** is the continued rubbing of a solid in a mortar with a pestle to reduce the size of the solid's particles to a desirable degree of fineness. The term is also used to describe the grinding together of two or more substances in a mortar to intimately mix them. Trituration is achieved by firmly holding the pestle and exerting a downward pressure with it while moving it in successively larger concentric circles, starting at the center of the mortar, moving outward to the sides of the mortar, then back again toward the center. To ensure adequate mixing and uniform particle size reduction, compacted powder is constantly removed from the sides of the mortar and the pestle by scraping with a spatula. Three different types of mortars are available for triturating drugs. Their properties and uses are described in Chapter 12.

    b. **Pulverization by intervention**

        (1) Some compounds do not lend themselves to direct trituration and must be handled in special ways. For example, some substances have hard crystalline structures that do not crush or triturate easily. The manner in which these drugs are handled depends on their ultimate use. If they are to be added to a liquid or semisolid preparation, and if they are soluble in a suitable solvent, they may be dissolved first and incorporated as a solution. If they are to be included in a powdered dosage form, the procedure is more complex. One possible technique is pulverization by intervention.

        (2) Pulverization by intervention uses recrystallization as a method of obtaining fine particles. The word "intervention" refers to the first step of the process, dissolving the drug in a suitable solvent, the solvent being the so-called intervening compound. In this process, the solid is first dissolved in a minimum volume of a volatile solvent such as alcohol.

        (a) If the volume of the liquid is small and the rest of the powder in the preparation is not soluble in the chosen solvent, the solution may be mixed directly with the other powdered ingredients. The powders are then mixed until the solvent has completely evaporated.

        (b) If the other powder ingredients are soluble in the chosen solvent, or if too much solvent is required to dissolve the drug, the solution of the drug in the solvent is spread in a thin layer on the sides of a glass mortar or on an ointment slab. The solvent is allowed to evaporate, and the thin film of fine, solid crystals is then scraped off the glass surface using a metal spatula. The solid can then be blended with the other ingredients in the product.

(3) The most common use of this technique is to obtain fine particles of Camphor. Camphor is a hard, chunky solid that does not reduce to a fine powder when triturated in a mortar. When fine crystals of Camphor are needed, pulverization by intervention is a useful method.

c. **Levigation** is the process of reducing the particle size of a solid by triturating it in a mortar or spatulating it on an ointment slab or pad with a small amount of a liquid in which the solid is not soluble. Optimally, the liquid is somewhat viscous and has a low surface tension to improve the ease of wetting the solid. Mineral Oil and Glycerin are examples of common levigating agents. Levigation and levigating agents are discussed in detail in Chapter 30, Ointments, Creams, Gels, and Pastes.

C. Blending

1. The goal in blending powders is to create a homogeneous mixture. This is essential for obtaining uniform doses when mixtures of solid drugs are involved.

2. Four methods—spatulation, trituration, sifting, and tumbling—are generally described in pharmacy textbooks as methods of blending in extemporaneous compounding. Pharmacists may also use newer technology, such as electric mixers and blenders.

a. **Spatulation** is the mixing of powders on an ointment slab or pad using a spatula. With this method there is no particle size reduction, so the powders to be mixed must be fine and of uniform size. Because no pressure is used, the resulting powder is usually light and is not compacted. This method should be used when hard trituration is to be avoided, such as when blending powders that have previously been coated to prevent the formation of a liquid eutectic mixture.

b. Trituration was described previously under particle size reduction. It is the preferred method of blending under most circumstances because it mixes powders more intimately than other methods. It should always be used when making mixtures that contain small quantities of potent drugs. Because trituration accomplishes two processes at the same time—namely, particle size reduction and blending—this method saves time when powders of unequal particle size are being combined.

c. Clear glass or plastic bottles and zipper-sealed polyethylene bags are useful for mixing powders by tumbling. These are especially useful when it is important to carefully contain the powders, such as hazardous or cytotoxic substances or lightweight powders that get into the air when mixed.

d. Pharmacists who do a lot of compounding use a variety of other equipment for blending. For example, blending moderate to large quantities of powders can be accomplished efficiently with an electric mixer. Special stainless steel sifters, available from vendors of compounding equipment and supplies, can also be used for blending powders.

e. Although visual inspection of the finished powder is important, it is not easy to determine when adequate mixing has been achieved. Because most drugs are white powders, visual determination of uniformity is nearly impossible.

(1) Some pharmacists add a small amount (approximately 0.1%) of a certified dye to the mixture so they can see visually when the powder is adequately mixed.

(2) Pharmacists who think it is unwise to add extra ingredients or who do not want to bother with this extra step may prefer using appropriate techniques and mixing for a length of time that they have found by experimentation will ensure proper blending of the powders. One technique that is useful in blending powders is geometric dilution; another is alternate addition by portions.

f. Geometric dilution is used when blending two or more powder ingredients of unequal quantities. It is a method designed to help ensure that small quantities of ingredients, usually potent drugs, are uniformly distributed throughout the powder mixture. Trituration usually is the blending method of choice with geometric dilution because it gives more intimate mixing than other methods. (The steps in geometric dilution are given here, and the technique is demonstrated with Sample Prescription 24.2 on the CD that accompanies this book. The compounding procedures in Samples Prescriptions 24.2 through 24.5 also illustrate the use of this method.)

    (1) Weigh all ingredients for the preparation.

    (2) Place the ingredient present in the smallest quantity in a mortar.

    (3) Select the ingredient present in the next largest quantity and place in the mortar an amount of this ingredient approximately equal in powder volume to that of the first ingredient.

    (4) Triturate the powders well until a uniform mixture is achieved.

    (5) Add a volume of powder of the second ingredient equal in size to the powder volume of the mixture in the mortar and triturate well.

    (6) Continue adding powder to the mortar in this fashion, always adding a volume of powder equal to the volume of powder mixture in the mortar, until all the powder ingredients have been added.

    g. When a formulation calls for combining relatively equal amounts of moderate to large quantities of two or more powdered ingredients, a uniform mixture can be obtained most easily by first combining and mixing small portions of each ingredient, then adding additional small portions of each alternately with adequate trituration or mixing with each addition. This process is sometimes referred to as alternate addition by portions.

D. Stability and Compatibility

    1. Although solids are generally quite stable physically, a few problems can be encountered with selected drugs and chemicals.

        a. The potential physical problems for solids include liquefaction of eutectic mixtures and deliquescent powders, loss of water of hydration for efflorescent powders, and absorption of water by hygroscopic and deliquescent powders. Definitions are given at the beginning of this chapter, and these processes are described in Chapter 34, Compatibility and Stability of Drug Products and Preparations Dispensed by the Pharmacist. Commonly used labile drugs are also listed in Chapter 34.

        b. Methods of handling these incompatibilities of solids are discussed below and in Chapter 34. (Examples are given in the current chapter with Sample Prescriptions 24.2 and 24.5, and the techniques are demonstrated on the CD using Sample Prescription 24.2.)

    2. Most solids are also quite stable chemically.

        a. Chemical stability of drugs and chemicals is addressed in Chapter 34, and a general discussion on assigning beyond-use dates for solid dosage forms can be found in Chapter 4, Expiration and Beyond-use Dating.

        b. Each sample prescription at the end of this chapter considers the chemical stability of each ingredient in the given dosage form and uses this information in assigning a beyond-use date to the preparation. Examples are given that illustrate the use of various reference resources to determine stability and beyond-use dates.

        c. Even though most solids are quite stable, it is important to check out ingredients before formulating a preparation. Sample prescriptions 24.4, 24.5, and 24.6 are all single drugs mixed with lactose for divided powder dosage forms. Although two of the drug preparations, Hydralazine and Mercaptopurine, are stable in this dosage form, the third drug, Carbamazepine, is relatively unstable even in a solid dosage form. It would be difficult to predict this without checking references.

VI. BULK POWDERS

A. Bulk Powders for External Use

1. Powders intended for topical application are called dusting powders.

2. Bulk powders often contain one or more active ingredients incorporated in a diluent powder. Powders most often chosen as diluents for external bulk powders are starch and talc.

3. When a bulk powder contains a potential eutectic mixture that needs protection, the pharmacist should, if possible, use as the protectant an ingredient already in the prescription. Sample Prescription 24.2 illustrates this principle. If the prescription order does not contain an ingredient that is suitable for this purpose, the pharmacist should consult with the prescriber to select a protectant. Because this may affect the final concentrations of the active ingredients, the prescriber should be made aware of this. Any added ingredients and their quantities must then be recorded, either on the face of the prescription order or in the compounding record kept for that purpose. As stated previously, eutectic mixtures are described in Chapter 34.

4. Containers for dusting powders

   a. Although dusting powders may be dispensed in a wide-mouth bottle or container, they are more easily applied by the patient when dispensed in a sifter-topped powder can or shaker canister. Although shaker canisters have been available in the past from vendors of compounding supplies, some companies have discontinued these items in favor of plastic bottles with flip spout, snap cap, or Yorker spouts. Some of these plastic bottle/closure systems have the advantage of being tight containers.

   b. Most shaker canisters are not tight containers, and bulk powder formulations that contain volatile ingredients can lose these components through evaporation when they are dispensed in these containers. Furthermore, moisture from the environment can permeate through these containers and into the contained powder. To avoid these problems, bulk powders that contain either volatile active ingredients or components that are sensitive to moisture should be dispensed when possible in tight containers. If this is not practical, a conservative beyond-use date should be assigned to the preparation. This is illustrated with Sample Prescription 24.2.

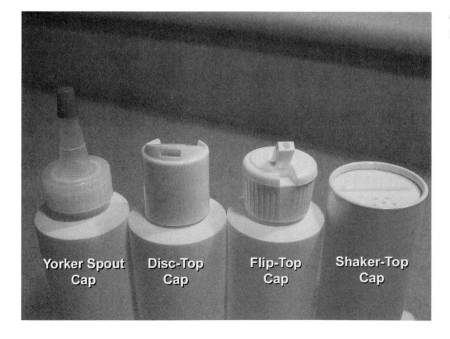

Containers for topical powders

5. For labeling the content of a topical bulk powder, the concentrations of active ingredients are expressed as percent weight-weight or as weight of active ingredient per gram of powder.

B. Bulk Powders for Internal Use

1. Bulk powders for internal use are dispensed in wide-mouth powder-squares, pharmaceutical rounds, or other wide-mouth containers. When the dose to be administered is a teaspoonful or tablespoonful, the container selected should, when possible, allow the patient or caregiver to insert the measuring spoon to withdraw the appropriate dose. As with external bulk powders, the nature of the powder components should be considered when selecting a container, and tight containers should always be used when the situation dictates.

2. If an internal bulk powder contains a potential eutectic mixture, the ingredients involved must be protected or the formed eutectic mixture must be adsorbed on an appropriate powder. As with external use powders, an ingredient already in the prescription is preferred for this purpose. If the prescription order does not contain a suitable adsorbent or protective ingredient, the pharmacist should consult with the prescriber to select an ingredient for this purpose. Agents commonly used as adsorbents for internal products include light or heavy magnesium oxide, magnesium carbonate, calcium carbonate, starch, and lactose. Because addition of any extra powder may affect the final concentration and therefore the dose of the product, such a change should be made in consultation with the prescriber. The volume to be administered will need adjustment. Any added ingredients must be recorded on the face of the prescription order or in the record of compounding.

3. Internal bulk powders are labeled with the weight of active ingredient per volume to be ingested or administered (e.g., teaspoonful, tablespoonful). To determine the content of active ingredients in this volume, the pharmacist must perform the following procedure to calibrate the powder content:
   a. Prepare the formulation as directed in the prescription order.
   b. Using the appropriate measuring device (e.g., teaspoon), measure the volume of powder to be taken or administered.
   c. Weigh this volume of powder.
   d. From the concentration or percent of active ingredient(s) in the prepared powder and the weight of the volume to be administered, calculate the weight(s) of active ingredient(s) in the volume to be administered. An example of this procedure is given in Sample Prescription 24.1, which follows.

VII. DIVIDED POWDERS OR CHARTULAE

A. Divided Powders, also known as Chartulae or Powder Papers, have individual doses of powder packaged in folded papers or plastic bags.

B. Preparing the Powder

1. Amount of powder
   a. Prepare enough powder for one extra dosage unit, because some powder will be lost in the blending process. If the prescription contains a controlled substance, this loss in compounding must be minimal and should be documented on the prescription order or compounding record sheet.
   b. If the amount of powder for each paper is less than the minimum weighable quantity (MWQ) for the balance being used, an inert diluent powder should be added and an aliquot method of measuring should be used. This procedure is described in Chapter 9, Aliquots Calculations, and is illustrated in Sample Prescription 24.4 in the current chapter.
   c. If the amount of powder is above the MWQ but is still small (for example, below 300 mg per unit), a diluent such as lactose may be added to bring the quantity of powder per unit to an amount that is convenient for handling and administration.

    (1) An intermediate amount of powder (300 to 500 mg) is desirable.

    (2) Smaller quantities are difficult to handle, and any amount left in the powder paper or bag or spilled by the patient or caregiver significantly affects the dose. In a recent study, Nifedipine divided powders were compounded using crushed Nifedipine tablets and lactose as a diluent. Each packet was formulated to contain 1 mg of Nifedipine in 500 mg of powder. An analysis showed that the delivered content was 0.92 mg Nifedipine per packet and that 3/4 of the loss was found on the powder papers (4). Obviously, the loss of active ingredient would have been greater if the drug had not been diluted with lactose.

    (3) Large quantities of diluent should also be avoided, since larger amounts of powder are more difficult to mix into soft food for administration.

  2. The techniques for preparing and mixing the powders are the same as for bulk powders.

C. Packaging the Divided Powders

  1. Divided Powders can be folded into powder papers or packaged in reclosable, so-called zip-lock, polybags, or heat-sealed in polyethylene or cellophane bags.

  2. Folded powder papers

    a. This method is used only when other packaging materials for Divided Powders are not available. Folded powder papers have the following disadvantages over Divided Powders packaged in polybags: time-consuming preparation, poor moisture barriers, and failure to meet safety packaging regulations.

    b. Types of paper most commonly used for folded powder papers include:

      (1) Glassine weighing papers, as described in the section on weighing

      (2) Powder papers made of vegetable parchment paper. These are available in a variety of sizes, ranging from 2½" × 3¾" to 4½" × 6½".

    c. Folding papers for Divided Powders: The dimensions given below are approximate because these depend on the size of the powder papers being used, the amount of the powder enclosed in each paper, and the dimensions of the powder box.

      (1) Place the paper on a clean, flat surface and fold toward you the long top edge of the paper with a uniform flap of 1/4" to 1/2". This fold should be creased sharply. The size of this first fold, together with the dimensions of the paper, determines the height of the finished paper. Because it is desirable to have uniform-sized papers for a given product, this first step should be done on all the required papers concurrently, using the first paper as a guide.

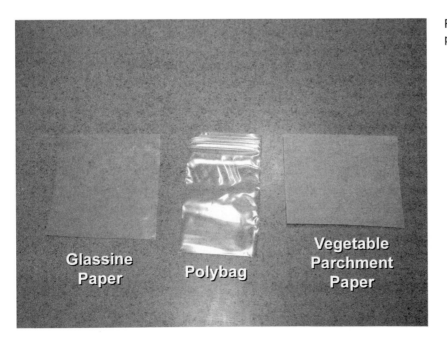

Polybags and powder papers

Glassine Paper   Polybag   Vegetable Parchment Paper

(2) Place the weighed portion of powder in the center of the paper. Some pharmacists use the powder paper as a weighing paper and weigh the powder directly on the powder paper that will contain the powder.

(3) Bring the bottom edge of the paper up and insert this edge under the top flap, with the bottom edge at the very top of the crease of the fold at the top of the paper. Press a gentle fold at the bottom of the paper. Do not make this bottom fold a sharp crease because powder will be present in this fold, and making a sharp crease could cause the paper to tear.

(4) Bring the top of the creased edge of the paper down toward you so that this edge is approximately halfway down to the bottom soft-creased edge of the paper. The exact position of this last fold may need to be adjusted so that the finished folded paper is slightly taller than the top inside lip of the powder box.

(5) Being careful not to disturb the powder in the paper, pick up the paper and center it lengthwise over a hinged powder paper box that has its lid open. Crease the outside flaps of the paper downward on the outside edges of the box while pressing slightly inward on the sides of the box. Pressing inward on the box sides will make the finished powder paper slightly smaller than the inside dimension of the box so that the papers will fit neatly in the box.

(6) Lift the paper from the box and finish folding the flaps backward along the crease marks made against the box edges.

(7) Place the finished paper in the box in an upright position with the flaps facing the back of the box.

(8) Repeat this procedure for all the doses. If the box is not full, place a tissue or piece of cotton in the back of the box so that the papers are held upright.

(9) Close the lid and position the prescription label and necessary auxiliary labels on the top of the box.

(10) Because this system does not meet child-resistant safety packaging standards, it is necessary to devise some method of bringing it into compliance. In any case, the patient or caregiver must be given adequate warnings about storing the product in a secure place, out of the reach of children. The system also does not meet the requirements for a tight container, so any compounded preparation containing a drug that has special recommendations for storage should either be protected or given an adequately conservative beyond-use date.

3. Polybags

   a. Polybags are available in various sizes and can be purchased either with reclosable zipper-type seals or as bags that require a heat-seal or adhesive tape seal. Amber or opaque polybags are also available for drugs that require protection from light.

   b. Preparing Divided Powders with polybags is much easier.

   (1) The weighed quantity of prepared powder for one dose is placed in each bag.

   (2) For reclosable bags, the closure is zipped shut. Plain polybags may be sealed by tape or heat-sealed with an impulse sealer.

   (3) The sealed bags may be dispensed in a hinged or telescoping box, or may be placed in a powder-square or other tight container with a screw top.

D. Miscellaneous Issues

   1. One of the main uses of Divided Powders is for supplying doses for patients who cannot swallow whole tablets or capsules.

      a. Always be sure that the manufactured dosage form is one that may be manipulated. The issue of oral solid dosage forms that should not be crushed is discussed in the section of Chapter 12 on compounding ingredients.

      b. If the dose needed is a **whole unit** of a tablet or capsule, there are some convenient alternatives:

         (1) For capsules, the powder can be emptied easily from the capsule shell by the patient or caregiver.

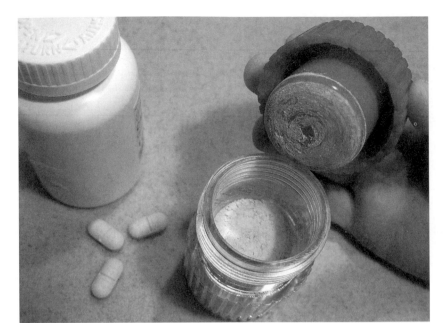

Tablet crusher

(2) Because tablets need to be crushed, other methods are required. Tablet crushers, intended for use by patients, nurses, or other caregivers, are available at various prices, ranging from under $10 to deluxe models that are over $50. One easy, inexpensive method is for the patient or caregiver to place the tablet in a small plastic bag, such as a sandwich bag, and crush the tablet with the back of a spoon.

c. When the dose needed is either customized with other ingredients or is a fractional part of a manufactured tablet or capsule, Divided Powders offer a convenient method of administration. Examples of this are shown in Sample Prescriptions 24.5 and 24.6.

d. When crushing tablets that contain cytotoxic or other hazardous drugs, special precautions are necessary. These tablets should be placed in a disposable plastic bag and crushed with a pestle. The bag should be thick enough to avoid being punctured. Sample Prescription 24.6 illustrates this technique.

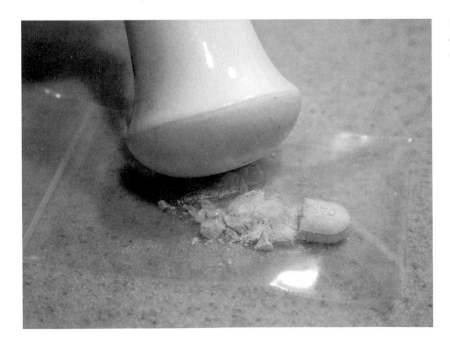

Pulverizing a tablet containing a hazardous drug in a polybag

SAMPLE PRESCRIPTIONS

➤ **Prescription 24-1**

Contemporary Physicians Group Practice
20 S. Park Street, Triturate, WI 53706
Tel: (608) 555-1333 Fax: (608) 555-1335

R # 022

Name *Roberta Fifrick*	Date *00/00/00*
Address *713 Reed Street*	Age Wt/Ht

R

Aluminum Hydroxide	*3.75 g*
Magnesium Trisilicate	*3.75 g*
Peppermint Oil	*qs*
Calcium Carbonate q s ad	*15 g*

J. Rivera   00/00/00

Sig: One level tsp in water tid pc

Refills   2   *H. G. Fedder*   M.D.

DEA No. _____

Ingredients Used

Ingredient	Quantity Used	Manufacturer Lot #-Exp Date	Solubility	Dose Comparison Given	Dose Comparison Usual	Use in the Prescription
Aluminum Hydroxide	3.75 g	JET Labs XY1143-mm/yy	insol in water and alcohol	0.4 g t.i.d.	0.3–0.6 g 4–6 X daily	antacid
Magnesium Trisilicate	3.75 g	JET Labs XY1144-mm/yy	insol in water and alcohol	0.4 g t.i.d.	1 g q.i.d.	antacid
Peppermint Oil	10 drops	JET Labs XY1145-mm/yy	immis w/water mis w/alcohol	—	—	flavor, scent
Calcium Carbonate	7.5 g	JET Labs XY1146-mm/yy	insol in water and alcohol	0.8 g t.i.d.	1 g 4–6 X daily	antacid

Compatibility–Stability/Beyond-Use Date

Stability–Compatibility: All ingredients in this preparation are compatible and very stable when in a solid dosage form.

Packaging and Storage and Beyond-use date: The *USP* monographs recommend storage in well-closed containers for all of these active ingredients when formulated into tablets (5). Pharmacist Rivera will use the maximum 6-month beyond-use date as specified in *USP* Chapter ⟨795⟩ for solid formulations made with USP ingredients (6).

Calculations

Dose/Concentration

Weight of powder in one level teaspoonful = 1.6 g

Weight of Aluminum Hydroxide and Magnesium Trisilicate per teaspoonful (1.6 g):

$$\frac{3.75 \ g \ Al/Mg}{15 \ g \ powder} = \frac{x \ g \ Al/Mg}{1.6 \ g \ powder}; \ x = 0.4 \ g \ Al/Mg$$

Weight of Calcium Carbonate per teaspoonful (1.6 g):

$$\frac{7.5 \ g \ CaCarb.}{15 \ g \ powder} = \frac{x \ g \ CaCarb.}{1.6 \ g \ powder}; \ x = 0.8 \ g \ CaCarb.$$

Ingredient Amounts

Aluminum Hydroxide and Magnesium Trisilicate: 3.75 g each

Calcium Carbonate: *15 g − (3.75 g + 3.75 g) = 7.5 g*

> **Note**: Weight of Peppermint Oil negligible

Compounding Procedure

All weighing is done on a Class 3 torsion or electronic balance. Weigh 3.75 g each of Magnesium Trisilicate and Aluminum Hydroxide and 7.5 g of Calcium Carbonate. Using either spatulation or trituration, mix the powders geometrically, spatulating or triturating well after each addition. Add Peppermint Oil dropwise until a desirable scent is obtained, and record the number of drops on the compounding record or on the face of the prescription order (e.g., 10 drops). Calibrate the dose by weighing the contents of one level teaspoonful—found to be 1.6 g. Using a paper funnel, transfer the powder into an appropriate-sized powder jar with child-resistant closure. Label the preparation appropriately.

Quality Control

Dosage form is a fine white powder. The actual weight is checked and matches the theoretical weight of 15 g.

Labeling

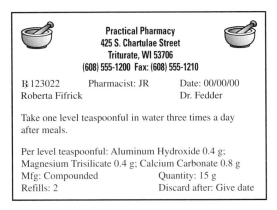

Practical Pharmacy
425 S. Chartulae Street
Triturate, WI 53706
(608) 555-1200 Fax: (608) 555-1210

℞ 123022   Pharmacist: JR   Date: 00/00/00
Roberta Fifrick   Dr. Fedder

Take one level teaspoonful in water three times a day after meals.

Per level teaspoonful: Aluminum Hydroxide 0.4 g;
Magnesium Trisilicate 0.4 g; Calcium Carbonate 0.8 g
Mfg: Compounded   Quantity: 15 g
Refills: 2   Discard after: Give date

Patient Consultation

Hello, Ms. Fifrick, I'm Juanita Rivera, your pharmacist. Do you have any drug allergies? What do you know about this medication? (Or, what did your doctor tell you about it?) Are you taking any prescription or non-prescription medications? This medicine is for your stomach problem. Take one level teaspoonful mixed very well in a glass of water three times a day after meals. If you continue to have discomfort, or if you become constipated or develop diarrhea, consult with Dr. Fedder. This medication should be stored at room temperature, tightly closed, in a cool dry place. Any unused portion should be discarded after 6 months. You may have this prescription refilled two more times. Do you have any questions?

► **Prescription 24.2**

Contemporary Physicians Group Practice
20 S. Park Street, Triturate, WI 53706
Tel: (608) 555-1333 Fax: (608) 555-1335

R # 009

Name *James Reisman*   Date *00/00/00*

Address *532 Minocqua Court*   Age   Wt/Ht

Rx

Benzocaine	0.75 g
Salicylic Acid	0.75 g
Benzoic Acid	1.5 g
Camphor	1 g
Methyl Salicylate	qs
Talc q s ad	30 g

J. Johnson 00/00/00

Sig: Apply to feet ut dict q AM and hs

Refills   3   *K. W. Shapiro*   M.D.

DEA No. _____

Ingredients Used

Ingredient	Quantity Used	Manufacturer Lot #-Exp Date	Solubility	Dose Comparison Given	Usual	Use in the Prescription
Benzocaine	0.75 g	JET Labs XY1147-mm/yy	1 g/2500 mL water, 5 mL alcohol	2.5%	1 to 20%	local anesthetic
Salicylic Acid	0.75 g	JET Labs XY1148-mm/yy	1 g/460 mL water, 2.7 mL alcohol	2.5%	1 to 20%	keratolytic
Benzoic Acid	1.5 g	JET Labs XY1149-mm/yy	1 g/300 mL water, 2.3 mL alcohol	5%	6%	antifungal
Camphor	1.0 g	JET Labs XY1150-mm/yy	1 g/800 mL water, 1 mL alcohol	3.3%	0.1–10%	antipruritic
Methyl Salicylate	6 drops	JET Labs XY1151-mm/yy	1 g/1500 mL water, mis w/alcohol	—	—	scent
Talc	26 g	JET Labs XY1152-mm/yy	insol in water and alcohol	86.7%	—	vehicle & absorbent

Compatibility–Stability/Beyond-Use Date

Stability–Compatibility: All ingredients are quite stable; however, the Benzocaine, Salicylic Acid, and Camphor have the potential to form a liquefied eutectic mixture if triturated together. In this case that would be an advantage because Camphor is available as hard crystals that do not reduce to a fine powder with direct trituration. Therefore, for this preparation, the preferred treatment would be to "force" the eutectic mixture by triturating the Benzocaine, Salicylic Acid, and Camphor together in a glass mortar to liquefy these solids. If the mixture does not liquefy adequately to dissolve the Camphor, a few drops of Alcohol may be added to complete the process. An alternate method of compounding is to first reduce the Camphor to a fine powder using pulverization by intervention. Then protect each of the eutectic-formers by separately triturating each with a small amount of Talc, then gently spatulating these portions together, finally adding the rest of the Talc by spatulation using geometric dilution.

Packaging and Storage and Beyond-use date: If this preparation is dispensed in a tight, light-resistant container as recommended in the *USP* monograph for Camphor USP (5), it would be acceptable to use the maximum 6-month beyond-use date as specified in *USP* Chapter ⟨795⟩ for solid formulations made with USP ingredients (6). In this example, Pharmacist Johnson has selected a shaker can to improve the ease of use for the patient. The shaker can is not a tight container, so a more conservative 3-month beyond-use date should be used.

Calculations

Dose/Concentration

$$\% \, Benzocaine \, \& \, Sal.\,Ac: \quad \frac{0.75 \, g \, Benz/S.A.}{30 \, g \, powder} = \frac{x}{100}; \; x = 2.5\%$$

$$\% \, Camphor: \quad \frac{1 \, g \, Camphor}{30 \, g \, powder} = \frac{x}{100}; \; x = 3.3\%$$

$$\% \, Benzoic \, Acid: \quad \frac{1.5 \, g \, Ben.\,Ac.}{30 \, g \, powder} = \frac{x}{100}; \; x = 5\%$$

$$\% \, Talc: \quad \frac{26 \, g \, Talc}{30 \, g \, powder} = \frac{x}{100}; \; x = 86.7\% \, \left(Optional, Talc \, is \, not \, an \, active \, Ingredient \right)$$

Ingredient Amounts

All ingredient weights are given on the prescription order except Talc.

$$Talc = 30 \, g - (wgts \, of \, other \, ingredients) = 30 \, g - (0.75 + 0.75 + 1.5 + 1) \, g$$
$$= 30 \, g - 4 \, g = 26 \, g$$

Compounding Procedure

On a Class 3 torsion or electronic balance, weigh 0.75 g of Benzocaine and 0.75 g of Salicylic Acid, 1.5 g of Benzoic Acid, 1 g of Camphor, and 26 g of Talc. Transfer the Benzocaine, Salicylic Acid, Benzoic Acid, and Camphor to a glass mortar and triturate these together, "forcing" the eutectic mixture. If the mixture does not liquefy adequately to dissolve the Camphor, add a few drops of Alcohol. Add the Talc to the mortar in portions with trituration using geometric dilution, adsorbing the liquid eutectic on the Talc. Add Methyl Salicylate drop-wise until a desired scent is achieved (e.g., 6 drops); record the number of drops on the document or compounding record. Place the finished product in a shaker-can and label appropriately.

Quality Control

Dosage form is a fine whitish-gray powder. The actual weight is checked and matches the theoretical weight of 30 g.

Labeling

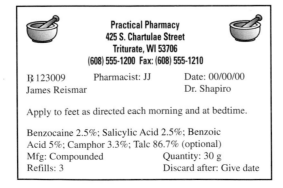

Auxiliary Labels: For External Use Only; Keep Out of Reach of Children;

Patient Consultation

Hello, Mr. Reismar, I'm your pharmacist, John Johnson. Do you have any drug allergies? What do you know about this medicine? (Or, what did your doctor tell you about it?) Are you taking any prescription or nonprescription drugs? This prescription is for a fungal infection. Apply to your feet as directed each morning and at bedtime. If the condition doesn't improve in a few days, or if it gets worse, discontinue use and contact Dr. Shapiro. Keep this in a cool, dry place, out of the reach of children. This is for external use only. Discard any unused contents after 3 months (give date). This prescription can be refilled three times. Do you have any questions?

➤ Prescription 24.3

Contemporary Physicians Group Practice
20 S. Park Street, Triturate, WI 53706
Tel: (608) 555-1333 Fax: (608) 555-1335

℞ # 025

Name *Jared Stone*   Date *00/00/00*

Address *2530 Lego Lane*   Age   Wt/Ht

℞

     Mix Nystatin Powder 1:10 with the following:
     Zinc Oxide
     Talc
     Starch
     Calcium Carbonate | *equal quantities to give 20 g*

    Sig: Apply to area with each diaper change

Called Dr. Schultz to confirm ratio interpretation and use of Nystatin Topical Powder   B. Bell   00/00/00

Refills   *3*   *Aleta Schultz*   , M.D.

              DEA No. _____

Ingredients Used

Ingredient	Quantity Used	Manufacturer Lot #-Exp Date	Solubility	Dose Comparison Given	Dose Comparison Usual	Use in the Prescription
Zinc Oxide	5 g	JET Labs XY1153-mm/yy	insol in water and alcohol	22.7%	any	astringent, adsorbent
Talc	5 g	JET Labs XY1152-mm/yy	insol in water and alcohol	22.7%	any	vehicle, adsorbent
Starch	5 g	JET Labs XY1155-mm/yy	insol in water and alcohol	22.7%	any	vehicle, adsorbent
Calcium Carbonate	5 g	JET Labs XY1146-mm/yy	practically insol in water	22.7%	any	astringent, adsorbent
Nystatin 100,000 units/g	2 g	BJF Generics XY1157-mm/yy	4 mg/mL water, 1.2 mg/mL alcohol	9090 units/g	100,000 units/g	antifungal

Compatibility–Stability/Beyond-Use Date

Stability–Compatibility: All ingredients are compatible and stable in a powder dosage form.

Packaging and Storage and Beyond-use date: The *USP* monographs for all ingredients, including Nystatin Topical Powder, allow storage in well-closed containers (5). If using a manufactured product form of Nystatin Topical Powder, use the recommended beyond-use date as specified in *USP* Chapter ⟨795⟩ for solid formulations made with active ingredients from manufactured drug products: not later than 25% of the time remaining until the product's expiration date or 6 months, whichever is earlier. If using all bulk active ingredients, it would be acceptable to use the maximum 6-month beyond-use date as specified in *USP* Chapter ⟨795⟩ for solid formulations made with USP ingredients (6).

Calculations

This order is an example of a ratio strength that can be interpreted in two ways, with the colon as a "plus" or as a "q.s. ad." We will assume for this exercise that the pharmacist called the prescriber and the intent is 2 g of Nystatin Powder **plus** 20 g of the bulk powder. This would also make sense anecdotally, given the quantity of bulk powder of 20 grams and the ratio strength of 1:10.

The other difficulty with interpreting this order is whether the "Nystatin Powder" should be taken to mean pure Nystatin USP or Nystatin Topical Powder USP. Both are powders and both are available. This is addressed below.

Dose/Concentration

ZnO, Talc, Starch, and Calcium Carbonate concentrations:

$$\% \text{ } ZnO, Talc, Starch, CaCarb.: \frac{5 \text{ } g \text{ } Ingred.}{22 \text{ } g \text{ } powder} = \frac{x}{100}; \text{ } x \text{ } 22.7\% \approx 23\%$$

Nystatin concentration:

If we assumed the Nystatin powder is Nystatin Topical Powder 100,000 units/g:

$$\left(\frac{100,000 \text{ } units \text{ } Nystatin}{g \text{ } Nys.Top.Powder}\right)\left(\frac{2 \text{ } g \text{ } Nys.Top.Powder}{22 \text{ } g \text{ } total \text{ } powder}\right) = 9,090 \text{ } units/g \text{ } \left(\approx 1/10 \text{ } the \text{ } normal \text{ } dose\right)$$

If we assumed the Nystatin Powder is pure Nystatin:
(**Note**: Pure Nystatin is 4,400 units/mg)

$$\left(\frac{4,400 \text{ } units \text{ } Nystatin}{mg \text{ } Nys. \text{ } powder}\right)\left(\frac{2,000 \text{ } mg \text{ } Nys. \text{ } powder}{22 \text{ } g \text{ } total \text{ } powder}\right) = 400,000 \text{ } units \text{ } Nystatin/g \text{ } \left(\approx 4\times \text{ } the \text{ } normal \text{ } dose\right)$$

For this exercise, we will assume that the pharmacist consulted with the physician and the first interpretation, Nystatin Topical Powder, is the desired one.

Ingredient Amounts

ZnO, Talc, Starch, Calcium Carbonate: *20 g/ 4 = 5 g of each*

Nystatin Topical Powder:

$$\frac{1 \text{ } part \text{ } Nystatin \text{ } powder}{10 \text{ } parts \text{ } other \text{ } powders} = \frac{x \text{ } g \text{ } Nystatin \text{ } powder}{20 \text{ } g \text{ } other \text{ } powders}; \text{ } x = 2 \text{ } g \text{ } Nystatin \text{ } powder$$

Compounding Procedure

On a Class 3 torsion or an electronic balance, weigh 2 g of Nystatin Topical Powder 100,000 units/g, and 5 g each of Zinc Oxide, Talc, Starch, and Calcium Carbonate. Mix the adsorbent powders together by spatulation or trituration, and then combine geometrically with the Nystatin Topical Powder. Alternatively, each of the adsorbent powders could be mixed geometrically with the Nystatin Topical Powder, using trituration. Dispense in a plastic cylinder bottle with a Yorker or flip spout cap, and label as shown below.

Quality Control

Dosage form is a fine white powder. The actual weight is checked and matches the theoretical weight of 22 g.

Labeling

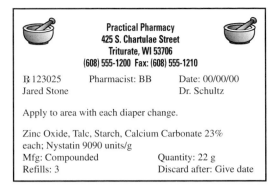

Practical Pharmacy
425 S. Chartulae Street
Triturate, WI 53706
(608) 555-1200 Fax: (608) 555-1210

| Ŗ 123025 | Pharmacist: BB | Date: 00/00/00 |
| Jared Stone | | Dr. Schultz |

Apply to area with each diaper change.

Zinc Oxide, Talc, Starch, Calcium Carbonate 23% each; Nystatin 9090 units/g

| Mfg: Compounded | Quantity: 22 g |
| Refills: 3 | Discard after: Give date |

Auxiliary Labels: For External Use Only

Patient Consultation

Hello, Mrs. Stone, I'm your pharmacist, Barbara Bell. Does Jared have any drug allergies? Is he currently using any nonprescription or prescription medications? What did your physician tell you about this or how to use it? This is a topical dusting powder for diaper rash. It will help keep the area dry and will treat any fungal or yeast infection in the diaper area. You should apply this to the affected area each time you change Jared's diaper, being careful not to get this in Jared's eyes, nose, or mouth. It is also very important to carefully cleanse the area first before applying the powder. If you don't notice any improvement in a few days, or if it appears that the area is getting worse, discontinue use and contact Dr. Schultz. This may be stored at room temperature, in an area away from moisture, and out of the reach of children. This prescription may be refilled three times. Any unused portion should be discarded after (give date). Do you have any questions?

➤ Prescription 24.4

Contemporary Physicians Group Practice
20 S. Park Street, Triturate, WI 53706
Tel: (608) 555-1333 Fax: (608) 555-1335

Ŗ # 042

| Name *Jacob Stone* | Date *00/00/00* | |
| Address *521 Lego Circle* | Age   *11 yr* Wt/Ht | *88 lb* |

Ŗ

Hydralazine 0.75 mg/kg/day in 4 divided doses

M & Ft Chartulae   #6

Sig: Take contents of one chart on Cool Whip or pudding qid

J. Jackson   00/00/00

Refills   2   R. Farrell   M.D.

DEA No. _____

Ingredients Used: *for seven doses*

Ingredient	Quantity Used	Manufacturer Lot #-Exp Date	Solubility	Dose Comparison Given	Usual	Use in the Prescription
Hydralazine HCl	120 mg weighed; 52.5 mg used	JET Labs XY1158-mm/yy	1 g/33 mL water, 500 mL alcohol	0.75 mg/kg/day or 7.5 mg q.i.d.	same	antihypertensive
Lactose	360 mg weighed for aliquot; 1890 mg used for extra diluent	JET Labs XY1159-mm/yy	1 g/5 mL water, v sl sol in alcohol	—	—	diluent

Compatibility–Stability/Beyond-Use Date

Stability–Compatibility: In a solid dosage form Hydralazine HCl is relatively stable.
Packaging and Storage and Beyond-use date: The *USP* monograph for Hydralazine Hydrochloride Tablets recommends storage in tight, light-resistant containers (5). Pharmacist Jackson is formulating this preparation with pure Hydralazine powder and Lactose and will use the recommended 6-month beyond-use date as specified in *USP* Chapter ⟨795⟩ for solid formulations made with USP ingredients (6).

Calculations

Dose/Concentration

$$Weight\ of\ child\ in\ kg: \frac{88\ lb}{2.2\ lb/kg} = 40\ kg$$

$$Dose\ in\ mg: \left(\frac{0.75\ mg}{kg/day}\right)\left(40\ kg\right)\left(\frac{day}{4\ doses}\right) = 7.5\ mg/dose$$

Ingredient Amounts (for seven doses)
Hydralazine:

$$\frac{7.5\ mg\ Hydralazine}{dose} \times 7\ doses = 52.5\ mg\ Hydralazine$$

Pure powder will be used and the amount calculated above is below the MWQ; therefore, an aliquot is needed. If the MWQ of 120 mg of Hydralazine is weighed and mixed with 360 mg of Lactose to give 480 mg of dilution, the amount of this dilution that will contain the needed 52.5 mg of Hydralazine can be calculated:

$$\frac{120\ mg\ Hydralazine}{480\ mg\ dilution} = \frac{52.5\ mg\ Hydralazine}{x\ mg\ dilution}; \ x = 210\ mg\ dilution$$

Extra Lactose diluent for the divided papers:
If you want the final contents of each packet to weigh 300 mg, extra Lactose must be added

300 mg × 7 = 2,100 mg total powder

2,100 mg total powder − 210 mg Hydralazine aliquot = 1,890 mg Lactose

Compounding Procedure

On a Class 3 torsion balance or an electronic digital balance, weigh 120 mg of Hydralazine HCl powder and 360 mg Lactose. Transfer the Hydralazine powder to a glass mortar and add the Lactose to the Hydralazine powder by geometric dilution, triturating well. Weigh 210 mg of this powder and transfer to a clean glass mortar. Weigh an additional 1,890 mg of Lactose and add the Lactose to the 210 mg of Hydralazine aliquot by geometric dilution, again triturating well. Weigh 300 mg of this powder for each dose and place each dose in a polyethylene zip-lock bag. Dispense the bags in a wide-mouth container with a child-resistant closure.

Quality Control

The preparation is a fine, white powder. Each powder packet is weighed to contain 300 mg of powder.

Labeling

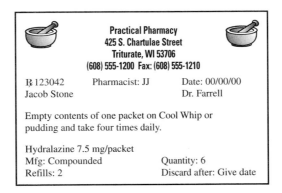

Practical Pharmacy
425 S. Chartulae Street
Triturate, WI 53706
(608) 555-1200 Fax: (608) 555-1210

R 123042   Pharmacist: JJ   Date: 00/00/00
Jacob Stone   Dr. Farrell

Empty contents of one packet on Cool Whip or
pudding and take four times daily.

Hydralazine 7.5 mg/packet
Mfg: Compounded   Quantity: 6
Refills: 2   Discard after: Give date

Auxiliary Labels: Keep Out of Reach of Children; Dizziness Warning

Patient Consultation

Hello, Mr. Stone (or caretaker), I'm your pharmacist, Jennie Jackson, and I have Jacob's prescription ready. Does Jacob have any drug allergies? Is he currently taking any nonprescription or prescription medication? Do you know (or did Dr. Farrell explain) what this medication is for? This is used to treat hypertension. You are to empty the contents of one packet onto Cool Whip or some kind of pudding or other soft food and have him eat the total portion prepared. He should do this four times a day. Some side effects that he could possibly experience include headache, dizziness, fast or irregular heartbeat, diarrhea, loss of appetite, nausea, or vomiting. These usually go away after Jacob has taken this for awhile. If he notices chest pain, joint pain, sore throat and fever, swelling of his arms or legs, skin rashes, or itching, consult with Dr. Farrell immediately. Store this in a cool, dry place, out of the reach of children. Discard any unused portion after the date given on the bottle, which is 6 months from now. This may be refilled two times. Since these powders must be custom-made, please call in advance when you need more so that I can prepare them and have them ready for you. Do you have any questions?

➤ Prescription 24.5

Contemporary Physicians Group Practice
20 S. Park Street, Triturate, WI 53706
Tel: (608) 555-1333 Fax: (608) 555-1335

R # 045

Name *Lawrence Bow*   Date *00/00/00*

Address *511 Academy Lane*   Age *2 yr*   Wt/Ht *25 lb*

R

30
Carbamazepine   ~~100~~ mg/powder packet

M & Ft Divided Powders #8   ***Bill Bailey 00/00/00***

Sig: Take contents of one powder packet qid, pc and hs

Changed dose to 30 mg/packet per telephone consult with Dr. Wurtz. BB

Refills   5   *Ozzie Wurtz*   M.D.

DEA No. _____

Ingredients Used: *for 9 packets*

Ingredient	Quantity Used	Manufacturer Lot #-Exp Date	Solubility	Dose Comparison Given	Usual	Use in the Prescription
Carbamazepine as 2 × 200 mg tablets	270 mg drug from 378 mg crushed tablet powder	BJF Generics XY1160-mm/yy	practically insoluble in water	35 mg/Kg/day – changed to ~10 mg/Kg/day	10–20 mg/Kg/day	Anticonvulsant
Lactose	2322 mg	JET Labs XY1159-mm/yy	1 g/5 mL water, v sl sol in alcohol	—	—	Diluent

Compatibility–Stability/Beyond-Use Date

Stability–Compatibility: Even when in a solid dosage form, Carbamazepine has some stability concerns, and its solid preparations require special packaging and storage for maximum stability. In two articles reported in the *American Journal of the Hospital Pharmacy* and reviewed in the Carbamazepine monograph in *Trissel's Stability of Compounded Formulations*, it is reported that the bioavailability of Carbamazepine, when in tablet form, can be reduced by one third if exposed to excess moisture. The reduction in bioavailability is reported to be caused by tablet hardening due to the uptake of water by the drug molecule with the formation of the dihydrate (7–9). This is the reason for the more restrictive packaging and storage conditions recommended by the USP, as given below.

Packaging and Storage and Beyond-use date: The *USP* monograph for Carbamazepine Tablets recommends storage in tight, preferably glass, containers. It also states that the product should be labeled for storage in a dry place, protected from moisture (5). Pharmacist Bailey checked the stability of Carbamazepine in *Trissel's Stability of Compounded Formulations* and found the information given above. Because of the stability problems with Carbamazepine, Pharmacist Bailey has decided to use a more conservative beyond-use date of 30 days rather than the usual allowable 25% of the time remaining until the product's expiration date or 6 months, whichever is earlier.

Calculations

Dose/Concentration

$$Weight\ of\ child\ in\ kg: \frac{25\ lb}{2.2\ lb/kg} = 11.4\ kg$$

$$Prescribed\ dose\ in\ mg/kg/day: \left(\frac{100\ mg\,Carbam.}{dose}\right)\left(\frac{4\ doses}{day}\right)\left(\frac{1}{11.4\ kg}\right) = 35\ mg/kg/day$$

Upon consultation with the patient, the pharmacist is told that this prescription order is for an initial dose. The *USP/DI* gives an initial dose of 10–20 mg/kg/day. The above dose exceeds this recommended dose. If the *USP/DI* recommended range is used, a daily dose would be: 10–20 mg/kg/day × 11.4 kg = 114–228 mg/day. With four doses per day, a range of 29–57 mg/dose is acceptable. The pharmacist then calls Dr. Wurtz and together they decide to change the order from 100 mg/packet to 30 mg/packet.

Ingredient Amounts (for nine doses)

If using 30 mg/dose:

30 mg/dose × 9 doses = 270 mg of Carbamazepine is needed for this order (including enough powder for one extra dose)

Carbamazepine is available as 200-mg tablets; two of these are needed, and it is determined that each tablet weighs 280 mg. The amount of crushed tablet powder is calculated to be:

$$\frac{200\ mg\,Carbam.}{280\ mg\,tablet\,powder} = \frac{270\ mg\,Carbam.}{x\ mg\,tablet\,powder}; x = 378\ mg\ crushed\ tablet\ powder$$

To make each powder packet weigh 300 mg:

300 mg/packet × 9 packets = 2,700 mg powder is needed.

The amount of lactose needed is:

2,700 mg—378 mg = 2,322 mg Lactose

Compounding Procedure

On a Class 3 torsion balance or an electronic digital balance, weigh two Carbamazepine 200-mg tablets. Each tablet weighs 280 mg (weights will vary with different manufacturers). Crush the two tablets and weigh 378 mg of crushed powder, containing 270 mg of active ingredient. Weigh 2,322 mg of Lactose and add to the Carbamazepine by trituration using geometric dilution. Weigh 300 mg of powder for each dose, and place each dose in an individual polyethylene zip-lock bag. Dispense the bags in a glass, wide-mouth, tight container with a child-resistant closure. Label appropriately.

Quality Control

The preparation is a fine, white powder. The Carbamazepine tablets used for the source of active ingredient were white tablets. Each powder packet is weighed to contain 300 mg of powder.

Labeling

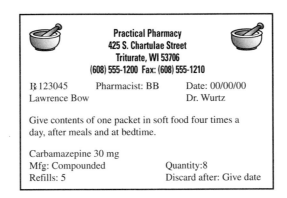

Practical Pharmacy
425 S. Chartulae Street
Triturate, WI 53706
(608) 555-1200 Fax: (608) 555-1210

℞ 123045   Pharmacist: BB   Date: 00/00/00
Lawrence Bow   Dr. Wurtz

Give contents of one packet in soft food four times a
day, after meals and at bedtime.

Carbamazepine 30 mg
Mfg: Compounded   Quantity:8
Refills: 5   Discard after: Give date

Auxiliary Labels: Drowsiness Warning; Photosensitivity Warning (optional);
Store in a Dry Place, Protect from Moisture; Keep Out of Reach of Childre

Patient Consultation

Hello, Mrs. Bow, I'm your pharmacist, Bill Bailey. Does Lawrence have any drug allergies? Does he take any other medications, either prescription or nonprescription drugs? What did Dr. Wurtz tell you about this medication? (Mrs. Bow replies that Larry is taking it to prevent seizures.) You should give the contents of one packet, mixed with food (e.g., pudding, applesauce) four times a day, after meals and at bedtime. This medication might cause some drowsiness or dizziness, especially initially. Larry should avoid exposure to direct sunlight as much as possible as it may cause a rash—be sure to apply sunscreen when he will be outdoors in the sunlight. Watch for changes in vision, darkened stool, behavioral changes, or seizures; contact Dr. Wurtz immediately if you notice any of these changes. Store this medication in a cool, dry place (protect from moisture), out of the reach of children. This may be refilled five times. Discard any unused portion after 1 month. Do you have any questions?

➤ **Prescription 24.6**

```
                Contemporary Physicians Group Practice
                   20 S. Park Street, Triturate, WI 53706
                  Tel: (608) 555-1333  Fax: (608) 555-1335

                                          R # 047

Name  John Denali                         Date   00/00/00

Address  296 Mountaineer Rd               Age     2½ yrs  Wt/Ht   30#/36"

   R
                Mercaptopurine              75 mg/m²/day

                  M et Ft. Divided Oral Powders  #8
                                        D. Alpine  00/00/00

        Sig:  Give the contents of one packet with breakfast and supper


Refills   1                            Patsy Heider              M.D.

                        DEA No. _____
```

Ingredients Used: *for 9 packets*

Ingredient	Quantity Used	Manufacturer Lot #-Exp Date	Solubility	Dose Comparison Given	Dose Comparison Usual	Use in the Prescription
Mercaptopurine as 5 × 50 mg tablets	225 mg drug from 1274 mg crushed tablet powder	BJF Generics XY1162-mm/yy	insol in water sol in hot alcohol	75mg/ m²/day	75mg/ m²/day	immunosuppressant
Lactose	1.426 g	JET Labs XY1159-mm/yy	1 g/5 mL water, v sl sol in alcohol	—	—	diluent

Compatibility–Stability/Beyond-Use Date

Stability–Compatibility: In a solid dosage form Mercaptopurine is relatively stable, but the FDA recommends consideration of proper handling and disposal of this drug as an antineoplastic agent.

Packaging and Storage and Beyond-use date: The *USP* monograph for Mercaptopurine Tablets recommends storage in well-closed containers (5). Pharmacist Alpine will use the recommended beyond-use date as specified in *USP* Chapter ⟨795⟩ for solid formulations made with active ingredients from manufactured drug products: no later than 25% of the time remaining until the product's expiration date or 6 months, whichever is earlier (6).

Calculations

Dose/Concentration

This patient has a body weight of 30 lbs and a height of 36". Based on this weight and height, the body surface area (BSA) from the nomogram in Appendix E is 0.57 m^2.

Daily dose: *75 mg/m²/day × 0.57 m² = 43 mg/day*

The dosage reference states to increase the daily dose to the nearest 25 mg; in this case increase the 43 mg to 50 mg per day.

$$Dose\ in\ mg: \frac{50\ mg}{2\ doses/day} = 25\ mg/dose$$

Ingredient Amounts (for nine doses)

Using 25 mg/dose:

25 mg/dose × 9 doses = 225 mg of Mercaptopurine is needed for this order (including enough powder for one extra dose)

Mercaptopurine is available as 50-mg tablets, each weighing 283 mg. For 225 mg of Mercaptopurine, we will need 4.5 or 5 tablets (*225 mg ÷ 50 mg/tablet = 4.5 tablets*)

Amount of crushed tablet powder:

$$\frac{50\ mg\ MP}{283\ mg\ tablet\ powder} = \frac{225\ mg\ MP}{x\ mg\ tablet\ powder}; x = 1274\ mg\ tablet\ powder$$

Amount of tablet powder to discard:

283 mg × 5 tablets = 1,415 mg

1,415 mg − 1,274 mg = 141 mg to be discarded

To make each powder packet weigh 300 mg:

300 mg/packet × 9 packets = 2,700 mg powder is needed

The amount of lactose needed is:

2,700 mg − 1,274 mg = 1,426 mg Lactose

Compounding Procedure

Pharmacist Alpine noted the following: the Mercaptopurine monograph in the 8th edition of *Drug Information Handbook* states that the FDA's current recommendations are for consideration of proper handling and disposal of antineoplastic drugs like Mercaptopurine. Therefore, the following procedure treats this material as a biohazard.

Using an electronic balance and wearing disposable gloves, tare a zip-lock bag and add one or more Mercaptopurine 50-mg tablets to determine an average weight per tablet. This is found to be 283 mg. Place a total of 5 tablets into the bag, close it, and using a pestle on the outside of the bag, crush the tablets to a fine powder. Withdraw 141 mg of this crushed powder and discard this in another zip-lock bag that has a Biohazard label on it. Weigh 1,426 g of Lactose and add to the bag containing 1,274 mg of crushed Mercaptopurine powder, and mix this well by shaking and manipulating the bag. Reopen the bag and withdraw and weigh 300 mg of the powder in a smaller tared zip-lock bag. Repeat this for eight 300-mg portions. Place the bags in a tight container with a child-resistant closure. Label and dispense. Leave any remaining powder in the zip-lock bag that was used for mixing, place a Biohazard warning label on it, and discard in a Biohazard container.

Quality Control

The preparation is a fine, white powder. The Mercaptopurine tablets used for the source of active ingredient were white tablets. Each powder packet is weighed to contain 300 mg of powder.

Labeling

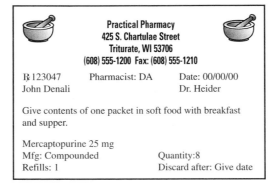

Practical Pharmacy
425 S. Chartulae Street
Triturate, WI 53706
(608) 555-1200 Fax: (608) 555-1210

℞ 123047   Pharmacist: DA   Date: 00/00/00
John Denali   Dr. Heider

Give contents of one packet in soft food with breakfast and supper.

Mercaptopurine 25 mg
Mfg: Compounded   Quantity:8
Refills: 1   Discard after: Give date

Auxiliary Labels: Keep Out of Reach of Children; Drowsiness Warning

Patient Consultation

Hello, I'm your pharmacist, David Alpine. Are you John Denali's mother? Does John have any drug allergies? What do you know about this medication (or what did Dr. Heider tell you about it)? Is John taking any other prescription or nonprescription medications? These packets contain Mercaptopurine, which is an agent used to treat leukemia. You are to give John the contents of one packet with some pudding or other soft food with breakfast and supper. Be sure that John drinks plenty of fluids while on this medication. Use caution when handling this medication, and be sure to wash your hands after giving John his dose. Possible side effects of this drug include nausea, loss of appetite, or diarrhea, and drowsiness or weakness. If John experiences any of these, you can call Dr. Heider or me for suggestions. Because this drug suppresses the immune system, have John practice good dental and hygiene habits, and protect him when possible from sources of infection. Be sure to contact the doctor if John experiences a rash or unusual bruising or bleeding or severe nausea. You should have John monitored closely by his physician. Store this medication in a dry, cool place, away from sunlight and out of the reach of children. Discard any unused contents after (give date); if you wish you can return it to our pharmacy for proper disposal. This prescription has one refill. Do you have any questions?

References

1. The 2002 United States Pharmacopeia 25/National Formulary 20. Rockville, MD: The United States Pharmacopeial Convention, Inc., 2001; 2220.
2. The 2002 United States Pharmacopeia 25/National Formulary 20. Rockville, MD: The United States Pharmacopeial Convention, Inc., 2001; 977.
3. The 2002 United States Pharmacopeia 25/National Formulary 20. Rockville, MD: The United States Pharmacopeial Convention, Inc., 2001; 2060.
4. Helin MM, Kontra KM, Naaranlahti TJ, Wallentius KJ. Content uniformity and stability of nifidipine in extemporaneously compounded oral powders. Am J Health-Syst Pharm 1998; 55: 1299-1301.
5. The 2002 United States Pharmacopeia 25/National Formulary 20. Rockville, MD: The United States Pharmacopeial Convention, Inc., 2001; Official Monographs.
6. The 2002 United States Pharmacopeia 25/National Formulary 20. Rockville, MD: The United States Pharmacopeial Convention, Inc., 2001; 2054-2055.
7. Trissel LA. Stability of compounded formulations, 2nd ed. Washington DC: The American Pharmaceutical Association, 2000; 60.
8. Moisture hardens carbamazepine tablets, FDA finds. Am J Hosp Pharm 1990; 47: 958.
9. Lowe MMJ. More information on hardening of carbamazepine tablets. Am J Hosp Pharm 1991; 48: 2130-2131.

CHAPTER 25

Capsules, Lozenges, and Other Solid Oral Dosage Forms

I. DEFINITIONS

A. **Capsules:** "Capsules are solid dosage forms in which the drug is enclosed within either a hard or soft soluble container or 'shell.' The shells are usually formed from gelatin; however, they also may be made from starch or other suitable substances" (1)—*USP*

B. **Lozenges:** "Lozenges are solid preparations, which are intended to dissolve or disintegrate slowly in the mouth. They contain one or more medicaments, usually in a flavored, sweetened base. They can be prepared by molding (gelatin and/or fused sucrose or sorbitol base) or by compression of sugar-based tablets . . . . They are usually intended for treatment of local irritation or infections of the mouth or throat but may contain active ingredients intended for systemic absorption after swallowing" (1)—*USP*

C. **Pastilles:** Some references make no distinction between lozenges and pastilles (2). However, the USP uses the term "pastille" for a subclass of lozenges; that is, molded lozenges (1). Secundum Artem differentiates the two terms by describing pastilles as lozenges that are softer and that contain a high concentration of sugar or sugar and gelatin (3).

D **Troches:** Although some references do not distinguish between lozenges and troches (2–4), the USP uses the term "troches" for a subcategory of lozenges; that is, compressed lozenges (1).

II. CAPSULES

A. Uses: As stated at the beginning of Chapter 24, powders for internal use are often formulated into capsules. Hard shell capsules offer a customized dosage form that can be made easily and conveniently in the pharmacy. Because the quantity of drug formulated into capsules can be measured accurately, this system is ideal for potent drugs and chemicals.

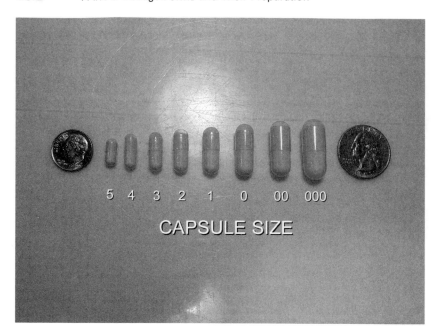

Range of capsule sizes

B. Hard Shell Capsules

1. Empty hard shell capsules are available in sizes that range from the largest size, 000, to the smallest size, 5. Larger bolus capsule shells are also available for veterinary use in large animals.

   a. Size 00 (double zero) is usually the largest capsule size used orally for humans. For some patients even size 00 capsules are too large to swallow.

   b. Size 000 (triple zero) capsules are sometimes used to encapsulate medication for rectal or vaginal use. The capsule is then used like a suppository. The capsule should be moistened with lubricating jelly or water before insertion.

2. The approximate capacities by capsule size for representative drugs and chemicals are given in Table 25.1. Notice that the weight capacity for a given capsule size is highly dependent on the density of the powder. The approximate volume capacities in milliliters are given in Table 25.2.

3. Empty hard shell capsules may be purchased from vendors of compounding supplies. They are available as clear, colorless gelatin capsules and in a variety of colors. Some capsule shells are made opaque by the addition of titanium oxide. These are especially useful when it is necessary or desirable to conceal the powder contents, such as when dispensing powders with an unappealing appearance or when making capsules for blind studies.

TABLE 25.1 Approximate Capacities of Gelatin Capsules for Representative Drugs and Chemicals (13)

| | Capsule Size | | | | | | | |
| | 5 | 4 | 3 | 2 | 1 | 0 | 00 | 000 |
Drug Substance	Capacity in grams of drug powder							
Acetaminophen	0.13	0.18	0.24	0.31	0.42	0.54	0.75	1.10
Aluminum hydroxide	0.18	0.27	0.36	0.47	0.64	0.82	1.14	1.71
Ascorbic acid	0.13	0.22	0.31	0.40	0.53	0.70	0.98	1.42
Aspirin	0.10	0.15	0.20	0.25	0.33	0.55	0.65	1.10
Bismuth subnitrate	0.12	0.25	0.40	0.55	0.65	0.80	1.20	1.75
Calcium carbonate	0.12	0.20	0.28	0.35	0.46	0.60	0.79	1.14
Calcium lactate	0.11	0.16	0.21	0.26	0.33	0.46	0.57	0.80
Corn starch	0.13	0.20	0.27	0.34	0.44	0.58	0.80	1.15
Lactose	0.14	0.21	0.28	0.35	0.46	0.60	0.85	1.25
Quinine sulfate	0.07	0.10	0.12	0.20	0.23	0.33	0.40	0.65
Sodium bicarbonate	0.13	0.26	0.32	0.39	0.52	0.70	0.97	1.43

Adapted from Narducci WA, Newton DW. Extemporaneous formulations. In: King RE, ed. Dispensing of medications, 9th ed. Easton, PA: Mack Publishing Co., 1984:268, and from Shaw MA. Capsules. In: King RE, ed. Dispensing of medications, 9th ed. Easton, PA: Mack Publishing Co., 1984:48.

TABLE 25.2   Approximate Volume Capacity by Capsule Size

Size	Milliliters
000	1.36
00	0.95
0	0.67
1	0.48
2	0.37
3	0.27
4	0.20
5	0.13

4. In addition to gelatin, capsule shells may also contain dispersing agents, hardening agents such as sucrose, or preservatives. A certain percentage of water, usually 10–15%, must be present in hard shell capsules (1). Lack of adequate moisture in these shells causes them to be hard and brittle, which makes them difficult to work with and which may affect their dissolution and bioavailability. For this reason, it is advisable to store capsules in tight containers that maintain a constant, adequate relative humidity. Capsules supplied by the manufacturer in paper boxes should be transferred to amber glass powder squares or other tight containers.

5. Hard shell capsules consist of two telescoping pieces, a body piece and a cap. In extemporaneous compounding, the two pieces are separated, the body piece is filled with the powder, then the cap is replaced on the body.

6. Selecting a capsule size for encapsulating a compounded powder
   a. General procedure
      (1) Determine the weight of the powder to be filled into each capsule.
      (2) Consult a capsule capacity table such as Table 25.1.
      (3) If you have a single capsule ingredient and that ingredient is a representative substance in the table, select the capsule size directly from the table.
      (4) Because most formulations are mixtures, selection of a capsule size usually requires judgment and sometimes trial and error. Try to pick a representative substance in the table that has a density similar to that of the ingredient in your formulation that is present in the greatest quantity. If you do not know this information, pick a capsule size that best fits your powder weight for the greatest number of representative drugs and chemicals.
      (5) In selecting a capsule size, you want the smallest size that will produce a filled capsule with no void space. For this reason, if your ingredient weight falls between two weights on the table, try the smaller capsule size first.
   b. Selecting a capsule size is something of a compromise. For best bioavailability of the powder, a loosely packed capsule is preferred because the powder disperses easily as the capsule shell dissolves. However, when filling capsules individually by hand, it is easier to fill capsules that are **slightly** packed because as you fill a number of capsules to a given weight, your fingers will be able to sense the packing pressure that corresponds to the desired weight of capsule ingredients. This

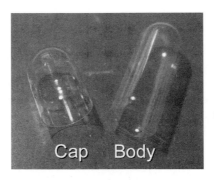

Parts of a capsule shell

makes it easier to achieve the appropriate capsule weight with a minimum number of balance checks. You do not have this sense of pressure with loosely packed capsules.

    c. If the amount of powder per unit necessitates a capsule size that is too large for the patient to comfortably swallow, divide the powder per dose in half and put each dose in two capsules. The number of capsules dispensed must then be doubled and the directions for use must be changed to double the number of units administered. The prescriber should be advised of any changes made in the prescription order.

    d. If the amount of powder for each capsule is less than the minimum weighable quantity for the balance being used, an inert solid diluent, such as lactose or cornstarch, should be added to the powder ingredients to give a desirable weight per capsule.

    e. Occasionally, the amount of powder per dose does not fit properly in any given capsule size—it is too much powder to fit in one size but gives void space in the next larger size. If this occurs, lactose, cornstarch, or another inert solid diluent may be added.

    f. When hand-filling capsules individually, a well-packing diluent may also be added to a granular powder to improve its ease of packing. Lactose Monohydrate (the non-spray-dried variety) and Starch are two diluents that work well for this purpose.

    g. The size and color of capsule used for compounding a prescription should be written on the prescription order or the compounding record so that any refills have the same appearance. When this information is recorded on the front of the prescription order, the number of the capsule size is usually put inside a triangle, Δ, and the capsule color is recorded beneath the triangle. (This is demonstrated for Sample Prescription 25.1 on the CD that accompanies this book.)

7. Procedure for hand-filling capsules with dry ingredients

    a. Prepare the powder using the techniques and procedures for particle size reduction and blending as described in Chapter 24. Make enough powder for one extra capsule because there will be some loss in the blending process. If the prescription contains a controlled substance, this loss in compounding must be minimal and should be documented on the prescription order or compounding record.

    b. Place the powder mixture for all the capsules on an ointment slab or pad. Using a spatula, arrange the powder into a compact, flat powder bed of uniform thickness. This is sometimes referred to as "blocking the powder bed." The height of the powder bed should be just slightly shorter than the long dimension of the body piece of the capsule shell. This allows for most efficient punching of powder into the shell. If the powder bed is even and uniformly packed, it is possible, after punching a few capsules, to get an idea of the number of times to punch powder into each shell body to give the approximate desired weight of powder per capsule.

    c. Although it is permissible to handle capsules with clean hands, the use of disposable gloves is preferred. In addition to being more sanitary, the use of gloves eliminates the problem of fingerprints on capsule shells; any dampness on bare fingers will cause a partial dissolution of the gelatin shell and a smudging of its surface. Furthermore, use of gloves protects the compounder from contact exposure to the drugs or chemicals being encapsulated.

    d. Separate the capsule cap from the body of the capsule shell and repeatedly press the open end of the body of the shell downward into the powder bed. This process is called "punching" capsules.

    e. Replace the cap on the body loosely and check the weight of the capsule. The weighing procedure for a double-pan balance is given in Figure 25.1 and for an electronic balance in Figure 25.2. Add to or empty powder from the capsule shell until the desired weight is achieved. A tolerance in final capsule weight of $\pm 5\%$ usually can be achieved without too much difficulty.

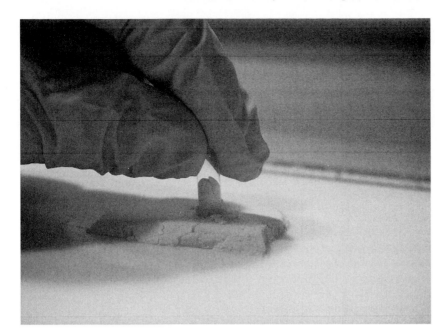

Hand-filling a capsule with dry powder

■ **Figure 25.1** Procedure for weighing capsules with a double-pan torsion balance.

**FIGURE 25.1 PROCEDURE FOR WEIGHING CAPSULES
WITH A DOUBLE-PAN TORSION BALANCE**

1. Place the balance on a smooth, level surface. Be sure the dial-in weights or rider are at zero. Release the balance pan arrest and check that the balance is operating properly with balance pans and index pointer moving freely.

2. Using the leveling feet at the front of the balance, bring the balance pans into equilibrium.

3. Put a weighing paper on each balance pan and re-establish equilibrium using the leveling feet. **After this step, do not touch the leveling feet again during this weighing operation.**

4. On the right-hand balance pan, place an empty capsule shell of the appropriate size plus weights to offset the weight of the powder per capsule. Adding weights on the dial at the front of the balance adds weight to the right side of the balance.
   Example: If a capsule is to contain 300 mg. of drug, place an empty capsule shell on the right balance pan and add 300 mg in fractional weights to the right balance pan **or** dial 0.3 g on the dial-in weights.

5. For each capsule, punch powder into an empty capsule shell and place it on the left balance pan. This will be offset by the weights added or dialed in plus the empty capsule shell placed on the right balance pan. Add or remove powder to the capsule shell until the index pointer is at the center of the index plate or until it moves an equal distance to the right and left of the center.

■ **Figure 25.2** Procedure for weighing capsules with an electronic balance.

---

1. Place the balance on a smooth, level surface. Press the tare button and observe the balance set at 000.0.

2. Place a weighing paper and an empty capsule shell of the appropriate size on the balance pan. Re-zero the balance by pressing the tare button. The digital display should read 000.0 **After this step, do not touch the tare button again during this weighing operation.**

3. Remove the empty capsule shell from the balance pan. The digital display will read a negative value which represents the weight of the capsule shell.

4. For each capsule, punch powder into an empty capsule shell and place it on the balance pan. Add or remove powder to the capsule shell until the digital display shows the desired weight of the capsule powder. The weight of the capsule shell will be offset by the negative value achieved when taring the empty shell at the beginning of the procedure.
   Example: If a capsule is to contain 300 mg of drug, the digital display should read 0.300 g when the completed capsule is on the balance pan.

---

8. Use of manufactured tablets and capsules in compounded hard shell capsules
   a. Manufactured tablets or capsules may be used as ingredients for compounded capsules. Review the discussion on using manufactured dosage forms in Chapter 12.
   b. Depending on the situation, one of the following techniques may be used:
      (1) The tablets may be crushed or the manufactured capsule contents emptied and the resulting powder used as would any powdered ingredient.
      (2) A whole tablet or capsule may be embedded in powder that has been punched into a capsule shell.
         (a) When making a customized combination preparation, if the dose of an ingredient per capsule is the exact quantity in a manufactured tablet or capsule, it may be easier to punch the correct amount of the other ingre-

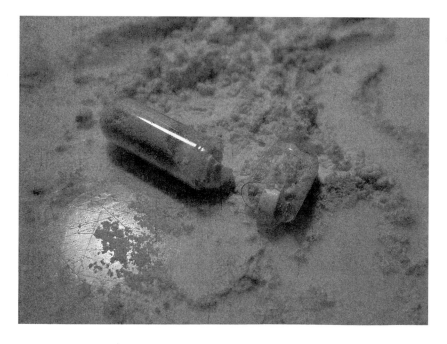

Embedding a tablet in
capsule powder

dients into the shell and then embed the manufactured tablet or capsule in this powder. This technique is particularly useful for protecting ingredients from each other when there is a question about compatibility.

(b) This method is also used when encapsulating tablets or capsules for blind studies. In this case the capsule shell is partially filled with Lactose or another inert diluent, and the tablet or capsule containing the active ingredient is concealed by embedding it in the diluent. If a tablet is concealed in this way, it may be split in two so that a smaller capsule shell can be used. This is especially important when making capsules for children and the elderly, who may have difficulty swallowing larger capsules.

9. Procedure for compounding capsules with liquid ingredients

   a. Liquid drugs or solutions or dispersions of drugs may be filled into capsule shells if the shell material is not soluble in the liquid.

   b. Care must be exercised to ensure that the liquid does not leak out of the capsule during storage or use.

      (1) Leakage can be minimized by sealing the capsule cap to the body of the capsule shell by moistening the inside edge of the cap before replacing it on the body. This can be done with a cotton applicator that has been dipped in water or a water/alcohol solution.

      (2) Several brands of capsule shells now are grooved so that the cap snaps in place on the body piece of the capsule. If possible, use capsule shells of this type to prevent leakage of liquid ingredients.

      (3) A third method is to mix the liquid drug with a melted miscible material that is a solid at room temperature but will melt at body temperature or will dissolve in the aqueous fluid in the stomach. The solution of the drug in this melted material is added in liquid form to the capsule shell. Because the material solidifies on standing, it will not leak out of the capsule shell during storage or use. Examples of such drug vehicles are the fatty bases and appropriate blends of polyethylene glycol polymers.

   c. Capsule shells may be filled with liquids volumetrically using a syringe or a graduated dropper or pipette.

   d. Liquids can also be filled in capsule shells by weight.

      (1) Insert the bodies of capsule shells in a holder (the holder may be as simple as the lid of a powder box with holes punched that are the size of the capsule bodies).

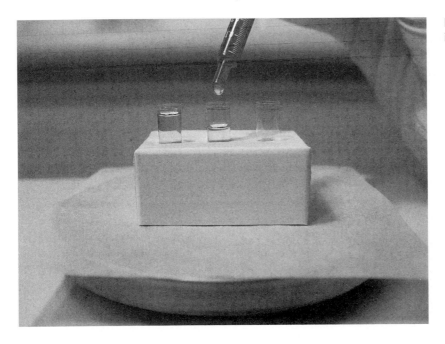

Filling capsules with liquid ingredients

(2) Place the holder containing the capsule bodies on an electronic balance and tare out the weight.

(3) Using a syringe, dropper, or pipette, add liquid to each shell body to the predetermined desired weight. This procedure is illustrated with Sample Prescription 25.5 later in this chapter.

10. Use of capsule-filling machines

    a. Pharmacists who compound capsules routinely or in larger quantities may want to invest in a capsule filler or capsule-filling machine. The non-automated fillers are available through pharmacy vendors at prices ranging from approximately $15 to over $1,000. There are also motorized capsule-loading machines in the $5,000 to $7,000 price range that can fill 300 capsules per batch. These fillers work on a principle of calibrated volume fill rather than weight, and their use requires good quality control procedures to ensure precise and accurate dose per capsule.

    b. When using a capsule-filling machine, the powder must be formulated so that its flow properties give capsules of uniform weight. If flow is a problem, one recommendation is to add a small quantity (less than 1% of the total powder weight) of Magnesium Stearate, a powdered excipient used as a lubricant in manufacturing tablets (5). Because an inert diluent is usually added to the powder when making capsules by volume, this ingredient should be selected carefully with flow properties in mind.

    (1) Lactose is a common inert diluent. It is commonly available as the monohydrate, and some suppliers sell the monohydrate in two forms, regular and spray-dried. The regular Lactose monohydrate packs well but does not have particularly good flow properties. Spray-dried Lactose monohydrate has been modified through processing to give a powder with improved flow characteristics. Anhydrous Lactose is also available, and it too has good flow properties. Spray-dried Lactose monohydrate and anhydrous Lactose are good diluents for capsule-filling machines. Check the type carefully when purchasing lactose for use as a diluent in capsule machines.

    (2) Microcrystalline Cellulose has been used successfully as a diluent for capsule-filling machines. It is a free-flowing powder classified by the NF as a tablet disintegrant and tablet and capsule diluent.

    (3) Some granular materials, such as Sodium Carboxymethylcellulose (CMC), have good flow properties, but depending on the other ingredients in the formulation, they may change the dissolution and absorption characteristics of

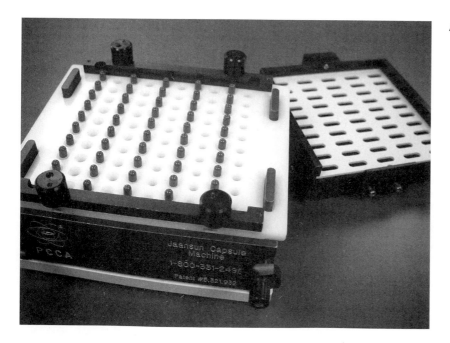

A capsule-filling machine

the drug. Unless specifically called for, natural and synthetic gum powders should be avoided as diluents because they may form thick viscous barriers around the drug particles when exposed to the aqueous fluid in the stomach and may prevent the drug from being released from the dosage form. Some sustained-release capsule formulations use synthetic gums to modify drug release, but these formulations should always be thoroughly tested before use.

c. As with capsules punched individually, capsules made using a filling machine should always be checked for accuracy and uniformity. A modification of the Weight Variation Test (6) given in Chapter ⟨905⟩ of the *USP* is useful when evaluating capsules made in this way.

(1) Select 10 capsules and weigh them individually.

(2) Calculate a mean, a standard deviation, and a relative standard deviation for this sample using these equations:

$$s = \left[\frac{\sum (x_i - \overline{X})^2}{n-1} \right]^{1/2}$$

$$RSD = \frac{100s}{\overline{X}}$$

where:

s = sample standard deviation.

RSD = relative standard deviation (the sample standard deviation expressed as a percentage of the mean).

$\overline{X}$ = mean of the values obtained from the units tested, expressed as a percentage of labeled amount of drug.

n = number of units tested.

x_i = individual values of the units tested, expressed as a percentage of the labeled amount of drug

(3) The capsules are satisfactory if all 10 units are within the range of 85% to 115% of the labeled amount of drug per capsule and if the relative standard deviation is less than or equal to 6%.

(4) If capsules fail to meet these standards, consult Chapter ⟨905⟩ of the *USP* for more detailed instructions. Basically, you select 20 extra capsules, and the specifications are met if none of the 30 capsules is outside 75% to 125% and not more than 3 of the 30 is outside 85% to 115% of label claim and the RSD of the 30 capsules does not exceed 7.8% (6).

(5) A quality control record with sample data that utilizes ⟨905⟩ standards is given in Figure 25.3.

d. Pharmacists who compound batches of capsules routinely should develop written formula and batch record sheets and written standard operating procedures (SOPs).

(1) Sample SOPs for capsule making have been published in the *International Journal of Pharmaceutical Compounding.* The quality control record as shown in Figure 25.3 is also useful to pharmacists who want to develop SOPs for their capsule compounding procedures.

(2) An additional control procedure that some pharmacists have found useful is to weigh the containers of formulation ingredients before and after the compounding procedure. The difference in the weight of each container should coincide with the calculated amount of that ingredient in the batch.

11. Handling incompatibilities

a. Proper handling of drugs and drug mixtures that liquefy when mixed is discussed in the section on bulk powders in Chapter 24 and in Chapter 34, Compatibility and Stability of Drug Products and Preparations Dispensed by the Pharmacist. The same principles apply when handling powders to be encapsulated.

■ **Figure 25.3** Sample quality control record for hard shell capsules.

---

1. Date: mm/dd/yy

2. Preparation/Quantity: Estradiol 10 mg Capsules   #100

3. Batch or Prescription Number: XXXX#####

4. Equipment: Handy Dandy Capsule Filling Machine, Model A689X

5. Capsule Size: 0

6. Diluent (Manufacturer/Lot #/Exp. Date):

      Anhydrous Lactose, JET Labs, #KYB4856-mm/yy

7. Formulation

   Calibrated powder weight for Anhydrous Lactose per capsule: 367 mg

   Capsules were made using the following formula:

   Weight of powder for 100 capsules: 36700 mg
   Weight of active ingredient for 100 capsules: 1000 mg
   Weight of Diluent for 100 capsules: 35700 mg

8. Randomly select 10 filled capsules. Weigh each capsule individually and record the weights in column (2) on the attached table.

9. Select ten empty capsule shells from the lot used to make the capsules. Weigh the shells on an electronic balance and calculate the average weight per shell. Record this weight in column (3) of the attached table.

10. Subtract the weight of a capsule shell from the weight of each capsule to determine the weight of powder in each shell and record this weight in column (4).

11. Using the formulation quantities above, and the true weight of powder in each capsule, calculate the amount of active ingredient in each capsule and record this in column (5). For example:

$$\frac{10 \; mg \; Estradiol}{367 \; mg \; capsule \; power} = \frac{x \; mg \; Estradiol}{343 \; mg \; capsule \; power} ; x = 9.3 \; mg \; Estradiol$$

12. For each capsule, express the amount of active ingredient as a percentage of label claim (LC) and record this in column (6).

$$\frac{9.3 \; mg \; actual \; Estradiol}{10 \; mg \; LC \; Estradiol} \times 100\% = 93\% \; of \; LC$$

13. Calculate the mean value of the units expressed as a percentage of label claim and record this as $\overline{X}$ in the last row of the table.

14. Calculate the range of 85% to 115% of label claim for this preparation.

      85% $\times$ 10 mg = 8.5 mg

      115% $\times$ 10 mg = 11.5 mg

15. Calculate the range of 75% to 125% of label claim for this preparation.

      75% $\times$ 10 mg = 7.5 mg

      125% $\times$ 10 mg = 12.5 mg

■ **Figure 25.3** Sample quality control record for hard shell capsules. *(Contd)*

16. Using the statistics function on a preprogrammed calculator, calculate the standard deviation (s) and the relative standard deviation (*RSD*) for this sample. (Note: Chapter <905> Uniformity of Dosage Units in the *USP* allows these values to be calculated with a preprogrammed calculator or computer or using the equations given in <905> (6) and reproduced in Chapter 25 of this text.)

$$s = 2.18 \qquad\qquad RSD = 2.35\%$$

17. Determine if the batch meets the tests as specified in <905>:

    a. If any unit is outside the 75% to 125% range, the batch fails.

    b. The batch passes if the amount of active ingredient in not less than 9 of 10 units is within the 85 to 115% range and no unit is outside the 75% to 125% range, and the RSD of the 10 units is less than or equal to 6%.

       Our batch passes this test because no capsule is outside the range of 8.5 to 11.5 mg (the range for our sample is 8.9 to 9.7 mg) and the RSD of our sample is less than 6% (our RSD is 2.35%).

    c. If 2 or 3 units are outside the 85% to 115% range, but none is outside the 75% to 125% range, and/or if the RDS is greater than 6%, 20 additional units may be tested. The requirements are met if not more than 3 units of the 30 are outside the 85% to 115% range and none is outside the 75% to 125% range and the RSD of the 30 units is not greater than 7.8%.

(1) Capsule Number	(2) Weight of Capsule (mg)	(3) Ave. Weight of Capsule Shell (mg)	(4) Weight of Capsule Contents (mg)	(5) Active Ingredient Weight (mg)	(6) Active Ingredient expressed as a percentage of label claim (x_i)
1	435	92	343	9.3	93
2	419	92	327	8.9	89
3	447	92	355	9.7	97
4	436	92	344	9.4	94
5	431	92	339	9.2	92
6	432	92	340	9.3	93
7	425	92	333	9.1	91
8	439	92	347	9.5	95
9	435	92	343	9.3	93
10	429	92	337	9.2	92
mean value of the units expressed as a percentage of label claim:				$\overline{X}$ =	92.9

b. Capsules provide a unique method of handling incompatibilities between ingredients. Two mutually incompatible ingredients can be contained in the same capsule shell by first punching one of the ingredients in a smaller shell. The other powder is punched into a larger capsule, and the smaller capsule is then embedded in this powder.

C. Soft Shell Capsules or Soft-gels
1. The principal material for the shells of these capsules is usually gelatin, but, as their name implies, the shell is a softer, more pliable material than that used for hard shell capsules. This is caused by the presence of glycerin and/or sorbitol, which act as plasticizers. The shells of soft-gels are also thicker than those of hard shell capsules (1).
2. These capsules are usually filled with liquids; either the physical form of the active ingredient is a liquid, or a solid active ingredient is dissolved or suspended in a liquid vehicle.
3. The liquid vehicle used in soft shell capsules must be approved for oral use. It is usually a vegetable oil or a nonaqueous, water-miscible liquid glycol, such as polyethylene glycol 400 or one of the other liquid polyethylene glycols (1).
4. The technology and equipment required for making soft shell capsules is more complex than that available to the compounding pharmacist, so this dosage form is not made extemporaneously.
5. Manufactured soft shell capsules are sometimes used as ingredient sources for compounding.
    a. In this case the capsules are punctured with a 16- to 20-gauge needle, the liquid contents of the capsules are withdrawn with a syringe or are squeezed into a graduate, and a suitable liquid vehicle is added.
    b. If the capsule contents are oleaginous, corn oil or another vegetable oil may be added and used directly, or an emulsion can be made with the addition of water and an emulsifying agent.
    c. If the contents have a liquid polyethylene glycol base, a water-miscible liquid or syrup vehicle may be used.

III. LOZENGES

A. Uses
1. Lozenges have traditionally been used for local effect—to administer topical anesthetics and demulcents for soothing irritated throat passages experienced with cough and sore throat, and to deliver antibacterial agents intended to promote healing of inflamed and abraded mouth and throat tissues.
2. More recently, lozenges are being used as a way to deliver drugs systemically. As the lozenge slowly dissolves in the mouth, drug is released for absorption in the mouth, either buccally or sublingually, and drug that is swallowed can be absorbed in the gastrointestinal tract.
3. Lozenges are especially useful for patients who have difficulty swallowing oral solid dosage forms. This includes some pediatric and geriatric patients and patients with gastrointestinal blockage.
4. Because lozenges dissolve slowly in the mouth, this dosage form is also useful for medications that give maximum benefit when in prolonged contact with local tissues. Examples include antifungals used for the treatment of candidiasis (thrush) and sodium fluoride used for the prevention of dental caries.
5. To enhance patient compliance, especially in children, lozenges are formulated to taste good. Because they may look and taste like candy, lozenges are a potential danger to children; households with children should be warned to keep these products out of the reach of children.

B. Types of Lozenges
1. Hard Lozenges
    a. Hard candy lozenges are mixtures of sucrose and other sugars and/or carbohydrates in an amorphous state. Although they are made from aqueous syrups, the water, which is initially present, evaporates as the syrup is boiled during processing so that the moisture content in the finished product is 0.5–1.5% (3).

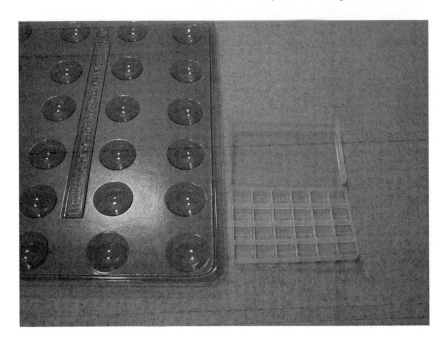

Sample lozenge molds

b. Because making hard lozenges is similar to candy making, helpful hints can be found by consulting a comprehensive cookbook or a candy-making reference. Flavorings, colors, and special molds can be purchased from some vendors of compounding supplies and from businesses that specialize in selling supplies for making candies and confectioneries. Hard candy lollipops have become an especially popular compounded dosage form in recent years, and special molds and sucker sticks and wrappers are available from various vendors.

c. Successful preparation of smooth hard lozenges depends on careful handling of the syrup and monitoring of temperatures. This is because the crystal-amorphous form of the sugar in the final product depends on these factors. If a formula states that the syrup should not be stirred until a particular temperature is reached, or if it states that the temperature of the syrup must reach 154°C, it is wise to follow these instructions precisely.

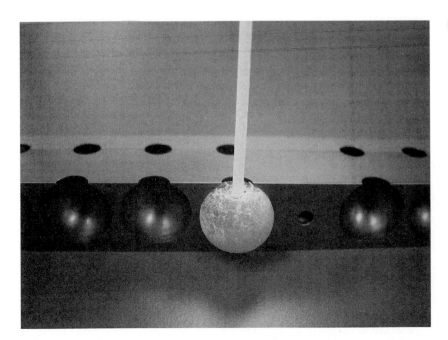

Molded hard candy lollipop

    d. The finished hardness of the candy depends partly on its water content. To obtain lozenges that are hard and not tacky, the temperature of the melt must reach 149–154°C (300–310°F). This is called the *hard crack* stage. This temperature is based on conditions at sea level and average relative humidity. At higher altitudes these temperatures are lower; on humid days the syrup should be heated 1°C higher than usual.

    e. Because of the high temperatures needed to make hard lozenges, drugs or chemicals that are unstable to heat should not be incorporated into this dosage form.

    f. Formulas for two hard lozenge bases are given in Table 25.3.

  2. Soft Lozenges

Soft lozenges can be made with a flavored fatty base (such as chocolate), a polyethylene glycol (PEG) base, or a sugar-acacia base.

TABLE 25.3   Lozenge Formulas

Clear, Hard Lozenge Base
This formula is modified from a hard candy formula available from the LorAnn Oil, Inc.
70 g Sucrose
40 g Light Corn Syrup
20 mL Purified Water
0.5 mL Flavoring Oil
q.s. Color (if desired)
q.s. Active Ingredients

Combine the Sucrose, corn syrup, and Purified Water in a beaker. Place on a hot plate at medium heat and stir until the sucrose dissolves. Bring to a boil and boil without stirring until the temperature reaches 154°C (310°F). A candy thermometer is useful for monitoring the temperature. Remove from heat. Stir in flavoring oil, active ingredients and the coloring (if desired). Pour into pre-calibrated molds that have been lubricated with vegetable spray or dusted with powdered sugar. Alternatively place mold(s) on an electronic balance and tare out the weight of the mold(s); then pour lozenge material into each mold cavity to the desired weight.

Opaque, Hard Lozenge Base (7)
This base has been used to make medicated lollipops.
150 g Sucrose
0.5 g Potassium bitartrate (Cream of Tartar)
50 mL Purified Water
The following should be dissolved in 5 mL of Purified Water
0.5 mL Flavoring Concentrate
q.s. Color (if desired)
q.s. Active Ingredients

Dissolve the Sucrose and Potassium bitartrate in the Purified Water in a beaker. Bring to a boil on a hot plate and heat until the temperature reaches 154°C (310°F). Remove from heat. Add the solution containing the active ingredients, but do not stir until the mixture has cooled to 125°C (257°F), then stir until uniform. Pour into a pre-calibrated mold that has been dusted with powdered sugar. If this is used for lollipops, insert a stick into each lozenge before allowing the product to cool.

Chocolate Lozenge Base (8)
30 g Dipping chocolate
10 g Vegetable oil (corn, soybean, etc.)
q.s. Active Ingredients

On an electronic balance tare out the weight of a 150 mL beaker. Add vegetable oil to the beaker to a weight of 10 grams. Set the beaker in a warm water bath. Break the chocolate into pieces and add to the heated oil in portions, melting the chocolate with each addition. Stir until completely melted and well mixed. Weigh the desired amount of chocolate base and active ingredient(s). Add the active ingredient(s) to the base and stir to mix well. Pour into mold cavities to a predetermined weight or volume. The chocolate base material can be stored in the refrigerator. Portions can be weighed and used as needed for preparing chocolate lozenges.

Fatty Base Soft Lozenges (3)
25 g Synthetic Cocoa Butter Base, e.g., Fattibase®
1 g Acacia
q.s. Flavor
q.s. Sweetener, e.g. sodium saccharin
q.s. Active Ingredient(s)

Melt the Fattibase® on a warm water bath to approximately 40°C. Gradually add the acacia powder, then the drug, stirring to form a uniform mixture. Add the flavor and the sweetener and stir well. Place a mold(s) on an electronic balance and tare out the weight of the mold(s); then pour lozenge material into each mold cavity to the desired weight.

(Continued)

TABLE 25.3	Continued

PEG Base Soft Lozenges (3, 9, 10, 11)
Bases of this type contain PEG 1000 (m.p. 37–40°C), PEG 1450 (m.p. 43–46°C), or a combination of solid and liquid PEGs. In some formulas Acacia is added, approximately 0.5 g per 20 g of PEG.

The PEG is placed in a beaker and melted on a warm water bath or a hot plate to

approximately 70°C. The acacia (if added) and the active ingredient(s) are added and the mixture stirred well. Flavoring and a heat-stable artificial sweetener, such as sodium saccharin, should be added. Color may be added if desired. Either pour the melted material into a pre-calibrated mold or use the tared mold method described above.

Hand-rolled Sugar Lozenges (3)
10 g Powdered sugar
0.7 g Acacia
q.s. Purified Water
q.s. Flavor
q.s. Color (if desired)
q.s. Active Ingredient(s)

Put the Acacia in a mortar and add sufficient Purified Water with trituration to form a mucilage. Using geometric dilution combine the active ingredient(s) and the powdered sugar and mix thoroughly by

spatulation. Put this powder into a sifter and sift together onto an ointment slab. Add the powders to the Acacia mucilage in portions to make a mass of a proper consistency for hand-rolling. Add the flavor and color (if desired). On the ointment slab, roll the mass into a cylindrical pipe. Using a ruler as a gauge, cut the pipe into equal portions. Check the weight of individual pieces; this should be the final weight of the ingredients divided by the number of doses of active ingredient added.

Glycerinated Gummy Gel Base
This base is similar to glycerinated gelatin suppository base. Here it is used as a base for chewable gummy gels. An alternative to making the base would be to purchase gummy bears or worms and melt them on a warm water bath.

18 g Gelation
70 mL Glycerin
12 mL Purified Water
q.s. Flavor
q.s. Color (if desired)
q.s. Active Ingredient(s)

Either weigh (87.5 g) or measure (70 mL) of Glycerin and pour into a 150 mL beaker. Add the Purified Water and stir to mix. Prepare a boiling water bath using a 600 mL beaker and a stirring hotplate. Heat the Glycerin-Water together for 4–5 minutes, then slowly and carefully sprinkle the gelatin onto the liquid. Continue stirring until it is a uniform mixture and is free of all lumps. Continue heating for about 40–45 minutes. Remove from heat and allow to cool. Portions of this gel can be weighed and used as a base for preparing gummy gel dosage forms.

---

   a. Fatty base soft lozenges
     (1) The chocolate lozenge base shown in Table 25.3 contains dipping chocolate melted together with a vegetable oil. These lozenges are easy to make and taste good.
       (a) The oil depresses the congealing point of the base to facilitate the homogeneous incorporation of active ingredients and the pouring of accurately measured doses.
       (b) After melting and mixing, this base can either be poured directly or drawn into a syringe and carefully squirted into tared mold cavities—all without congealing. Plastic medication cups work well as extemporaneous molds.
       (c) The finished lozenges should be placed in a freezer to harden for ease of removal from the mold cavities. The removed lozenges should be placed in individual polyethylene bags and stored in the freezer. Because of the presence of oil, these lozenges are too soft to be stored at room temperature. Sample Prescription 25.6 illustrates a compounding procedure for chocolate lozenges.
     (2) Table 25.3 also shows a formula for a fatty base soft lozenge made with a synthetic cocoa butter base and artificial flavor and sweetener. These have a less appealing taste than the chocolate base. Perhaps the chocolate flavor is a needed complement for the oily feel of such a base.

    b. PEG base soft lozenges

      (1) These bases are similar to PEG suppository bases except they are formulated to be less firm. Most commonly, PEG 1000, with a melting point of 37–40°C, or PEG 1450, with a melting point of 43–46°C, is used alone or with added Acacia, approximately 0.5 g per 20 g of PEG base. Some formulas are more complex and use a combination of solid and liquid PEGs to give a particular desired consistency.

      (2) To make these soft lozenges palatable, flavoring and a heat-stable artificial sweetener, such as sodium saccharin, should be added. Color may be added if desired. Even with added flavor and sweetener, these lozenges would not be considered tasty. If this sort of base is used, considerable experimentation with flavoring and sweetener must be done to formulate a product with a satisfactory taste.

    c. Hand-rolled acacia-sugar lozenges

      (1) The base material for this lozenge is powdered sugar held together by an Acacia mucilage.

      (2) These lozenges are one of the simplest to make. A sample formula and procedure is given in Table 25.3 and is illustrated in Sample Prescription 25.8. The general compounding procedure is given below in section C2 on compounding methods for hand-rolled lozenges.

3. Chewable Gummy Gel Lozenges

    a. This lozenge base is similar to the old-fashioned glycerinated gelatin, which was used for many years as a base for vaginal suppositories. It made its appearance as a base for chewable oral drug preparations after a candy for children, so-called *gummy worms* or *gummy bears,* was introduced and became popular.

    b. A gummy gel base such as that shown in Table 25.3 can be made from scratch in the pharmacy. This requires time and patience because the material must be heated carefully for 40 to 45 minutes. This is only the beginning. To make a palatable product, appropriate flavoring and sweetening must be added; citric acid is sometimes added to improve the taste—the tartness it provides takes away from the acrid taste of the glycerin. In addition, Acacia may be added to provide smoothness. If the active ingredient or ingredients are insoluble, a small amount of a suspending agent, such as bentonite, may also be added (12). In short, making this base is a time-consuming process.

    c. An alternative to making the gummy gel base is to purchase gummy candy. It can be heated in a beaker on a warm water bath until a fluid is obtained. This gives a flavorful base of a desirable consistency.

C. General Compounding Methods for Lozenges

    1. Lozenges are similar to suppositories in that they are made either by hand-rolling or by fusion. Depending on the compounding method selected, special calculations, compounding techniques, and equipment may be required to give accurate doses of lozenges.

    2. Hand-rolled lozenges

      a. Advantages

        (1) Hand-rolled lozenges do not require special calculations.

        (2) Special equipment is not required for this method. A pill roller is useful, but a broad-bladed spatula or any stiff, flat piece of nonreactive material can be used for this purpose.

      b. Disadvantages

        (1) Preparing and forming hand-rolled lozenges requires experience and good technique.

        (2) Even when well made, hand-rolled lozenges do not have an elegant appearance.

      c. General compounding method (This method is used in Sample Prescription 25.8 near the end of this chapter.)

(1) Check the doses of the active ingredients.

(2) Decide on the desired finished weight per lozenge, usually 1–2 grams.

(3) Calculate the quantity of each ingredient needed for compounding the product. Make enough material for two extra lozenges.

    (a) Multiply the dose per unit times the number of units to determine the quantity of each active ingredient.

    (b) Multiply the finished weight per unit times the desired number of units.

    (c) Subtract the weight of the active ingredients from the total weight of the lozenges to determine the amount of base material.

(4) Weigh and prepare the active ingredients and base materials.

(5) Combine the ingredients to form a cohesive mass.

(6) Place the mass on an ointment slab and roll into a cylindrical pipe of an appropriate length.

(7) Using a clean razor blade and a ruler for a gauge, cut the pipe into equal pieces of the desired number of dosage units.

(8) Weigh each piece and shave off extra material if needed to achieve lozenges of the approximate correct weight.

  3. Molded lozenges, fusion method (using heat)

    a. Advantages

      (1) Some of the better-tasting lozenges, such as hard candy, chocolate, and gummy gel chewable lozenges, can only be made using heat and molding.

      (2) When well made, the products have a finished, professional appearance. Special molds, including those to make lollipops, are available from some vendors of compounding supplies and from confectioneries.

    b. Disadvantages

      (1) Special molds are usually required to make lozenges by molding. It is possible to improvise by using the caps of items like vials, or plastic medication cups for mold forms.

      (2) Handling some types of base materials requires special skill, experience, and care to obtain satisfactory preparations.

      (3) Caution must be used when incorporating drugs sensitive to heat.

      (4) While the dosage units of molded lozenges may be determined either by weight or by volume, both methods require special equipment, calculations, or procedures.

    c. General compounding methods

      (1) By weight (This method is illustrated with Sample Prescription 25.6.)

        (a) When lozenges are compounded to a final weight, an electronic digital balance is nearly a necessity.

        (b) Follow steps (1) through (4) as given above for hand-rolled lozenges.

        (c) Using heat, prepare the lozenge base material.

        (d) Add the active ingredient(s) to the molten base.

        (e) Place the lozenge mold(s) on an electronic balance and tare out the weight of the mold(s).

        (f) Pour melted lozenge material into each mold cavity to the calculated desired weight per lozenge, using the balance weight readout as the gauge. In some cases it is easier to first draw the lozenge material into a syringe and use this to add the molten material to the mold cavities.

      (2) By volume

        (a) If volume is used, density calculations, mold calibrations, double-casting, or other procedures are required to give accurate doses.

        (b) Because lozenges are solid at room temperature, most of the base components and active ingredients are solids and are measured by weight.

        (c) The components are then combined, melted, and poured into mold cavities. This means that the dosage unit is determined by volume—the volume of the mold cavity. The final amount of drug in a dosage unit therefore depends on two factors: the w/w concentration of active ingredient in the base material, and the weight of the mixture contained in each mold cavity. The weight of mixture in the mold cavity depends on the volume of the cavity and the density (ρ) of the molten mixture. Obviously, the density of the material has a significant effect on the final weight of the dosage unit.

(d) To determine the quantity of base and active ingredients(s) to weigh when using this method, it is necessary to either calibrate the mold cavities for the desired material or use a double-casting procedure. Descriptions of these procedures are given in Chapter 31, Suppositories.

IV. MISCELLANEOUS SOLID DOSAGE FORMS

A. Pharmacists have used their imaginations and ingenuity to create a variety of methods for delivering solid oral dosage forms. The lozenges just described give some examples. In recent years lollipops, which in essence are hard molded lozenges on a stick, have become a popular compounded dosage form. Sample Prescription 25.7 later in this chapter shows a Popsicle formula; other variations of this include added flavored gelatin (e.g., Jell-O®) or Kool-Aid®.

B. Keeping abreast of ideas and materials in this rapidly changing and innovative area of practice requires reading the pharmaceutical literature. As stated in Chapter 12, information is also available from vendors of compounding supplies and on various sites on the Internet.

SAMPLE PRESCRIPTIONS

➤ **Prescription 25-1**

Contemporary Physicians Group Practice
20 S. Park Street, Triturate, WI 53706
Tel: (608) 555-1333 Fax: (608) 555-1335

R # 834

Name *Jack Heller*	Date *00/00/00*	
Address *802 Arbor Street*	Age	Wt/Ht

R

Theophylline	118 mg
Ephedrine Sulfate	24 mg
Phenobarbital	8 mg
Dispense Capsules #6	

J. Jacobson 00/00/00

Sig: 1 - 2 caps q 4 hr prn breathing

Refills 4   E. S. Clyde   M.D.

DEA No. _____

Ingredients Used (for 7 doses, 1 extra)

Ingredient	Quantity Used	Manufacturer Lot #-Exp Date	Solubility	Dose Comparison Given	Dose Comparison Usual	Use in the Prescription
Theophylline	826 mg	JET Labs XY 1162-mm/yy	sl. sol. water sp. sol. in alcohol	118–236 mg q 4 h	max. 900 mg/day	bronchodilator
Ephedrine Sulfate	168 mg.	JET Labs XY 1163-mm/yy	v. sol. water sp. sol. in alcohol	24 mg	24 mg	bronchodilator decongestant
Lactose	240 mg weighed 112 mg used	JET Labs XY 1159-mm/yy	fr. sl. water v. sl. sol. in alcohol	—	—	diluent
Phenobarbital	120 mg weighed 56 mg used	JET Labs XY 1165-mm/yy	v. sl. sol. in water fr. sol. in alcohol	8 mg	*6–20 mg	sedative

*While the normal dose of Phenobarbital when used as a sedative hypnotic is 15–100 mg, Phenobarbital has a lower dosage level when used to counteract the stimulant effects of drugs like Theophylline and Ephedrine.

Compatibility–Stability/Beyond-Use Date

Stability–Compatibility: All ingredients in this preparation are compatible and quite stable when in a solid dosage form.

Packaging and Storage and Beyond-use date: The *USP* monographs for Phenobarbital Tablets and Theophylline Tablets recommend storage in well-closed containers, but the monograph for Ephedrine Sulfate Capsules recommends a tight, light-resistant container (14). Pharmacist Jacobson will use the maximum 6-month beyond-use date as specified in *USP* Chapter ⟨795⟩ for solid formulations made with USP ingredients (15).

Calculations

Dose/Concentration

All doses are OK, but the maximum daily adult dose of Theophylline is 900 mg, so the patient should be instructed to take no more than 7 capsules in 24 hours.

Ingredient Amounts

Calculations are for 7 doses, 1 extra

Theophylline: *118 mg/dose × 7 doses = 826 mg*

Ephedrine Sulfate: *24 mg/dose × 7 doses = 168 mg*

Phenobarbital: *8 mg/dose × 7 doses = 56 mg*

> This amount is below the minimum weighable quantity (MWQ); therefore, an aliquot is needed. If the MWQ of 120 mg of Phenobarbital is weighed and mixed with 240 mg of Lactose to give 360 mg of dilution, the amount of this dilution that will contain the needed 56 mg of Phenobarbital can be calculated as shown here.

$$\frac{120\ mg\ Pb}{360\ mg\ dilution} = \frac{56\ mg\ Pb}{x\ mg\ dilution}; x = 168\ mg\ dilution$$

Because Phenobarbital powder is a C-IV substance, we must account for the amount weighed, dispensed, and discarded in making the aliquot and the extra dose to allow for the loss in compounding.

Amount weighed: *120 mg*
Amount dispensed: *8 mg/capsule × 6 capsules dispensed = 48 mg*
Amount discarded: *120 mg — 48 mg = 72 mg*

Capsule Content Weight

$$\frac{826 \ mg \ Theop. + 168 \ mg \ Eph. + 168 \ mg \ Pb \ aliquot}{7 \ capsules} = \frac{1162 \ mg \ powder}{7 \ capsules} = 166 \ mg \ / \ capsule$$

With 166 mg of mixed powder per capsule, try a size **#4** capsule shell (See Table 25.1 for approximate capsule shell capacities in grams of various powders).

(An alternative procedure for this prescription is demonstrated on the CD that accompanies this book. With this method, Pharmacist Jacobsen wants to use a slightly larger capsule shell [for some people the very small capsules, such as **#4** and **#5**, are difficult to handle], so she adds additional Lactose to give a powder weight per unit that will fit in a preferred shell size. View the procedure on the CD for details and calculations for this method.)

Compounding Procedure

All weighing is done on a Class 3 torsion balance or an electronic balance. Weigh 120 mg of Phenobarbital and 240 mg of Lactose and triturate well together. Weigh 168 mg of this mixture and place in a mortar. Weigh 168 mg Ephedrine SO_4 and add to the mixture in the mortar with trituration. Weigh 826 mg of Theophylline and add to the mixture in the mortar with trituration using geometric dilution. Punch powder into size **#4** capsules. Tare out the weight of an empty capsule shell and weigh each filled capsule and adjust to a powder content weight of 166 mg. Place capsules in a capsule vial with a child-resistant closure and label the vial appropriately.

Quality Control

The powder in the capsules appears as fine, white powder. The size **#4** clear gelatin capsules are full, with no dead space. Each capsule has been individually weighed to contain 166 mg of powder.

Labeling

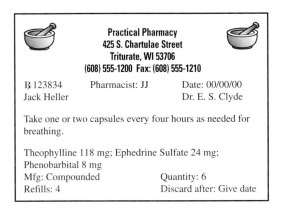

Practical Pharmacy
425 S. Chartulae Street
Triturate, WI 53706
(608) 555-1200 Fax: (608) 555-1210

R 123834   Pharmacist: JJ   Date: 00/00/00
Jack Heller   Dr. E. S. Clyde

Take one or two capsules every four hours as needed for breathing.

Theophylline 118 mg; Ephedrine Sulfate 24 mg;
Phenobarbital 8 mg
Mfg: Compounded   Quantity: 6
Refills: 4   Discard after: Give date

Auxiliary Labels: Drowsiness-alcohol-driving warning

Patient Consultation

Hello Mr. Heller, I'm your pharmacist, Julia Jacobsen. Do you have any drug allergies? What do you know about this medication (or did your doctor tell you anything about it)? Are you taking any over-the-counter or prescription medication? This medicine will help your breathing. You are to take one or two capsules every 4 hours when needed for breathing. Is Dr. Clyde monitoring your theophylline levels? If not, you should not take any more than seven capsules in a 24-hour period. This medication can cause some excitement, difficulty sleeping, headaches, or a jittery feeling. It contains some Phenobarbital to help offset these side effects, but the Phenobarbital could cause drowsiness. See how you react to this combination therapy before operating a motor vehicle, machinery, and so on. This may cause some stomach upset because it contains Theophylline. If this occurs, it might be helpful to take with food or milk. If you experience diarrhea or pounding heart, call Dr. Clyde. Store this in a cool, dry place and discard any unused contents after 6 months (give beyond-use date). You may refill this four times. Do you have any questions?

➤ **Prescription 25-2**

Contemporary Physicians Group Practice
20 S. Park Street, Triturate, WI 53706
Tel: (608) 555-1333 Fax: (608) 555-1335

R # 822

Name *Shanna Woodruff*   Date *00/00/00*

Address *863 Wildwood Circle*   Age *7 y.o.* Wt/Ht

R

For Blind Study:
1)   *Methylphenidate   5 mg*
        Lactose   qs
        Dispense #14 Caps
Sig: i po at 7 am and 11 am during weeks 1 & 2
        Label: Methylphenidate A 5 mg

2)   *Lactose   qs*
        Dispense #14 Caps
Sig: i po at 7 am and 11 am during weeks 3 & 4
        Label: Methylphenidate B 5 mg

B. Badger 00/00/00

Refills   *0*   *Adolph Runnel*   M.D.

DEA No. *AR 3938745*

Ingredients Used

Ingredient	Quantity Used	Manufacturer Lot #-Exp Date	Solubility	Dose Comparison		Use in the Prescription
				Given	Usual	
Methylphenidate 5 mg tabs	14 × 5 mg	BJF Generics XY1166-mm/yy	freely sol in water; sol in alcohol	5 mg bid	5–20 mg 2–3 × daily	hyperactivity ADD
Lactose	qs	JET Labs XY1159-mm/yy	1 g/5 mL water; v.sl.sol. in alcohol	—	—	diluent/placebo

Compatibility–Stability/Beyond-Use Date

Stability–Compatibility: In a solid dosage form Methylphenidate is quite stable.
Packaging and Storage and Beyond-use date: The *USP* monograph for Methylphenidate Tablets recommends storage in tight containers (14). Pharmacist Badger will use the recommended beyond-use date as specified in *USP* Chapter <795> for solid formulations made with active ingredients from manufactured drug products: no later than 25% of the time remaining until the product's expiration date or 6 months, whichever is earlier (15).

Calculations

Dose/Concentration

OK

Ingredient Amounts

No calculations are needed. One 5-mg tablet is put in each capsule for Methylphenidate A.

Compounding Procedure

To avoid mixing up the active and placebo capsules, make the vial labels and label the vials first. Punch a small quantity of Lactose into a size #3 capsule. If available, use opaque capsule shells. Break a Methylphenidate 5-mg tablet in half and embed the two halves into the Lactose in the capsule, and then punch more Lactose into the capsule, concealing the broken tablet halves. Place this capsule in the capsule vial labeled Methylphenidate A 5 mg. Repeat this procedure for 13 more capsules. Then punch 14 #3 capsules with Lactose only, and make sure that these approximate the size and appearance of the "A" capsules. Place these capsules in the capsule vial labeled Methylphenidate B 5 mg. Dispense the vials with child-resistant closures.

Quality Control

The powder in the capsules appears as fine, white powder. The size #3 clear gelatin capsules are full, with no dead space. Each capsule has been inspected so be sure that in no instance is an edge of a pale-yellow hidden Methylphenidate tablet visible.

Labeling

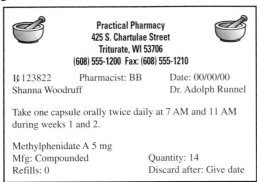

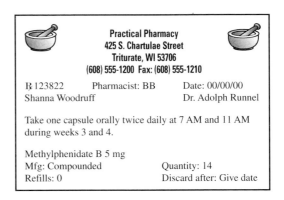

Practical Pharmacy
425 S. Chartulae Street
Triturate, WI 53706
(608) 555-1200 Fax: (608) 555-1210

Rx 123822   Pharmacist: BB   Date: 00/00/00
Shanna Woodruff   Dr. Adolph Runnel

Take one capsule orally twice daily at 7 AM and 11 AM during weeks 1 and 2.

Methylphenidate A 5 mg
Mfg: Compounded   Quantity: 14
Refills: 0   Discard after: Give date

Auxiliary Labels: Federal Do not transfer label

Practical Pharmacy
425 S. Chartulae Street
Triturate, WI 53706
(608) 555-1200 Fax: (608) 555-1210

Rx 123822   Pharmacist: BB   Date: 00/00/00
Shanna Woodruff   Dr. Adolph Runnel

Take one capsule orally twice daily at 7 AM and 11 AM during weeks 3 and 4.

Methylphenidate B 5 mg
Mfg: Compounded   Quantity: 14
Refills: 0   Discard after: Give date

Auxiliary Labels: Federal Do not transfer label

Patient Consultation

Hello Mrs. Woodruff, I'm your pharmacist, Barry Badger, and I have Shanna's prescription ready. Does she have any drug allergies? Are you giving her any other medicine, either over-the-counter or prescription? I'm sure your doctor has discussed that this is a double-blind study to determine if Shanna needs to take this drug. Neither you, your daughter, nor your doctor should know which of these vials contains capsules with the drug and which has capsules with no drug. If Shanna exhibits any unusual behavior while taking this medication, contact your doctor immediately, because the study might have to be discontinued. Give her one capsule at 7 AM and one at 11 AM every morning for 4 weeks. Notice you give the capsules from vial A on weeks 1 and 2 and switch to giving the capsules from vial B on weeks 3 and 4. Note that the bottles tell you which weeks to give capsules from that bottle. DO NOT MIX UP THE BOTTLES. Store in a dry place, at room temperature, away from the reach of children. Discard any unused portion after 6 months (or 25% of expiration date of tablets). This prescription may not be refilled. Be sure to report to your physician as he has requested. Don't give this medication to anyone else. Do you have any questions?

➤ **Prescription 25-3**

Contemporary Physicians Group Practice
20 S. Park Street, Triturate, WI 53706
Tel: (608) 555-1333 Fax: (608) 555-1335

R # 828

Name *Wayne John*	Date *00/00/00*
Address *2530 Blackhawk Estates*	Age Wt/Ht

R

Acetaminophen	*325 mg*
Diphenhydramine HCl	*25 mg*
Atropine sulfate	*0.12 mg*
Caffeine	*30 mg*

M et Ft Capsules #6

Sig: 1-2 caps po q 8 hr prn headache and congestion

B. Boggs   00/00/00

Refills   *3*   *Lance Smitby*   M.D.

DEA No. _____

Ingredients Used (for 7 doses, 1 extra)

Ingredient	Quantity Used	Manufacturer Lot #-Exp Date	Solubility	Dose Comparison Given	Dose Comparison Usual	Use in the Prescription
Acetaminophen (APAP)	2275 mg	JET Labs XY1168-mm/yy	1 g/70 mL water, 10 mL alcohol	325–650 mg q 8 h	0.3–1 g 3–4 x daily	antipyretic analgesic
Diphenhydramine (DPH) 50 mg capsules	175 mg in 893 mg powder	BJF Generics XY1168-mm/yy	1 g/1 mL water, 2 mL alcohol	25–50 mg q 8 h	25–50 mg 3–4 x daily	antihistamine
Atropine Sulfate	120 mg weighed/ 0.84 mg used	JET Labs XY1170-mm/yy	1 g/0.5 mL water, 5 mL alcohol	0.12–0.24 mg q 8 h	0.3–1.2 mg q 4–6 h	anticholinergic, antispasmodic
Lactose	5040 mg weighed/ 133 used	JET Labs XY1159-mm/yy	fr sol in water, v sl sol in alcohol	—	—	diluent
Caffeine	210 mg	JET Labs XY1172-mm/yy	1 g/50 mL water, 70 mL alcohol	30–60 mg q 8 h	100–500 mg prn	counteracts drowsiness of CNS depressants & active for vascular headache

Compatibility–Stability/Beyond-Use Date

Stability–Compatibility: All ingredients in this preparation are compatible and quite stable when in a solid dosage form.

Packaging and Storage and Beyond-use date: The *USP* monographs for Atropine Sulfate Tablets and Caffeine recommend storage in well-closed containers, but the monographs for Diphenhydramine HCl Capsules and Acetaminophen Tablets are more restrictive and recommend storage in tight containers (14). Because the source of one of the active ingredients, Diphenhydramine HCl, is a manufactured capsule, Pharmacist Boggs will use the recommended beyond-use date as specified in *USP* Chapter ⟨795⟩ for solid formulations made with active ingredients from manufactured drug products: no later than 25% of the time remaining until the product's expiration date or 6 months, whichever is earlier (15).

Calculations

Dose/Concentration

All doses OK

Ingredient Amounts

Calculations are for 7 doses, 1 extra
Acetaminophen (APAP): *325 mg/dose × 7 doses = 2,275 mg*

Caffeine: *30 mg/dose × 7 doses = 210 mg*

Diphenhydramine HCl (DPH): *25 mg/dose × 7 doses = 175 mg*

DPH is available as 50-mg capsules with capsule content weight of 255 mg/capsule. For 175 mg of DPH, 4 capsules are needed and the weight of capsule powder is calculated as:

$$\frac{50 \, mg \, DPH}{255 \, mg \, capsule \, powder} = \frac{175 \, mg \, DPH}{x \, mg \, capsules \, powder}; \, x = 893 \, mg \, capsule \, powder$$

Atropine Sulfate: *0.12 mg/dose × 7 doses = 0.84 mg*

This amount is below the MWQ, and because it is such a small amount, a serial dilution is required.
Dilution A: Weigh the MWQ of 120 mg of Atropine Sulfate and mix with an intermediate amount of Lactose, 4,680 mg, to give 4,800 mg of Dilution A. Weigh the MWQ of this dilution. The amount of Atropine Sulfate in Dilution A is calculated as:

$$\frac{120 \, mg \, Atropine}{4800 \, mg \, Dilution \, A} = \frac{x \, mg \, Atropine}{120 \, mg \, Dilution \, A}; \, x = 3 \, mg \, Atropine$$

To the 120 mg of Dilution A (which contains 3 mg of Atropine Sulfate) add 360 mg of Lactose to give 480 mg of Dilution B. Calculate the amount of Dilution B that will contain 0.84 mg of Atropine Sulfate:

$$\frac{3 \, mg \, Atropine}{480 \, mg \, Dilution \, B} = \frac{0.84 \, mg \, Atropine}{x \, mg \, Dilution \, B}; \, x = 134 \, mg \, Dilution \, B$$

Capsule Content Weight

$$\frac{2275 \, mg \, APAP + 210 \, mg \, Caf + 134 \, mg \, Atr \, Alq + 893 \, mg \, DPH}{7 \, capsules} = \frac{3512 \, mg \, powder}{7 \, capsules} = 502 \, mg \, / \, capsules$$

With 502 mg of powder per capsule, try size #1 capsules. If that is too small, use size #0 capsules (see Table 25.1).

Compounding Procedure

All weighing is done on a Class 3 torsion or an electronic digital balance. Weigh 120 mg of Atropine Sulfate and place in a glass mortar. Weigh 4,680 mg of Lactose and mix with the Atropine by trituration using geometric dilution. Weigh 120 mg of this first dilution, transfer to a clean glass mortar and add 360 mg of Lactose by trituration using geometric dilution. Weigh 134 mg of this second dilution and transfer it to a clean mortar. Weigh 210 mg of Caffeine and add it to the second dilution and triturate the powders well. Weigh the contents of a Diphenhydramine 50-mg capsule to determine the total powder weight per capsule (255 mg). Weigh 893 mg of powder from four capsules and add to the Atropine aliquot–Caffeine mixture by geometric dilution with trituration. Weigh 2,275 mg of Acetaminophen and add to above by geometric dilution with trituration. Punch powder in size **#1** capsules so that contents of each capsule weigh 502 mg; use an empty capsule shell as a tare. Dispense in a capsule vial with a child-resistant closure and label.

Quality Control

The powder in the capsules appears as fine, white powder. The size **#1** clear gelatin capsules are full, with no dead space. Each capsule has been individually weighed to contain 502 mg of powder.

Labeling

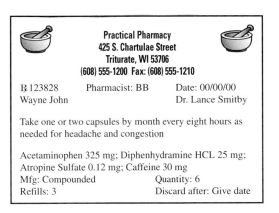

Practical Pharmacy
425 S. Chartulae Street
Triturate, WI 53706
(608) 555-1200 Fax: (608) 555-1210

℞ 123828   Pharmacist: BB   Date: 00/00/00
Wayne John   Dr. Lance Smitby

Take one or two capsules by month every eight hours as
needed for headache and congestion

Acetaminophen 325 mg; Diphenhydramine HCL 25 mg;
Atropine Sulfate 0.12 mg; Caffeine 30 mg
Mfg: Compounded   Quantity: 6
Refills: 3   Discard after: Give date

Auxiliary Labels: Drowsiness-alcohol-driving warning

Patient Consultation

Hello, Mr. John, I'm your pharmacist, Brenda Boggs. Do you have any drug allergies? Are you taking any over-the-counter or prescription medications? Do you know what this prescription is for? (What did your doctor tell you about this medication?) This is a pain medication combined with an antihistamine and a drying agent. You may take one or two capsules every 8 hours as needed. Some side effects include drowsiness and dry mouth, but these capsules also contain some caffeine, which may make you jittery. See how you react to this combination therapy before operating a motor vehicle, machinery, and so on. Don't exceed the prescribed dose, because large doses of Acetaminophen can cause kidney and liver problems. If you don't get relief, if your condition gets worse, or if you develop a skin rash, contact your physician. It is best not to consume alcoholic beverages or at least be very moderate in their use while taking this medication. Keep out of the reach of children. This may be refilled three times. Discard any unused portion after 6 months or 25% of DPH expiration date, whichever is less (give date). Do you have any questions?

➤ **Prescription 25-4**

Contemporary Veterinarian Group Practice
22 S. Park Street, Triturate, WI 53706
Tel: (608) 555-1334 Fax: (608) 555-1336

R # 890

Name *Letta Mae Draheim (dog)*   Date *00/00/00*
         owner: G. W. Draheim

Address *15805 Mercury Drive*   Age   Wt/Ht *15 lb*

R

         Doxycycline   5 mg/kg/dose

     M & Ft Capsules for 21 days–Put in small capsules

     Sig: Give one cap bid for 21 days

                            W. Thompson 00/00/00

Refills *0*   *Peter Janssen*   D.V.M.

                 DEA No. _____

Ingredients Used (amounts are for 44 capsules, 2 extra doses)

Ingredient	Quantity Used	Manufacturer Lot #-Exp Date	Solubility	Dose Comparison		Use in the Prescription
				Given	Usual	
Doxycycline 50 mg Capsules	30 × 50 mg	BJF Generics Y067G-mm/yy	sol in water; sl.sol in alcohol	5 mg/kg bid	Dogs: 5-10 mg/kg/day	broad-spectrum antibiotic
Lactose	623 mg	JET Labs XY1159-mm/yy	1 g/5 mLwater; v.sl.sol. in alcohol	—	—	diluent

Compatibility–Stability/Beyond-Use Date

Stability–Compatibility: Doxycycline in manufactured capsules is in the hydrate form, Doxycycline Hyclate. In a solid dosage form Doxycycline Hyclate is quite stable.

Packaging and Storage and Beyond-use date: The *USP* monograph for Doxycycline Capsules recommends storage in tight, light-resistant containers (14). Because the source of the active ingredient is manufactured capsules, Pharmacist Thompson will use the recommended beyond-use date as specified in *USP* Chapter ⟨795⟩ for solid formulations made with active ingredients from manufactured drug products: no later than 25% of the time remaining until the product's expiration date or 6 months, whichever is earlier (15).

Calculations

Dose/Concentration

Note: Dose of Doxycycline in dogs confirmed by pharmacist Thompson in *The Veterinary Formulary*, 5th ed., edited by Yolande Bishop, published by Pharmaceutical Press in association with the British Veterinary Association.

$$Weight\ in\ kg\ of\ dog: \frac{15\ lb}{2.2\ lb/kg} = 6.8\ kg$$

$$Dose\ in\ mg: \left(\frac{5\ mg\ Doxycycline}{kg/dose} \right) \left(\frac{6.8\ kg}{} \right) = 34\ mg\ Doxycycline/dose$$

Ingredient Amounts

Calculations are for two extra capsules.

Doxycycline: *34 mg/capsule × 44 capsules = 1,496 mg*

Active ingredient available: Doxycycline Hyclate capsules, USP 50 mg (BJF Generics; Lot Y067G; Exp mm/yy)

Number of 50-mg capsules needed:

$$\frac{50\ mg\ Doxycycline}{cap} = \frac{1496\ mg\ Doxycycline}{x\ caps}; x = 29.92\ or\ 30\ capsules$$

Average content weight for each 50-mg capsule is 288 mg. Weight of doxycycline capsule powder needed for 44 doses:

$$\frac{50\ mg\ Doxycycline}{288\ mg\ capsule\ powder} = \frac{1496\ mg\ Doxycycline}{x\ mg\ capsule\ powder}; x = 8617\ mg\ capsule\ powder$$

Capsule Content Weight

Weight of doxycycline capsule powder needed for each capsule:

8,617 mg/44 caps =   196 mg/cap

After consulting Table 25.1, Pharmacist Thompson tried capsule sizes #5 and #4. There was too much powder for size #5 and too little for size #4, so he decided to add a small amount of extra Lactose. The table gives 210 mg of Lactose per capsule for size #4 capsules. For 44 capsules, the amount of extra Lactose is calculated:

210 mg/capsule × 44 capsules = 9,240 mg

9,240 mg powder − 8,617 mg powder from Doxycycline caps = 623 mg Lactose

Compounding Procedure

Weigh all ingredients on a Class 3 torsion or digital balance. Weigh the capsule powder for Doxycycline Hyclate 50-mg capsules. Each 50-mg capsule contains 288 mg of Doxycycline capsule powder. Empty 30 Doxycycline capsules, weigh 8,617 mg of the Doxycycline capsule powder, and transfer it to a glass mortar. Each capsule is to weigh 210 mg (size 4 capsules). Therefore, weigh 623 mg of Lactose and combine the Lactose and Doxycycline capsule powder and triturate well. Transfer the powder mixture to an ointment pad and punch 42 capsules using size 4 capsule shells. Tare out the weight of an empty size #4 capsule shell and weigh each filled capsule so that the powder contents weigh 210 mg. Label and dispense the capsules in a capsule vial with a child-resistant closure.

Quality Control

The powder in the capsules appears as fine, white powder. The size #4 clear gelatin capsules are full, with no dead space. Each capsule has been individually weighed to contain 210 mg of powder.

Labeling

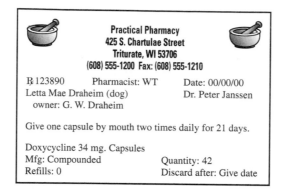

> **Practical Pharmacy**
> **425 S. Chartulae Street**
> **Triturate, WI 53706**
> **(608) 555-1200 Fax: (608) 555-1210**
>
> ℞ 123890   Pharmacist: WT   Date: 00/00/00
> Letta Mae Draheim (dog)   Dr. Peter Janssen
>   owner: G. W. Draheim
>
> Give one capsule by mouth two times daily for 21 days.
>
> Doxycycline 34 mg. Capsules
> Mfg: Compounded   Quantity: 42
> Refills: 0   Discard after: Give date

Patient Consultation

Hello, Mr. Draheim, I'm Wayne Thompson, your pharmacist. What did your veterinarian tell you about this medication? This medication is an antibiotic called doxycycline; it is used to treat infections. You should give Letta Mae one capsule twice a day for 21 days. You will need to open her mouth and put the capsule in the very back of her mouth at the top of her throat. Make sure she swallows the capsule and doesn't spit it out. It often helps to close her mouth and gently hold it shut while massaging her throat. It is important that you complete the full course of therapy. If her symptoms don't start to clear up within a few days, call your veterinarian. Try not to miss any doses. If you should miss a dose, give it as soon as possible. However, if it is almost time for her next dose, skip the missed dose and go back to her regular dosing schedule. This medication should be stored in a cool, dry place away from children. Discard any unused portion after 6 months or 25% of Doxycycline date, whichever is less (give date), although you should not have any capsules left because you will be giving Letta Mae all of the capsules. There are no refills with this prescription. Do you have any questions or concerns?

➤ Prescription 25-5

> # Contemporary Physicians Group Practice
> ## 20 S. Park Street, Triturate, WI 53706
> ### Tel: (608) 555-1333 Fax: (608) 555-1335
>
> ℞ # 881
>
> Name   *Tammy Gruber*   Date   *00/00/00*
>
> Address   *3075 Vallarta Court*   Age   *48*   Wt/Ht
>
> ℞
>
>   *For 50 capsules:*
>   *Estradiol*   *0.025 g*
>   *Estriol*   *0.1 g*
>   *Peanut Oil*   *qs to   10 mL*
>   *M. et div.*   *Dispense 30 Capsules*
>
>   ***J. Hutter   00/00/00***
>
>   *Sig: 1 cap po q day ut dict*
>
> Refills   2   *K. W. Shapiro*   M.D.
>
>   DEA No. _____

Ingredients Used (for 50 capsules, 20 extra doses)

Ingredient	Quantity Used	Manufacturer Lot #-Exp Date	Solubility	Dose Comparison		Use in the Prescription
				Given	Usual	
Estradiol	25 mg	JET Labs XY1133-mm/yy	pr insol in water; sol in alcohol	500 mcg daily	500 mcg – 2 mg daily ut dict	estrogen therapy
Estriol	100 mg	JET Labs XY1134-mm/yy	insol in water; sp.sol in alcohol	2 mg qd	2 mg qd	estrogen therapy
Peanut Oil	qs to 10mL	JET Labs XY1135-mm/yy	immis. with water; v. sl. sol in alcohol	—	—	solvent, vehicle

Compatibility–Stability/Beyond-Use Date

Stability–Compatibility: All ingredients in this preparation are compatible and quite stable when in a non-aqueous, oil-based dosage form.

Packaging and Storage and Beyond-use date: The *USP* monograph for Estriol recommends storage in a tight container, and the monograph for Estradiol recommends storage in a tight, light-resistant container (14). A beyond-use date of 6 months is recommended for a similar compounded preparation described in *Allen's Compounded Formulations* (16). Pharmacist Hutter will use a 6-month beyond-use date as specified in *USP* Chapter ⟨795⟩ for solid formulations made with USP ingredients (15). A 1-month beyond-use date recommended for "Other Formulations" may also be used in <795>.

Calculations

Dose/Concentration

Estriol: *100 mg/50 capsules = 2 mg/capsule OK*

Estradiol: *25 mg/50 capsules = 0.5 mg/capsule = 500 mcg/capsule OK*

Ingredient Amounts

This example assumes the use of an electronic balance with an MWQ of 20 mg. Because of the small quantities of active ingredients needed and the sensitivity limitations of the balance, the entire quantity for 50 capsules is made.

Estradiol: 0.025 g = 25 mg   Estriol: 0.1 g = 100 mg

Peanut Oil:

   Volume: Assume a volume of 10 mL with a zero powder volume for the Estradiol and Estriol because of the very small quantities of powder.

   Weight: Peanut Oil has a density of 0.919 g/mL. The weight of Peanut Oil can be calculated:

$$\frac{1 \, mL \, Peanut \, Oil}{0.919 \, g \, Peanut \, Oil} = \frac{10 \, mL \, Peanut \, Oil}{x \, g \, Peanut \, Oil}; x = 9.19 \, g \, Peanut \, Oil$$

Capsule Content Weight

Total weight of capsule contents:

9.19 g Peanut Oil
0.1 g Estriol
0.025 g Estradiol
9.315 g

Weight per capsule: *9.315 g ÷ 50 capsules = 0.186 g/capsule*

Compounding Procedure

Weigh 100 mg Estriol and 25 mg of Estradiol on an electronic balance with an MWQ of 20 mg. Place the powders in a glass mortar and add approximately 6 mL Peanut Oil slowly with trituration to form a smooth slurry.

Transfer mixture to a graduated cylinder and add sufficient Peanut Oil to make 10 mL. Use some of the oil to rinse out the mortar to ensure complete transfer of the estrogen mixture. Stir mixture thoroughly using a glass stirring rod. Draw into a 1-mL syringe an amount of the estrogen mixture. Using either an improvised or manufactured capsule holder, place the bodies of size #1 capsules (use type with snap-closure feature) on the electronic balance and tare out the weight. Fill each capsule body with 186 mg of the liquid and replace the capsule caps. Place capsules in a vial with a child-resistant closure, label, and dispense.

Quality Control

The oil in the capsules appears as straw-colored. The size #1 clear gelatin capsules are approximately one-third full. Each capsule has been individually weighed to contain 186 mg of oil solution. Each capsule has been inspected to ensure that the cap is snapped securely in place.

Labeling

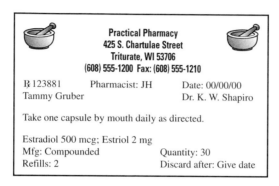

Practical Pharmacy		
425 S. Chartulae Street		
Triturate, WI 53706		
(608) 555-1200 Fax: (608) 555-1210		

℞ 123881   Pharmacist: JH   Date: 00/00/00
Tammy Gruber   Dr. K. W. Shapiro

Take one capsule by mouth daily as directed.

Estradiol 500 mcg; Estriol 2 mg
Mfg: Compounded   Quantity: 30
Refills: 2   Discard after: Give date

Auxiliary Labels: Keep in the refrigerator

Patient Consultation

Hello, Ms. Gruber, I'm your pharmacist, Julie Hutter. Are you using any other prescription or nonprescription medications? Are you allergic to any medication? What has Dr. Shapiro told you about this medication? This is an Estrogen replacement medication. You are to take one capsule by mouth daily as directed. You will want to report to Dr. Shapiro your response to the medication as well as any adverse effects; sometimes the dosage needs to be adjusted for maximum benefit. The capsules should be stored in the refrigerator. Discard any unused capsules after 6 months (give date). This may be refilled two times. Do you have any questions?

➤ Prescription 25-6

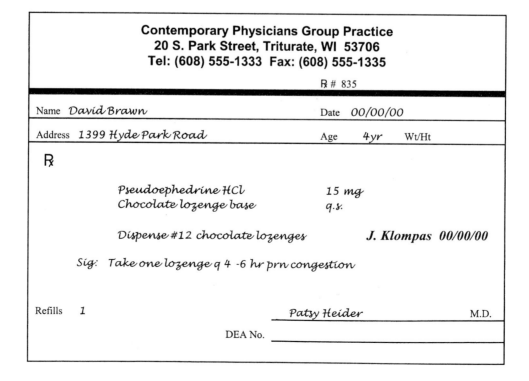

Contemporary Physicians Group Practice
20 S. Park Street, Triturate, WI 53706
Tel: (608) 555-1333 Fax: (608) 555-1335

℞ # 835

Name *David Brawn*   Date *00/00/00*

Address *1399 Hyde Park Road*   Age *4yr*   Wt/Ht

℞

         Pseudoephedrine HCl   15 mg
         Chocolate lozenge base   q.s.

       Dispense #12 chocolate lozenges   *J. Klompas 00/00/00*

    Sig: Take one lozenge q 4 -6 hr prn congestion

Refills   1   *Patsy Heider*   M.D.

          DEA No. _____

Ingredients Used (for 14 doses, 2 extras)

Ingredient	Quantity Used	Manufacturer Lot #-Exp Date	Solubility	Dose Comparison		Use in the Prescription
				Given	Usual	
Pseudoephedrine HCI	210 mg	JET Labs XY1175-mm/yy	v sol in water fr sol in alcohol	15 mg q 4–6 hr	15 mg q 4–6 hr	decongestant
Chocolate lozenge base made from:	27.79 g		immis. w/water and alcohol	—	—	flavored, sweetened base
Dipping Chocolate	30 g	Evon T54H-mm/yy	immis. w/water and alcohol	—	—	flavored, sweetened base
Corn Oil	10 g	Westle BR72-mm/yy	immis. w/water and alcohol	—	—	m.p/viscosity reducer

Compatibility–Stability/Beyond-Use Date

Stability–Compatibility: In a solid dosage form Pseudoephedrine HCl is quite stable.

Packaging and Storage and Beyond-use date: The *USP* monograph for Pseudoephedrine Hydrochloride Tablets recommends storage in a tight container (5). Pharmacist Klompas will use the recommended 6-month beyond-use date as specified in *USP* Chapter ⟨795⟩ for solid formulations made with USP ingredients (6).

Calculations

Dose/Concentration

Pediatric (2- to 6-year-old) pseudoephedrine dose: 15 mg q 4–6h—OK

Ingredient Amounts

Calculations are for 14 lozenges, two extra doses.

Pseudoephedrine HCl: *15 mg/dose × 14 doses = 210 mg*

Base: The formula for the base is 30 g of dipping chocolate plus 10 g of vegetable oil. This is made first, then the desired amount of base material is weighed for use. The lozenges are made to a weight of 2 g/lozenge.

Total weight of lozenges: *2 g/lozenge × 14 lozenges = 28 g*

Base: *28 g − 0.210 g Pseudoephedrine = 27.79 g chocolate base*

Compounding Procedure

All weighing is done on an electronic balance. Weigh 210 mg of Pseudoephedrine HCl. Prepare chocolate lozenge base by melting together 30 g of dipping chocolate and 10 g of corn oil. On the balance, tare out the weight of a 150-mL beaker and add melted chocolate base to a weight of 27.79 g. Place the Pseudoephedrine into a glass mortar and triturate to get a powder of smooth consistency. Transfer the powder completely to the beaker containing the melted chocolate base and stir well to mix. Place a lozenge mold on a piece of weighing paper on the balance and tare out this weight. Pour molten chocolate-drug material into each mold cavity to a weight of 2 g per lozenge. When all 12 lozenges are poured, place the mold in the freezer to cool and solidify. When solid, remove lozenges from the mold with a double-ended nickel spatula. Place each lozenge in a small zipper-closure bag and put the bags in a suitable outer container. Label and dispense. Lozenges are best when stored in the freezer. If lozenge molds are not available, use plastic medication cups. Weight per lozenge will vary with the mold used.

Quality Control

The lozenges are chocolate-brown in color with a smooth surface. Each appears uniform in size with a depth of 0.5 cm. Each lozenge has been individually weighed to contain 2 g of total material.

Labeling

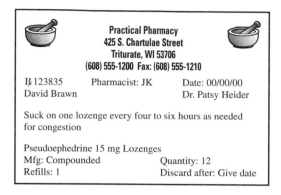

> **Practical Pharmacy**
> **425 S. Chartulae Street**
> **Triturate, WI 53706**
> **(608) 555-1200 Fax: (608) 555-1210**
>
> ℞ 123835   Pharmacist: JK   Date: 00/00/00
> David Brawn   Dr. Patsy Heider
>
> Suck on one lozenge every four to six hours as needed
> for congestion
>
> Pseudoephedrine 15 mg Lozenges
> Mfg: Compounded   Quantity: 12
> Refills: 1   Discard after: Give date

Auxiliary Labels: Store in freezer; Keep out of the reach of children

Patient Consultation

Hello, Mrs. Brawn, I'm your pharmacist, Jack Klompas, and I have David's prescription ready. Does David have any drug allergies? Is he currently taking any nonprescription or prescription medications? What did Dr. Heider tell you about this medication? These chocolate lozenges should help control David's congestion and runny nose. David may suck on one lozenge every 4 to 6 hours as needed for his congestion. If these lozenges do not help, or if the situation gets worse, contact Dr. Heider. Store these in the freezer. Be sure to keep out of the reach of children. This is especially important because they could be mistaken for candy. Discard any unused contents after 6 months (give date). You may have one refill. Do you have any questions?

➤ Prescription 25-7

> ### Contemporary Physicians Group Practice
> ### 20 S. Park Street, Triturate, WI 53706
> ### Tel: (608) 555-1333 Fax: (608) 555-1335
>
> ℞ # 865
>
> Name *Pat Schoenfeld*   Date *00/00/00*
>
> Address *2227 Pine Crest Colony Rd.*   Age   *2 yr*   Wt/Ht
>
> ℞
>
> Nystatin   2,000,000 units
> Sorbitol 70% Solution USP   10 mL
> Syrup NF   30 mL
> Purified Water   q s ad 100 mL
>
> M et Div. to make #10 popsicles
>
>   *A. Berg   00/00/00*
>
> Sig: Eat one popsicle q 8 hr for thrush
>
> Refills   2   *Patsy Heider*   M.D.
>
>   DEA No. _____

Ingredients Used

Ingredient	Quantity Used	Manufacturer Lot #-Exp Date	Solubility	Dose Comparison		Use in the Prescription
				Given	Usual	
Nystatin Powder 6050 units/mg	330 mg (2,000,000 units)	JET Labs XY1178-mm/yy	4 mg/mL water; 1.2 mg/mL alcohol	200,000 units q 8 hrs	200,000–400,000 units q 8 hrs	antifungal
Sorbitol 70% solution	10 mL	JET Labs XY1179-mm/yy	misc. with water	—	—	vehicle, sweetener, suspending agent
Syrup NF	30 mL	JET Labs XY1180-mm/yy	misc. with water	—	—	vehicle, flavor, sweetener
Purified water	60 mL	Sweet Springs AL0529-mm/yy		—	—	vehicle

Compatibility–Stability/Beyond-Use Date

Stability–Compatibility: Nystatin has some major stability concerns, which are described in some detail in the Nystatin monograph in *Trissel's Stability of Compounded Formulations* (17). Common flavored syrups with low pH (e.g., 2–4) should be avoided since the pH range for official USP Nystatin formulations is 4.5–7.0. The measured pH of the prescribed preparation is an acceptable 5. A flavoring concentrate that does not alter the pH may be added to improve the taste. The Nystatin monograph in the 11th edition of *The Merck Index* states that aqueous solutions and suspensions of Nystatin start to lose activity shortly after preparation. Suspensions that were tested at elevated temperature were found to be most stable at pH 7.0 and in moderately alkaline media. They were unstable at pH 2 and pH 9. A formulation similar to the one for this prescription was described in a *Hospital Pharmacy* journal article, and a 2-month beyond-use date was suggested for that preparation by the drug manufacturer Squibb (18).

Packaging and Storage and Beyond-use date: Based on the above information, Pharmacist Berg has decided to use a conservative beyond-use date of 30 days with storage in polybags in the freezer.

Calculations

Dose/Concentration

Nystatin: *2,000,000 units ÷ 10 doses = 200,000 units/dose—OK*

Amounts

Nystatin powder from JET Labs, Lot #XY1178, is 6,050 units/mg, so the amount of this powder needed is:

$$\frac{6050 \; units \; Nystatin}{mg \; Nystatin} = \frac{2,000,000 \; units \; Nystatin}{x \; mg \; Nystatin}; x = 330 \; mg \; Nystatin$$

The other ingredient amounts are all stated on the order, except for the Purified Water. Assuming a zero powder volume for the Nystatin, the volume of Purified Water needed is:

100 mL − 30 mL Syrup − 10 mL sorbitol = 60 mL Purified Water

Compounding Procedure

On a Class 3 torsion or an electronic balance, weigh 330 mg (2,000,000 units) of Nystatin powder. In a 50-mL graduated cylinder, measure 30 mL of Syrup NF, and in a 10-mL graduate, measure 10 mL of Sorbitol 70% Solution. Put the Nystatin in a glass mortar, add the Sorbitol 70% Solution to the Nystatin, and triturate well. Add the Syrup NF in portions while triturating. Using a 100-mL graduated cylinder, measure 60 mL of Purified Water. Slowly add to the mortar with trituration. Some of the water may be used if needed to first rinse out the graduates used for the Syrup and Sorbitol Solution with the rinsings added to the mortar. Using a 10-mL disposable syringe or a 10-mL graduated cylinder, measure 10-mL portions of the liquid and pour or squirt each portion into one cavity of an ice cube tray. Place in the freezer. When the Popsicles are semisolid, insert a Popsicle stick into each Popsicle. Put the ice cube tray back into the freezer. When the Popsicles are completely frozen, remove them from the tray and package in a large zipper-closure bag, label, and dispense.

Quality Control

The Popsicles appear as ice cubes with a slight pale-yellow opaque color. All are uniform in depth at 1.5 cm and each has been individually measured volumetrically to contain 10 mL of liquid.

Labeling

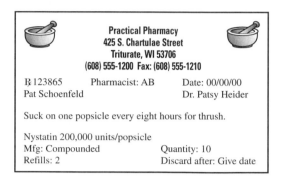

Practical Pharmacy
425 S. Chartulae Street
Triturate, WI 53706
(608) 555-1200 Fax: (608) 555-1210

℞ 123865	Pharmacist: AB	Date: 00/00/00
Pat Schoenfeld		Dr. Patsy Heider

Suck on one popsicle every eight hours for thrush.

Nystatin 200,000 units/popsicle

Mfg: Compounded	Quantity: 10
Refills: 2	Discard after: Give date

Auxiliary Labels: Keep out of the reach of children; Store in freezer

Patient Consultation

Hello, Mrs. Schoenfeld, I'm your pharmacist, Alec Berg. Does Pat have any drug allergies? Is she currently taking any other medications? What do you know about this medication? What sort of instructions did Dr. Heider give you about using this medication? These are Nystatin Popsicles to treat Pat's oral thrush. You should have her suck on one Popsicle every 8 hours. If they do not taste good at first, they may taste better after the cold Popsicle numbs her taste buds. If these do not help, or the situation worsens, contact Dr. Heider. Store these in the freezer, and be sure to keep them out of the reach of children. This is especially important because they look tempting to children. Discard any unused contents after 1 month. You may have two refills. Do you have any questions?

➤ Prescription 25-8

Contemporary Physicians Group Practice
20 S. Park Street, Triturate, WI 53706
Tel: (608) 555-1333 Fax: (608) 555-1335

℞ # 834

Name	*Jay Riemenschneider*	Date	*00/00/00*	
Address	*187 Enurese St.*	Age		Wt/Ht

℞

Lorazepam	24 mg
Diphenhydramine HCl	600 mg
Haloperidol	96 mg
Acacia	1.65 g
Powdered Sugar	21.63 g
Flavoring	q s
Purified Water	q s

S. White 00/00/00

M et Div. for 24 Lozenges

1" Red C

Sig: Suck on one lozenge q 8 hr prn N & V

Refills	2	*Linus Ashman*	M.D.

DEA No.   *AA4436677*

Ingredients Used (for 26 doses, 2 extra)

Ingredient	Quantity Used	Manufacturer Lot #-Exp Date	Solubility	Dose Comparison		Use in the Prescription
				Given	Usual	
Lorazepam 2 mg tablets	26 mg drug 13 tablets	BJF Generics XY1170-mm/yy	insol. water, sl sol in alcohol	1 mg q 8 hrs	2–6 mg/day	anti-emetic; amnesiac
Diphenhydramine HCl	650 mg	JET Labs XY1183-mm/yy	1 g/1 mL water, 2 mL alcohol	25 mg q 8 hrs	25–50 mg q 6 hrs	anti-emetic; sedative
Haloperidol 10 mg tablets & 2 mg tablets	104 mg drug 10 × 10 mg 2 × 2 mg	BJF Generics XY1171-mm/yy	1 g/78 mL cold water	4 mg q 8 hrs	0.5–5 mg q 8 hrs	anti-emetic; tranquillizer
Acacia	1.788 g	JET Labs XY1186-mm/yy	sol in water	—	—	binder
Powdered sugar	23.433 g	G & H M86J5-mm/yy	sol in water	—	—	sweetener, vehicle
Orange flavor	5 drops	JET Labs XY1184-mm/yy	miscible	—	—	flavoring
Purified water	2.5 mL	Sweet Springs AL0529-mm/yy	—	—	—	vehicle, wetting agent

Compatibility–Stability/Beyond-Use Date

Stability–Compatibility: All ingredients in this preparation should be quite stable when in a solid dosage form. For this prescription, Pharmacist White was asked to prepare ABH Troches for this patient. The letters ABH stand for Ativan® (Lorazepam), Benadryl® (Diphenhydramine HCl), and Haldol® (Haloperidol). Pharmacist White found the formula used here on page 27 of the Jan./Feb. 1997 (Vol. 1, No.1) issue of the *International Journal of Pharmaceutical Compounding*. Unfortunately, the article stated that no stability studies have been reported on this specific formulation.

Packaging and Storage and Beyond-use date: The *USP* monograph for Diphenhydramine HCl Capsules recommends storage in a tight container, but the monographs for both Lorazepam Tablets and Haloperidol Tablets recommend tight, light-resistant containers (14). Because water has been added to this preparation, Pharmacist White has decided to use a conservative 14-day beyond-use date as specified in *USP* Chapter ⟨795⟩ for water-containing formulations (15).

Calculations

Dose/Concentration

Lorazepam: *24 mg ÷ 24 doses = 1 mg/dose OK*

Haloperidol: *96 mg ÷ 24 doses = 4 mg/dose OK*

Diphenhydramine: *600 mg ÷ 24 doses = 25 mg/dose OK*

Ingredient Amounts

Calculations for are for 26 lozenges, 2 extra dosage units.

Lorazepam: *1 mg/dose × 26 doses = 26 mg needed.*

Available as 2-mg tablets; 13 tablets needed; Weight of 13 tablets = 1,469 mg

Haloperidol: *4 mg/dose × 26 doses = 104 mg needed*

Available as 0.5-, 1-, 2-, 5-, and 10-mg tablets; use ten 10-mg tablets and two 2-mg tablets for the 104 mg needed. Weight of these tablets = 2,560 mg

Diphenhydramine HCl: *25 mg/dose × 26 doses = 650 mg needed*

Powdered Sugar:

$$\frac{21.63 \ g \ powdered \ sugar}{24 \ lozenges} = \frac{x \ g \ powdered \ sugar}{26 \ lozenges}; x = 23.433 \ g \ powdered \ sugar$$

Acacia:

$$\frac{1.65 \ g \ Acacia}{24 \ lozenges} = \frac{x \ g \ Acacia}{26 \ lozenges}; x = 1.788 \ g \ Acacia$$

Lozenges Content Weight

Total weight of lozenges:

23.433 g powder sugar
1.469 g Lorazepam
2.560 g Haloperidol
1.788 g Acacia
0.650 g Diphenhydramine
2.500 g Purified Water
32.400 g

Weight per lozenge: 32.4 g ÷ 26 lozenge = 1.246 g/lozenge

Compounding Procedure

All weighing is done on a Class 3 torsion or an electronic balance. Weigh 650 mg of Diphenhydramine HCl powder and place in a mortar. Take ten Haloperidol 10-mg tablets and two Haloperidol 2-mg tablets and weigh them—2,560 mg. Transfer them to a glass mortar, crush and triturate the tablets to a fine powder, and add this powder to the Diphenhydramine powder by geometric dilution. Weigh 13 Lorazepam 2-mg tablets—1,469 mg. Crush the 13 Lorazepam tablets and add this to the Haloperidol/Diphenhydramine powder in portions; triturate well after each addition. Weigh 1.788 g of Acacia and 23.433 g of powdered sugar. Add the Acacia to a clean glass mortar and add 2.5 mL of Purified Water and five drops of orange flavoring, then triturate to form a mucilage. Using spatulation, combine the powdered sugar with the powdered drugs, then put the powders in a flour sifter and sift the powder onto an ointment pad. Gradually add the mix of drugs and powdered sugar to the acacia mucilage in the mortar. Triturate and mix until a firm but pliable solid forms. Roll the mass into a cylindrical shape on a glass ointment slab and cut into 24 equal portions. Each should weigh approximately 1.246 g. Place each lozenge in its own zipper-closure bag, and place in a suitable container with a child-resistant closure. Label.

Quality Control

The lozenges are buff in color. They are coin-shaped with a diameter of 1.5 mm and a depth of 0.5 cm. The weight of each lozenge has been individually checked and is within the range of ±10%, 1,122 mg to 1,370 mg.

Labeling

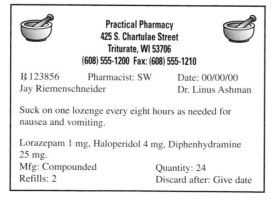

Auxiliary Labels: Keep out of the reach of children

Patient Consultation

Hello, Mr. Riemenschneider, I'm your pharmacist, Slappy White. Do you have any drug allergies? What other medications are you currently taking? What did Dr. Ashman tell you about this medication? These are lozenges that should help control your nausea from the chemotherapy you are receiving. You should suck on one lozenge every 8 hours as needed for nausea and vomiting. These lozenges will probably make you drowsy, so do not drive or do anything requiring mental alertness if you have taken a lozenge. If this medication does not help with your nausea, call me or Dr. Ashman and we will try some other medications. Also, if you notice any uncontrolled body movements while taking these, contact Dr. Ashman immediately. Do not drink any alcohol while taking this medication, as it can make you more drowsy. Store these in the refrigerator, out of the reach of children. Discard any unused contents after 2 weeks. You may have two refills. Do you have any questions?

References

1. The 2002 United States Pharmacopeia 25/National Formulary 20. Rockville, MD: The United States Pharmacopeial Convention, Inc., 2001; 2216-2218.
2. Rudnic E, Schwartz JB. Oral solid dosage forms. In: Gennaro AR, ed. Remington: The science and practice of pharmacy, 19th ed. Easton, PA: Mack Publishing Co., 1995; 1648.
3. Allen Jr LV. Troches and lozenges. Secundum Artem, Vol. 4, No. 2. Minneapolis, MN: Paddock Laboratories, Inc.
4. Sadik F. Tablets. In: King RE, ed. Dispensing of medications, 9th ed. Easton, PA: Mack Publishing Co., 1984; 56.
5. Allen Jr LV. Pharmaceutical Compounding Tips and Hints. Secundum Artem, Vol. 5, No.12. Minneapolis, MN: Paddock Laboratories, Inc.
6. The 2002 United States Pharmacopeia 25/National Formulary 20. Rockville, MD: The United States Pharmacopeial Convention, Inc., 2001; 2082-2084.
7. Allen Jr LV, ed. Tetracaine 20-mg lollipops. IJPC 1997; 1: 112.
8. Allen Jr LV, ed. Pediatric chocolate troche base. IJPC 1997; 1: 106.
9. Allen Jr LV, ed. ABH soft troche base. IJPC 1997; 1: 27.
10. Allen Jr LV, ed. HDDM soft troche base. IJPC 1997; 1: 30.
11. Allen Jr LV, ed. Tetracycline compound troche. IJPC 1997; 1: 113.
12. Allen Jr LV, ed. Pediatric chewable gummy gels. IJPC 1997; 1: 107.
13. Shaw MA, Narducci WA, Newton DW. Extemporaneous formulations. In: King RE, ed. Dispensing of medications, 9th ed. Easton, PA: Mack Publishing Co., 1984; 48, 268.
14. The 2002 United States Pharmacopeia 25/National Formulary 20. Rockville, MD: The United States Pharmacopeial Convention, Inc., 2001; Official Monographs.
15. The 2002 United States Pharmacopeia 25/National Formulary 20. Rockville, MD: The United States Pharmacopeial Convention, Inc., 2001; 2054-2055.
16. Allen, Jr LV. Allen's Compounded Formulations. Washington DC: American Pharmaceutical Association, 1999; 76-77.
17. Trissel LA. Stability of compounded formulations, 2d ed. Washington DC: The American Pharmaceutical Association, 2000; 276-278.
18. Dobbins JC. A frozen nystatin preparation. Hosp Pharm 1983; 18: 452-453.

CHAPTER 26

Solutions

I. GENERAL DEFINITION

"Solutions are liquid preparations that contain one or more chemical substances dissolved, i.e., molecularly dispersed, in a suitable solvent or mixture of mutually miscible solvents." (1)—*USP*

II. USES AND DESIRED PROPERTIES OF SOLUTIONS

Solutions are used pharmaceutically in a wide variety of ways. Specific desired or required properties depend on the intended route of administration and/or the solvent or solvent system. Below are descriptions of various classes of pharmaceutical solutions. More detailed information can be found in Chapters ⟨1151⟩ Pharmaceutical Dosage Forms and ⟨1⟩ Injections of the *USP*.

A. Solutions Classified by Solvent System (1)
  1. Spirits
   a. These are alcoholic or hydroalcoholic solutions of volatile substances. They are usually made by direct dissolution.
   b. Some spirits are used as flavoring agents; others contain therapeutically active ingredients. Two examples of spirits are Camphor Spirit USP and Peppermint Spirit.
   c. The high alcoholic content of a spirit is usually necessary for solubility of the ingredient(s). Addition of water may cause turbidity or precipitation.
   d. These solutions should be stored and dispensed in tight, light-resistant containers to retard evaporation of the volatile ingredients and the alcohol and to minimize oxidation of labile active ingredients.
  2. Tinctures
   a. Tinctures contain vegetable materials or chemical substances in alcoholic or hydroalcoholic solutions.
   b. Some tinctures, such as Iodine Tincture USP, are made by direct dissolution. Other tinctures, such as those containing vegetable materials, are made by special percolation (called Process P) or maceration (called Process M) processes, outlined in Chapter ⟨1151⟩ of the *USP*. Compound Benzoin Tincture, which is used as an ingredient in Sample Prescription 26.4, is an example of a tincture made using Process M.
  3. Aromatic waters
   a. These are clear, saturated solutions of volatile oils or other aromatic or volatile substances. As with spirits, they should be stored in tight, light-resistant containers.
   b. The solvent is usually water.

4. Elixirs

    a. This term is commonly used for oral solutions that use a sweetened hydro-alcoholic vehicle.

    b. In addition to active ingredients, elixirs may contain additive ingredients as described below under oral solutions.

5. Syrups

    a. Oral solutions that contain a high concentration of sucrose or other sugars are often called syrups, but this term is also used in a more general sense to describe sweet, viscous, oral liquid preparations, including suspensions.

    b. In addition to active ingredients, syrups may contain additive ingredients as described below under oral solutions.

B. Solutions by Route of Administration

    1. Oral solutions (1)

        a. These are liquid preparations intended for oral administration.

        b. They contain one or more therapeutically active ingredients dissolved in water or a water-cosolvent system. Solutions are most often made by direct dissolution. Factors that affect this process are described later in this chapter. Sample Prescriptions 26.2, 26.3, and 26.10 illustrate principles and techniques used in making oral solutions.

        c. Oral solutions may contain inactive ingredients to improve their palatability, stability, and/or esthetic appeal. Examples of such ingredients include flavors, sweetening or coloring agents, viscosity-increasing agents, buffers, antioxidants, and preservatives.

        d. As described above, syrups are oral solutions containing high concentrations of sugars. Oral solutions may contain other polyols such as glycerin or sorbitol, which prevent "cap-lock" by inhibiting crystallization of the sugars in the cap and adjacent areas of the container. Depending on the polyol, these additives may also serve as sweetening agents, preservatives, cosolvents, and viscosity-increasing agents to improve mouth feel.

    2. Topical solutions (1)

        a. These are solutions intended for topical application to the skin or oral mucous membranes.

        b. They are usually aqueous but may also contain other solvents, such as alcohols and/or polyols or other solvents approved for topical use.

        c. They may also contain additives, such as preservatives, antioxidants, buffers, humectants, viscosity-increasing agents, colors, or scents.

        d. The term **lotion** is used for topical liquid preparations, but a lotion may be either a solution or a dispersion.

        e. Specialized containers for topical preparations are available from vendors of compounding supplies. Bottles with glass applicators, with dauber or roller tops, with sprayer assemblies, and with specialized spout or disc caps are convenient administration aids for topical solutions.

    3. Otic solutions (1)

        a. These are intended for instillation in the outer ear.

        b. The vehicle may be water or glycerin, or a cosolvent system containing water, alcohol, and/or polyols.

        c. Otic solutions may also contain additives such as preservatives, antioxidants, buffers, viscosity-increasing agents, or surfactants. Sample Prescription 26.9 illustrates use of various additive ingredients in an otic preparation.

        d. Bottles with dropper closures are available to facilitate administration of otic solutions.

    4. Nasal solutions

        a. These solutions are sprayed or instilled into the nose. Although they are not specifically mentioned as a class in Chapter ⟨1151⟩, there are official USP nasal solutions such as Naphazoline Hydrochloride Nasal Solution. While nasal solutions

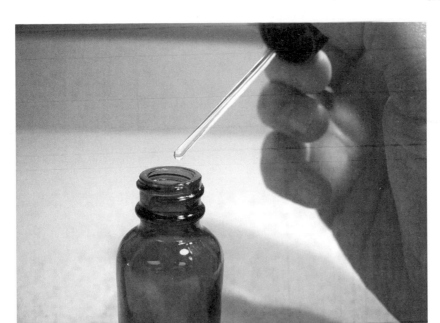

Applicator bottle

are most often used for local action, this dosage form is being investigated for administration of drugs for systemic effect.

b. The vehicle for nasal solutions is usually water, but it may be a cosolvent system.

c. Nasal solutions may also contain preservatives, buffers, antioxidants, surfactants, and/or tonicity-adjusting additives.

d. The cilia in nasal passages are sensitive to osmotic pressure, so nasal solutions should be as close to isotonic as possible.

  (1) Nasal solutions with osmolarity comparable to aqueous 0.5–2% Sodium Chloride solutions are relatively comfortable and should not harm nasal cilia.

  (2) Sodium Chloride and Dextrose are recommended tonicity adjustors (2).

e. The effect of tonicity and the specific effects of various drugs, salts, surfactants, cosolvents, oils, and preservatives were investigated in the late 1940s and early 1950s by Proetz. A summary of this work can be found in the 7th edition of *Dispensing of Medication*, pages 913–915. Some findings helpful in formulating

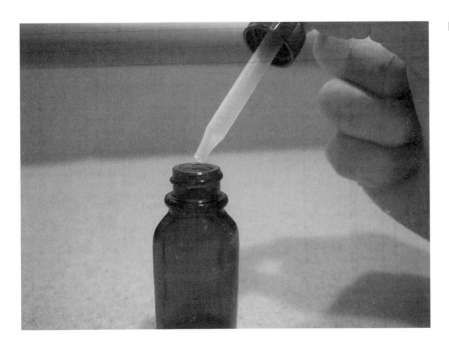

Dropper bottle

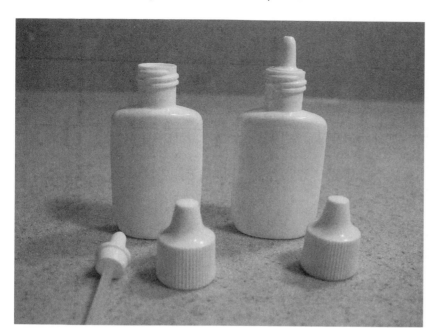

Nasal spray bottle

compounded nasal solutions are given here. Sample Prescription 26.8 uses a formula developed by Proetz for a nasal preparation.

    (1) Although nasal passages can tolerate a relatively wide range of tonicity without pain, isotonicity is important. Highly hypertonic solutions (4-4.5% Sodium Chloride solutions) and hypotonic solutions (0.3% or less Sodium Chloride solutions) were found to cause damage to nasal cilia.

    (2) Alcohol in concentrations up to 10%, when in an isotonic solution, caused no problems.

    (3) Benzalkonium Chloride in concentrations up to 0.1%, if incorporated into an isotonic saline solution, showed no damage to cilia.

    (4) Anionic surfactants such as Sodium Lauryl Sulfate and Docusate Sodium could be used in concentrations of 0.01% without pain or a burning sensation, but concentrations of 0.05% caused some discomfort. Nonionic surfactants were acceptable at much higher concentrations (3).

f. Normal nasal secretions have a pH in the range of 5.5 to 6.5. Because nasal secretions lack significant natural buffer capacity, highly buffered solutions, especially outside the normal pH range, should be avoided (2).

    (1) If a buffer is desired with a pH in the neutral range, a dilute phosphate buffer at pH 6.5 is recommended (2). The isotonic Sorenson's Modified Phosphate Buffer Solution at pH 6.5, as given in Chapter 17 of this book, would be a good choice.

    (2) If a buffer is needed for purposes of drug stability or solubility with a pH that is outside of the normal range, a buffer or pH adjusting agent that has low buffer capacity should be selected. See Chapter 17 for more information on this subject.

g. Preservatives are required by the USP for solutions in multidose containers such as nasal dropper or spray bottles. Preservatives that are approved for ophthalmic solutions (listed and described in Chapter 15 of this book) are suitable for preserving nasal solutions. When selecting a preservative, check for compatibility with active ingredients and other necessary added excipients. Also check to be sure that the preservative is active at the pH of the finished nasal solution.

h. Nasal solutions should be sterile when dispensed.

    (1) The FDA Center for Drug Evaluation and Research (CDER) has issued a "Guidance for Industry, Nasal Spray and Inhalation Solution, Suspension, and Spray Drug Products." This guidance is available on the Internet at www.fda.gov.cder/guidance/2836dft/htm Section 2.f. states, "All inhalation solutions, suspensions, and spray drug products should be sterile." This guidance, which is intended for the industry, requires both sterile products and validation of the sterilization process. This guidance took effect May 26, 2002, and applies to single- or multiple-dose nasal sprays and inhalation solutions and suspensions that are sold outside the state of manufacture. It does not apply to pressurized metered-dose inhalers (4). While this guidance does not legally apply to pharmacists who compound, the FDA has found this to be an important safety issue, so pharmacists who compound nasal or inhalation solutions or suspensions should render them sterile.

(2). Sterilization of compounded nasal solutions can be fairly easily accomplished by sterile filtration with a 0.2- or 0.45-μ bacterial filter and use of a sterile container. Sterile containers can be purchased from vendors of compounding supplies. The sterilization process and packaging should be done in a sterile environment such as a laminar airflow hood or a barrier isolator. If an autoclave is available, terminal steam sterilization of the preparation in its dispensing container is another alternative. With either method, compatibility and stability of the preparation ingredients should be considered. Some bacterial filters adsorb certain types of drug molecules; large molecules such as peptides or proteins are particularly vulnerable. Because steam sterilization uses elevated temperature and pressure, this method may not be acceptable for some drugs that have stability concerns.

i. Compounding and dispensing nasal solutions for systemic administration should be done with the greatest of caution. Although procedures have been described in the literature for calibration of droppers and nasal sprays, results in practice have not been encouraging. In one study of nasal droppers, 10 physicians acted as the test subjects; all 10 overused the drug by a range of 41% to 338% (5). Similar results were found during an informal study conducted by pharmacy students using a procedure recommended for calibration of nasal spray bottles in which nasal solution was sprayed into plastic bags. For systemic nasal drug administration, metered-dose drug delivery systems are recommended, especially when potent drugs are involved.

5. Inhalations (1)

    a. Inhalations may be drugs, solutions, or suspensions.

    b. They are administered either by the nasal or oral route with the respiratory tract as the intended site for local effect or for systemic absorption of an active ingredient.

    c. For proper delivery of solution to the respiratory tract, inhalation solutions must first be nebulized to form very small, uniform droplets that will pass through the

Nebulizer

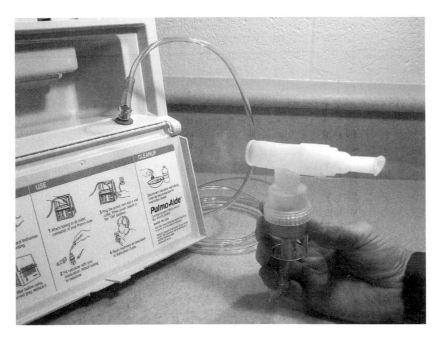

mouth or nose, throat, and bronchial tree to the bronchioles and alveoli of the lungs. Hand-held nebulizers and intermittent positive-pressure breathing (IPPB) machines are available for this purpose.

   d.   The usual vehicles for inhalation solutions are sterile water and sterile isotonic sodium chloride solution. Small quantities of cosolvents such as alcohol or glycerin may be added when needed (6).

   e.   Inhalation solutions may contain additives similar to those used in nasal solutions, but agents such as preservatives, antioxidants, buffers, and surfactants should be used only as necessary, and the concentration of these additives should be as low as possible. These solutions are delivered to very sensitive tissues in the lungs, and this should always be considered in formulating a solution for inhalation.

   f.   Inhalation solutions are also similar to nasal solutions in that they should be sterile and they should be as close to isotonic as is possible. A preservative is required for any inhalation solution dispensed in a multidose container.

6. Ophthalmic solutions (1)

   a.   These are sterile, particle-free solutions formulated for instillation in the eye.

   b.   The vehicle for ophthalmic solutions is sterile water or sterile isotonic sodium chloride solution.

   c.   In addition to the active ingredients and water, ophthalmic solutions may also contain buffers, preservatives, antioxidants, tonicity adjustors, and viscosity-increasing agents.

   d.   Because of the delicate nature of the eye and surrounding membranes, special consideration must be given to isotonicity, buffering, and preservation. These issues and sample calculations are given in Chapter 10, Isotonicity Calculations, Chapter 15, Preservatives, Chapter 16, Antioxidants, Chapter 17, Buffers and pH Adjusting Agents, Chapter 27, Ophthalmic Solutions, and in the *ASHP Technical Assistance Bulletin on Pharmacy-Prepared Ophthalmic Products*, which is available on the ASHP Internet site (www.ashp.org).

7. Irrigating solutions (1)

   a.   These are sterile solutions used to soak, flush, or irrigate wounds or body cavities, such as the bladder. They are not for parenteral use and should be labeled "Not for injection" and "For irrigation only."

   b.   The usual vehicle for irrigating solutions is water.

   c.   Because irrigating solutions come in contact with open wounds and delicate body tissues and membranes, special consideration must be given to the isotonicity and pH of the solution. Additives may be necessary to achieve these objectives.

8. Parenteral solutions (1,7)

   a.   These are solutions injected through the skin or a boundary membrane or directly into a blood vessel, muscle, organ, or other tissue.

   b.   Because these solutions are injected into delicate body tissues, special consideration must be given to osmolarity and pH of the solution.

   c.   Parenteral solutions must meet the standards given in Chapter ⟨1⟩ Injections of the *USP*, including requirements for sterility, pyrogens, particulates, and contaminants.

   d.   Additional guidelines have been established for preparing, handling, and storing parenteral solutions that are manipulated in some way by the pharmacist before being administered to the patient. One of these guidelines, *NABP Model Rules for Sterile Pharmaceuticals,* is available in the Appendices section of the CD that accompanies this book; a second, *ASHP Technical Assistance Bulletin on Pharmacy-prepared Sterile Products* is on the ASHP Internet site described above; and a third guideline, Chapter ⟨1206⟩ Sterile Drug Products for Home Use, can be found in the *USP*. Chapter ⟨1206⟩ is being considered for significant changes and a change of chapter number to ⟨797⟩; this may affect how pharmacists process sterile preparations. (*USP* informational chapters numbered below 1,000 are potentially legally enforceable.) Consult the *USP* and any guidances that may be issued by FDA for current standards in handling sterile preparations.

> **e.** Vehicles and extra ingredients, such as preservatives, for these solutions must be approved for parenteral use.
>
> **f.** Methods of preparation and handling parenteral solutions are discussed in Chapter 32, Parenteral Products, and in Chapter 33, Parenteral Nutrition.

III. ADVANTAGES OF SOLUTIONS

A. Because solutions are molecularly dispersed systems, they offer these advantages:
  1. Completely homogenous doses
  2. Immediate availability for absorption and distribution

B. Solutions also provide a flexible dosage form.
  1. They may be used by any route of administration.
  2. They can be taken or administered to patients who cannot swallow tablets or capsules.
  3. Doses are easily adjusted.

IV. DISADVANTAGES OF SOLUTIONS

A. Drugs and chemicals are less stable when in solution than when in dry form.

B. Some drugs are not soluble in solvents that are acceptable for pharmaceutical use.

C. Drugs with objectionable taste require special additives or techniques to mask the taste when in solution.

D. Because solutions are more bulky and heavy than dry solid dosage forms, they are more difficult to handle, package, transport, and store.

E. Oral solutions in bulk containers require measurement by the patient or caregiver. This is often less accurate than individual solid dosage forms, such as tablets and capsules.

V. PRINCIPLES OF COMPOUNDING SOLUTIONS

A. When making a solution of a drug or chemical, consider the following:
  1. Will the drug or chemical dissolve in the desired solvent?
  2. How long will it take to dissolve the drug or chemical?
  3. Will the drug or chemical stay in solution?
  4. Will the drug or chemical be stable in solution? For how long?
  5. Is a preservative needed to prevent the growth of microorganisms inadvertently introduced at the time of preparation or during use by the patient?

B. Questions 1 and 2 concern the making of solutions (that is, dissolving drug or chemical in a solvent). Methods and factors affecting dissolution are discussed below.

C. Questions 3, 4, and 5 are considerations of stability and compatibility of drug preparations once they are made. Questions 3 and 4 concern the chemical and physical stability of drugs and drug products; these topics are the focus of Chapter 34, but appropriate consideration of these issues is illustrated in each of the sample prescriptions in this chapter. Question 5, which concerns the need for and use of preservatives, is considered in Chapter 15, but this topic is also addressed with each of the sample prescriptions presented here. Additional information on stability can also be found in Chapter 4, Expiration and Beyond-use Dating.

D. Will the drug or chemical dissolve in the desired solvent?
  1. Dissolution of solids
      a. Pharmaceutical solvents
          (1) Water is the most commonly used and most desirable solvent.
          (2) Other common solvents include Alcohol, Isopropyl Alcohol, Glycerin, Propylene Glycol, Polyethylene Glycol 400, and various oils. These and other USP solvents are described in Chapter 14, Pharmaceutical Solvents.
          (3) Some solvents, such as Isopropyl Alcohol, are approved for topical solutions but may not be used internally because of their systemic toxicity.
      b. To make a solution of a solid in a solvent, the concentration of the solid in the solvent must be at or below the solubility of the solid in that solvent. Obviously, a solid will not dissolve above its solubility.
      c. When predicting solubility very generally, the old saying "Like dissolves like" is a useful guide, where **like** refers to similarity of functional group or molecular structure.
      d. Usually more precise information on solubility is required, so the first step in making a drug solution is to check the solubility of the drug. Suitable references for this purpose include *The Merck Index, Remington: The Science and Practice of Pharmacy,* and the *USP DI Volume III.*
          Example: Boric Acid   10%
                      Sterile Water q.s. ad.   60 mL
          On checking the solubility of Boric Acid, the pharmacist finds it to be 1 g/18 mL water, or approximately 5%. The above preparation cannot be made because the prescribed concentration, 10%, is above the solubility of the Boric Acid in water.
          (1) Remember that solubilities are given in grams of solute per milliliter of **solvent,** not per milliliter of solution, so unless you know the density of the saturated solution, you cannot know the precise amount of solution that will result. Therefore, the 5% given above is a rough estimate.
          (2) A useful table of information on saturated solutions of many chemicals and drugs can be found in the miscellaneous tables section of *The Merck Index.*
          (3) Many times solubility is given in descriptive terms, such as soluble, slightly soluble, and sparingly soluble. The numerical equivalents of these terms can be found in the *USP* and other references. They are also given in Appendix D of this text.
      e. If possible, always dissolve the drug in pure solvent. For example, although Syrup NF contains a lot of water, these solvent molecules are tied up through hydrogen bonding with the sucrose and are unavailable for the purposes of interacting with and dissolving additional solute.
      f. Beware of dissolving drugs or chemicals in boiling water (a useful technique to speed up dissolution), because the drug may precipitate when the preparation cools to room temperature if its concentration is above its solubility at room temperature. In the example with Boric Acid, the solubility of Boric Acid is 1 g/4 mL of boiling water, or approximately 25%. The 10% solution could easily be made using hot or boiling water, but the Boric Acid will precipitate out on cooling to room temperature.
      g. If the solution is to be stored or used at a temperature other than room temperature, the solubility of the drug at that temperature must be considered.
      h. The following are several useful compounding strategies when a drug solution is prescribed if the desired concentration is above the drug's solubility:
          (1) Make as a suspension. You may need to add a suspending agent. Remember to use a "Shake Well" label.
          (2) Use a different solvent or a cosolvent system. To calculate the approximate volume fraction of each solvent needed in a cosolvent system for the drug, use the equation:
          $$\log S_T = vf_{water}\log S_{water} + vf_{sol}\log S_{sol}$$

where:

S_T = total concentration of drug in solution
S_{water} = solubility of the drug in water
S_{sol} = solubility of the drug in the chosen cosolvent
vf_{water} = volume fraction of water in the solution
vf_{sol} = volume fraction of the cosolvent in the solution

Use of this equation is illustrated in the section on alcohol calculations in Chapter 7 and in Sample Prescription 26.5 in this current chapter.

(3) Decrease the concentration of the prescribed drug or chemical. For systemic medications, the volume of the dose to be administered must be adjusted to give the prescribed amount of drug per dose. Two examples of this are illustrated in Sample Prescriptions 26.2 and 26.4.

(4) In all cases where changes are required, consult with the prescriber.

2. Miscibility of liquids

   a. You know that oil and water don't mix, but consider the miscibility of the following examples:

- Alcohol and Water?   Yes
- Glycerin and Water?   Yes
- Glycerin and Alcohol?   Yes
- Glycerin and Mineral Oil?   No
- Alcohol and Mineral Oil?   No

  (Mineral Oil is miscible with chloroform, ether, benzene, and many other oils, but not with Alcohol and not with Glycerin.)

- Alcohol and Cottonseed Oil?   No
- Alcohol and Castor Oil?   Yes (in equal parts)

  (Castor Oil is the only fixed oil that is miscible with Alcohol.)

- Cottonseed Oil and Mineral Oil? Yes
- Castor Oil and Mineral Oil?   No

  (Castor Oil is the only fixed oil not miscible with Mineral Oil.)

   b. Obviously, miscibility is not always easily predicted. Therefore, if you don't know the miscibility of two liquids, consult a suitable reference, such as *The Merck Index, Remington: The Science and Practice of Pharmacy,* or the *USP DI Volume III.*

   c. Useful compounding strategies when it is necessary to combine immiscible liquids:

     (1) Make an emulsion by adding an emulsifying agent. Be sure to use a "Shake Well" label.

     (2) Use a different solvent or an appropriate cosolvent system.

     (3) In all cases in which changes are required, consult with the prescriber.

E. How long will it take to dissolve the drug or chemical?

In other words, what is the rate of dissolution? In practical terms, what we often want to know is, how can we speed up the rate of dissolution? This can be analyzed in terms of the Noyes-Whitney equation, which was given in Chapter 24, Powders, and which is repeated below.

$$\frac{dC}{dt} = K\,S(C_s - C)$$

1. From Fick's First Law of Diffusion, it can be shown that the dissolution rate constant, K, is equal to D/hV, where D is the diffusion coefficient, h is the thickness of the unstirred layer around the particle, and V is the volume of the solvent into which the drug is dissolved.

2. The diffusion coefficient D is actually composed of several factors expressed in the Stokes-Einstein equation given below. A knowledge of these factors will help the pharmacist to understand conditions that can be changed or controlled to increase the rate of dissolution.

$$D = \frac{kT}{6\pi\eta r}$$

where: k is the Boltzmann constant (the gas constant, R, divided by Avogadro's number),

T is absolute temperature,

η is viscosity of the medium,

r is the radius of the drug molecule.

From the Noyes-Whitney and Stokes-Einstein equations, it can be seen that some factors can be controlled or modified to increase the rate of dissolution and some cannot.

dC/dt, the rate of dissolution, is dependent on:

a. T: Temperature is an important factor that can be altered by the pharmacist. As temperature increases, D increases, so diffusion and the rate of dissolution increase. In practical terms, we can use warm solvents or can heat solutions to increase the rate of dissolution. Care must be exercised when using heat because increasing the temperature also increases the rate of degradation of drug molecules.

b. η: Increasing the viscosity of the medium has the opposite effect on diffusion and dissolution rate; increasing viscosity decreases the diffusion coefficient and the rate of dissolution. For this reason, drugs dissolve more slowly in viscous vehicles like syrups. This is one reason why it is best to dissolve drugs in pure solvents, like water or alcohol, which have lower viscosity, then add the more viscous necessary liquids, such as glycerin, syrups, or gels. This is illustrated in Sample Prescription 26.2.

c. r: Even though we cannot control the radius of the drug molecule, it is important and helpful to understand how it affects diffusion and the rate of dissolution. The larger the radius (r), the smaller D becomes and the slower the rate of dissolution. This means that, all other things being equal, large drug molecules dissolve more slowly than do smaller molecules. This is especially important when working with macromolecules, such as Erythromycin Lactobionate and Amphotericin B. When making solutions of these drugs, it is necessary to give them sufficient time to dissolve. This is illustrated with Sample Prescription 26.6, a Clindamycin topical solution. This factor will have increasing importance as pharmacists handle more peptide and protein drugs, because these are very large molecules.

d. The factor h, which is the thickness of the unstirred layer around the particle, can be affected by stirring. The dissolution rate is faster if the drug-solvent-solution system is agitated or stirred. By stirring, the dissolved drug molecules are moved away from the surface of the solid to the bulk of the solution. This has the effect of decreasing h, which increases K and therefore increases the rate of dissolution.

e. The surface area of the solid, S: As was stated in the discussion on powders, because, for a given weight of solid, the surface area of a solid increases as the particle size is decreased, the smaller the particle size, the larger the surface area and the faster the rate of dissolution.

(1) Although important, this principle has limited practical application in compounding solutions. Most drugs and chemicals are purchased in a fine state of subdivision. Unless a solid ingredient is in large pieces, any mechanical manipulation, such as trituration, by the pharmacist has only a minor effect on the rate of dissolution. The amount of time saved in speeding the rate of dissolution by decreasing the particle size is usually more than offset by the time lost in the extra steps of weighing, triturating, transferring, and reweighing before dissolving the drug or chemical.

(2) For a few drugs, like sulfurated potash (used to make White Lotion, as shown in Sample Prescription 28.3), that are available in large chunks or "rocks," particle size reduction is useful for increasing the rate of dissolution.

f. The solubility of the solid, C_s: Although the solubility of the solid is a given property of the drug, it is important to know that poorly soluble drugs may dissolve slowly.

g. *C*, the concentration of the drug or chemical in solution at time = t. As the solution approaches saturation, the quantity $(C_s - C)$ gets smaller and smaller until $C_s = C$. At this point, $(C_s - C) = 0$, saturation is reached, and dissolution stops. As saturation is approached, the rate of dissolution may become very slow. This is one reason for making saturated solutions ahead of time, because getting that last little amount to dissolve may take a long time. Some pharmacists maintain stock bottles of saturated solutions with excess drug or chemical on the bottom of the vessel and then decant the saturated solution when it is needed.

VI.   STABILITY

A. Physical stability of the system: The major concern with regard to physical stability of solutions is the issue of precipitation. This subject is discussed in some detail in Chapter 34, Compatibility and Stability of Drug Products and Preparations.

B. Chemical stability of the ingredients
  1. Check references such as *Trissel's Stability of Compounded Formulations, Chemical Stability of Pharmaceuticals, Extemporaneous Formulations, Pediatric Drug Formulations,* the *USP/DI Vol I,* or professional pharmacy journals such as the *International Journal of Pharmaceutical Compounding,* or the *American Journal of Health-System Pharmacy.* Chemical stability in general is also discussed in Chapter 34 and in Chapter 4, Expiration and Beyond-use Dating, and this topic is considered for the prescription ingredients in each of the sample prescriptions that follow in this chapter.
  2. The *USP* chapter on pharmacy compounding, Chapter ⟨795⟩, recommends a maximum 14-day dating for all water-containing preparations made with ingredients in solid form when the stability of the ingredients in the formulations is not known (8). Concerns for the chemical stability of known labile drugs may limit beyond-use dates even more.
  3. While technically it is very easy to make solutions, care should always be used in checking and validating the stability and the beyond-use date of the compounded preparation.

C. Microbiological stability: The *USP* states that for oral solutions, antimicrobial agents are generally added to protect against bacteria, yeasts, and molds (1). Preservatives should also be considered for topical solutions. If antimicrobial ingredients are prescribed as part of the formulation, extra preservatives are not needed. Antimicrobial agents and their proper use are discussed in Chapter 15, and consideration of preservatives is presented in each of the following sample prescription formulations.

SAMPLE PRESCRIPTIONS

➤ **Prescription 26.1**

Contemporary Physicians Group Practice
20 S. Park Street, Triturate, WI 53706
Tel: (608) 555-1333 Fax: (608) 555-1335

℞ # 178

Name *Ashley Fingerhut*   Date *00/00/00*

Address *5487 Social Avenue*   Age _____   Wt/Ht _____

℞

KMnO4   1:6000

Dispense 6 oz.

J. Jones 00/00/00

Sig: Apply 2 - 3 times daily as a wet dressing

Refills   *0*   M. Q. Attles   M.D.

DEA No. _____

Ingredients Used

Ingredient	Quantity Used	Manufacturer Lot #-Exp Date	Solubility	Dose Comparison		Use in the Prescription
				Given	Usual	
Potassium Permanganate	120 mg weighed, 30 mg used	JET Labs SN2611-mm/yy	1 g/4 mL	0.017%	0.004%–1%	antibacterial, antifungal, germicidal
Purified Water	q.s. 180 mL	Sweet Springs AL0529-mm/yy	—	—	—	vehicle

Compatibility–Stability/Beyond-Use Date

Stability–Compatibility: With regard to physical stability, this solution should be very stable because Potassium Permanganate is very water-soluble, and this is a very dilute solution. Chemical stability is a very different matter. Potassium Permanganate is a very strong oxidizing agent and is not very stable chemically. This is apparent as solutions turn from purple to brown with the formation of manganese dioxide.

Preservative: No additional preservative is needed because Potassium Permanganate is an antimicrobial agent. Packaging and Storage and Beyond-use date: This solution should be dispensed in a tight container. Although it would be possible to use the beyond-use dating recommended in Chapter ⟨795⟩ in the *USP*, that is, a maximum 14-day beyond-use date for compounded water-containing formulations prepared from ingredients in solid form (7); Pharmacist Jones has decided to use a more conservative 7-day dating because of the labile nature of Potassium Permanganate. Because this is a topical product, controlled room temperature will be the recommended storage condition.

Calculations

Dose/Concentration
Concentration OK for intended use.

Ingredient Amounts

Potassium Permanganate ($KMnO_4$) :

$$6\ oz = 180\ mL;\quad \frac{1\ g\ KMnO_4}{6000\ mL\ solution} = \frac{x\ g\ KMnO_4}{180\ mL\ solution};\ x = 0.03\ g = 30\ mg\ KMnO_4$$

This amount is below the MWQ; a solid–liquid aliquot is needed:

Weigh 120 mg $KMnO_4$ and dissolve in 12 mL H_2O:

120 mg/12 mL = 10 mg/mL.

Because 30 mg is needed, measure 3 mL of this solution: *10 mg/mL × 3 mL = 30 mg*
The 1:6,000 ratio strength may be expressed on the label as a w/v percent:

$$\frac{1\ g\ KMnO_4}{6000\ mL\ solution} = \frac{x\ g}{100\ mL};\ x = 0.017\ g/100\ mL = 0.017\%$$

Compounding Procedure

Rinse equipment well with **Purified Water.** On a class 3 torsion or an electronic balance, weigh 120 mg of Potassium Permanganate. Dissolve this in 12 mL of Purified Water measured in a 25-mL graduated cylinder. Measure 3 mL of this solution in a 10-mL graduate, and transfer to a 6-oz graduated prescription bottle with a child-resistant closure. Add Purified Water to the 180-mL graduation mark. Replace closure, close tightly, and agitate to mix. Label and dispense.

Quality Control

The preparation is a clear purple solution with no brown coloration. The actual volume is checked and matches the theoretical volume of 180 mL.

Labeling

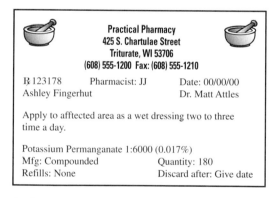

Auxiliary Labels: For External Use Only;
Keep out of the reach of children

Patient Consultation

Hello, Ms. Fingerhut, I'm your pharmacist, Jack Jones. Are you allergic to any drugs? Are you taking or using any prescription or nonprescription medications? What did your physician tell you about this prescription? This product is usually used as an antibacterial or antifungal agent. Apply sterile gauze to the affected areas and carefully pour this solution on the gauze and let it soak as directed. Do this 2 or 3 times a day. If the condition worsens, or doesn't improve, discontinue use and contact your physician. Keep this out of reach of children. This product will stain clothing, sheets, and so on, so be careful. Any unused portion should be discarded after 1 week (give date), or if the product turns brown. Dr. Attles has not authorized refills. Did he tell you how long to continue therapy? This solution should be stored at room temperature, away from light. Do you have any questions?

➤ **Prescription 26.2**

Contemporary Physicians Group Practice
20 S. Park Street, Triturate, WI 53706
Tel: (608) 555-1333 Fax: (608) 555-1335

R # 182

Name *Fred Flynn Stone*   Date *00/00/00*

Address *983 Bronto Lane*   Age *72 y.o.* Wt/Ht

R

> *Potassium Gluconate* ~~*10 mEq/5 mL*~~ *Change to 10 mEq/15 mL*
>
> *M & Ft. Flavored Sugar-free syrup*
>
> *Dispense* ~~*120 mL*~~ *Change to 360 mL*
>
> *Change to 45 mL*
> *Sig:* ~~*15 mL*~~ *bid in juice or water*

Per consult with with Dr. Behling, changed concentration, dose volume, and dispensed volume because of solubility issues.   *J. Juarez 00/00/00*

Refills 5   *F. Behling*   M.D.

DEA No. _____

Ingredients Used

Ingredient	Quantity Used	Manufacturer Lot #-Exp Date	Solubility	Dose Comparison Given	Dose Comparison Usual	Use in the Prescription
Potassium Gluconate	56.16 g	JET Labs SN2621-mm/yy	1 g/3 mL water prac insol in alcohol	30 mEq bid	20–80 mEq per day	potassium supplement
Grape Flavor	10 drops	JET Labs SV2622-mm/yy	miscible	—	—	flavor
Sodium Saccharin	30 mg	JET Labs SN2623-mm/yy	fr sol in water sp sol in alcohol	—	—	sweetener
Paraben-Propylene Glycol Stock Solution	7.2 mL	Prac. Pharm. JT6814-mm/yy	miscible	0.18% MP 0.02% PP 2% Pr Gly	0.18% MP 0.02% PP 2% Pr Gly	Preservative System
Sodium Carboxymethyl-cellulose Solution 1%	q.s. 360 mL	Prac. Pharm. JT6803-mm/yy	miscible	—	—	vehicle
Purified Water	170 mL	Sweet Springs AL0529-mm/yy	—	—	—	vehicle

Note: MP = Methylparaben; PP = Propylparaben; Pr Gly = Propylene Glycol

Compatibility–Stability/Beyond-Use Date

Stability–Compatibility: Before compounding this prescription, Pharmacist Juarez checked the solubility of the Potassium Gluconate at the concentration prescribed and found that it was not sufficiently soluble. It is necessary to change the volumes of the solution (see calculations below). This means that both the total volume and dose volume must be changed; the final strength will be 10 mEq per 15 mL, rather than per 5 mL. The dose volume will become 45 mL instead of 15 mL, and the total volume dispensed will be 360 mL so the same number of doses will be dispensed.

With regard to chemical stability, Potassium Gluconate is very stable; there are numerous official USP solution and elixir monographs for Potassium Gluconate (9).

For the sugar-free syrup, Methylcellulose 1% gel would be a preferred vehicle, but this gum is incompatible with the high electrolyte content of the Potassium Gluconate solution. Sodium Carboxymethylcellulose (CMC) is more stable to concentrated salts solutions, so a 1% gel of medium viscosity CMC, flavored with grape concentrate and sweetened with Sodium Saccharin, is the selected vehicle.

Preservative: Pharmacist Juarez realizes that Sodium Benzoate and Potassium Sorbate are not effective preservatives at the alkaline pH of this solution. She will use the paraben stock preservative solution described in Chapter 15, which contains 9% Methylparaben and 1% Propylparaben in Propylene Glycol. At a concentration of 2 mL of the stock solution per 100 mL of preparation solution, it provides Methylparaben 0.18%, Propylparaben 0.02%, and Propylene Glycol 2%.

Packaging and Storage and Beyond-use date: The *USP* monographs for similar preparations recommend storage in tight containers (9). Although manufactured versions of this formulation are given expiration dates of several years, Pharmacist Juarez will use a more conservative 30-day beyond-use date as recommended in *USP* Chapter ⟨795⟩ for "other formulations" (8) and will label the product to be stored in the refrigerator.

Calculations

Dose/Concentration

Dose of 60 mEq/day is within the usual adult prescribing limits as given in the *USP DI*, but potassium blood levels should be monitored.

Ingredient Amounts

Grams of Potassium Gluconate required for this preparation:

(K Gluconate MW = 234, 1 mEq/mmol)

$$\left(\frac{234\ mg\ KGluc}{mmol\ KGluc}\right)\left(\frac{mmol\ KGluc}{1\ mEq\ K^+}\right)\left(\frac{10\ mEq\ K^+}{5\ mL}\right)\left(\frac{120\ mL}{}\right) = 56160\ mg = 56.16\ g\ KGluc$$

The solubility of Potassium Gluconate is 1 g/3 mL of water. To dissolve the needed 56.16 g of K Gluconate, the amount of Purified Water can be calculated:

$$\frac{1\ g\ KGluc}{3\ mL\ water} = \frac{56.16\ g\ KGluc}{x\ mL\ water}; x = 168\ mL\ water—too\ much\ water$$

If we multiply all the volumes by three, the drug is sufficiently soluble. In this case, the new dose volume is 15 mL (10 mEq/15 mL) and the dispensing volume is 360 mL. The prescriber must be called and the patient advised of the change.

The prescription content should be labeled both in terms of mEq/dose and grams or milligrams of the salt per dose. It can be observed that with a molecular weight of 234 mg/mmol, a 1 mEq/mmol equivalence, and 10 mEq/dose, each dose will contain 2,340 mg or 2.34 g per 15-mL dose.

Volume of paraben stock solution:

The paraben–propylene glycol stock solution that is described in Chapter 15 will be used as the preservative system. This solution contains 9% Methylparaben and 1% Propylparaben in Propylene Glycol. If 2 mL of the stock solution is added per 100 mL of preparation solution, the final concentrations provided are Methylparaben 0.18%, Propylparaben 0.02%, and Propylene Glycol 2%. Calculate the volume of the stock solution needed for this preparation:

2 mL stock solution/100 mL preparation × 360 mL preparation = 7.2 mL stock solution

Compounding Procedure

On a class 3 torsion or electronic digital balance, weigh 56.16 g of Potassium Gluconate and put in a clean 400-mL beaker. Add 168 to 170 mL Purified Water and stir to dissolve. With stirring, add 120 to 150 mL of Sodium Carboxymethylcellulose (CMC) 1% solution, 7.2 mL of the paraben stock solution, 30 mg of Sodium Saccharin, and 10 drops of grape flavoring concentrate. (Any flavor is acceptable; however, if the flavor concentrate is an oil, a small amount of alcohol should be added to render it water-miscible.) Transfer the solution from the beaker into a precalibrated 360-mL or 12-oz prescription bottle (if not available, use a pint bottle), and q.s. to the 360-mL mark with the Sodium CMC 1% solution. Agitate well to mix, label, and dispense.

Quality Control

The preparation is a clear, colorless viscous solution. The pH of the preparation is checked and recorded; pH = 7.5. The actual volume is checked and matches the theoretical volume of 360 mL.

Labeling

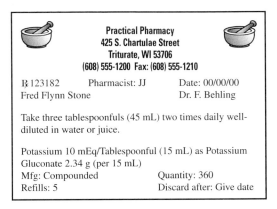

Practical Pharmacy
425 S. Chartulae Street
Triturate, WI 53706
(608) 555-1200 Fax: (608) 555-1210

R 123182   Pharmacist: JJ   Date: 00/00/00
Fred Flynn Stone   Dr. F. Behling

Take three tablespoonfuls (45 mL) two times daily well-diluted in water or juice.

Potassium 10 mEq/Tablespoonful (15 mL) as Potassium Gluconate 2.34 g (per 15 mL)

Mfg: Compounded   Quantity: 360
Refills: 5   Discard after: Give date

Auxiliary Labels: Keep in the Refrigerator

Patient Consultation

Hello, Mr. Stone, I'm your pharmacist, Juanita Juarez. Do you have any drug allergies? Are you taking any other medications? What did your doctor tell you about this medication? This is a potassium supplement that is used to keep your electrolytes in balance. You are to take three tablespoonfuls (**not 3 teaspoonfuls,** as Dr. Behling may have said; we had to make an adjustment because of some formulation issues) twice a day in juice or water. It is very important that you dilute this adequately so as to improve its taste and to avoid any stomach problems. To minimize any stomach upset, take it with food or after meals. Other side effects include light-headedness, weakness, or irregular heartbeat. If any of these occur, contact Dr. Behling immediately. When did your doctor tell you to have your electrolytes checked? This is very important. Be sure to store this in a refrigerator, out of the reach of children, and discard any unused portion after 30 days. Check the solution in the bottle when you take a dose; if you notice that any of the drug has formed crystals in the solution, bring the bottle back into the pharmacy so that we can make some adjustments in the formulation; that won't cost you anything extra, so don't hesitate to do that. Dr. Behling has authorized five refills. Do you have any questions?

➤ **Prescription 26.3**

```
┌─────────────────────────────────────────────────────────────────────┐
│                  Contemporary Physicians Group Practice               │
│                  20 S. Park Street, Triturate, WI 53706               │
│                  Tel: (608) 555-1333  Fax: (608) 555-1335             │
│                                                    ℞ #  721           │
│  ──────────────────────────────────────────────────────────────────  │
│  Name  Chelsea Liegel                        Date  00/00/00           │
│  ──────────────────────────────────────────────────────────────────  │
│  Address  1290 Hoopster Lane              Age          Wt/Ht          │
│  ──────────────────────────────────────────────────────────────────  │
│   ℞                                                                    │
│                    Hydrochloric Acid    2.5%                          │
│                                                                       │
│                    Dispense 30 mL                                     │
│                                                                       │
│         Sig:    Add one teaspoonful to 4 oz of fruit juice and sip    │
│                    through a straw. Take with each meal.              │
│                                                                       │
│                                      J. Jackson 00/00/00              │
│                                                                       │
│   Refills   1                    P. V. Heider              M.D.       │
│                                                                       │
│                          DEA No.  _____                 │
└─────────────────────────────────────────────────────────────────────┘
```

Ingredients Used

Ingredient	Quantity Used	Manufacturer Lot #-Exp Date	Solubility	Dose Comparison Given	Dose Comparison Usual	Use in the Prescription
Hydrochloric Acid NF 37% w/w	1.72mL	JET Labs SN2631-mm/yy	miscible with water and alcohol	5 mL of 2.5% or 0.125 g	1–10 mL of 10% or 0.1–1 g	digestion; Vit. B-12 absorption
Purified Water	q.s.30 mL	Sweet Springs AL0529-mm/yy	—	—	—	vehicle

Compatibility–Stability/Beyond-Use Date

Stability–Compatibility: This preparation is very similar to an official formulation, Diluted Hydrochloric Acid NF, which is known to be very stable (9).

Preservative: No additional preservative is needed because Hydrochloric Acid has a pH unfavorable to microbial growth.

Packaging and Storage and Beyond-use date: The *NF* monograph for Diluted Hydrochloric Acid recommends storage in tight containers (9). Although this preparation is known to be very stable, Pharmacist Jackson will use a conservative 6-month beyond-use date for this compounded preparation. It may be stored either in the refrigerator or at room temperature.

Calculations

Dose/Concentration

The interpretation of the 2.5% should be checked with the prescriber. It could be interpreted as % v/v of the concentrated acid in water (that is, 2.5 mL of Hydrochloric Acid NF with sufficient water to give 100 mL of solution) or as % w/v of the pure HCl in water. This order was done using the % w/v interpretation.

Hydrochloric Acid NF is 37% w/w HCl specific gravity = 1.18 MW = 36.5

Number of grams of HCl: $2.5\% \times 30\ mL = 0.75\ g\ HCl$

Number of mL of Hydrochloric Acid NF:

$$\left(\frac{mL\ HCl\ NF}{1.8\ g\ HCl\ NF}\right)\left(\frac{100\ g\ HCl\ NF}{37\ g\ HCl}\right)\left(\frac{0.75\ g\ HCl}{}\right) = 1.72\ mL\ HCl$$

If using a 10-mL graduated cylinder to measure this, the amount is below the MMQ and a liquid-liquid aliquot is needed. For example, if a multiple factor of two is used, measure *2 × 1.72 mL = 3.4 mL.* Dilute this by adding it to a small amount of water (always add concentrated acids **to** water); then q.s. to a convenient volume (e.g., 10 mL) and take half of this (e.g., 5 mL). An easier method would be to use a 3-mL syringe and measure the 1.72 mL directly.

Sometimes Hydrochloric Acid is prescribed by normality. Below are the calculations to find the normality of this solution:

$$\left(\frac{1\ eq\ HCl}{mol\ HCl}\right)\left(\frac{mol\ HCl}{36.5\ g\ HCl}\right)\left(\frac{2.5\ g\ HCl}{100\ mL}\right)\left(\frac{1000\ mL}{L}\right) = 0.68\ eq\ /\ L = 0.68\ N$$

Compounding Procedure

Use safety glasses when handling acid!

Pour approximately 15 mL of Purified Water into a 1-oz prescription bottle with a child-resistant closure. Measure 1.7 mL of Hydrochloric Acid NF (37% w/w) using a 3-mL syringe. Carefully transfer the HCl to the prescription bottle and q.s. to the 30-mL calibration mark with Purified Water. Agitate the bottle to ensure a homogeneous solution. Label and dispense.

Quality Control

The preparation is a clear, colorless solution with apparent viscosity approximately that of water. The pH of the preparation is checked with pH paper with a 0–14 range; the value shown is pH = 0, but since this is the end of the range, the pH is recorded as less than or equal to 0. The actual volume is checked and matches the theoretical volume of 30 mL.

Labeling

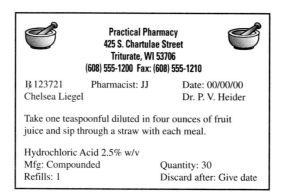

Practical Pharmacy
425 S. Chartulae Street
Triturate, WI 53706
(608) 555-1200 Fax: (608) 555-1210

℞ 123721   Pharmacist: JJ   Date: 00/00/00
Chelsea Liegel   Dr. P. V. Heider

Take one teaspoonful diluted in four ounces of fruit
juice and sip through a straw with each meal.

Hydrochloric Acid 2.5% w/v
Mfg: Compounded   Quantity: 30
Refills: 1   Discard after: Give date

Auxiliary Labels: Keep out of the reach of children

Patient Consultation

Hello, Miss Liegel, I'm Joe Jackson, your pharmacist. Are you allergic to any drugs? Are you currently taking any other medications? Do you know, or did your Dr. Heider tell you, what this medicine is for? This is a dilute acid to aid with problems of digestion and absorption of vitamin B_{12}. It is very important that you dilute this well before taking it. Never take it directly from the bottle without diluting it first. Measure one teaspoonful and put it in 4 ounces of fruit juice, then sip the solution through a straw. Do this at each meal. Never use less than 4 ounces of juice to dilute this. Try to avoid getting this solution on your teeth, because this may etch enamel. Don't take with antacids because they will neutralize the effect of this medication. If your symptoms persist, contact your physician. Discard any unused contents after 6 months. Store at room temperature, out of the reach of children. Do you have any questions?

► **Prescription 26.4**

Contemporary Veterinarian Group Practice
22 S. Park Street, Triturate, WI 53706
Tel: (608) 555-1334 Fax: (608) 555-1336

R # 780

Name   *Pam Perfect*   Date   *00/00/00*

Address   *285 Polly Point*   Age   Wt/Ht

R

Podophyllum	*12%*
Salicylic Acid	~~*25%*~~ ***Changed to 15%***
Compound Benzoin Tincture	*q s ad 7.5 mL*

   Sig: *Apply to warts q hs*

Changed concentration of Salicylic Acid to 15% in consultation with
Dr. Parker because of insufficient solubility of 25%. Billie Burke 00/00/00

Refills   *1*   *J. L. Parker*   D.V.M.

                          DEA No. _____

Ingredients Used

Ingredient	Quantity Used	Manufacturer Lot #-Exp Date	Solubility	Dose Comparison Given	Usual	Use in the Prescription
Salicylic Acid	1.125 g	JET Labs SN2641-mm/yy	1 g/3 mL alcohol 1 g/460 mL water	15% (changed from 25%)	2–60%	keratolytic
Podophyllum	0.9 g	JET Labs SN2642-mm/yy	sol in alcohol insol in water	12%	12–25%	caustic for warts
Compound Benzoin Tincture	q.s. 7.5 mL	JET Labs SN2643-mm/yy	miscible with alcohol immis with water	—	—	vehicle, demulcent

Compatibility–Stability/Beyond-Use Date

Stability–Compatibility: With regard to chemical stability, all ingredients in this preparation are known to be very stable in this alcohol medium. Podophyllum Resin Topical Solution is an official USP formulation that contains Podophyllum Resin in an alcoholic extract of Benzoin. Compound Benzoin Tincture is also an official USP preparation.

With regard to physical properties, Pharmacist Burke checked the prescribed concentrations of Salicylic Acid and Podophyllum against their solubility in an alcoholic medium such as Compound Benzoin Tincture and determined that the content of Salicylic Acid would have to be lowered because of inadequate solubility. The supporting calculations are shown below.

Preservative: No added preservative is needed due to the high alcoholic content of the preparation and the presence of ingredients that are toxic to microbes.

Packaging and Storage and Beyond-use date: The *USP* monographs for similar preparations recommend storage in tight, light-resistant containers (9). Although this formulation is quite stable, it does contain a volatile solvent with concentration of ingredients near the saturation point. Pharmacist Burke will use a 1-month beyond-use date for this compounded preparation. Storage should be at room temperature.

Calculations

Dose/Concentration

Podophyllum is used in a concentration range of 12–25%—OK

Salicylic Acid is used in a range of 2–60%—OK

Ingredient Amounts

Podophyllum: *12% × 7.5 mL = 0.12 × 7.5 mL = 0.9 g*

Salicylic Acid: *25% × 7.5 mL = 0.25 × 7.5 mL = 1.875 g*

Solubility:

The solvent here is Compound Benzoin Tincture (Compd. Tr. Benzoin), which is 74–80% alcohol. The number of milliliters of alcohol available for dissolving the Podophyllum and Salicylic Acid depends on the final volume of Compd. Tr. Benzoin in the product. Because the tincture is used to q.s. ad 7.5 mL and the powder volume of the Podophyllum and Salicylic Acid is unknown, the volume of Compd. Tr. Benzoin can only be estimated. If we assume a powder volume of 2 mL for the 2.775 g (0.9 + 1.875) of powder, the amount of Compd. Benzoin Tr. would be *7.5 mL—2 mL* = 5.5 mL. The amount of alcohol available for dissolution would be approximately *77% × 5.5 mL = 4.23 mL.*

   Podophyllum: Although Podophyllum is listed as soluble in alcohol (1 g/10–30 mL), it should be satisfactory at the 12% concentration because its usual recommended concentration in alcoholic vehicles is 12–25%. In this preparation, the high concentration of Salicylic Acid may tie up solvent and limit the amount of alcohol available for dissolving the Podophyllum.

   Salicylic Acid: The solubility of Salicylic Acid in alcohol is given as 1 g/3 mL. In this prescription, we have 1.875 g Salicylic Acid, so we need *1.875 g × 3 mL/g = 5.63 mL* of alcohol. Because we have only about 4.23 mL of alcohol in this preparation, we have too little to dissolve the Salicylic Acid. If the Salicylic Acid concentration is changed to 15%, then we would reduce the amount of Salicylic Acid to *0.15 × 7.5 = 1.125 g* and we would then need only *1.125 g × 3 mL/g = 3.375 mL* of alcohol for dissolution. Because this concentration is still in the therapeutically effective range for Salicylic Acid, it would be acceptable to request a change of concentration of Salicylic Acid to 15%. Because the above is based on estimates, the product should be observed for proper dissolution.

Compounding Procedure

Note: It is advisable to use a face mask when preparing this preparation, as the Salicylic Acid and the Podophyllin are highly irritant powders that should not be inhaled. The *USP* also warns that Podophyllum Resin is highly irritating to the eye and mucous membranes (9).

   On a class 3 or an electronic balance, weigh 1.125 g Salicylic Acid and place in a small clean beaker. Add about 4.5 mL of Compound Benzoin Tincture to dissolve the Salicylic Acid. Weigh 0.9 g of Podophyllum and dust it on top of the solution in the beaker and stir gently. Repeat until all is dissolved. Premark an applicator bottle at 7.5 mL, using alcohol as the calibration liquid (water is incompatible with this preparation). Transfer the prepared solution to the bottle and q.s. to the final volume with Compound Benzoin Tincture. Use some of this Compound Benzoin Tincture to rinse the beaker into the applicator bottle to effect a complete transfer of active ingredients. Place the applicator cap on the bottle and close tightly. Agitate the solution to ensure complete mixing. Label and dispense.

Quality Control

The preparation is a dark-brown viscous solution. It has the characteristic odor of Compound Benzoin Tincture. The actual volume is checked and matches the theoretical volume of 7.5 mL.

Labeling

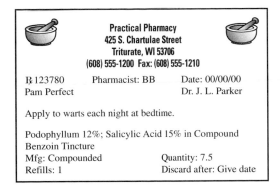

> **Practical Pharmacy**
> **425 S. Chartulae Street**
> **Triturate, WI 53706**
> **(608) 555-1200 Fax: (608) 555-1210**
>
> ℞ 123780   Pharmacist: BB   Date: 00/00/00
> Pam Perfect   Dr. J. L. Parker
>
> Apply to warts each night at bedtime.
>
> Podophyllum 12%; Salicylic Acid 15% in Compound
> Benzoin Tincture
> Mfg: Compounded   Quantity: 7.5
> Refills: 1   Discard after: Give date

Auxiliary Labels: Caution: Flammable; For External Use Only
Keep out of the reach of children

Patient Consultation

Hello, Ms. Perfect, I'm your pharmacist, Billie Burke. Do you have any drug allergies? Are you taking or using any prescription or over-the-counter medications? This medication is to treat your warts. Apply it each night at bedtime, using the applicator provided in the bottle and being careful not to get this near your eyes or mouth. You may want to cover the skin surrounding the wart with Vaseline® for protection of the healthy skin. Be sure to wash your hands carefully after handling this solution, as it is very irritating to healthy skin. If the treated area becomes irritated or the condition worsens, discontinue use and contact your physician. Store at room temperature, away from heat, and out of reach of children. It is a flammable liquid that should be kept away from any open flame, lighted smoking materials, or anything else that may ignite it. Discard any unused portion after 1 month. You may get one refill. Do you have any questions?

➤ Prescription 26.5

Contemporary Physicians Group Practice
20 S. Park Street, Triturate, WI 53706
Tel: (608) 555-1333 Fax: (608) 555-1335

℞ # 772

Name   *Ronnie Snax*   Date   *00/00/00*

Address   *425 Instinct Lane*   Age   *32*   Wt/Ht

℞

Benzocaine	*3%*
Benzethonium Chloride	*0.1%*
Alcohol	*qs*
Methyl Salicylate	*qs*
Purified Water	*qs ad* *30 mL*

Fernie Bohunting
00/00/00

Sig: Apply bid prn ut dict

Refills   2   *Roberta Barksen*   M.D.

DEA No. _____

Ingredients Used

Ingredient	Quantity Used	Manufacturer Lot #-Exp Date	Solubility	Dose Comparison		Use in the Prescription
				Given	Usual	
Benzocaine	900 mg	JET Labs SN2651-mm/yy	1 g/2500 mL water or 5 mL alcohol	3%	1–20%	local anesthetic
Benzethonium Chloride	120 mg weighed, 30 mg used	JET Labs SV2652-mm/yy	v sol in water sol in alcohol	0.1%	0.1%	antimicobial, antiseptic
Alcohol	22 mL	JET Labs SN2653-mm/yy	miscible with water	—	—	solvent, preservative
Methyl Salicylate	5 drops	JET Labs SN2654-mm/yy	sl sol in water sol in alcohol	—	—	scent
Purified Water	q.s. 30 mL	Sweet Springs AL0529-mm/yy	—	—	—	vehicle

Compatibility–Stability/Beyond-Use Date

Stability–Compatibility: The Benzethonium Chloride, Alcohol, and Methyl Salicylate in this preparation are compatible and very stable when in a hydroalcoholic solution. In an aqueous solution, the Benzocaine presents some concerns for both physical compatibility and chemical stability.

With regard to physical compatibility, Benzocaine is quite insoluble in water and a cosolvent system containing alcohol is required for dissolution. Calculations for the relative amounts of water and alcohol are shown below.

With regard to chemical stability, Benzocaine is an ester that undergoes hydrolysis in aqueous solution. Pharmacist Bohunting found information on the stability of Benzocaine in the reference *Chemical Stability of Pharmaceuticals* (10). Benzocaine undergoes both acid- and base-catalyzed hydrolysis, and it is most stable at neutral pH. The half-life at pH 9 and 30°C is 127 days. This translates to a shelf-life under those conditions of about 19 days. This preparation has a neutral pH, so this would provide more stable conditions.

Preservative: No extra preservative is needed because Benzethonium Cl is an antimicrobial agent. In addition, the alcohol content is 70%.

Packaging and Storage and Beyond-use date: This preparation should be stored in a tight container. Using the literature cited above as a guide, Pharmacist Bohunting will use a 14-day beyond-use date for this preparation. Because this is a topical preparation, controlled room temperature will be the recommended storage conditions.

Calculations:

Dose/Concentration

The concentrations are OK for the intended use.

Ingredient Amounts

Benzocaine: *3% × 30 mL = 0.9 g*

Benzethonium Cl: *0.1% × 30 mL = 0.03 g = 30 mg*

The 30 mg of Benzethonium Cl is below the MWQ, so an aliquot is needed. A solid–liquid aliquot would be the most convenient. If we weigh the MWQ of 120 mg of Benzethonium Cl and dissolve it in 4 mL water, we get a solution of 120 mg/4 mL = 30 mg/mL. One mL of this measured with a 1-mL syringe will be the amount needed.

Benzocaine has very limited solubility in water (1 g/2,500 mL), but it is very soluble in Alcohol (1 g/5 mL). Therefore, a cosolvent system is needed and the alcohol content can be calculated using the log Solubility equation given in this chapter and shown here:

log Solubility equation: $\log S_T = vf_{water} \log S_{water} + vf_{alc} \log S_{alc}$

To use this equation, all concentrations must be expressed using the same units.

Total required solution concentration (S_T) of Benzocaine in mg/mL:

$3\% = 3\ g/100\ mL = 3,000\ mg/100\ mL = 30\ mg/mL$

Water solubility (S_{water}) of Benzocaine in mg/mL:

$1\ g/2,500\ mL = 1,000\ mg/2,500\ mL = 0.4\ mg/mL$

Alcohol solubility (S_{alc}))of Benzocaine in mg/mL:

$1\ g/5\ mL = 1,000\ mg/5\ mL = 200\ mg/mL$

The sum of the volume fractions is 1: $vf_{water} + vf_{alc} = 1$

   Therefore: $vf_{water} = 1 - vf_{alc}$

Substituting: $log\ 30 = (1 - vf_{alc})\ log\ 0.4 + vf_{alc}\ log\ 200$

Solving for the volume fraction of alcohol (vf_{alc}) :
$log\ 30 = log\ 0.4 - vf_{alc}\ log\ 0.4 + vf_{alc}\ log\ 200$
$log\ 30 - log\ 0.4 = vf_{alc}\ log\ 200 - vf_{alc}\ log\ 0.4 = vf_{alc}\ (log\ 200 - log\ 0.4)$

$$f_{alc} = \frac{(log\,30 - log\,0.4)}{(log\,200 - log\,0.4)} = \frac{1.87506}{2.69897} = 69.5\% \approx 70\%$$

Based on an alcohol-water cosolvent system with 70% alcohol, we can calculate the volume of ethyl alcohol (C_2H_5OH) needed for our preparation: $70\% \times 30\ mL = 21\ mL$. Using Alcohol USP 95%, we can calculate the number of milliliters of this cosolvent needed:

$$\frac{21\ mL\ C_2H_5OH}{x\ mL\ Alcohol\ USP} = \frac{95\ mL\ C_2H_5OH}{100\ mL\ Alcohol\ USP}; x = 22\ mL\ Alcohol\ USP$$

Compounding Procedure

All weighing is done on a class 3 torsion or electronic balance. Weigh 900 mg of Benzocaine and transfer to a clean beaker. Measure 22 mL of Alcohol USP in a 25-mL graduated cylinder and add to the Benzocaine to dissolve it. Weigh 120 mg of Benzethonium Chloride and dissolve this in 4 mL of Purified Water, which has been measured in a 10-mL graduated cylinder. With a 1-mL disposable syringe, measure 1 mL of the Benzethonium Chloride solution and add this to the Benzocaine solution. Add 5 drops of Methyl Salicylate and transfer the solution to a 50-mL graduated cylinder and q.s. to the 30-mL mark using Purified Water. Pour this solution into a 1-oz dauber bottle, label, and dispense.

Quality Control

The preparation is a clear, colorless solution with apparent viscosity approximately that of Alcohol. It has the characteristic odor of Alcohol. The pH of the preparation is checked and recorded as pH = 5.5. The actual volume is checked and matches the theoretical volume of 30 mL

Labeling

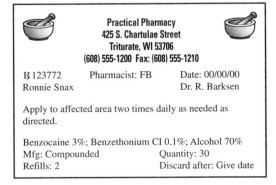

Auxiliary Labels: Caution: Flammable; For External Use Only
Keep out of the reach of children

Patient Consultation

Hello, Mr. Snax, I'm Pharmacist Fernie Bohunting. I have your prescription for your skin irritation ready. Are you taking or using any other prescription or nonprescription medications currently? Do you have any allergies? What did Dr. Barksen tell you about this medication? You are to dab this on the affected area of your skin two times daily as needed and directed by Dr. Barksen. It should give you relief from the itching, but if your skin condition does not improve or gets worse, discontinue using this solution and contact Dr. Barksen so we can try something else. Store this at room temperature and away from sunlight. This is for external use only and should be kept out of the reach of children. It does contain a fairly large percentage of alcohol, so be careful not to get it near your eyes and wash your hands after applying it. It is a flammable liquid that should be kept away from any open flame, lighted smoking materials, or anything else that may ignite it. Discard any unused portion after 2 weeks (give date). If needed, you may have this refilled two times. Do you have any questions?

► **Prescription 26.6**

Contemporary Physicians Group Practice
20 S. Park Street, Triturate, WI 53706
Tel: (608) 555-1333 Fax: (608) 555-1335

R # 756

| Name *Lilly La Lane* | Date *00/00/00* |

| Address *592 Pirate Cove Apts.* | Age *16 y.o.* Wt/Ht |

R

Clindamycin HCl	*1%*
Propylene Glycol	*1.5 mL*
Isopropyl Alcohol 50%	
Purified Water	*aa qs ad* *15 mL*

B. Bilder 00/00/00

Sig: Apply as directed to acne q am and hs

Refills   3   *Ozzie Wurtz*   M.D.

DEA No. _____

Ingredients Used

Ingredient	Quantity Used	Manufacturer Lot #-Exp Date	Solubility	Dose Comparison Given	Usual	Use in the Prescription
Clindamycin HCl as 150 mg capsules	150 mg (1 capsule)	JET Labs SN2661-mm/yy	freely sol in water and alcohol	1%	1%	antibiotic
Propylene Glycol	1.5 mL	JET Labs SV2662-mm/yy	miscible with water and alcohol	10%	varies	solvent, humectant, antiseptic
Isopropyl Alcohol (IPA) 70%	7.1 mL to make 10 mL 50% IPA	JET Labs SN2663-mm/yy	miscible with water	22.5%	varies	solvent, antiseptic
Purified Water	q.s. 15 mL	Sweet Springs AL0529-mm/yy	—	—	—	vehicle

Compatibility–Stability/Beyond-Use Date

Stability–Compatibility: With regard to chemical stability, topical Clindamycin solutions in this type of solvent system have been evaluated and reported in the literature. A good review of this subject can be found in the Clindamycin monograph in *Trissel's Stability of Compounded Formulations*. At 25°C these formulations were stable for at least 6 months, but a 6- to 8-week beyond-use date was recommended (11).

With regard to solubility and physical stability, Clindamycin HCl is freely soluble (1 g/1–10 mL) in water and soluble (1 g/10–30 mL) in alcohol. This means that the 0.15 g of Clindamycin HCl in this product should dissolve in 0.15–1.5 mL water or 1.5–4.5 mL of alcohol. This information is important because capsule contents are being used for this product, and there may be insoluble materials in the capsule contents. If a solution is to be made, the preparation should be filtered. Although we want to filter out the inert ingredients, we don't want to filter any drug. Therefore, we want to be certain to dissolve all the drug from the capsule contents. To ensure complete dissolution of this large molecule, it is recommended that the capsule contents be put in a sufficient amount of the solvent system (approximately 30 mL for 4 capsules) and the liquid shaken for 30-second time intervals and repeated several times over a 10- to 15-minute period before filtering out the excipients. Additional solvent is then added to the remaining solids and the process repeated, rinsing this portion through the same filter (11).

Preservative: No additional preservative is needed for this preparation because the formula contains the antibacterial Clindamycin and 23% Isopropyl Alcohol.

Packaging and Storage and Beyond-use date: Because the *USP* monographs for Clindamycin solutions recommend storage in tight containers, this would be recommended for this preparation (9). Using the literature cited above as a guide, Pharmacist Bilder will use a 1-month beyond-use date for this preparation.

Calculations

Dose/Concentration

Clindamycin: 1% concentration of Clindamycin is appropriate for the intended use.

Propylene Glycol (PG): % v/v concentration is calculated to be:

$$\frac{1.5\ mL\ PG}{15\ mL\ solution} = \frac{x\ mL\ PG}{100\ mL\ solution}; x = 10\ mL\ PG\,/\,100\ mL\ solution = 10\%$$

Isopropyl Alcohol (IPA): % v/v concentration is calculated here.

Assuming a zero powder volume for the Clindamycin and additive volumes for the liquids, the volume of the 1:1 mixture of Water and 50% IPA in the final solution is:

$$\frac{(15\ mL - 1.5\ mL)}{2} = \frac{13.5\ mL}{2} = 6.75\ mL$$

The amount of pure IPA in 6.75 mL of 50% IPA is: *50% × 6.75 mL = 3.38 mL*
The %v/v IPA in the finished product is:

$$\frac{3.38\ mL\ IPA}{15\ mL\ solution} = \frac{x\ mL\ IPA}{100\ mL\ solution}; x = 22.5\ mL\ IPA\,/\,100\ mL\ solution = 22.5\% \approx 23\%$$

Ingredient Amounts

Clindamycin HCl: *1% × 15 mL = 0.150 g Clindamycin HCl (Contents of one capsule)*

50% Isopropyl Alcohol (IPA): Need to make this from the 70% IPA available in the pharmacy. The amount made may be any reasonable amount that is greater than or equal to the amount actually needed in the product, which is calculated above to be 6.75 mL. It is decided that 10 mL of a 50% solution will be made. The amount of pure IPA needed is:

50% × 10 mL = 5 mL

The volume of 70% IPA to give 5 mL of IPA is:

$$\frac{70 \; mL \; IPA}{100 \; mL \; of \; 70\% \; solution} = \frac{5 \; mL \; IPA}{x \; mL \; of \; 70\% \; solution}; x = 7.1 \; mL \; of \; 70\% \; solution$$

Measure 7.1 mL of 70% IPA and q.s. to 10 mL with Purified Water

Compounding Procedure

Make 10 mL (see calculations above) of 50% IPA by measuring 7.1 mL of 70% IPA and q.s. ad. 10 mL with Purified Water. Add 10 mL of Purified Water to this to make a 50/50 solution of Purified Water and 50% IPA. Empty the contents of one Clindamycin 150-mg capsule into a beaker and add 7 mL of the 50/50 solvent mixture to dissolve the drug. Allow it to dissolve with intermittent stirring over 10 to 15 minutes. Filter this solution into a 25-mL graduated cylinder or a graduated prescription bottle. Add the 1.5 mL of Propylene Glycol to the drug solution. Using another 7-mL portion of the 50/50 solvent mixture. rinse the beaker and filter into the drug solution to ensure complete transfer of the drug. Then q.s. to 15 mL with the 50/50 mixture of Purified Water and 50% IPA. If the final solution was made in a graduated cylinder, transfer the solution to a prescription bottle or, if available, a dauber bottle. Agitate the solution to ensure homogeneity. Label and dispense.

Quality Control

The preparation is a clear, colorless solution with apparent viscosity approximately that of a water–alcohol solution. It has the characteristic odor of Isopropyl Alcohol. The pH of the preparation is checked and recorded as pH = 5.5. The actual volume is checked and matches the theoretical volume of 15 mL.

Labeling

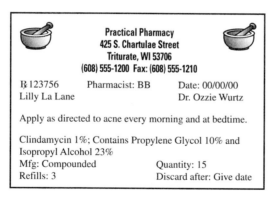

Practical Pharmacy
425 S. Chartulae Street
Triturate, WI 53706
(608) 555-1200 Fax: (608) 555-1210

℞ 123756   Pharmacist: BB   Date: 00/00/00
Lilly La Lane   Dr. Ozzie Wurtz

Apply as directed to acne every morning and at bedtime.

Clindamycin 1%; Contains Propylene Glycol 10% and
Isopropyl Alcohol 23%
Mfg: Compounded   Quantity: 15
Refills: 3   Discard after: Give date

Auxiliary Labels: For External Use only.

Patient Consultation

Hello, Ms. La Lane, I'm your pharmacist, Becky Bilder. Do you have any drug allergies? Are you taking any prescription or over-the-counter medications? This is to treat your acne. Apply to the acne every morning and every evening at bedtime. Wash and rinse the area carefully before applying. Apply to entire area, not just to pimples. (If dispensed in a dauber bottle, show how to use. If dispensed in a prescription bottle, instruct how to apply with a pledget of cotton.) This solution contains alcohol, so keep it away from your eyes or other sensitive parts, and wash your hands after applying the solution. Because it is a flammable liquid, it should be kept away from any open flame, lighted smoking materials, or anything else that may ignite it. If your skin condition does not improve or worsens, contact your doctor. This preparation is for external use only and should be stored at room temperature, out of the reach of children. You may have three refills. Discard any unused portion after 1 month or 25% rule (give date). Do you have any questions?

➤ **Prescription 26.7**

```
┌─────────────────────────────────────────────────────────────┐
│              Contemporary Physicians Group Practice           │
│              20 S. Park Street, Triturate, WI 53706           │
│              Tel: (608) 555-1333  Fax: (608) 555-1335         │
│                                          R # 745              │
├─────────────────────────────────────────────────────────────┤
│  Name  Lindy Infamous            Date  00/00/00              │
├─────────────────────────────────────────────────────────────┤
│  Address  689 Lombardi Blvd.         Age    62 yr   Wt/Ht    │
├─────────────────────────────────────────────────────────────┤
│   R                                                          │
│           Acetic Acid              5%                         │
│           Lactic Acid                                         │
│           Salicylic Acid       │      aa  10%                 │
│           Flexible Collodion   q s ad  30 mL                 │
│                                                              │
│                                    B. Block  00/00/00        │
│        Sig:   Apply to affected area on toe q hs x 1 wk      │
│                                                              │
│   Refills   1                     Ralph Nock          M.D.   │
│                          DEA No. _____            │
└─────────────────────────────────────────────────────────────┘
```

Ingredients Used

Ingredient	Quantity Used	Manufacturer Lot #-Exp Date	Solubility	Dose Comparison Given	Dose Comparison Usual	Use in the Prescription
Glacial Acetic Acid	1.4 mL	JET Labs SN2671-mm/yy	miscible with water and alcohol	5%	2–100%	caustic, keratolytic
Lactic Acid	2.8 mL	JET Labs SV2672-mm/yy	miscible with water and alcohol	10%	5–20%	caustic, keratolytic
Salicylic Acid	3 g	JET Labs SN2641-mm/yy	1 g/460 mL water or 2 mL alcohol	10%	5–20%	caustic, keratolytic
Flexible Collodion	q.s. 30 mL	JET Labs SN2673-mm/yy	misc with alcohol immis with water	—	—	vehicle, protectant

Compatibility–Stability/Beyond-Use Date

Stability–Compatibility: This product is similar to Salicylic Acid Collodion USP (9), and the following procedure is patterned after that monograph. The Salicylic Acid and other organic acid ingredients in this preparation are quite stable in this liquid solvent formulation. Collodion preparations should not be made in open containers because the Flexible Collodion contains very volatile solvents such as ether, acetone, and alcohol. Furthermore, Flexible Collodion is very incompatible with water, so it is best to make these preparations directly in the dispensing container. Flexible Collodion should not be put in graduated cylinders, beakers, mortars, or sinks!

Preservative: No added preservative is needed for this preparation because the formulation ingredients are sufficiently hostile to microorganisms.

Packaging and Storage and Beyond-use date: The *USP* monograph for Salicylic Acid Collodion recommends storage in tight containers, at controlled room temperature, and away from fire (9). These conditions would be recommended for this preparation. Because this formulation contains no water and is made from USP ingredients, a 6-month beyond-use date would be acceptable; however, because of the volatile solvents in Flexible Collodion, a more conservative 1-month date will be used.

Calculations

Dose/Concentration

All OK

Ingredient Amounts

Note: The percent concentration of the Acetic Acid and Lactic Acid can be interpreted in several ways. (This is discussed in the Concentrated Acid section of Chapter 7.) If a % v/v interpretation is used, the gram amounts given below would be in milliliters; that is, 1.5 mL Acetic Acid and 3 mL Lactic Acid. The alternate interpretation of % w/v of pure chemical in solution is shown here and is used in this prescription order. For these ingredients, the difference in amounts is negligible, but that is not always the case; it depends on the w/w percent of the concentrated acid and its density.

Acetic Acid in grams: *5% × 30 mL = 1.5 g Acetic Acid*

Salicylic Acid and Lactic Acid in grams: *10% × 30 mL = 3 g of each*

Volume of Glacial Acetic Acid:
  Glacial Acetic Acid USP is 100% w/w with a density of 1.05 g/mL.

$$\left(\frac{1\,mL\ Gl.\ AA}{1.05\,g\ Gl.\ AA} \right)\left(\frac{100\,g\ Gl.\ AA}{100\,g\ AA} \right)\left(\frac{1.5\,g\ AA}{} \right) = 1.4\,mL\ Glacial\ Acetic\ Acid$$

Volume of Lactic Acid:
  Lactic Acid USP is 90% w/w with a density of 1.2 g/mL.

$$\left(\frac{1\,mL\ L.A.\,USP}{1.2\,g\ L.A.\,USP} \right)\left(\frac{100\,g\ L.A.\,USP}{90\,g\ L.A.} \right)\left(\frac{3\,g\ L.A.}{} \right) = 2.8\,mL\ Lactic\ Acid\ USP$$

Compounding Procedure

On a class 3 or a digital balance, weigh 3 g of Salicylic Acid. Calibrate a 1-oz applicator bottle at 30 mL using Alcohol. Using a 3-mL syringe, measure 1.4 mL of Glacial Acetic Acid. Using a 10-mL graduate (or 3-mL syringe), measure 2.8 mL of Lactic Acid. Place all of the above in the applicator bottle and add approximately 3/4 of the needed volume of Flexible Collodion and swirl to mix and dissolve the Salicylic Acid. Add the remainder of the Flexible Collodion to q.s. to the calibration mark on the applicator bottle. Replace the applicator cap and carefully tighten, then agitate to thoroughly mix the solution. Label and dispense.

Quality Control

The preparation is a clear, colorless or slightly yellow, viscous solution with the odor of ether. The actual volume of the preparation is checked and matches the theoretical volume of 30 mL. (Note: Because this is not an aqueous solution, pH has no meaning and is not measured.)

Labeling

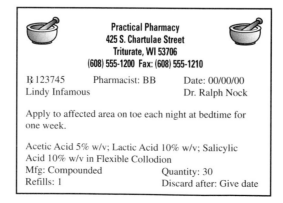

Practical Pharmacy
425 S. Chartulae Street
Triturate, WI 53706
(608) 555-1200 Fax: (608) 555-1210

R 123745   Pharmacist: BB   Date: 00/00/00
Lindy Infamous   Dr. Ralph Nock

Apply to affected area on toe each night at bedtime for one week.

Acetic Acid 5% w/v; Lactic Acid 10% w/v; Salicylic Acid 10% w/v in Flexible Collodion
Mfg: Compounded
Refills: 1
Quantity: 30
Discard after: Give date

Auxiliary Labels: Caution: Flammable; For External Use Only
Keep out of the reach of children

Patient Consultation

Hello, Mr. Infamous, I'm your pharmacist, Ben Block. Do you have any drug allergies? Are you using any other medications? What did you see your physician for? This medicine can be used for warts, corns, and so on. You are to apply this to the affected area on your toe each night at bedtime for 1 week only. To increase its effectiveness, you might want to soak the toe in warm water for about 5 minutes before application, and put a covering, such as an adhesive bandage, over the area during the night. Wash off the medication in the morning. Be very careful not to get this near eyes, mucous membranes, or genital areas, and apply in a well-ventilated area (don't inhale the fumes). Keep away from flames or lighted pipes, cigars, or cigarettes; this is a very flammable mixture. Wash your hands immediately after applying this solution, and be sure to immediately replace the container cap tightly. This product is for external use only and should be stored at room temperature, out of the reach of children. You may get one refill if necessary, but don't use for longer than the prescribed time (1 week) unless your doctor advises you to continue. Discard any unused contents after 1 month.

➤ Prescription 26.8

Contemporary Physicians Group Practice
20 S. Park Street, Triturate, WI 53706
Tel: (608) 555-1333 Fax: (608) 555-1335

℞ # 705

Name *Andrea Gill* Date *00/00/00*

Address *1593 Michigan Lake Drive* Age Wt/Ht

℞

Proetz Nasal Solution:
Glycerin *20 mL*
Ethanol 70% *40 mL*
Normal Saline Sol'n *q s ad 500 mL*

Pat Butler
Dispense 60 mL **00/00/00**

Sig: Put 3 drops in each nostril qid and prn for irritation
and dryness
Please label as Proetz Nasal Solution O.Q.

Refills *prn* *Olive Quacky* M.D.

DEA No. _____

Ingredients Used

Ingredient	Quantity Used	Manufacturer Lot #-Exp Date	Solubility	Dose Comparison Given	Usual	Use in the Prescription
Glycerin	2.4 mL	JET Labs SS2813-mm/yy	miscible with water and alcohol	4%	varies	humectant, vehicle, preservative
Alcohol USP 95% v/v	3.5 mL to make 4.8 mL 70% ethanol	JET Labs SN2653-mm/yy	miscible with water	5.6%	varies	vehicle, preservative, antiseptic
Sodium Chloride	540 mg to make 60 mL NSS	JET Labs SN2681-mm/yy	1 g/2.8 mL water 10 mL Glycerin v sl sol in alcohol	0.9%	0.9%	tonicity adjustor
Purified Water	q.s. 60 mL	Sweet Springs AL0529-mm/yy	—	—	—	vehicle

Compatibility–Stability/Beyond-Use Date

Stability–Compatibility: All ingredients in this preparation are compatible and very stable when in an aqueous solution.

Preservative: No extra preservative is needed because the Glycerin (4%) and Alcohol (5.6%) act as preservatives.

Packaging and Storage and Beyond-use date: Because the ingredients in this preparation are known to be very stable, Pharmacist Butler can use a longer beyond-use date than the 14-day dating recommended by *USP* for compounded water-containing formulations prepared from ingredients in solid form when there is no stability information for the formulation (8). Because this is a nasal solution that should be sterile, a conservative 30-day beyond-use date will be used. Controlled room temperature will be the recommended storage conditions.

Calculations

Dose/Concentration

Glycerin in v/v percent:

$$\frac{20 \; mL \; Glycerin}{500 \; mL \; solution} = \frac{x \; mL \; Glycerin}{100 \; mL \; solution} ; x = 4\% \quad OK$$

Alcohol in v/v percent: *70% × 40 mL = 28 mL*

$$\frac{28 \; mL \; C_2H_5OH}{500 \; mL \; solution} = \frac{x \; mL \; C_2H_5OH}{100 \; mL \; solution} ; x = 5.6\% \quad OK$$

Ingredient Amounts

Glycerin in mL:

$$\frac{20 \; mL \; Glycerin}{500 \; mL \; solution} = \frac{x \; mL \; Glycerin}{60 \; mL \; solution} ; x = 2.4 \; mL \; Glycerin$$

The 70% Ethanol must be made using Alcohol USP, which is 95% Ethyl Alcohol. The amount of Alcohol USP needed is calculated in the following steps.

70% Ethanol in mL needed for 60 mL of preparation:

$$\frac{40 \; mL \; 70\% \; Ethanol}{500 \; mL \; solution} = \frac{x \; mL \; 70\% \; Ethanol}{60 \; mL \; solution} ; x = 4.8 \; mL \; 70\% \; Ethanol$$

Ethyl Alcohol (C_2H_5OH) contained in this volume of 70% Ethanol:

70% × 4.8 mL = 3.36 mL

Alcohol USP in mL that will contain this amount of Ethyl Alcohol:

$$\frac{95 \; mL \; C_2H_5OH}{100 \; mL \; Alcohol \; USP} = \frac{3.36 \; mL \; C_2H_5OH}{x \; mL \; Alcohol \; USP} ; x = 3.5 \; mL \; Alcohol \; USP$$

Sodium Chloride for 60 mL of Normal Saline Solution (NSS) if Sterile NSS is unavailable:

$$\frac{0.9 \; g \; NaCl}{100 \; mL \; NSS} = \frac{x \; g \; NaCl}{60 \; mL \; NSS} ; x = 0.54 \; g \; NaCl$$

Compounding Procedure

If possible, perform this compounding procedure in a sterile environment such as a laminar airflow hood or a barrier isolator. Measure 3.5 mL of Alcohol USP in a 10-mL graduated cylinder and q.s. to 4.8 mL with sterile water or Purified Water. Transfer this solution to a 100-mL graduated cylinder. Measure 2.4 mL of Glycerin with a 3-mL syringe or a 10-mL graduated cylinder. Add to the alcohol solution. If possible, use Sterile Sodium Chloride for Injection or Inhalation to q.s. the alcohol-glycerin solution to the 60 mL mark. Although there are various manufactured sterile saline nasal solutions, all have Sodium Chloride concentrations of less than 0.9% and most contain the preservative Benzalkonium Chloride. If sterile saline is unavailable, make 60 mL of this as follows: Weigh 540 mg of Sodium Chloride, put in a 100-mL graduate, and q.s. with sterile water or Purified Water to 60 mL. Stir to dissolve. Then use the sodium chloride solution to q.s. the alcohol-glycerin solution to the 60-mL mark. Using a sterile syringe that is fitted with a 0.45-μ or 0.2-μ bacterial membrane filter, transfer the completed solution to a 60 mL-sterile dropper bottle. Label and dispense.

Quality Control

The preparation is a clear, colorless solution with apparent viscosity approximately that of water. It may have a slight characteristic odor of Alcohol. The pH of the preparation is checked and recorded as pH = 5. The actual volume is checked and matches the theoretical volume of 60 mL.

Labeling

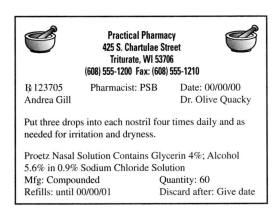

Practical Pharmacy
425 S. Chartulae Street
Triturate, WI 53706
(608) 555-1200 Fax: (608) 555-1210

℞ 123705   Pharmacist: PSB   Date: 00/00/00
Andrea Gill   Dr. Olive Quacky

Put three drops into each nostril four times daily and as needed for irritation and dryness.

Proetz Nasal Solution Contains Glycerin 4%; Alcohol 5.6% in 0.9% Sodium Chloride Solution
Mfg: Compounded   Quantity: 60
Refills: until 00/00/01   Discard after: Give date

Auxiliary Labels: For the Nose

Patient Consultation

Hello, Ms. Gill, I'm your pharmacist, Pat Butler. Are you currently using any other medications? Are you allergic to any drugs? What has your doctor told you about this medication? This is a nasal solution used for nasal stuffiness caused by low humidity. The directions are to put three drops into each nostril four times a day and as needed for irritation and dryness. You may put the drops into your nostrils by tilting your head back and depressing the dropper bulb. Try to avoid contaminating the dropper tip by not touching the inside of your nostril with it. I am giving you this instruction sheet on using nose drops to give you some extra guidance (Fig. 26.1). If your condition seems to show no improvement or seems to get worse, contact your doctor. Although this solution is very stable, you may eventually contaminate it because you are putting drops into your nostrils, so discard any unused portion after 1 month. This prescription may be refilled anytime for a year. Do you have any questions?

■ **Figure 26.1. *HOW TO USE NOSE DROPS***

1. Blow your nose gently.
2. Wash your hands with soap and warm water.
3. Draw up a small amount of medication into the medicine dropper.
4. Lie down on your back and place a pillow under your shoulders. Tilt your head back so that it is hanging lower than your shoulders.
   Note: If putting drops into the nose of a child, lay the child on his or her back over your lap. The head should be tilted back.
5. Breathe through your mouth.
6. Place the **tip** of the medicine dropper just inside the nostril. Avoid touching the dropper against the nostril or anything else.
7. Squeeze the directed number of drops into the nostril.
8. Repeat steps 3–7 for the other nostril.
9. Remain lying down for about 5 minutes, so that the medication has a chance to spread throughout your nasal passages.
10. Replace the cap tightly on the bottle.

NOTE:

• Some of the solution may drain down into your mouth. If the taste is unpleasant, you may cough the excess solution into a handkerchief or tissue.

• It may be much easier to have someone help you instill your nose drops.

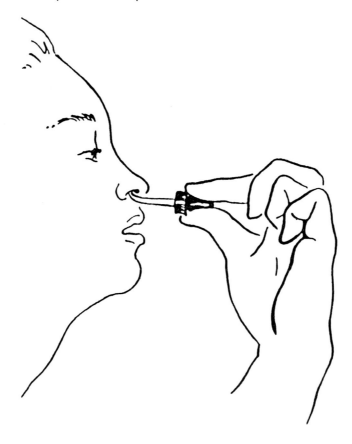

➤ **Prescription 26.9**

```
┌─────────────────────────────────────────────────────────────┐
│           Contemporary Physicians Group Practice             │
│           20 S. Park Street, Triturate, WI  53706            │
│           Tel: (608) 555-1333  Fax: (608) 555-1335           │
│─────────────────────────────────────────────────────────────│
│                          ℞ #  714                            │
│─────────────────────────────────────────────────────────────│
│  Name  Beavus Budhead            Date  00/00/00              │
│─────────────────────────────────────────────────────────────│
│  Address  931 Dumbdy Lane        Age    16     Wt/Ht         │
│                                                              │
│   ℞                                                          │
│              Antipyrine              5%                      │
│              Hydrocortisone          0.5%                    │
│              Neomycin sulfate        5 mg/mL                 │
│              Na metabisulfite        0.1%                    │
│              Glycerin                25%                     │
│              Propylene Glycol        25%                     │
│              Purified Water      q s ad  30 mL               │
│                                    Al Bungy  0/00/00         │
│       Sig:   Instill 4 gtt. in left ear 3-4 times daily     │
│                                                              │
│   Refills   0              Norace Osgood          M.D.       │
│                     DEA No. _____                 │
└─────────────────────────────────────────────────────────────┘
```

Ingredients Used

Ingredient	Quantity Used	Manufacturer Lot #-Exp Date	Solubility	Dose Comparison Given	Dose Comparison Usual	Use in the Prescription
Antipyrine	1500 mg	JET Labs SN2691-mm/yy	1 g/mL water or 1.3 mL alcohol	5%	5%	antipyretic, analgesic
Hydrocortisone	150 mg	JET Labs SN2692-mm/yy	v sl sol in water 1 g/40 mL alcohol	0.5%	0.5–2.5%	anti-inflammatory
Neomycin Sulfate	150 mg	JET Labs SN2693-mm/yy	1 g/mL water v sl sol alcohol	5 mg/mL (0.5%)	5 mg/mL	antibiotic
Sodium Metabisulfite	120 mg weighed, 30 mg used	JET Labs SN2694-mm/yy	1 g/2 mL water v sl sol alcohol	0.1%	0.1%	antioxidant
Glycerin	7.5 mL	JET Labs SS2813-mm/yy	miscible with water or alcohol	25%	varies	humectant, preservative, vehicle
Propylene Glycol	7.5 mL	JET Labs SV2662-mm/yy	miscible with water or alcohol	25%	varies	humectant, preservative, vehicle
Purified Water	q.s. 30 mL	Sweet Springs AL0529-mm/yy	—	—	—	vehicle

Compatibility–Stability/Beyond-Use Date

Stability–Compatibility: Because of the multiple ingredients in this formulation, this is a more difficult order to evaluate. The Antipyrine in aqueous solution has been evaluated and found to be reasonably stable, although storage in tight, light-resistant containers is recommended (12). Aqueous solutions of Neomycin Sulfate are reported to be stable over a fairly wide pH range (pH 2 to 9), but the drug is subject to oxidation, and tight, light-resistant containers should be used (13). The Hydrocortisone is somewhat more difficult to assess. It undergoes oxidation and other complex degradation reactions. It is most stable at pH 3.5 to 4.5, and its stability is quite dependent on pH, with steep slopes for its pH profile in both the acidic and basic regions (14). No stability data for this specific formulation are available.

Preservative: No extra preservative is needed because 50% of the preparation is a Glycerin–Propylene Glycol cosolvent, and both of these ingredients act as preservatives at this concentration.

Packaging and Storage and Beyond-use date: Pharmacist Bungy will use the *USP* recommended maximum 14-day beyond-use date for compounded water-containing formulations prepared from ingredients in solid form when there is no stability information for the formulation (8). Packaging should be in a tight, light-resistant container with recommended storage at controlled room temperature.

Calculations

Dose/Concentration

All concentrations are OK.

If a % w/v concentration is desired for labeling the Neomycin Sulfate, this can be calculated as follows:

$$\frac{0.005 \ g \ Neomycin}{mL \ solution} = \frac{x \ g \ Neomycin}{100 \ mL \ solution} ; x = 0.5\% \ Neomycin \ Sulfate$$

Ingredient Amounts

Antipyrine: *5% × 30 mL = 1,500 mg*

Hydrocortisone: *0.5% × 30 mL = 150 mg*

Neomycin Sulfate: *5 mg/mL × 30 mL = 150 mg*

Sodium Metabisulfite: *0.1% × 30 mL = 30 mg*

Glycerin and Propylene Glycol: *25% × 30 mL = 7.5 mL of each*

Sodium Metabisulfite aliquot:

Weigh 4 times the amount needed, 120 mg, dissolve in 8 mL of water and take ¼ that volume, 2 mL, to give 30 mg. The validity of this may be checked as follows:

120 mg/8 mL = 15 mg/mL × 2 mL = 30 mg

Compounding Procedure

This solution can be made in a variety of ways. An Aliquot is required for the Sodium Metabisulfite. One example is provided above, but keep in mind that there are many ways to do this. When syringes are available they may be used to measure small quantities. The Sodium Metabisulfite is very soluble in water, so solid-liquid aliquots with water would be the likely choice. One limitation is the amount of water available in the formula. Assuming zero powder volumes and additive liquid volumes, the amount of available water is 15 mL. This will affect the aliquot volumes selected. The Hydrocortisone is soluble in Glycerin and Propylene Glycol, but it is not easily wetted by these viscous liquids. It could be partially dissolved or wetted with a small amount of alcohol first. It requires 6 mL of alcohol to be fully dissolved, and this is probably too much alcohol for this type of formulation.

All weighing is done on a class 3 torsion or an electronic balance. One procedure is to weigh 150 mg of Neomycin Sulfate and dissolve in 4 mL of Purified Water and transfer to a clean beaker. Weigh 150 mg of Sodium Metabisulfite and dissolve in 8 mL of Purified Water. Measure 2 mL of this solution and add it to the beaker containing the Neomycin. Next weigh 1,500 mg of Antipyrine and add this to the beaker. It should dissolve in the 6 mL of water present, but you may add a small amount of additional water if it doesn't readily dissolve. Weigh 150 mg of Hydrocortisone and place in a clean beaker. Wet the Hydrocortisone with a few drops of Alcohol. Add 7.5 mL each of Glycerin and Propylene Glycol and swirl to mix. Put the beaker in a warm water bath and heat gently to dissolve the Hydrocortisone (a few seconds in a microwave oven also works, but there may be concern about drug degradation). Transfer all the drug solutions to a ½-oz dropper bottle that has been precalibrated with water and marked at 30 mL. Use Purified Water to rinse the beakers to ensure complete transfers of the solutions and to q.s. to the 30-mL mark. Agitate to mix. Label and dispense.

Quality Control

The preparation is a clear, colorless or slightly yellowish solution with apparent viscosity slightly greater than that of water. The pH of the preparation is checked and recorded to be pH = 6. The actual volume is checked and matches the theoretical volume of 30 mL.

Labeling

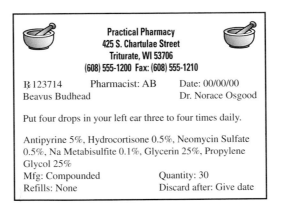

Practical Pharmacy
425 S. Chartulae Street
Triturate, WI 53706
(608) 555-1200 Fax: (608) 555-1210

℞ 123714   Pharmacist: AB   Date: 00/00/00
Beavus Budhead   Dr. Norace Osgood

Put four drops in your left ear three to four times daily.

Antipyrine 5%, Hydrocortisone 0.5%, Neomycin Sulfate 0.5%, Na Metabisulfite 0.1%, Glycerin 25%, Propylene Glycol 25%
Mfg: Compounded   Quantity: 30
Refills: None   Discard after: Give date

Auxiliary Labels: For the Ear

Patient Consultation

Hello, Mr. Budhead, I'm your pharmacist, Al Bungy. Are you currently using any over-the-counter or prescription medication? Are you allergic to any drugs? What has your doctor told you about this medication? This is used to treat your ear infection. Place four drops into the left ear three or four times daily. I am giving you this instruction sheet on using ear drops to give you some extra guidance (Fig. 26.2). If your condition shows no improvement or gets worse, contact Dr. Osgood. If any intense reaction, such as inflammation or pain in the ear, occurs, discontinue use and immediately contact Dr. Osgood. Keep the container tightly closed in a cool dry place out of the reach of children. Discard any unused portion after 2 weeks. This prescription does not have any refills, so you will need to contact your physician if you need a refill. If you are not relieved in 2 weeks, you should see Dr. Osgood again anyway. Do you have any questions?

■ Figure 26.2. *HOW TO USE EAR DROPS*

1. Wash your hands with soap and warm water.
2. Draw up a small amount of medication into the medicine dropper.
3. Lie on your side so that the affected ear points toward the ceiling.
4. Position the **tip** of the medicine dropper just inside the affected ear canal. Avoid touching the dropper against the ear or anything else. For adults, hold the earlobe up and back; for children, hold the earlobe down and back.
5. Squeeze the directed number of drops into your ear canal and allow the drops to run in.
6. Remain lying down for 3 to 5 minutes so that the medication has a chance to spread throughout the ear canal; you may gently massage the area around your ear to aid the spreading and distribution of the ear drops in the canal.
7. Place a clean cotton pledget just inside your ear to prevent leakage of the solution when your head is held in an upright position.
8. Replace the cap tightly on the bottle.

IMPORTANT:

1. Never use ear drops if your eardrum has been damaged.
2. Avoid using very hot or very cold ear drops. The medication should be at room temperature or slightly warmer. If necessary, warm the drops by holding the bottle in your hand for a few minutes.

NOTE:

It may be much easier to have someone else instill your ear drops.

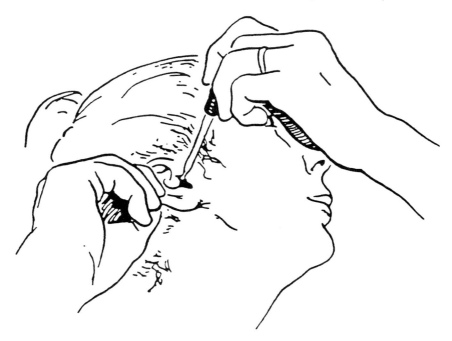

► **Prescription 26.10**

Contemporary Physicians Group Practice
20 S. Park Street, Triturate, WI 53706
Tel: (608) 555-1333 Fax: (608) 555-1335

R # 215

Name *Merry Math*   Date *00/00/00*

Address *6525 Division Lane*   Age   4   Wt/Ht *36 lbs*

R

Hydralazine HCl Oral Solution   1 mg/mL

Dispense 60 mL

Susie Gretsky 00/00/00

Change to 0.75 mg/kg/day
Sig: Give *0.75 mcg/kg/day* po in four divided doses

Per phone consult with Dr. Barksen, dose was changed as indicated here. S.G.

Refills   2   *R. Barksen*   M.D.

DEA No. _____

Ingredients Used

Ingredient	Quantity Used	Manufacturer Lot #-Exp Date	Solubility	Dose Comparison Given	Dose Comparison Usual	Use in the Prescription
Hydralazine HCl	120 mg weighed, 60 mg used	JET Labs SN2611-mm/yy	sol in water sl sol alcohol	0.75 mcg/kg/day changed to 0.75 mg/kg/day	0.75 mg/kg/day	anti-hypertensive
Sorbitol Solution 70%	24 g	JET Labs SV2612-mm/yy	miscible with water or alcohol	—	—	sweetened vehicle
Propylene Glycol	6 g	JET Labs SV2662-mm/yy	miscible with water or alcohol	10% w/v	varies	solvent, preservative
Methylparaben	21 mg	JET Labs SN2613-mm/yy	sl sol in water fr sol in alcohol	0.035%	0.05–0.25%	preservative
Propylparaben	39 mg	JET Labs SN2614-mm/yy	v sl sol in water fr sol in alcohol	0.065%	0.02–0.04%	preservative
Aspartame	30 mg	JET Labs SN2615-mm/yy	sp sol in water sl sol alcohol	0.05%	0.05%	sweetener
Purified Water	q.s. 60 mL	Sweet Springs AL0529-mm/yy	—	—	—	vehicle

Compatibility–Stability/Beyond-Use Date

Stability–Compatibility: The is an official USP formulation with known stability. This solution is made according to the compounding formula for Hydralazine Hydrochloride Oral Solution USP. The formula is given below. Hydralazine has compatibility and stability problems with some sugars and aldehydes, so it should not be made with sucrose-based syrups, and flavors should be avoided except at the time of administration (15).
Preservative: The formulation contains the paraben preservatives.
Packaging and Storage and Beyond-use date: The *USP* monograph for this preparation recommends storage in a light-resistant glass or plastic bottle with a child-resistant closure and storage in the refrigerator. The monograph gives a beyond-use date of 30 days for this formulation (15).

Calculations

Dose/Concentration

Hydralazine HCl: The dose in the *USP/DI* for this drug is 0.75 mg/kg/day in four divided doses rather than the 0.75 **mcg**/kg/day given in this prescription. Pharmacist Gretsky calls Dr. Barksen, who thanks Gretsky for noticing the error and agrees to change the dose to the recommended amount.

$$Weight\ of\ child\ in\ kg: \frac{36\ lb}{2.2\ lb/kg} = 16.4\ kg$$

$$Dose\ in\ mg: \left(\frac{0.75\ mg}{kg/day}\right)\left(\frac{16.4\ mg}{}\right)\left(\frac{day}{4\ doses}\right) = 3\ mg/dose$$

Ingredient Amounts

The USP formula for Hydralazine Hydrochloride Oral Solution is given here (15):

Hydralazine Hydrochloride	
for 0.1% Oral Solution	100 mg
for 1.0% Oral Solution	1.0 g
Sorbitol Solution (70%)	40 g
Methylparaben	65 mg
Propylparaben	35 mg
Propylene Glycol	10 g
Aspartame	50 mg
Purified Water, a sufficient quantity to make	100 mL

Note—Hydralazine reacts with many flavors; do not add flavors when compounding.

Reducing the formula above to make 60 mL of the 0.1% solution (1 mg/mL = 100 mg/100 mL), we need the following:

Hydralazine HCl: 100 mg/100 mL × 60 mL = 60 mg

Sorbitol Solution: 40 g/100 mL × 60 mL = 24 g

Methylparaben: 65 mg/100 mL × 60 mL = 39 mg

Propylparaben: 35 mg/100 mL × 60 mL = 21 mg

Aspartame: 50 mg/100 mL × 60 mL = 30 mg

Propylene Glycol: 10 g/100 mL × 60 mL = 6 g

Aliquots

Hydralazine HCl: Weigh 2 times the amount needed, 120 mg, dissolve in 20 mL of water and take ½ that volume, 10 mL, to give 60 mg. The validity of this may be checked as follows: *120 mg/20 mL = 6 mg/mL × 10 mL = 60 mg*

Aspartame: Weigh 4 times the amount needed, 120 mg, dissolve in 12 mL of water and take ¼ that volume, 3 mL, to give 30 mg. The validity of this may be checked as follows: *120 mg/12 mL = 10 mg/mL × 3 mL = 30 mg*

Methylparaben and Propylparaben: The pharmacy has a paraben–propylene glycol stock solution, which has the following formula:

Methylparaben	0.65 g
Propylparaben	0.35 g
Propylene Glycol	100.0 g
	101.0 g

By taking 6.06 g of this stock solution, you will have exactly the 6 g of Propylene Glycol, 39 mg of Methylparaben, and 21 mg of Propylparaben. This can be checked by performing the following calculation:

$$\left(\frac{650 \ mg \ Methylparaben}{101 \ g \ stock \ solution} \right)\left(\frac{6.06 \ g \ stock \ solution}{} \right) = 39 \ mg \ Methylparaben$$

Compounding Procedure

All weighing is done on a class 3 torsion or an electronic balance. Weigh 120 mg of Hydralazine HCl and dissolve in 20 mL of water in a 25-mL graduated cylinder. Measure 10 mL of this and transfer to a clean beaker. Weigh 120 mg of Aspartame and dissolve in 12 mL of water. Measure 3 mL of this solution and add it to the beaker containing the Hydralazine. Next, weigh in a tared beaker 24 g of Sorbitol 70% Solution and add this to the beaker containing the Hydralazine solution. Weigh 6.06 g of the Propylene Glycol–paraben stock solution and add this to the beaker. Some Purified Water may be used to completely rinse the Sorbitol Solution and the Propylene Glycol–paraben stock solution into the beaker for complete transfer. Transfer the solution to a 2-oz amber prescription bottle and add sufficient Purified Water to make the preparation measure 60 mL. Agitate the bottle to mix completely. Label and dispense.

Quality Control

The preparation is a clear, colorless solution with apparent viscosity slightly greater than that of water. The pH of the preparation is checked and recorded as pH = 5. The actual volume is checked and matches the theoretical volume of 60 mL.

Labeling

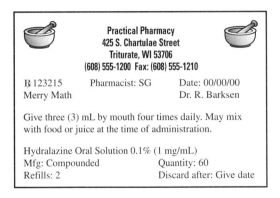

Auxiliary Labels: Keep in the refrigerator

Patient Consultation

Good afternoon, Mrs. Math, I'm your pharmacist, Susie Gretsky. Here is the prescription for Merry. Is Merry allergic to any drugs? Is she currently taking any other medications? What did Dr. Barksen tell you about this drug? This medication is to help control her blood pressure. You are to give Merry 3 mL four times a day. Do you have an oral syringe to measure this amount? Do you feel comfortable with measuring this, or would you like to go over that just to make sure? You may mix this with some fruit juice or applesauce just prior to giving it to Merry. If you forget to give a dose, give it as soon as you remember, but if it's close to the next dose, just skip it; do not double doses. This medication could make Merry a little dizzy or give her a headache. If this becomes a problem, I suggest you call Dr. Barksen. I assume that Merry will be getting regular checkups to make sure everything is going well. Store this in the refrigerator and discard any unused contents after 1 month;

I have put that date on this bottle. Keep this out of the reach of children. This may be refilled 2 times; because this takes a little time to prepare, I suggest that you call ahead when you need a refill. Do you have any questions?

References

1. The 2002 United States Pharmacopeia 25/National Formulary 20. Rockville, MD: The United States Pharmacopeial Convention, Inc., 2001; 2218-2222.
2. Cadwallader DE. EENT preparations. In: King RE, ed. Dispensing of medication, 9th ed. Easton, PA: Mack Publishing Co., 1984; 157-158.
3. Riegelman S, Sorby DL. EENT medications. In: Martin EW, ed. Dispensing of medication, 7th ed. Easton, PA: Mack Publishing Co., 1971; 913-915.
4. News. Am J Health-Syst Pharm 2001;58:2369.
5. Gallagher G. Doctors and drops. Br Med J 1991;303:761.
6. Allen Jr. LV. The Art, Science and Technology of Pharmaceutical Compounding. Washington, DC: Amercan Pharmacetical Association, 1998;244-245.
7. The 2002 United States Pharmacopeia 25/National Formulary 20. Rockville, MD: The United States Pharmacopeial Convention, Inc., 2001;1833-1836.
8. The 2002 United States Pharmacopeia 25/National Formulary 20. Rockville, MD: The United States Pharmacopeial Convention, Inc., 2001;2054.
9. The 2002 United States Pharmacopeia 25/National Formulary 20. Rockville, MD: The United States Pharmacopeial Convention, Inc., 2001; Official Monographs.
10. Connors KA, Amidon GL, Stella VJ. Chemical Stability of Pharmaceuticals, 2d ed. New York: John Wiley & Sons, 1986;264-273.
11. Trissel LA. Trissel's Stability of Compounded Formulations, 2d ed. Washington, DC: Amercan Pharmacetical Association, 2001;95-98.
12. Trissel LA. Trissel's Stability of Compounded Formulations, 2d ed. Washington, DC: Amercan Pharmacetical Association, 2001;28-29.
13. Trissel LA. Trissel's Stability of Compounded Formulations, 2d ed. Washington, DC: Amercan Pharmacetical Association, 2001;268-270.
14. Connors KA, Amidon GL, Stella VJ. Chemical Stability of Pharmaceuticals, 2d ed. New York: John Wiley & Sons, 1986;483-490.
15. The 2002 United States Pharmacopeia 25/National Formulary 20. Rockville, MD: The United States Pharmacopeial Convention, Inc., 2001;847-848.

CHAPTER 27

Ophthalmic Solutions

I. DEFINITION

"Ophthalmic solutions are sterile solutions, essentially free from foreign particles, suitably compounded and packaged for instillation into the eye" (1)—*USP*

II. REFERENCES

The references listed below give useful information on making ophthalmic solutions. The ASHP technical assistance bulletin is available on the ASHP Internet site at www.ashp.org. This resource provides a good overall guide on proper procedures for compounding ophthalmic solutions. For pharmacists who work in ophthalmology, the book by Reynolds and Closson is an important resource. This book contains a general introductory section and over 300 pages of ophthalmic formulations, including information on stability.

Deardorff DL. Ophthalmic solutions. In: Hoover JE, ed. Remington's pharmaceutical sciences, 14th ed. Easton, PA: Mack Publishing Co., 1970;1545–1577.

Hecht G. Ophthalmic preparations. In: Gennaro AR, ed. Remington: The science and practice of pharmacy, 20th ed. Philadelphia: Lippincott Williams & Wilkins, 2000;821-835.

Cadwallader DE. EENT preparations. In: King RE. Dispensing of medication, 9th ed. Easton, PA: Mack Publishing Co., 1984;140–152.

Reynolds LA, Closson RG. Extemporaneous ophthalmic preparations. Vancouver, WA: Applied Therapeutics, Inc., 1993.

The 1995 United States Pharmacopeia XXI-National Formulary XVI. Rockville, MD: The United States Pharmacopeial Convention, Inc., 1985;1338–1339.

ASHP Technical Assistance Bulletin on pharmacy-prepared ophthalmic products. Am J Hosp Pharm 1993;50:1462–1463.

The following sections are intended to give some basic information on making ophthalmic solutions.

III. CAUTIONS

A. As stated in the definition, ophthalmic solutions must be sterile and free from particulates. Because of the inherent danger of causing serious eye infection and even loss of eyesight through the use of contaminated ophthalmic solutions, the pharmacist must use the greatest care in preparing these drug preparations.

B. Ophthalmic solutions should be made extemporaneously only if:
1. There are no available commercial product alternatives.
2. The pharmacist possesses the appropriate knowledge and technique.
3. The necessary equipment and supplies are available to make sterile solutions.

C. Compounded ophthalmic solutions should be given conservative beyond-use dates. For information on this, read the portion on beyond-use dating at the end of this section and in Chapter 4, Expiration and Beyond-use Dating.

IV. DESIRED PROPERTIES OF OPHTHALMIC SOLUTIONS

The properties of an ideal ophthalmic solution are given below. Achieving all of these objectives simultaneously is sometimes impossible; in these cases, appropriate compromises can be made, or another therapeutic option may necessary.

A. Sterility and clarity are not just desired properties but absolute requirements for ophthalmic solutions. The preparation and packaging should be done in a sterile environment such as a laminar airflow hood or a barrier isolator. A sterile, particle-free solution can be achieved by one of the following methods:
1. Prepare the solution as you would a parenteral preparation, using aseptic technique with sterile parenteral drug products as the solution ingredients, and packaging the solution in a clean, particle-free, sterile container.
2. Prepare the solution using nonsterile but high-quality ingredients, and filter the solution using a 0.2- or 0.45-μ bacterial filter into a dispensing container that is clean, particle-free, and sterile.
3. If an autoclave is available, terminal steam sterilization can be used. In this case, the solution may be prepared using nonsterile but high-quality ingredients and packaged in an appropriate clean, particle-free container that is stable to the elevated temperature and pressure needed for steam sterilization. The preparation is then autoclaved in the dispensing container.
   a. Usual quality control procedures for steam sterilization must be used. Monitoring devices that track and record time, temperature, and pressure are used, as is validation of the autoclave cycle through use of biological and other indicators. For pharmacies that have access to autoclaves in institutional settings such as hospitals, the methods are well controlled and documented as required by accreditation standards. Pharmacists using their own equipment should employ standard oper-

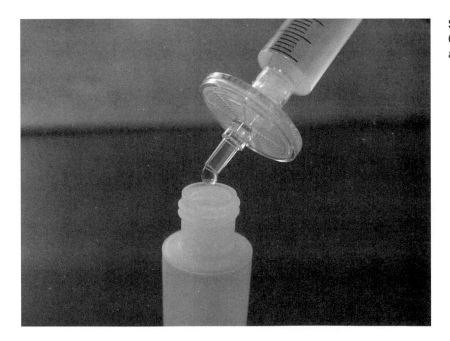

Sterilization of an
Ophthalmic Solution Using
a Bacterial Membrane Filter

ating procedures that ensure that the equipment and methods give preparations that are sterile. Unfortunately, there have been a number of accidents in recent years in which a preparation prepared by a pharmacy that was intended to be sterile was not processed properly and was not sterile. In one case the preparations were ophthalmic solutions; several patients were injured and two patients lost eyes.

    b. Because steam sterilization uses elevated temperature and pressure, consideration of drug stability is important before using this method.

B. When the solution is dispensed in a multidose container that is to be used over a period of time longer than 24 hours, a preservative must be added to ensure microbiologic safety over the period of use.

C. Although solutions with the same pH as lacrimal fluid (7.4) are ideal, the outer surfaces of the eye tolerate a larger range, 3.5 to 8.5 (1). The normal useful range to prevent corneal damage is 6.5 to 8.5 (2). The final pH of the solution is often a compromise, because many ophthalmic drugs have limited solubility and stability at the desired pH of 7.4. Buffers or pH adjusting agents or vehicles can be added to adjust and stabilize the pH at a desired level.

D. Solutions that are isotonic with tears are preferred. An amount equivalent to 0.9% NaCl is ideal for comfort and should be used when possible. The eye can tolerate within the equivalent range of 0.6–2% NaCl without discomfort (1). There are times when hypertonic ophthalmic solutions are necessary therapeutically or when the addition of an auxiliary agent, required for reasons of stability, supersedes the need for isotonicity.

E. As with all pharmaceutical solutions, ophthalmics must be chemically and physically stable. This is discussed in the chapter on stability and compatibility of drug products and preparations, Chapter 34.

F. The active ingredient(s) should be present in the most therapeutically effective form. This goal must often be compromised for reasons of solubility or stability of the active ingredient or patient comfort. For example, while most drugs are most active in their undissociated form, they are least soluble in this form. They may also be less stable at pH values that favor the undissociated form.

G. Ophthalmic solutions should be free of chemicals or agents that cause allergy or toxicity to the sensitive membranes and tissues of the eye. Auxiliary agents, such as preservatives and antioxidants, should be added with care because many patients are sensitive to these substances. Before adding an auxiliary agent, check with the patient about allergies and sensitivities.

V. ACTIVE INGREDIENTS AND AUXILIARY AGENTS

A. Active Ingredients
    1. Active ingredients are available as pure powder, as sterile powder manufactured for parenteral administration, or as a sterile, parenteral solution of the desired ingredient.

B. Auxiliary Agents
In deciding what auxiliary ingredients to add, the pharmacist must use knowledge of chemistry, pharmaceutics, bacteriology, and therapeutics. Auxiliary agents added to ophthalmic solutions include buffers, tonicity adjustors, preservatives, antioxidants, and viscosity-inducing agents.
    1. Buffers

a. Formulas for a variety of ophthalmic buffering vehicles are given in Chapter 17, Buffers and pH Adjusting Agents. The most widely used ophthalmic buffer solutions are Boric Acid Vehicle and Sorensen's Modified Phosphate Buffer.

b. Boric Acid Vehicle

(1) Boric Acid Vehicle is a 1.9% solution of Boric Acid in Purified Water or preferably sterile water. It is isotonic with tears. This solution is not iso-osmotic with red blood cells because the membrane on these cells is permeable to Boric Acid. Although Boric Acid is a common ingredient in ophthalmic products, it may not be used parenterally.

(2) Boric Acid Vehicle has a pH of approximately 5. Although this vehicle does not possess large buffer capacity, it will stabilize the pH of a drug solution close to pH 5. This, of course, depends on the pH generated by the drug itself and on the buffer capacity of the drug.

(3) Because Boric Acid Vehicle does not have strong buffering capacity, it is useful when extemporaneously compounding ophthalmic solutions of drugs that are most stable at acid pH. Boric Acid Vehicle will stabilize the pH of the solution at approximately 5 for the short expiratory periods used for compounded solutions. At the same time, its weak buffer capacity is easily overcome by the natural buffers in lacrimal fluid, so its acidic solutions are not uncomfortable when instilled in the eye. A vehicle with strong buffer capacity should not be used below pH 6.5.

(4) Boric Acid is available as crystals and powder. The crystals are preferred for making Boric Acid Vehicle because they give more crystal-clear solutions than does the powder. Air often is entrapped on the surface of Boric Acid powder, which causes incomplete dissolution and gives floating aggregates of powder.

(5) According to the *USP XXI*, Boric Acid Vehicle is useful for making ophthalmic solutions of the salts of the following drugs: Benoxinate, Cocaine, Dibucaine, Phenylephrine, piperocaine, Procaine, Proparacaine, Tetracaine, and Zinc (3). King's *Dispensing of Medication* adds ethylmorphine, Neostigmine, ethylhydrocupreine, and phenacaine to the list (4).

(6) A modified Boric Acid Vehicle can be made for drugs that are especially sensitive to oxidation. The antioxidants Sodium Bisulfite and Sodium Metabisulfite in a concentration of 0.1%, or the chelating agent Disodium Edetate in a concentration of 0.1%, may be added to retard oxidation. This modified vehicle is useful for drugs prone to oxidation. Examples include Physostigmine and Epinephrine (4).

c. Sorensen's Modified Phosphate Buffer

(1) Sorensen's Phosphate Buffer is made using two stock solutions: one acidic, containing NaH_2PO_4, and one basic, containing Na_2HPO_4. The formulas for the stock solutions are given in Table 17.8 of Chapter 17. Each solution is 1/15 or 0.067 M. The stock solutions are mixed in an appropriate ratio to give a desired pH. Table 17.8 also shows the volume ratios to mix to give a desired pH.

(2) When mixed as directed, these buffer solutions are not isotonic. If an isotonic buffer is desired, a solute must be added for tonicity adjustment. Examples of possible solutes include sodium chloride, sodium nitrate, and dextrose. The choice of a tonicity-adjusting solute depends on the compatibility of the solute with the other ingredients in the formulation. Table 17.8 shows the weight in grams of sodium chloride that must be added to 100 mL of buffer solution to give an isotonic buffer. If a different solute is desired, the amount of this solute can be calculated using its sodium chloride equivalent.

(3) Sorensen's Modified Buffer has a large buffer capacity and should not be used outside the pH range of 6.5–8.0.

(4) According to the *USP XXI*, Sorensen's Phosphate Buffer is useful for making ophthalmic solutions of the salts of the following drugs: Pilocarpine, Eucatropine, Scopolamine, and Homatropine (3). King's *Dispensing of Medication* adds Atropine, Ephedrine, and Penicillin to this list (4).

d. An alternative way of adding a buffering vehicle is to choose a manufactured artificial tears preparation that contains an appropriate buffer. Caution must be exercised in using these products because they may also contain other ingredients, such as viscosity-inducing agents and preservatives, that could cause compatibility problems. *Drug Facts and Comparisons*, the *PDR for Ophthalmology*, and the product package insert list the ingredients of artificial tears products.

e. Amount of buffer solution to use

(1) The buffer solution is often used as the tonicity adjustor for the ophthalmic solution. Under these circumstances, isotonicity calculations determine the amount of buffer solution to use.

(2) A minimum amount of buffer is needed to provide a buffering effect.

(a) One general rule states that the concentration of the buffer should be 10 times that of the drug, the concentrations of both expressed in molar quantities (5).

(b) Another recommendation states that a concentration of 0.05 to 0.5 M of buffer gives sufficient buffering capacity (6).

(c) Both of these general rules are somewhat arbitrary; they are based on buffer solutions that are made from conjugate pairs with a pK_a within one unit of the desired pH. Although Boric Acid Vehicle has a higher molar concentration (approximately 0.3 M) than Sorenson's Modified Phosphate Buffer (0.067 M), Sorensen's buffer has significantly greater buffering capacity because it consists of a conjugate pair, whereas Boric Acid Vehicle is merely a solution of a mild acid.

(3) Because the above general rules require a bit of calculation, a more simplified recommendation that gives a "ballpark" figure is for the volume of the buffer solution to be one third of the volume of the finished product. If isotonicity calculations show that less than one third of the final volume should be buffer solution, a compromise between isotonicity and buffering is needed. The one third of the volume is an oversimplified but convenient figure (5).

2. Tonicity adjustor

a. As indicated above, the buffer solution is convenient to use as the tonicity adjustor.

b. In circumstances when an ophthalmic solution without a buffer is desired, any compatible salt or nonelectrolyte that is approved for ophthalmic products may be used. Sodium Chloride, Sodium Nitrate, Sodium Sulfate, and Dextrose are common neutral tonicity adjustors.

3. Preservatives

a. Chapter ⟨1151⟩ in the *USP* states the following concerning the use of preservatives in ophthalmic solutions: "Each solution must contain a suitable substance or mixture of substances to prevent the growth of, or to destroy, microorganisms accidentally introduced when the container is opened during use. Where intended for use in surgical procedures, ophthalmic solutions, although they must be sterile, should not contain antibacterial agents, since they may be irritating to the ocular tissues." (1)

b. The authors of *Extemporaneous Ophthalmic Preparations* give the following advice on the use of preservatives in ophthalmic solutions (7):

(1) Because of preservative toxicity, especially following ocular surgery, avoid preservatives if possible and use either unpreserved Sterile Water for Injection or Sterile 0.9% Sodium Chloride Injection as vehicles for ophthalmic drugs. This means that the solution should be discarded after 24 hours because of the danger of contamination by microorganisms. This practice is practical only in a hospital or institutional setting where fresh solution can be furnished every day, so it is useful primarily for inpatients.

(2) For ambulatory patients and when hospitalized patients are discharged, it can be assumed that the eye has sufficiently healed so that it is less vulnerable to irritation and toxicity due to preservatives. At this time the solution vehicle can be changed to Bacteriostatic Water for Injection or Bacteriostatic Sodium

Chloride Injection. The beyond-use date is then based on the chemical stability of the active ingredient(s).

(3) Manufactured artificial tears products contain a preservative(s); they provide another alternative ophthalmic vehicle for ambulatory patients. When using these products for vehicles, consideration must be given to the volume of any added solution so that the preservative in the product is not diluted beyond its effective concentration.

c. Agents: Although there are over a dozen preservatives approved for ophthalmic solutions, there is no ideal ophthalmic preservative.

(1) Benzalkonium Chloride (BAC), Phenylmercuric Acetate (PMA) or Phenylmercuric Nitrate (PMN), Thimerosal, and Chlorobutanol are the most commonly used ophthalmic preservatives. Information on each of these agents, including official articles, solubilities, effective concentrations, and information on incompatibilities, can be found in Chapter 15, Preservatives.

(2) Benzyl Alcohol and the parabens are not often used in manufactured ophthalmic products, but they are approved for ophthalmic use (8). They are the preservatives most commonly found in Bacteriostatic Water for Injection and Bacteriostatic Sodium Chloride Injection.

d. Before adding a preservative, always check on patient sensitivity, on compatibility of the preservative with all other ingredients in the formulation, and on recommended preservative concentration. *Martindale: The Complete Drug Reference* (formerly *The Extra Pharmacopoeia*) is an excellent resource of compatibility information.

e. Table 27.1 gives the maximum concentrations of preservatives approved for use in nonprescription ophthalmic products.

4. Antioxidants

a. Check references or use your general knowledge of chemistry to decide if the active ingredient(s) are subject to oxidation. If oxidation is a problem, an antioxidant may be necessary or recommended. If an antioxidant is recommended, check references for compatibility information. Maximum concentrations of antioxidants approved for use in nonprescription ophthalmic products are given in Table 27.2.

b. Agents: Although several antioxidants are approved for ophthalmic solutions, as with preservatives, they all have some disadvantages. Sodium Bisulfite, Sodium Metabisulfite, and Disodium Edetate are commonly used antioxidants for ophthalmic products. Information on each of these agents, including descriptions of official articles, solubilities, and effective concentrations, can be found in Chapter 16, Antioxidants.

(1) Sodium bisulfite and sodium metabisulfite

(a) Both are available as the pure powders. Only the metabisulfite is official in the *USP 25-NF 20*, (Sodium Metabisulfite NF), but sodium bisulfite is available as FCC (Food Chemical Codex) grade, which is acceptable for use in drug preparations.

TABLE 27.1	Maximum Concentrations of Preservatives Approved for Use in Ophthalmic Products* (9)
Agent	Maximum Level
Benzalkonium chloride	0.013%
Benzethonium chloride	0.01%
Chlorobutanol	0.5%
Phenylmercuric acetate	0.004%
Phenylmercuric nitrate	0.004%
Thimerosal	0.01%

Maximum levels are for direct contact with eye tissues and not for ocular devices such as contact lens products.

TABLE 27.2 Maximum Concentrations of Ophthalmic Additives for Use in Ophthalmic Products* (9)

Agent	Maximum Level
ANTIOXIDANTS	
Sodium bisulfite	0.1%
Sodium metabisulfite	0.1%
Thiourea	0.1%
Ethylenediaminetetraacetic acid	0.1%
WETTING/CLARIFYING AGENTS	
Polysorbate 80	1.0%
Polysorbate 20	1.0%
VISCOSITY AGENTS	
Polyvinyl alcohol	1.4%
Polyvinylpyrrolidone	1.7%
Methylcellulose	2.0%
Hydroxypropyl methylcellulose	1.0%
Hydroxyethylcellulose	0.8%

*Maximum levels are for direct contact with eye tissues and not for ocular devices such as contact lens products.

    (b) Descriptions and solubilities: See Chapter 16.

    (c) In ophthalmic products, both are used in a concentration of 0.1%.

    (d) Incompatibilities: Even though they have been used as antioxidants in solutions of epinephrine, they are reported to inactivate this compound. The reaction is pH-dependent, and Boric Acid has a stabilizing effect (10).

    (e) As reported in Chapter 16, sulfites must be used with caution because of reported incidents of allergic reactions to these compounds.

  (2). Disodium Edetate (Note: Although Edetic Acid is also an effective antioxidant, it is not often used in compounding ophthalmic solutions because of its poor water solubility)

    (a) Available as a pure powder

    (b) Description and solubility: See Chapter 16.

    (c) In ophthalmic products, Disodium Edetate is used in a concentration of 0.1%.

    (d) As discussed in Chapter 16, Disodium Edetate is technically not an antioxidant, but a chelator of heavy metal ions. It serves as an antioxidant for drugs that have their oxidation catalyzed by heavy metals. Edetate has a synergistic effect on the preservative effectiveness of BAC (11). This may be an added reason for its presence in many commercial ophthalmic products preserved with BAC.

VI. METHODS FOR CALCULATING ISOTONICITY

Ophthalmic solutions that are isotonic with tears are ideal for comfort and should be used when possible. Although the eye will tolerate some deviation from isotonicity without obvious discomfort, pharmacists attempt to compound solutions that are as close as possible to isotonic with tears. There are several methods useful for calculating isotonicity. These are described and illustrated in Chapter 10, Isotonicity Calculations.

VII. COMPOUNDING PROCEDURES

A. Check dose/concentration of the drug carefully.

B. Check on general stability and compatibility of the formulation ingredients.

C.   Amount of solution to make: If the solution must be sterilized by bacterial filtration, a slight excess, 2–5 mL, may be prepared to allow for loss on filtration.

D.   Compounding Procedures and Packaging
1. See the ASHP technical assistance bulletin on pharmacy-prepared ophthalmic products, described at the beginning of this chapter. It is available on ASHP's Internet site. This reference gives good general instructions on preparing ophthalmic solutions.
2. The easiest way to compound an ophthalmic solution is to use sterile water or sterile isotonic saline solution to dissolve sterile, solid drug or to dilute a sterile, concentrated, aqueous solution of the drug. The manipulation of these sterile ingredients should be accomplished using aseptic technique in a sterile environment such as a laminar airflow hood or a barrier isolator.
3. If the active ingredient is not available in a sterile form, a nonsterile but high-quality pure powder may be used.
4. If the resulting solution does not possess the desired properties with respect to comfort, therapeutics, or physical, chemical, or microbiological stability, an appropriate auxiliary agent or agents may be added. An ophthalmic ingredient checklist is shown in Table 27.3. A checklist like this is useful when creating a formulation for a preparation as complex as an ophthalmic solution.
5. If any of the formulation ingredients is not available in sterile form, the compounded preparation requires terminal sterilization, either steam sterilization or bacterial membrane filtration. If bacterial filtration is used, this process should be done in a sterile environment using aseptic technique.
6. Packaging must be in a sterile container. These containers are available for purchase from vendors of compounding supplies. An alternative is to empty the contents of a manufactured ophthalmic product such as artificial tears, rinse the sterile container with sterile water, and use this container for the compounded preparation.

VIII.   BEYOND-USE DATING

A.   Shorter beyond-use datings should be used for these preparations than for other topical solutions because of the danger of contamination during use and the serious consequences of using a nonsterile product. Research has been done and papers have been published on loss of sterility of ophthalmic solutions under conditions of use (12). As a result, some hospitals and nursing homes use a policy of discarding ophthalmic products 30 days after unsealing. The nurse or caregiver dates the sealed ophthalmic container when the seal is broken and the bottle is entered for the first time, and any unused portion is discarded in 30 days. This policy is for sterile, manufactured, preserved solutions used under controlled conditions by health care professionals.

TABLE 27.3 Ophthalmic Ingredient Checklist

Ingredient	Concentration/ Dose	Quantity	Incompatibilities	Water Solubility
Drug:	Rx: Usual:			
Buffer:				
Preservative:				
Antioxidant:				

B. For compounded ophthalmic preparations, especially for preparations used by outpatients, a more conservative beyond-use date is recommended. The *USP* chapter on pharmacy compounding of nonsterile preparations recommends a maximum 14-day dating for all water-containing preparations made with ingredients in solid form when the stability of the ingredients in the formulations is not known (13). With sterile preparations like ophthalmic solutions, an even more conservative approach is advisable. A beyond-use date of 1 to 2 weeks is a reasonable guideline for relatively stable drugs in sterile, preserved solutions. For drugs sensitive to degradation and for those of uncertain stability, a more limited beyond-use date should be considered.

C. Unpreserved ophthalmics should be dispensed in single-dose quantities and should be treated essentially like unpreserved parenteral products. If possible they should be made immediately before use. If use is delayed, they may be stored under refrigeration and warmed to room temperature just before use. A 24-hour dating is recommended for unpreserved ophthalmic solutions (7).

IX. PATIENT CONSULTATION ON USE OF OPHTHALMIC PRODUCTS

A. For outpatient use, be sure to give the patient or caregiver good instructions on how to administer the solution, including techniques to avoid contamination of the top or dropper and the solution.

B. Guides for instructing a patient on the proper administration and use of ophthalmic solutions and ointments are given in Figures 27.1 and 27.2.

■ **Figure 27.1.** HOW TO USE EYE DROPS

1. Wash your hands carefully with soap and warm water.
2. If the product container is transparent, check the solution before use. If it is discolored or has changed in any way since it was purchased (e.g., particles in the solution, color change), do not use the solution. Return it to the pharmacy.
3. If the product container has a depressible rubber bulb, draw up a small amount of medication into the eye dropper by first squeezing, then relieving pressure on the bulb.
4. Place the head back with chin tilted up and look toward the ceiling.
5. With both eyes open, gently draw down the lower lid of the affected eye with your index finger (see illustration A).
6. In the "gutter" formed, drop the directed number of drops.
   IMPORTANT: The dropper or administration tip should be held as near as possible to the lid without actually touching the eye. DO NOT allow the dropper or administration tip to touch any surface.
7. If possible, hold the eyelid open and do not blink for 30 seconds.
8. You may want to press your finger against the inner corner of your eye for one minute. This will keep the medication in your eye (see illustration B).
9. Tightly cap the bottle.
   REMEMBER:

   • This is a **sterile** solution. Contamination of the dropper or eye solution can lead to a serious eye infection. If you accidentally touch the dropper to any surface, wipe the dropper with a clean tissue. If you think you have contaminated the dropper or solution, consult your physician or pharmacist for instructions.

   • If irritation persists or increases, discontinue use, and consult your physician immediately.

   • Generally, eye makeup should be avoided while using eye solutions. If you have questions about this, consult your pharmacist or physician.

   • You may want to use a mirror when applying the drops, or it may be much easier to have someone help you instill your eye drops.

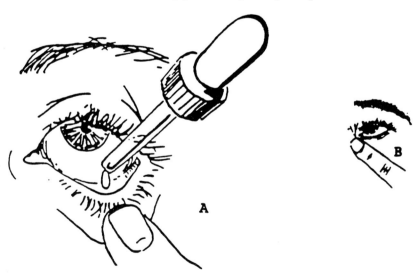

■ **Figure 27.2.** HOW TO USE EYE OINTMENT

1. Wash your hands carefully with soap and warm water.
2. You may want to hold the ointment tube in your hand for a few minutes to warm and soften the ointment.
3. Gently cleanse the affected eyelid with warm water and a soft cloth before applying the ointment.
4. This procedure should be done in front of a mirror.
5. With the affected eye looking upward, gently pull the lower eyelid downward with your index finger to form a pouch.
6. Squeeze a thin line (approximately 1/4–1/2 inch) of ointment from the tube along the pouch.
   IMPORTANT: Be very careful when applying this ointment. DO NOT allow the tip of the ointment tube to touch the eyelid, the eyeball, your finger, or any surface.
7. Close the eye gently and rotate the eyeball to distribute the ointment. You may blink several times to evenly spread the ointment.
8. Replace the cap on the ointment tube.
9. After you apply the ointment, your vision may be blurred temporarily. Do not be alarmed. This will clear up in a short while, but do not drive a car or operate machinery until your vision has cleared.
   REMEMBER:
   • This is a **sterile** ointment. Contamination of the tip or the cap of the tube can lead to a serious eye infection. If you accidentally touch the tip to any surface, wipe it with a clean tissue. If you think you have contaminated the tip or the ointment, consult your physician or pharmacist for instructions.
   • If irritation persists or increases, discontinue use and consult your physician immediately.
   • Generally, eye makeup should be avoided while using eye ointments. If you have questions about this, consult your pharmacist or physician.
   • It may be much easier to have someone help you apply your eye ointment.

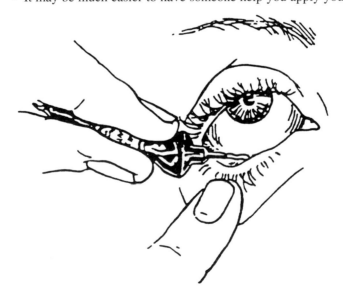

SAMPLE PRESCRIPTIONS

➤ **Prescription 27-1**

Note: Epinephrine HCl 1% Ophthalmic Solution is available as a manufactured product from various sources. It would, therefore, not normally be compounded in the pharmacy. In this case, a sulfite-free solution is needed, and because all of the manufactured products contain sodium metabisulfite as an antioxidant, a compounded preparation is made by the pharmacist.

Contemporary Physicians Group Practice
20 S. Park Street, Triturate, WI 53706
Tel: (608) 555-1333 Fax: (608) 555-1335

℞ # 237

Name *Chelsea Von Katrinca*   Date *00/00/00*

Address *512 Poodle Lane*   Age   Wt/Ht

℞

      Epinephrine HCl   *1%*

      Buffer, preserve and make isotonic, but make sulfite-free
        Dispense 30 mL

                                    J. Jorge 00/00/00

      Sig: 1 drop in left eye q hs

Refills 5   *Paque*   M.D.

                  DEA No. _____

Ingredients Used (Amounts are for 35 mL, 5 mL extra)

Ingredient	Quantity Used	Manufacturer Lot #-Exp Date	Solubility	Dose Comparison		Use in the Prescription
				Given	Usual	
Epinephrine HCl	350 mg	JET Labs OS2711-mm/yy	Readily sol in water	1%	0.25–2%	lower intraocular pressure
BAC 17%	170 mg measured; 3.5 mg used	JET Labs OS2712-mm/yy	v. sol in water & alcohol	0.01%	0.01%	preservative
Disodium Edetate	120 mg weighed; 35 mg used	JET Labs OS2713-mm/yy	soluble in water	0.1%	0.1%	antioxidant
Boric Acid	426 mg	JET Labs OS2714-mm/yy	soluble in water or alcohol	1.2%	—	buffer & isotonicity adjuster
Sterile Water	q.s. ad 35 mL.	Sterile Labs PP2715-mm/yy	—	—	—	vehicle-solvent

Compatibility–Stability/Beyond-Use Date

Stability–Compatibility: Epinephrine is an old, established ophthalmic drug that has been well studied (10,14). When in aqueous solution, the drug is subject to oxidation, racemization, and reactions with bisulfite, an antioxidant often added to epinephrine solutions to retard oxidation of the drug. Epinephrine is most stable at pH = 3–4. It should be protected from light and, as much as possible, from oxygen. Boric Acid has a protective effect against oxidation and bisulfite reactions. When these conditions are met, the drug is quite stable in solution. For this prescription preparation, which is to be made sulfite-free, Disodium Edetate has been added as a chelating agent to protect against oxidation and to enhance the effectiveness of the preservative Benzalkonium Chloride.

Preservative: Benzalkonium Chloride 0.01% is chosen as the preservative.

Packaging and Storage and Beyond-use date: The *USP* monograph for Epinephrine Ophthalmic Solution recommends storage in tight, light-resistant containers (15). The monograph also states that manufactured Epinephrine Ophthalmic Solutions should be labeled to indicate that the solution should not be used if it is pinkish or darker than slightly yellow or if it contains a precipitate. Although properly prepared Epinephrine solutions are quite stable, Pharmacist Jorge will use a conservative 14-day beyond-use date for this compounded ophthalmic solution. Storage at controlled room temperature will be recommended.

Calculations

Dose/Concentration

Concentration is OK for intended use.

Ingredient Amounts

Amounts are for 35 mL of solution to allow for loss in the filtering process.

Active ingredient: Epinephrine HCl (EPI): *1% × 35 mL = 0.35 g*

Preservative: Benzalkonium chloride (BAC) 0.01% is used to preserve this solution. The amount needed to preserve the solution: *0.01% × 35 mL = 0.0035 g = 3.5 mg*

This pharmacy has BAC as the 17% w/v concentrate. Expressed in more convenient units, this is: 17 g/100 mL = 17,000 mg/100 mL = 170 mg/mL. This solution is too concentrated to measure the needed amount, 3.5 mg, directly. A liquid-liquid aliquot is needed. If 1-mL syringes are available for measurement, one possible aliquot would be as follows. Measure 1 mL (170 mg) of the 17% BAC in a syringe, put in a 25-mL graduate, and q.s. to 17 mL with sterile water. This gives a solution with a concentration of 170 mg/17 mL = 10 mg/mL. Using a 1-mL syringe, measure 0.35 mL for the 3.5 mg needed. This can be verified by this calculation:

$$10 \ mg/mL \times 0.35 \ mL = 3.5 \ mg$$

Antioxidant: As stated above, an antioxidant is usually added to Epinephrine solutions because the drug is labile to oxidation. Sodium Metabisulfite is the usual antioxidant used, but in this case the patient is allergic to that compound. Pharmacist Jorge has decided to use the chelating agent Disodium Edetate (EDTA) in a concentration of 0.1% to enhance the stability of the epinephrine. The calculations for obtaining the required amount of this chelating agent are as follows:

$$0.1\% \times 35 \ mL = 0.035 \ g = 35 \ mg$$

This amount is below the MWQ, so a solid-liquid aliquot is needed. Weigh 120 mg (the MWQ) and dissolve in 12 mL of sterile water = 120 mg/12 mL = 10 mg/mL. Take 3.5 mL of this for the 35 mg needed. This can be verified by this calculation:

$$10 \ mg/mL \times 3.5 \ mL = 35 \ mg$$

Isotonicity Calculation

Note: For this prescription the Sodium Chloride Equivalent method is used to determine the amount of tonicity adjustor needed. Boric acid crystals are used as both the tonicity adjustor and the buffering agent. Because of their small concentrations in this preparation, the contributions to isotonicity of the BAC and Disodium Edetate are disregarded. The Sodium Chloride Equivalent values can be found in Appendix H.

The Sodium Chloride (NaCl) Equivalent for Epinephrine HCl (EPI) = 0.29

Amount of NaCl equivalent to 350 mg EPI:

$$\frac{0.29 \ g \ NaCl}{1 \ g \ EPI} = \frac{x \ g \ NaCl}{0.35 \ g \ EPI} ; x = 0.102 \ g \ NaCl$$

The amount of NaCl needed to make 35 mL of sterile water isotonic:

$$0.9\% \times 35\ mL = 0.315\ g$$

Amount of NaCl needed to make 1% EPI solution isotonic:

$$0.315\ g - 0.102\ g = 0.213\ g\ NaCl$$

Boric Acid (BA) will be used as the tonicity adjustor. The Sodium Chloride Equivalent of BA = 0.5

Amount of BA osmotically equivalent to 0.213 g NaCl:

$$\frac{0.5\ g\ NaCl}{1\ g\ B.A.} = \frac{0.213\ g\ NaCl}{x\ g\ B.A.}; x = 0.426\ g\ B.A.$$

This is the amount of BA that needs to be added to the 0.35 g of EPI to make 35 mL of solution isotonic. This should be sufficient for buffering. BA has a MW of 62, so that a solution that is 0.426 g/35 mL is approximately 0.2 M.

Compounding Procedure

Using sterile water, calibrate a small beaker at 35 mL. On a class 3 torsion or electronic balance, weigh 350 mg of Epinephrine HCl and 436 mg of Boric Acid crystals, and place both in the beaker. Weigh 120 mg of Disodium Edetate and place in a 25-mL graduated cylinder. Place the beaker and the graduated cylinder, the bottle of BAC concentrated solution, another 25-mL graduated cylinder, needles, syringes, bacterial membrane filter, and sterile dropper bottle in the LAF hood. Using a 1- or 3-mL syringe, measure 1 mL of BAC 17% and put this in the clean 25-mL graduate; q.s. to 17 mL with sterile water. Agitate to mix and measure 0.35 mL of this dilution using a 1-mL syringe (may either use a fresh syringe or carefully flush out the concentrated BAC solution from the first syringe with diluted BAC solution). Add this dilution to the beaker containing the EPI and Boric Acid. Add 12 mL of sterile water to the graduate containing the EDTA and measure 3.5 mL of this solution (contains 35 mg of Disodium Edetate) and add to the beaker. Q.s. to the 35 mL mark on the beaker with sterile water. Attach a 5-micron filter needle to a 30-mL syringe and use to draw up the 35 mL of solution. Remove the filter needle and apply a 0.22-micron bacterial filter to the syringe tip. With the syringe in an upright position (syringe tip up and plunger down), wet and fill the filter unit until a bead of solution is visible at the end of the filter unit. Now position the syringe with tip down and plunger upward and expel solution in excess of 30 mL onto sterile gauze or into a beaker used for waste solution. Finally push out the desired 30 mL of solution into the sterile dropper bottle. Carefully apply the ophthalmic bottle tip and cap to the bottle and tighten the bottle cap to ensure that the dropper tip is snapped securely in place. Agitate to completely mix the solution. Remove the preparation from the LAF hood; label and dispense.

Quality Control

The preparation is a clear, colorless solution with an apparent viscosity of water. The pH of the preparation is checked and recorded; pH = 5. The final actual volume is checked and matches the theoretical volume of 30 mL plus approximately 4 mL of excess waste solution.

Labeling

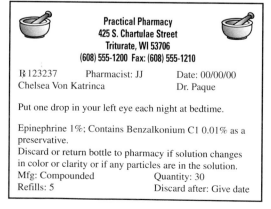

Practical Pharmacy
425 S. Chartulae Street
Triturate, WI 53706
(608) 555-1200 Fax: (608) 555-1210

R 123237   Pharmacist: JJ   Date: 00/00/00
Chelsea Von Katrinca   Dr. Paque

Put one drop in your left eye each night at bedtime.

Epinephrine 1%; Contains Benzalkonium Cl 0.01% as a preservative.
Discard or return bottle to pharmacy if solution changes in color or clarity or if any particles are in the solution.
Mfg: Compounded   Quantity: 30
Refills: 5   Discard after: Give date

Auxiliary Labels: For the Eye

Patient Consultation

Hello, Ms. Von Katrinca, I'm your pharmacist Jennie Jorge. Do you have any drug allergies? Are you currently using any other medications? Do you wear contact lens? Do you know, or has your physician told you, what this medicine is for? This is usually used to reduce the pressure in your eye in conditions such as glaucoma. Place one drop in your left eye each night at bedtime. I am giving you a sheet that describes proper use of eye drops. Would you like me to go over it with you? Use these drops until your physician tells you to stop or for the length of time he has told you. Discontinue and call Dr. Paque if you develop any eye irritation that doesn't go away. This medication should be stored in a cool place, away from the reach of small children. It should be discarded after 2 weeks or if you notice any change in color or clarity or any particles in the solution. This prescription may be refilled five times. Do you have any questions?

➤ Prescription 27-2

Note: Pilocarpine Nitrate 2% Ophthalmic Solution is available as a manufactured product. It would, therefore, not normally be compounded in the pharmacy. This sample prescription is given here to illustrate the use of other auxiliary ingredients and methods for determining isotonicity. A pilocarpine ophthalmic solution that is occasionally prescribed and that must be compounded is for a concentration, usually a more dilute concentration, that is not commercially available. In that case, a manufactured pilocarpine (either the hydrochloride or nitrate) ophthalmic solution may be diluted with an appropriate commercial artificial tears solution. In selecting an artificial tears product, choose one that uses the same preservative system as the product containing the pilocarpine. This will avoid the problem of diluting the preservative beyond its effective concentration. Also check any other auxiliary agents in both products to be sure there are no incompatibility problems.

Contemporary Physicians Group Practice
20 S. Park Street, Triturate, WI 53706
Tel: (608) 555-1333 Fax: (608) 555-1335

R # 248

Name *Shelby Richards*	Date *00/00/00*	
Address *982 Schweppe Road*	Age	Wt/Ht

R

      Pilocarpine Nitrate 2%

      Buffer, preserve and make isotonic

         Dispense 15 mL   *Bernie Brewer 00/00/00*

      Sig: One drop ou qid

Refills 2   *P. V. Heider*   M.D.

         DEA No.

Ingredients Used (Amounts to make 20 mL, 5 mL excess)

Ingredient	Quantity Used	Manufacturer Lot #-Exp Date	Solubility	Dose Comparison Given	Dose Comparison Usual	Use in the Prescription
Pilocarpine Nitrate	0.4 g	JET Labs OS2721-mm/yy	1 g/4 mL water	2%	0.5–6%	glaucoma
PMN 1 : 10,000 Solution	8 mL	Prac. Pharmacy JD8422-mm/yy	v. sl. sol. in water	0.004%	0.002–0.004%	preservative
Sorensen's acid stock soln	14 mL (6.8 mL in prod)	Prac. Pharmacy JD8423-mm/yy	miscible with water	—	—	buffering agent, vehicle
Sorensen's base stock soln	6 mL (2.9 mL in prod)	Prac. Pharmacy JD8424-mm/yy	miscible with water	—	—	buffering agent, vehicle
Sodium Nitrate	0.147 g (71 mg in prod)	JET Labs OS2725-mm/yy	1 g/1.1 mL water	—	—	isotonicity adjustor
Sterile water	2.3 mL	Sterile Labs PP2715-mm/yy	—	—	—	vehicle

Compatibility–Stability/Beyond-Use Date

Stability–Compatibility: Pilocarpine is an old, established ophthalmic drug that has been well studied (16,17). It is most stable at about pH = 5. Pilocarpine is quite stable, even when autoclaved. Protection from light is recommended.

Preservative: Phenylmercuric Nitrate (PMN) 0.004% is chosen as the preservative. Pilocarpine Nitrate is incompatible with Benzalkonium Chloride.

Packaging and Storage and Beyond-use date: The *USP* monograph for Pilocarpine Nitrate Ophthalmic Solution recommends storage in tight, light-resistant containers (15). Although this preparation is known to be very stable, Pharmacist Brewer will use a conservative 14-day beyond-use date for this compounded ophthalmic solution. Storage at controlled room temperature will be recommended.

Calculations

Dose/Concentration

Concentration OK for intended use.

Ingredient Amounts

Note: Calculate for 5 mL excess: *15 mL + 5 mL = 20 mL*

Active Ingredient: Pilocarpine NO$_3$: *2% × 20 mL = 0.4 g*

Preservative: Phenylmercuric Nitrate (PMN) 0.004% is chosen as the preservative (BAC is incompatible with Pilocarpine Nitrate). The amount needed to preserve the solution is calculated: *0.004% × 20 mL = 0.0008 g*

The pharmacy has a 1:10,000 stock solution of PMN. The amount of this solution needed is calculated:

$$\frac{1\ g\ PMN}{10,000\ mL\ solution} = \frac{0.0008\ g\ PMN}{x\ mL\ solution}; x = 8\ mL\ solution$$

Buffer: Sorensen's Modified Phosphate Buffer at pH 6.5 is chosen as the buffer. The pharmacy has the acid and basic stock solutions. Pharmacist Brewer has decided to make 20 mL of the buffer and will make it isotonic with Sodium Nitrate since Sodium Chloride is incompatible with PMN. Upon consulting with Table 17.7 in Chapter 17 for the formula of Sorensen's Modified Phosphate Buffer, it is determined that to obtain a pH of 6.5, the acid and basic stock solutions should be mixed in a ratio of 7:3.

Acid solution (Monobasic Sodium Phosphate solution):   *20 mL × 0.7 = 14 mL*
Basic solution (Dibasic Sodium Phosphate solution):   *20 mL × 0.3 = 6 mL*

From Table 17.7, the amount of NaCl needed to make 100 mL of this buffer solution isotonic is 0.5 g. For 20 mL, the amount is:

$$\frac{0.5 \ g \ NaCl}{100 \ mL \ solution} = \frac{x \ g \ NaCl}{20 \ mL \ solution}; x = 0.1 \ g \ NaCl$$

Sodium Nitrate has a Sodium Chloride Equivalent of 0.68. The amount of Sodium Nitrate equivalent to 0.1 g of NaCl is:

$$\frac{0.68 \ g \ NaCl}{1 \ g \ NaNO_3} = \frac{0.1 \ g \ NaCl}{x \ g \ NaNO_3}; x = 0.147 \ g \ NaNO_3$$

Isotonicity Calculation

With a mixed buffer system like Sorenson's Modified Phosphate Buffer, the easiest method for calculating isotonicity is the USP (also called the Sprowls or White-Vincent) Method. Using values in Appendix H, the volume of water needed to make 1 g of Pilocarpine NO_3 isotonic is 25.7 mL. The volume of water needed to make 0.4 g isotonic is:

$$\frac{1 \ g \ Pilocarpine}{25.7 \ mL \ water} = \frac{0.4 \ g \ Pilocarpine}{x \ mL \ water}; x = 10.3 \ mL \ water$$

The approximate volume of isotonic Sorenson's Modified Phosphate Buffer needed:

$$20 \ mL - 10.3 \ mL = 9.7 \ mL$$

REMEMBER: From an isotonicity point of view, the PMN aliquot solution is like water because the PMN content is so small, so 8 mL of the 10.3 mL of water to make the 0.4 g of Pilocarpine isotonic comes from the PMN aliquot solution.

The following calculations are not required. They are here should you prefer to use Boric Acid (BA) as the tonicity adjustor-buffer. This example uses the freezing point depression method for isotonicity calculations. Isotonicity values are given in Appendix H.

Freezing point depression of a 1% solution of Pilocarpine Nitrate = 0.14°C.

Freezing point depression of a 2% solution of Pilocarpine Nitrate is calculated to be:

$$\frac{1\% \ Pilocarpine \ NO_3}{0.14°C} = \frac{2\% \ Pilocarpine \ NO_3}{x°C}; x = 0.28°C$$

Amount of additional freezing point depression needed for isotonicity:

$$0.52°C - 0.28°C = 0.24°C$$

BA 1.9% solution has a freezing point depression of 0.52°C. The percent BA needed to give a freezing point depression of 0.24°C is calculated to be:

$$\frac{1.9\% \ B.A.}{0.52°C} = \frac{x\% \ B.A.}{0.24°C}; x = 0.88\% \ B.A.$$

Number of grams of BA needed at this concentration for 20 mL of solution is calculated to be:

$$\frac{0.88 \ g \ B.A.}{100 \ mL \ solution} = \frac{x \ g \ B.A.}{20 \ mL}; x = 0.176 \ g \ Boric \ Acid$$

Compounding Procedure

On a class 3 torsion or electronic balance, weigh 0.147 g Sodium Nitrate and place in a clean beaker. Measure 14 mL Sorensen's acid stock solution and 6 mL Sorensen's base solution and add both to the Sodium Nitrate. Swirl to dissolve. Using sterile water, calibrate a small beaker at 20 mL. Weigh 0.4 g Pilocarpine Nitrate and place in the calibrated beaker. Measure 8 mL PMN 1:10,000 in a clean 10-mL graduate and add this to the Pilocarpine in the beaker. Swirl to mix. Measure 2.3 mL sterile water and add this to the Pilocarpine Nitrate solution. Swirl to mix. Use the previously prepared buffer solution to q.s. the Pilocarpine Nitrate solution to 20 mL. Swirl to mix. Inspect for precipitation. For the filtration steps of this procedure, use aseptic technique and perform this part of the procedure in a sterile environment such as an LAF hood or a barrier isolator. Place the drug solution, a bacterial membrane filter, the sterile dropper bottle, and any needed syringes and needles in the LAF hood. Attach a 5-micron filter needle to a 30-mL syringe and draw the 20 mL of drug solution into the syringe. Remove the filter needle and apply a 0.22-micron bacterial filter to the syringe tip. With the syringe in an upright position (syringe tip up and plunger down), wet and fill the filter unit until a bead of solution is visible at the end of the filter unit. Now position the syringe with tip down and plunger upward, and expel solution in excess of 15 mL onto sterile gauze or into a beaker used for waste solution. Finally push out the desired 15 mL of solution into the sterile dropper bottle. Carefully apply the ophthalmic bottle tip and cap to the bottle and tighten the bottle cap to ensure that the dropper tip is snapped securely in place. Agitate to completely mix the solution. Remove the preparation from the LAF hood; label and dispense.

Quality Control

The preparation is a clear, colorless solution with an apparent viscosity of water. The pH of the preparation is checked and recorded; pH = 6.5. The final actual volume is checked and matches the theoretical volume of 15 mL plus the approximately 4 mL of residual excess waste solution.

Labeling

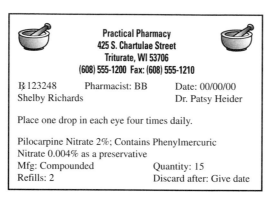

<table>
<tr><td colspan="3" style="text-align:center">Practical Pharmacy
425 S. Chartulae Street
Triturate, WI 53706
(608) 555-1200 Fax: (608) 555-1210</td></tr>
</table>

R 123248   Pharmacist: BB   Date: 00/00/00
Shelby Richards   Dr. Patsy Heider

Place one drop in each eye four times daily.

Pilocarpine Nitrate 2%; Contains Phenylmercuric
Nitrate 0.004% as a preservative
Mfg: Compounded   Quantity: 15
Refills: 2   Discard after: Give date

Auxiliary Labels: For the Eye

Patient Consultation

Hello, Ms. Richards, I'm your pharmacist, Bernie Brewer. Do you have any drug allergies? (If so, what reaction did you have to the medication?) What do you know about this medication (or did your doctor tell you anything about it)? Are you taking or using any other medications? Are you using any other eye drops? Do you wear contact lenses? This medication is Pilocarpine Nitrate eye drops and it is used for glaucoma (or other uses). Place one drop in each eye four times daily. I will give you an instruction sheet that will help you use these drops, and I will be happy to go over the procedure with you. Use this medication until your physician tells you to stop, or for length of time that he has told you. These drops may sting briefly. If they become too irritating or cause severe redness or swelling in your eyes, discontinue use and contact your doctor. Because these drops will contract your pupils, you may notice reduced night or poor light vision. These drops will cause blurred vision. Store at room temperature with the bottle tightly closed. Keep out of reach of children. Protect from freezing. Each time you use the solution, check it to be sure it is still clear and contains no particles. If you notice anything, do not use it, but return it to the pharmacy. Discard any unused portion after 2 weeks (give date). This may be refilled two times. Do you have any questions?

➤ **Prescription 27-3**

Note: This sample prescription is typical of orders for fortified antibiotic ophthalmic solutions, which are made using a manufactured ophthalmic solution and a more concentrated injectable solution of the same antibiotic.

Contemporary Physicians Group Practice
20 S. Park Street, Triturate, WI 53706
Tel: (608) 555-1333 Fax: (608) 555-1335

R # 255

Name _Melvin Dean_   Date _00/00/00_

Address _777 Highland Avenue_   Age _____   Wt/Ht _____

R

Tobramycin Fortified Ophthalmic Solution 1%

Dispense 5 mL

Sig: Put 1 drop in right eye q 4 hr x 7 days

P. Wineswig 00/00/00

Refills _0_   _Lance Smitby_   M.D.

DEA No. _____

Ingredients Used (for 5 mL, no excess made)

Ingredient	Quantity Used	Manufacturer Lot #-Exp Date	Solubility	Dose Comparison		Use in the Prescription
				Given	Usual	
Tobramycin Ophthalmic Solution 0.3%	4 mL	BJF Generics OB2726-mm/yy	misc with water	1% (Tobramycin)	0.3–1.4% (Tobramycin)	antibiotic
Tobramycin Injection 40 mg/mL	1 mL	Sterile Labs PP2715-mm/yy	misc with water	1% (Tobramycin)	0.3–1.4% (Tobramycin)	antibiotic

Compatibility–Stability/Beyond-Use Date

Stability–Compatibility: Fortified Tobramycin ophthalmic solutions are usually made with commercial Tobramycin Ophthalmic Solution and Tobramycin Injection. In a concentration range of 9.1 to 13.6 mg/mL (0.91 to 1.36% w/v), these have been reported in the literature to be stable for at least 91 days when at 8°C (18,19). Preservative: Tobramycin Ophthalmic Solution is available from various manufacturers; all are preserved with 0.01% Benzalkonium Chloride and contain Boric Acid. The injection products contain Phenol, sodium bisulfite, and EDTA.

Packaging and Storage and Beyond-use date: The *USP* monograph for Tobramycin Ophthalmic Solution recommends storage in tight containers and avoiding exposure to excessive heat (15). Although this preparation has been tested to be stable for 91 days, Pharmacist Wineswig will use a conservative 14-day beyond-use date for this compounded ophthalmic solution. Storage at controlled room temperature will be recommended.

Calculations

Dose/Concentration

Although the concentration of the commercial ophthalmic solution is 0.3%, there have been numerous reports of successful use of this antibiotic at this higher concentration.

Ingredient Amounts

The available ingredients for this fortified solution are Tobramycin Ophthalmic Solution 0.3% and Tobramycin Injection 40 mg/mL. The volume of each is calculated using either algebra or alligation. Both methods are shown here. In either case, the concentrations of the solutions must be expressed in a single format, either as percent or as mg/mL. This conversion is shown first.

Tobramycin Ophthalmic Solution: $0.3\% = 0.3 \, g/100 \, mL = 300 \, mg/100 \, mL = 3 \, mg/mL$

Tobramycin Injection 40 mg/mL: $40 \, mg/mL = 0.04 \, g/mL = 4 \, g/100 \, mL = 4\%$

By algebra:

First, the volumes of the two solutions add to the final preparation volume 5 mL:

$$V_I + V_O = 5 \, mL \text{ or } V_I = 5 \, mL - V_O$$

where V_I = volume of the injection (4% or 40 mg/mL)

V_O = volume of the 0.3% ophthalmic solution

Second, the sum of the percent of each solution times its volume is equal to the final percent desired times the final volume desired (this example uses concentration in percent):

$$0.3\% \, (V_O) + 4\% \, (5 - V_O) = 1\% \, (5)$$

$$0.003 \, V_O + 0.2 - 0.04 V_O = 0.05$$

$$0.037 \, V_O = 0.15$$

$$V_O = 4.05 \approx 4 \, mL$$

$$V_I = 5 \, mL - 4 \, mL = 1 \, mL$$

By alligation:

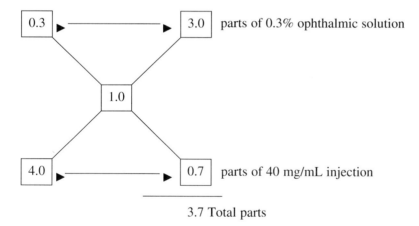

3.7 Total parts

The volume of the 0.3% Tobramycin Ophthalmic Solution is calculated to be:

$$\frac{3 \, parts \, 0.3\% \, Oph.}{3.7 \, parts \, total} = \frac{x \, mL \, 0.3\% \, Oph.}{5 \, mL \, total}; x = 4.05 \, mL \approx 4 \, mL \, of \, 0.3\% \, Oph. \, Solution$$

The volume of the Tobramycin Injection 40 mg/mL (4%) is calculated to be:

$$\frac{0.7 \, parts \, Injection}{3.7 \, parts \, total} = \frac{x \, mL \, Injection}{5 \, mL \, total}; x = 0.95 \, mL \approx 1 \, mL \, Injection$$

Compounding Procedure

Use aseptic technique and perform the procedure in a sterile environment such as an LAF hood or a barrier isolator. Place the drug solutions and any needed syringes and needles in the LAF hood. Remove the cap and dropper tip from the commercial bottle of Tobramycin Ophthalmic Solution. The tip should be removed carefully to avoid contamination; this can be done by using the loosened bottle cap to bend the tip until it dislodges from the bottle. Let the dropper tip rest in the bottle cap in the LAF hood so as to avoid contaminating any part of the tip. (Note: an alternative method is to use a fine-gauge needle to make the transfers through the dropper tip, but with this method, care must be used to avoid enlarging the dropper tip orifice.) Using a 1- or 3-mL syringe, withdraw 1 mL of the ophthalmic solution from its bottle and discard. Attach a 5-micron filter needle to a 3-mL syringe and withdraw a slight excess of 1 mL of drug solution from the Tobramycin Injection vial. Remove the filter needle and apply a regular needle. With the syringe positioned with the needle pointing upward, express any air bubbles and fill the new needle; then, with the needle pointing downward, express any excess drug solution onto sterile gauze or into a waste container so that the volume in the syringe is 1 mL. Transfer the 1 mL of injection to the ophthalmic bottle. Carefully, using the ophthalmic bottle cap, replace the ophthalmic bottle tip onto the bottle and snap the tip in place. Secure the bottle cap and agitate to completely mix the solution. Remove the preparation from the LAF hood; label and dispense.

Quality Control

The preparation is a clear, colorless solution with an apparent viscosity of water. Check the pH of the preparation by expressing a drop of the finished solution from the dropper tip onto pH paper while the finished container is still in the LAF hood; pH = 7.5. The volume from the injection vial in the syringe is verified at 1 mL and the volume remaining in the 2-mL injection vial is approximately 1 mL. This matches the theoretical volume that should remain. The amount withdrawn from the ophthalmic solution bottle is verified at 1 mL and the amount of final solution in the 5-mL ophthalmic bottle appears at the appropriate level.

Labeling

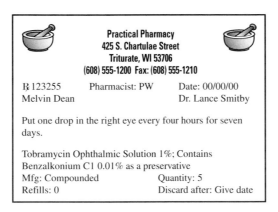

Practical Pharmacy
425 S. Chartulae Street
Triturate, WI 53706
(608) 555-1200 Fax: (608) 555-1210

℞ 123255   Pharmacist: PW   Date: 00/00/00
Melvin Dean   Dr. Lance Smitby

Put one drop in the right eye every four hours for seven days.

Tobramycin Ophthalmic Solution 1%; Contains
Benzalkonium Cl 0.01% as a preservative
Mfg: Compounded   Quantity: 5
Refills: 0   Discard after: Give date

Auxiliary Labels: For the Eye; Keep in the Refrigerator, Do not Freeze

Patient Consultation

Hello, Mr. Dean, I'm your pharmacist, Patsy Wineswig. Do you have any drug allergies? (If so, what reaction did you have to the medication?) What do you know about this medication (or did your doctor tell you anything about it)? Are you taking or using any other medications? Are you using any other eye drops? Do you wear contact lenses? Has your doctor told you when you can start using them again? This medication is Tobramycin eye drops, which is being used to treat your eye infection. Place one drop in your right eye every 4 hours for 7 days. We would like to have you use these drops as much as possible around the clock without your waking especially to put drops in your eye, so put a drop in your eye as soon as you arise in the morning and space out the doses approximately every 4 hours so that you put a drop in your eye just before you go to bed at night. If you do get up in the night and it has been about 3 or 4 hours since your last dose, put one in at that time. Do you understand my meaning? I will give you an instruction sheet that will help you use these drops, and I will be happy to go over the procedure with you. You want to make sure that you do not contaminate the dropper tip on the bottle by touching it to your eye or skin. Use this medication for the full 7 days of therapy. These drops may sting briefly. If they become too irritating or cause severe redness or swelling in your eyes, discontinue use and contact your doctor. Store these in the refrigerator, but protect from freezing. Take them out of the refrigerator a little while before you use them so they warm up a bit closer to room temperature. Keep them out of reach of children. Discard any unused portion as soon as your 7-day therapy is finished and certainly after 2 weeks (give date). You cannot save any leftover drops for future infections as they are not that stable and besides, you may unintentionally get some contamination in them, which grows over time. There are no refills; when did Dr. Smitby want to see you for a recheck? Do you have any questions?

➤ **Prescription 27-4**

Contemporary Physicians Group Practice
20 S. Park Street, Triturate, WI 53706
Tel: (608) 555-1333 Fax: (608) 555-1335

R # 229

Name *Jon Dropp*   Date *00/00/00*

Address *7685 Turkish Lane*   Age   24   Wt/Ht

R

    Cefazolin Ophthalmic Solution   0.33%

    Make isotonic but preservative-free

    Dispense 10 mL

                                    Steve Hunter
                                    00/00/00
    Sig: 1 gtt ou qid

Refills   2   *R. Barksen*   M.D.

DEA No. _____

Ingredients Used (for 10 mL, no excess made)

Ingredient	Quantity Used	Manufacturer Lot #-Exp Date	Solubility	Dose Comparison		Use in the Prescription
				Given	Usual	
Cefazolin Sterile Powder for Injection 250 mg vial	33 mg as 0.26 mL	Sterile Labs PP2728-mm/yy	sol in water	0.33% (Cefazolin)	0.3–1.3% (Cefazolin)	antibiotic
Sodium Chloride 0.9% Injection	2 mL for reconstitution; 9.74 to qs ad 10 mL	Sterile Labs PP2716-mm/yy	misc with water	—	—	vehicle

Compatibility–Stability/Beyond-Use Date

Stability–Compatibility: This sample prescription is typical of antibiotic ophthalmic solutions that are made using a manufactured sterile powder for injection. This preparation is prescribed to be made preservative-free. A *USP* formulation, Cefazolin Ophthalmic Solution, is also 0.33% Cefazolin, but it contains the preservative Thimerosal. That preparation is stated to be stable for 5 days when stored in the refrigerator. Another similar ophthalmic preparation that is 0.5% Cefazolin and that is preservative-free is reported in *Extemporaneous Ophthalmic Preparations* to be stable for 10 days at 2° to 8°C (20). A preparation identical to this one (preservative-free, 0.33% Cefazolin in Sterile Sodium Chloride Injection) is described in *Extemporaneous Ophthalmic Preparations*, and the recommended beyond-use date is 24 hours because of use in an uncontrolled home environment (20). It is obvious from these various sources that Cefazolin has both issues of chemical stability and concerns about contamination of a nonpreserved ophthalmic solution.

Preservative: The preparation below is preservative-free, which would be recommended during and immediately following ocular surgery and at certain other times. When the eye can tolerate a preservative, a preserved version of this solution could also be made by using Bacteriostatic Sodium Chloride Injection. Alternatively, Thimerosal 0.002% could be added, as indicated in the *USP* formulation.

Packaging and Storage and Beyond-use date: The *USP* monograph for Cefazolin Ophthalmic Solution requires storage in a sterile ophthalmic container (15). Pharmacist Hunter will use a conservative 24-hour beyond-use date for this nonpreserved compounded ophthalmic solution and will make fresh solution daily for this patient until the patient's eye can tolerate a preserved solution. Storage will be in the refrigerator. If a preservative is added to the preparation, the beyond-use date can be extended to 5 days when stored in the refrigerator.

Calculations

Dose/Concentration

Concentrations of Cefazolin in topical ophthalmic solutions in the range of 33 mg/mL (0.33%) to 133 mg/mL (1.33%) have been reported.

Ingredient Amounts

Cefazolin: *0.33% × 10 mL = 0.0033 × 10 mL = 0.033 g = 33 mg*

Cefazolin is available as the sodium salt in vials containing the powder for reconstitution. The 250-mg and 500-mg vials may be reconstituted with Sterile Water for Injection, Bacteriostatic Water for Injection, or Sodium Chloride Injection. The 250-mg vial is reconstituted with 2 mL of diluent to give 2 mL of solution with a concentration of 125 mg/mL (that is, zero powder volume). The 500-mg vial is reconstituted with 2 mL of diluent to give 2.2 mL of solution with a concentration of 225 mg/mL (that is, 0.2 mL powder volume).

Using a 250-mg vial and reconstituting it with 2 mL of diluent, we can calculate the volume of the injection to contain the 33 mg of Cefazolin that is needed:

$$\frac{250\ mg\ Cefazolin}{2\ mL\ solution} = \frac{33\ mg\ Cefazolin}{x\ mL\ solution}; x = 0.26\ mL\ solution$$

Add 9.74 mL of sterile diluent to the 0.26 mL of the above solution to give 10 mL of solution with a concentration of 33 mg/10 mL or 0.33%.

In selecting whether to use Sterile Water for Injection or Sodium Chloride 0.9% Injection as the diluent, our selection is made based on obtaining a solution that is as close as possible to isotonic. Either of the following methods can be used. The Sodium Chloride Equivalent, Freezing Point Depression, and USP Method values can be found in Appendix H. Note that the values in the table are for Cefazolin **Sodium**, which is the form of the drug we are using, and Cefazolin Sodium contains 2 mg of sodium/33 mg of cefazolin. Therefore, for these calculations we will use the content of Cefazolin Sodium in our preparation, 35 mg rather than 33 mg, and a percent concentration of 0.35% rather than 0.33%.

The easiest and most intuitive method to use in this case is the USP method. The V^{1g} value gives the volume of water that will make 1 g of the drug or chemical isotonic. The V^{1g} value for Sodium Cefazolin is 14.4 mL. The volume for 35 mg or 0.035 g is calculated to be:

14.4 mL/1 g Sodium Cefazolin × 0.035 g Sodium Cefazolin = 0.5 mL water

Obviously, from an isotonicity point of view, 0.5 mL out of a 10-mL preparation is a negligible amount of water needed, so Sodium Chloride Injection could be used entirely as the diluent for this preparation.

Sodium Chloride Equivalent Method:

The Sodium Chloride Equivalent for Sodium Cefazolin = 0.13

Amount of NaCl equivalent to 35 mg Sodium Cefazolin:

$$\frac{0.13\ g\ NaCl}{1\ g\ Na\ Cefazolin} = \frac{x\ g\ NaCl}{0.035\ g\ Na\ Cefazolin}; x = 0.0046\ g\ NaCl$$

The amount of NaCl needed to make 10 mL of sterile water isotonic:

0.9% × 10 mL = 0.009 × 10 mL = 0.09 g NaCl needed

Amount of NaCl needed to make Sodium Cefazolin solution isotonic:

0.09 g − 0.0046 g = 0.0854 g NaCl needed

As we can see, 0.0854 g is very close to 0.09 g, and the contribution of the 35 mg of Sodium Cefazolin to isotonicity for our 10-mL preparation is negligible. We can use Sodium Chloride Injection for our diluent.

Freezing Point Depression Method:

Freezing point depression of a 1% solution of Sodium Cefazolin = 0.07°C

Freezing point depression of a 0.35% solution of Sodium Cefazolin is calculated to be:

$$\frac{0.07°C}{1\% \, Na\,Cefazolin} = \frac{x°C}{0.35\% \, Na\,Cefazolin}; x = 0.024°C$$

Amount of additional freezing point depression need for isotonicity:

$$0.52°C - 0.024°C = 0.496°C \approx 0.50°C$$

Again, we can see that 0.50° is very close to 0.52°, and the contribution of the 35 mg of Sodium Cefazolin to isotonicity for our preparation is negligible. We can use Sodium Chloride Injection for our diluent.

Compounding Procedure

Use aseptic technique and perform the procedure in a sterile environment such as an LAF hood or a barrier isolator. Place the drug and diluent vials and any needed syringes and needles in the LAF hood. Using a 3-mL syringe, withdraw 2 mL of Sodium Chloride 0.9% Injection (could also use Sterile Water for Injection for this part) from its vial and inject into the Cefazolin Sodium vial. Shake the vial to dissolve the drug and mix the solution. Attach a 5-micron filter needle to a 1-mL syringe and withdraw a slight excess of 0.26 mL of drug solution from the Cefazolin Sodium vial. Remove the filter needle and apply a regular needle. With the syringe positioned with the needle pointing upward, express any air bubbles and fill the new needle; then, with the needle pointing downward, express any excess drug solution onto sterile gauze or into a waste container so that the volume in the syringe is 0.26 mL. Transfer the 0.26 mL of injection to a sterile ophthalmic bottle. Using a 10-mL syringe, transfer 9.74 mL of Sodium Chloride 0.9% Injection to the ophthalmic bottle. Carefully apply the ophthalmic bottle tip and cap to the bottle and tighten the bottle cap to ensure that the dropper tip is snapped securely in place. Agitate to completely mix the solution. Remove the preparation from the LAF hood; label and dispense.

Quality Control

The preparation is a clear, colorless solution with an apparent viscosity of water. Check the pH of the preparation by expressing a drop of the finished solution from the dropper tip onto pH paper while the finished container is still in the LAF hood; pH = 5. The volume from the injection vial that was drawn into the syringe is verified at 0.26 mL, and the volume remaining in the 2 mL injection vial is approximately 1.7 mL. This matches the theoretical volume that should remain. The amount of final solution in the ophthalmic bottle appears at the appropriate level for the bottle size.

Labeling

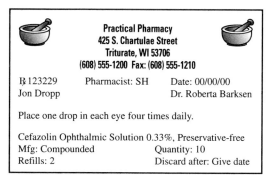

Practical Pharmacy
425 S. Chartulae Street
Triturate, WI 53706
(608) 555-1200 Fax: (608) 555-1210

R 123229   Pharmacist: SH   Date: 00/00/00
Jon Dropp   Dr. Roberta Barksen

Place one drop in each eye four times daily.

Cefazolin Ophthalmic Solution 0.33%, Preservative-free
Mfg: Compounded   Quantity: 10
Refills: 2   Discard after: Give date

Auxiliary Labels: For the Eye, Keep in the Refrigerator, Do not Freeze

Patient Consultation

Hello, Mr. Dropp, I'm your pharmacist, Steve Hunter. Do you have any drug allergies? (If so, what reaction did you have to the medication?) What do you know about this medication (or did your doctor tell you anything about it)? Are you taking or using any other medications? Are you using any other eye drops? Do you wear contact lenses? Has your doctor discussed with you when you can start using them again? This medication is

Cefazolin eye drops, which is being used to prevent an eye infection following your eye surgery. Place one drop in each eye four times a day. We would like to have you space out your doses as much as possible, so put a drop in each eye as soon as you arise in the morning and space out the doses so that you put drops in your eyes just before you go to bed at night. I will give you an instruction sheet that will help you use these drops, and I will be happy to go over the procedure with you. You want to make sure that you do not contaminate the dropper tip on the bottle by touching it to your eye or skin. These drops should be comfortable to use, but if they become irritating or cause redness or swelling in your eyes, discontinue use and contact your doctor. Store these in the refrigerator, but take them out of the refrigerator a little while before you use them so they warm up a bit. Keep them out of reach of children. Because these drops do not contain a preservative, bacteria, viruses, or molds could grow in the solution if it should be contaminated during use. Because you eye is so sensitive to infection right now, we want to guard against this, so I will make a fresh solution for you every day. Discard any unused portion as soon as you pick up you new bottle. At the end of 3 days, Dr. Barksen has told me she wants to see you. We will then evaluate your situation, and we may give you the same type of drops with a preservative so you don't have to get a fresh solution every day. Do you have any questions?

References

1. The 2002 United States Pharmacopeia 25/National Formulary 20. Rockville, MD: The United States Pharmacopeial Convention, Inc., 2001;2219–2220.
2. Gonnering R, et al. The pH tolerance of rabbit and human corneal endothelium. Invest Ophthalmol Vis Sci 1979;18: 373–390.
3. The 1985 United States Pharmacopeia XXI-National Formulary XVI. Rockville, MD: The United States Pharmacopeial Convention, Inc., 1985;1338–1339.
4. Cadwallader DE. EENT preparations. In: King RE. Dispensing of medication, 9th ed. Easton, PA: Mack Publishing Co., 1984;149–150.
5. Hanson AL. A practical guide to the compounding and dispensing of basic dosage forms. Madison, WI: University of Wisconsin, 1982;97.
6. Martin A, Bustamante P. Physical pharmacy, 4th ed. Philadelphia: Lea & Febiger, 1993;178.
7. Reynolds LA, Closson RG. Extemporaneous ophthalmic preparations. Vancouver, WA: Applied Therapeutics, Inc., 1993;6–7.
8. Kibbe AH. Handbook of Pharmaceutical Excipients, 3rd ed. Washington DC: American Pharmaceutical Association and Pharmaceutical Press, 2000.
9. FDA Advisory Review Panel on OTC Ophthalmic Drug Products. Final report, December 1979.
10. Connors KA, Amidon GL, Stella VJ. Chemical stability of pharmaceuticals, 2nd ed. New York: John Wiley & Sons, 1986;438–447.
11. Deardorff DL. Ophthalmic solutions. In: Hoover JE, ed. Remington's pharmaceutical sciences, 14th ed. Easton, PA: Mack Publishing Co., 1970;1545–1577.
12. Ford JL, Brown MW, Hunt PB. A note on the contamination of eye-drops following use by hospital outpatients. J Clin Hosp Pharm 1985;10: 203–209.
13. The 2002 United States Pharmacopeia 25/National Formulary 20. Rockville, MD: The United States Pharmacopeial Convention, Inc., 2001;2054.
14. Trissel LA. Trissel's Stability of Compounded Formulations, 2nd end. Washington DC: American Pharmaceutical Association, 2001;140-142.
15. The 2002 United States Pharmacopeia 25/National Formulary 20. Rockville, MD: The United States Pharmacopeial Convention, Inc., 2001; Official Monographs.
16. Connors KA, Amidon GL, Stella VJ. Chemical stability of pharmaceuticals, 2nd ed. New York: John Wiley & Sons, 1986;675-684.
17. Trissel LA. Trissel's Stability of Compounded Formulations, 2nd ed. Washington DC: American Pharmaceutical Association, 2001;302-304.
18. Reynolds LA, Closson RG. Extemporaneous ophthalmic preparations. Vancouver, WA: Applied Therapeutics, Inc., 1993;304–305.
19. McBride HA, et al. Stability of gentamicin sulfate and tobramycin sulfate in extemporaneously prepared ophthalmic solutions at 8°C. Am J Hosp Pharm. 1991;48: 507–509.
20. Reynolds LA, Closson RG. Extemporaneous ophthalmic preparations. Vancouver, WA: Applied Therapeutics, Inc., 1993;81–84.

CHAPTER 28

Suspensions

I. DEFINITIONS

A. **Suspensions:** "Suspensions are liquid preparations that consist of solid particles dispersed throughout a liquid phase in which the particles are not soluble." (1)—*USP*

B. **Surfactants:** As stated in Chapter 19, surfactants are molecules that are adsorbed at interfaces (2). Their molecular structures contain both a hydrophilic and a hydrophobic portion. They orient themselves at interfaces so as to reduce the interfacial free energy produced by the presence of the interface (3). For a detailed discussion of surfactants, see Chapter 19.

C. **Wetting Agents:** Wetting agents are surfactants that, when dissolved in water, lower the contact angle between a surface and the liquid and aid in displacing the air phase at the surface and replacing it with liquid phase (4).

II. USES OF SUSPENSIONS

A. Oral Products
   1. There is often a need to administer solid drugs orally in liquid form to patients \ cannot swallow tablets or capsules. These patients include adults who cannot swallow solid dosage forms, infants or children who have not yet learned how to swallow whole tablets or capsules, nonambulatory patients with nasogastric (NG) tubes, and geriatric patients who no longer have the ability to swallow solid oral dosage units.
   2. A manufactured liquid product should be used if available because the manufacturer has conducted stability and bioavailability testing on the product. Although a fairly large number of oral liquid drug products are now manufactured by pharmaceutical companies, many therapeutic agents are still not available in liquid dosage forms. Furthermore, in recent years there have been significant problems with product shortages, including oral liquids. When a manufactured product is unavailable, pharmacists are often asked to compound oral liquid preparations for their patients who need them.
   3. Liquid preparations can be made as solutions, suspensions, or emulsions, depending on the physical state and solubility properties of the active ingredients. For drugs that are soluble in water or a cosolvent system that is appropriate for oral use, oral solutions are made; oral and topical solutions are discussed in Chapter 26. If the active ingredient is an immiscible liquid, a liquid emulsion may be formulated; liquid emulsions are described in Chapter 29. When a liquid preparation is needed for a drug that is an insoluble solid, a suspension is formulated. In some cases, an insoluble form of a drug is made intentionally because the drug in soluble form has a bad taste.

B.   Topical Products

1. As with oral liquids, a manufactured liquid product should be used if available.

2. Often, topical liquid preparations require compounding by the pharmacist because dermatologists and other prescribers like to create their own unique formulas customized for a specific patient with a particular skin condition. As stated above, topical solutions are discussed in Chapter 26; liquid emulsions, including those for topical administration, are described in Chapter 29.

III.   DESIRED PROPERTIES OF A SUSPENSION

A.   Fine, Uniform-Sized Particles

1. Very fine particles are desirable for both topical and oral suspensions. Particles in suspensions usually range from 0.5 to 3 microns (micrometers) in diameter.

    a. Uniform, finely divided particles give optimal dissolution and absorption. This is particularly important for suspensions that are intended for systemic use.

    b. A smooth, nongritty product is essential for patient acceptance. This is true for both topical and internal-use preparations.

    c. As discussed below, small, uniform-sized particles are needed to give suspensions with acceptable sedimentation rates.

2. Solid powders used for making suspensions should be in the finest state of subdivision possible. This is achieved through choice of drug form, through proper selection of compounding equipment, and through use of good compounding techniques.

    a. Choice of drug form

        (1) If a prescription order specifies a certain form of a drug, that form must be used unless the prescriber is consulted. For example, if the prescription lists Precipitated Sulfur as an ingredient, that form should be used in the formulation.

        (2) In general, if a drug or chemical is available in more than one form and no form is specified on the prescription order, choose the form that has the finest particle size (e.g., Boric Acid powder rather than Boric Acid crystals, Colloidal Sulfur rather than Precipitated Sulfur). Remember, however, that very fine particles have a high degree of surface free energy, and very fine particles have an increased tendency to aggregate and eventually fuse together into a non-dispersible cake (5). For a complete discussion of this subject and factors to consider and control, consult a book on physical pharmacy.

        (3) The form of drug or chemical used in compounding should be specified on the face of the prescription document or on the record of compounding. This ensures product uniformity with each prescription refill.

    b. Compounding equipment and technique

        (1) Suspensions are made in the pharmacy using mortars and pestles. Choice of mortar type depends both on the characteristics of the ingredients and the volume of the preparation.

        (2) Proper technique for reducing particle size is discussed in Chapter 24, Powders.

        (3) Some pharmacists have found that they can ensure more uniform particles of the desired size for dispersions by passing the prepared powder through a sieve. A mesh size of the range 35–45 is considered adequate for suspensions. An example of this is in the *USP* compounding monograph for Ketoconazole Oral Suspension, which states, "If Tablets are used, finely powder the Tablets such that they pass through a 40-mesh or 45-mesh sieve." (6) Pharmaceutical sieves and mesh sizes are described and discussed in Chapter 24. Small sieve nests with mesh sizes suitable for compounding can be ordered from some vendors of compounding supplies.

Sieving a powder

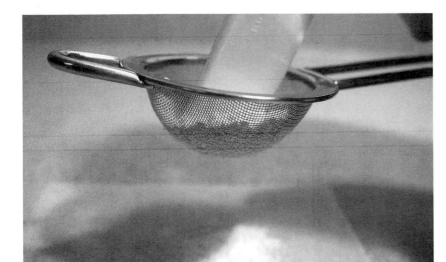

B. Uniform Dispersion of the Particles in the Liquid Vehicle
Because, in a suspension, the solid does not dissolve, the solid should be evenly dispersed in the liquid vehicle. This ensures a uniform mixture and a uniform dose. To accomplish this, the insoluble powder must be properly "wet": that is, the air on the surface of the powder particles must be displaced by liquid.

1. If the liquid vehicle is one with a low surface tension, this is not a problem; the liquid will easily wet the solid.

2. In most situations, however, water constitutes all or part of the dispersing liquid; water has a high surface tension and does not easily wet many solids, especially hydrophobic drugs or chemicals. When the liquid vehicle contains water, special additives, techniques, or order of mixing may be needed to create a uniform suspension. The ingredients and procedure depend on the nature of the solid phase, the other ingredients in the formulation, and the intended route of administration.

    a. If the insoluble powders are **hydrophilic**, they will be wet easily by water or any other liquid used for pharmaceutical preparations. In this case, no special additives or procedures are necessary.

       (1) Two common examples of powders in this class are Zinc Oxide and Calamine. Even though these ingredients are easily wet by the suspending liquid, they should be initially mixed with a small amount of that liquid to form a thick paste. In compounding, this is usually done by trituration using a mortar and pestle. This facilitates the desired efficient shearing of the solid particles and intimate mixing with the vehicle to give a nice, smooth suspension. This procedure is illustrated with Calamine Lotion USP, which is described in Sample Prescription 28.1.

       (2) Most manufactured tablets, when used as ingredients for suspensions, are also easily wet by water. They have been formulated with disintegrants, which absorb water to enhance the breakup of the tablet in the gastrointestinal tract. Tablet material is readily wet by a small amount of water or Glycerin. (This is illustrated in Sample Prescription 28.5, which is described in this chapter and demonstrated on the CD that accompanies this book.)

    b. Many water-insoluble drugs are **hydrophobic**; these powders are not easily wet by water. To wet such a solid, either a water-miscible liquid with a low surface tension may be used, or a wetting agent may be added to the water to reduce its surface tension. In both cases, remember to consider the route of administration when selecting an additive to improve wetting; additives to oral suspensions must be approved for internal use.

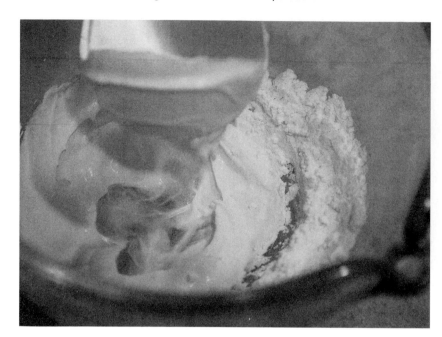

Wetting of a hydrophobic powder with Glycerin

(1) Use of water-miscible liquids with low surface tension for wetting solids: Although water has a surface tension of 72.8 dynes/cm at 20°C, Glycerin has a surface tension of 63.4 dynes/cm; therefore, glycerin is a better wetting medium for hydrophobic drugs than is water. Examples of liquids used for wetting hydrophobic solids include Glycerin, Alcohol, Propylene Glycol, Polyethylene Glycol, any liquid surfactant, or an ingredient containing a surfactant. The use of liquids of this type for wetting a hydrophobic powder is illustrated with the compounding procedure in Sample Prescription 28.4.

(2) Use of wetting agents: A wetting agent is a surfactant that, when added to water, improves its ability to wet hydrophobic powders. Examples include soaps such as Sodium Stearate, detergents such as Sodium Lauryl Sulfate and dioctyl sodium sulfosuccinate (Docusate Sodium), and nonionic surfactants such as Polysorbate 80. These are discussed and described in Chapter 19, Surfactants and Emulsifying Agents.

c. If possible, an ingredient that is already in the prescription order should be used for wetting the insoluble solid. If there are no suitable liquids or surfactants in the formulation, use professional judgment to decide what, if anything, should be added. A small amount of Glycerin, Alcohol, or Propylene Glycol is often helpful. A convenient source of surfactant in a pharmacy is the stool softener Docusate Sodium. Docusate Sodium is available formulated both in a liquid and in soft-gelatin capsules. To use a capsule, cut through the soft gelatin with a razor blade and express the contents into a small amount of water.

C. Slow Settling of the Particles (That Is, Slow Sedimentation Rate)

Although it is impossible to completely prevent settling of solid particles in a suspension, the rate of sedimentation can be controlled. Stoke's Law provides useful information in determining what parameters of a suspension should be controlled to retard the sedimentation rate of particles in a suspension.

$$v = \frac{2r^2(\rho_s - \rho_l)g}{9\eta}$$

where: v = velocity of sedimentation

g = gravitational acceleration

ρ_s = density of the solid

ρ_l = density of the liquid

r = radius of the particles

η = viscosity of the liquid

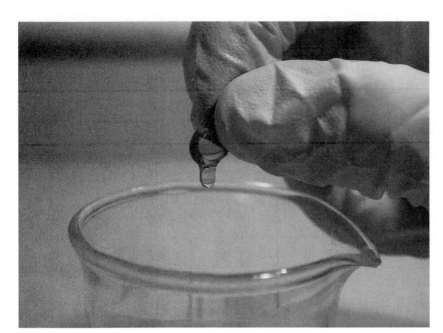

Extracting surfactant Docusate Na from a soft shell capsule.

Although gravitational acceleration (g) is a constant and the density of the solid (ρ_s) cannot be changed, the other factors in Stoke's Law can be manipulated to minimize sedimentation rate (v):

1. r: The particle size should be as small and uniform as possible. As discussed previously, this is controlled through choice of drug form and through proper use of compounding equipment and technique.

2. ρ_l: The density of the liquid may be increased. If the density of the liquid could be made equal to the density of the solid, the term ($\rho_s - \rho_l$) becomes zero, the sedimentation rate becomes zero, and the suspended particles do not settle. Although this is rarely achieved (e.g., Zinc Oxide has a density of 5.6, whereas water has a density of 1.0), the density of the medium can be manipulated to improve the sedimentation rate.

   a. For oral suspensions, the density of the liquid can be increased by adding Sucrose, Glycerin, Sorbitol, or other soluble or miscible, orally acceptable additives. Glycerin has a density of 1.25, Syrup NF has a density of 1.3, and Sorbitol 70% has a density of 1.285.

   b. For topical suspensions, any nontoxic soluble or miscible ingredient that is approved for topical use and that would increase density is acceptable.

3. η: The viscosity of the liquid medium may be increased by adding a viscosity-inducing agent, such as Methylcellulose, Sodium Carboxymethylcellulose, Acacia, Tragacanth, Carbomer, Colloidal Silicon Dioxide, Bentonite, or Veegum®. Detailed information on viscosity-inducing agents and their use is given in Chapter 18.

D. Ease of Redispersion When the Product Is Shaken

1. Solids should not form a hard "cake" on the bottom of the bottle when the preparation is allowed to stand.

   a. As stated previously, very fine particles have an increased tendency to aggregate and eventually fuse together into a non-dispersible cake because of the high surface free energy associated with very fine particles. This factor should be considered in selecting ingredients for suspensions.

   b. Because caking requires time to develop, a conservative beyond-use date should be considered for suspensions at risk for this problem.

2. The preparation should be sufficiently fluid so that redispersion of settled particles is easily accomplished with normal shaking of the container. The liquid should also pour freely from the container when a dose is to be administered or applied. Judicious use

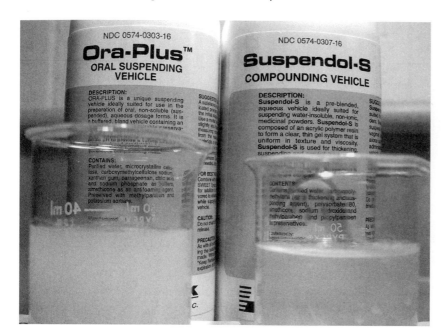

A sample of manufactured suspension vehicles for compounding

of viscosity-increasing ingredients when formulating suspensions is important in achieving this goal.

3. One special formulation technique, **flocculation**, is useful in producing suspensions that readily redisperse.

   a. Flocculation gives a controlled lacework-like structure of particles held together by weak bonds. These weak bonds hold the particles in the structure when the suspension is at rest, but break apart easily when the suspension is shaken.

   b. This technique is often used in the pharmaceutical industry for manufactured suspension products. Some viscosity-inducing agents, such as Bentonite and Xanthan Gum, form flocculated systems; these are available to the pharmacist and are useful as suspending agents in compounding.

   c. Various manufactured suspending vehicles, such as Ora-Plus® and Suspendol-S®, and the official NF suspending vehicles, Bentonite Magma, Suspension Structured Vehicle, and Sugar-Free Suspension Structured Vehicle, are examples of flocculated systems that are helpful in making suspensions that settle slowly, but that are easily redispersed on shaking.

IV. COMPOUNDING SUSPENSIONS

A. Calculate the amount of each ingredient required in the prescription or formulation.

B. Select the desired form for each solid ingredient. In some cases, this form depends on availability. For example, some drugs may be available only as manufactured tablets or capsules.

C. If tablets or capsules are used as an ingredient source for an active ingredient, the procedure varies depending on the need for either a whole number or a fractional number of units. Remember that tablets and capsule powder contain added formulation ingredients, and this must be considered when determining the amount of tablet or capsule material to use in making the suspension.

   1. If a whole number of tablets or capsules is needed, determine the correct number of dosage units to add, crush the tablets or empty the capsule contents in a mortar, and proceed with making the suspension. There is no need to first weigh the tablets or capsule contents. For an illustration of this procedure, see Sample Prescription 28.5.

2. If a fractional number of dosage units is needed, follow the steps given here. See also Sample Prescriptions 24.5 and 24.6 in Chapter 24 and Sample Prescription 28.6 in this chapter for examples of this procedure.

   a. Determine the average weight of a tablet or the contents of a capsule. If only one unit is needed, weigh that unit or, for a capsule, the contents of that unit. Remember, for capsules you will not be adding the capsule shell to the suspension, so this should not be weighed.

   b. Determine the amount of crushed tablet or capsule content needed for the suspension:

   $$\frac{mg \; of \; drug / tablet \; or \; capsule}{wt. \; of \; a \; tablet \; or \; capsule} = \frac{mg \; of \; drug \; needed}{x \; wt. \; tablet \; or \; capsule \; material \; needed}$$

   $$x = mg \; or \; g \; of \; tablet \; or \; capsule \; material \; needed$$

   c. Crush a sufficient number of tablets or empty a sufficient number of capsules and weigh the amount calculated above.

D. Use the techniques described in Chapter 24, Powders, for reducing particle size and mixing the powders.

E. Using the principles just described, wet the powders. When doing this, use a small amount of liquid so that a thick paste is obtained for efficient shearing of the solid particles in the mortar.

F. Add liquid vehicle in portions with trituration until a smooth, uniform preparation is obtained.

G. To ensure complete transfer of the suspended solid active ingredient to the dispensing container, use some of the remaining vehicle to rinse the material from the mortar into the dispensing container.

H. Add sufficient vehicle to the dispensing container to make the preparation the desired volume.

I. Some pharmacists recommend that suspensions be homogenized for maximum uniformity and improved physical stability. This can be accomplished by passing the suspension through a hand homogenizer or by using a high-speed blender or homogenizer. If this is done, you may need to make extra suspension to allow for loss of some preparation in the equipment.

V. STABILITY

A. Physical stability of the system: Both maintenance of small particles and ease of redispersion are essential to the physical stability of the system. Because suspensions are by nature physically unstable systems, beyond-use dates for these preparations should be conservative. This is discussed in Chapter 4, Expiration and Beyond-use Dating.

B. Chemical stability of the ingredients

   1. Check references such as *Trissel's Stability of Compounded Formulations, Chemical Stability of Pharmaceuticals, Extemporaneous Formulations, Pediatric Drug Formulations,* the *USP/DI Vol I,* or professional pharmacy journals such as the *International Journal of Pharmaceutical Compounding,* or the *American Journal of Health-System Pharmacy.* Chemical stability in general is discussed in Chapter 34 and in Chapter 4, Expiration and Beyond-use Dating, and this topic is considered for the prescription ingredients in each of the sample prescriptions in this chapter.

2. The *USP* chapter on pharmacy compounding, Chapter ⟨795⟩, recommends a maximum 14-day dating for all water-containing preparations made with ingredients in solid form when the stability of the ingredients in the formulations is not known (7). Concerns for chemical stability of known labile drugs may limit expiration time even more.
3. The *USP* requires that suspensions be stored and dispensed in tight containers (1).
4. While technically it is very easy to make suspensions from crushed tablets and available suspending vehicles, care should always be used in checking and validating the stability and the beyond-use date of the compounded preparation.

C. Microbiological stability
1. The USP states that suspensions should contain preservatives to protect against bacteria, yeasts, and molds (1). If antimicrobial ingredients are prescribed as part of the formulation, extra preservatives are not needed.
2. Remember that for suspensions, precipitation of the preservative is less of a concern because you are dealing with a disperse system, not a solution. A saturated solution of the preservative will be maintained, and this should be sufficient for preservation.
3. Antimicrobial agents and their proper use are discussed in Chapter 15, and consideration of preservatives is presented in each of the following sample prescription formulations.

VI.   LABELING

A.   All suspensions are disperse systems and require a "Shake Well" auxiliary label.

B.   External use suspensions should be labeled "For External Use Only."

SAMPLE PRESCRIPTIONS

➤ **Prescription 28.1**

Contemporary Physicians Group Practice
20 S. Park Street, Triturate, WI 53706
Tel: (608) 555-1333 Fax: (608) 555-1335

R # 655

Name *Deborah Summit*   Date *00/00/00*

Address *857 Triangle Parkway*   Age   Wt/Ht

R

    Calamine Lotion USP

    Dispense 180 mL

                                 J. Joyous 00/00/00

    Sig: Apply to poison ivy q 4 hr prn

Refills *3*   ___*Marcy Dacy*___   M.D.

DEA No. _____

Ingredients Used

Ingredient	Quantity Used	Manufacturer Lot #-Exp Date	Solubility	Dose Comparison		Use in the Prescription
				Given	Usual	
Calamine	14.4 g	JET Labs SS2811-mm/yy	insol in water and alcohol	8%	5–20%	astringent, antiseptic; protective
Zinc Oxide	14.4 g	JET Labs SS2812-mm/yy	insol in water and alcohol	8%	5–20%	astringent, antiseptic; protective
Glycerin	3.6 mL	JET Labs SS2813-mm/yy	misc w/ water and alcohol	2%	—	humectant, wetting, levigating agent
Bentonite Magma	45 mL	JET Labs SS2814-mm/yy	Bentonite insoluble	—	—	suspending medium
Calcium Hydroxide Solution	q.s. 180 mL	Prac. Pharm. JT1143-mm/yy	—	—	—	astringent, vehicle

Compatibility–Stability/Beyond-Use Date

Stability–Compatibility: This is an official USP formulation that is known to be very stable.

Packaging and Storage and Beyond-use date: The *USP* monograph for this preparation recommends storage in tight containers (8). Although manufactured versions of this formulation are given expiration dates of several years, Pharmacist Joyous will use a more conservative 6-month beyond-use date for this compounded preparation.

Calculations

Dose/Concentration

USP formula − All concentrations OK

Ingredient Amounts

The formula for Calamine Lotion USP is (8):

Calamine	80 g
Zinc Oxide	80 g
Glycerin	20 mL
Bentonite Magma	250 mL
Calcium Hydroxide Topical Solution a sufficient quantity to make	1,000 mL

Reducing this formula to make 180 mL:

Calamine and Zinc Oxide:

$$\frac{80\ g}{1000\ mL} = \frac{x\ g}{100\ mL}; x = 14.4\ g$$

Glycerin:

$$\frac{20\ mL\ Glycerin}{1000\ mL\ lotion} = \frac{x\ mL\ Glycerin}{180\ mL\ lotion}; x = 3.6\ mL\ Glycerin$$

Bentonite Magma:

$$\frac{250\ mL\ Bentonite\ Magma}{1000\ mL\ lotion} = \frac{x\ mL\ Bentonite\ Magma}{180\ mL\ lotion}; x = 45\ mL\ Bentonite\ Magma$$

Calcium Hydroxide Topical Solution: This saturated solution, also known as Lime Water, is usually made in the pharmacy using Calcium Hydroxide and Purified Water. The clear supernatant solution is decanted at the time of use. The formula is in the USP but is also given in Chapter 29 of this book under the topic of Nascent Soap Emulsions. For this prescription, the Calcium Hydroxide Topical Solution was available in the pharmacy.

Compounding Procedure

Measure 45 mL of Bentonite Magma and dilute with an equal volume of Calcium Hydroxide Topical Solution. On a class 3 or electronic balance, weigh 14.4 g each of Calamine and Zinc Oxide and triturate together in a mortar. Add the 3.6 mL of Glycerin and about 18 mL of the diluted Bentonite Magma to the powders in the mortar; triturate until a smooth paste is formed. Gradually add the rest of the diluted Bentonite Magma with trituration. Add about 20 or 30 mL of Calcium Hydroxide Solution to the mortar to dilute to a pourable lotion. Pour into a 6-oz prescription bottle and use the rest of Calcium Hydroxide Solution to rinse the mortar and q.s. to the 180-mL mark. Shake well; label and dispense.

Quality Control

The preparation is a pink suspension with a viscosity similar to a thick syrup. The dispersed particles settle minimally on standing, and the preparation is easily redispersed with shaking. The pH of the preparation is checked; pH = 12.

Labeling

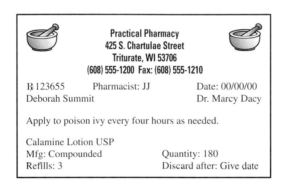

<table>
<tr><td colspan="3" align="center">Practical Pharmacy
425 S. Chartulae Street
Triturate, WI 53706
(608) 555-1200 Fax: (608) 555-1210</td></tr>
<tr><td>℞ 123655</td><td>Pharmacist: JJ</td><td>Date: 00/00/00</td></tr>
<tr><td>Deborah Summit</td><td></td><td>Dr. Marcy Dacy</td></tr>
<tr><td colspan="3">Apply to poison ivy every four hours as needed.</td></tr>
<tr><td colspan="3">Calamine Lotion USP</td></tr>
<tr><td>Mfg: Compounded</td><td colspan="2">Quantity: 180</td></tr>
<tr><td>Refills: 3</td><td colspan="2">Discard after: Give date</td></tr>
</table>

Auxiliary Labels: Shake well; For external use only

Patient Consultation

Hello, Ms. Summit, I'm Jerilyn Joyous, your pharmacist. Do you have any drug allergies? Are you currently using any other medication products, orally or topically? This prescription is for your poison ivy. It will help combat the itching and irritation. Apply it to the poison ivy every 4 hours as needed. If the rash seems to be getting worse, or if this is very irritating to your skin, discontinue use and contact your physician. You may want to pour this on a cotton ball and use that to dab the lotion on the affected areas. Be careful not to get this in your eyes or mouth. Wash your hands thoroughly before and after application. Shake this suspension well before using; store at room temperature out of the reach of children, and keep this container tightly closed. Discard any unused contents after 6 months (give date). This may be refilled three times. Do you have any questions?

➤ **Prescription 28.2**

Contemporary Physicians Group Practice
20 S. Park Street, Triturate, WI 53706
Tel: (608) 555-1333 Fax: (608) 555-1335

R # 687

Name	*Laura Lovely*	Date	*00/00/00*	
Address	*9856 Pinion Pine Way*	Age		Wt/Ht

R̡

Hydrocortisone		1%	
Menthol		1/8%	
Calamine		3 g	
Isopropyl Alcohol		10%	
Cetaphil		40 mL	
Purified Water	q s ad	60 mL	

J. Junco 00/00/00

Sig: *Apply to affected areas q.i.d.*

Refills   1   *O. P. Quacky*   M.D.

DEA No. _____

Ingredients Used

Ingredient	Quantity Used	Manufacturer Lot #-Exp Date	Solubility	Dose Comparison Given	Dose Comparison Usual	Use in the Prescription
Hydrocortisone	0.6 g	JET Labs SS2821-mm/yy	v sl sol water 1 g/40 mL alcohol	1%	0.5 to 2.5%	anti inflammatory
Menthol	150 mg weighed-75 mg used	JET Labs SS2822-mm/yy	sl sol water v sol alcohol	0.125%	1–3%	antipruritic local analgesic
Calamine	3 g	JET Labs SS2823-mm/yy	insol in water and alcohol	5%	1–20%	protective
IPA 70%	8.6 mL	JET Labs SS2824-mm/yy	misc with water	10%	varies	disinfectant, solvent drying agent
Cetaphil®	40 mL	Galderma JN9636-mm/yy	misc w/water, alcohol	67%	—	emollient vehicle
Purified Water	q.s. 60 mL	Sweet Springs AL0529-mm/yy	—	—	—	vehicle

Compatibility–Stability/Beyond-Use Date

Stability–Compatibility: Topical shake lotions of this type that contain Hydrocortisone have been evaluated and reported in the literature. A good review of this subject can be found in the Hydrocortisone monograph in *Trissel's Stability of Compounded Formulations*. Hydrocortisone lotions like this that contain Zinc Oxide-type ingredients (Calamine is essentially Zinc Oxide with 0.5-1% Ferric Oxide to impart the pink color) have a limited stability. One study showed a 7% loss of Hydrocortisone in 1 week and a 10% loss in 2 weeks (9). The other ingredients in this preparation are quite stable in a liquid suspension formulation.

Preservative: No additional preservative is needed for this preparation because the formula contains 10% Isopropyl Alcohol; also, Cetaphil contains paraben preservatives.

Packaging and Storage and Beyond-use date: Because the *USP* monographs for Hydrocortisone Lotion and Calamine Lotion both recommend storage in tight containers, this would be recommended for this preparation (10). Using the literature cited above as a guide, Pharmacist Junco will use a 14-day beyond-use date for this preparation.

Calculations

Dose/Concentration

Calamine concentration in percent:

$$\frac{3\,g\,Calamine}{60\,mL} = \frac{x\,g\,Calamine}{100\,mL}; x = 5\,g/100mL = 5\%$$

All concentrations OK

Ingredient Amounts

Hydrocortisone in grams: $1\% \times 60\,mL = 0.6\,g$

Menthol in grams and milligrams: $0.125\% \times 60\,mL = 0.075\,g = 75\,mg$

This amount is below the MWQ. Since Menthol is soluble in one of the prescription ingredients, Isopropyl Alcohol, a solid-liquid aliquot would be most convenient. One possible aliquot is made by weighing two times the amount of Menthol needed, $75\,mg \times 2 = 150\,mg$, dissolving this in a portion of the 70% IPA volume that is calculated below (4 mL would be a good amount), and taking ½ of this (2 mL in this case).

Isopropyl Alcohol (IPA) in mL: $10\% \times 60\,mL = 6\,mL$

IPA is available in the pharmacy as a 70% v/v solution. Below are the calculations for obtaining 6 mL of IPA from the 70% solution:

$$\frac{70\,mL\,IPA}{100\,mL\,70\%\,IPA} = \frac{6\,mL\,IPA}{x\,mL\,70\%\,IPA}; x = 8.6\,mL\,of\,70\%\,IPA$$

Compounding Procedure

On a class 3 torsion or electronic balance, weigh 150 mg of Menthol, 600 mg of Hydrocortisone, and 3 g of Calamine. Dissolve the Menthol in 4 mL of IPA 70% measured in a 10-mL graduate. Place the Hydrocortisone in a mortar, and add the Calamine geometrically. Take 2 mL of the Menthol-IPA solution and an additional 6.6 mL of IPA 70% and gradually add this to the powders in the mortar with trituration to form a smooth paste. Gradually with trituration, add about 10 mL of Purified Water to the paste. This is to dilute the alcohol content of the IPA in the mortar before adding the Cetaphil because Cetaphil has components that are soluble in alcohol, and a high concentration of IPA could break down the Cetaphil product. Gradually add 40 mL of Cetaphil (measured in a 100-mL graduate) in small portions with trituration. Do not over-triturate the preparation because the Cetaphil contains surfactants that facilitate the introduction of excess air bubbles into the preparation. Use additional small portions of Purified Water to rinse the graduate used to measure the Cetaphil, and add the rinsings to the mortar to dilute the preparation to give a pourable lotion. Transfer the lotion to a 2-oz prescription bottle that has calibration markings. Use a little more Purified Water to rinse the mortar and to facilitate transfer to the prescription bottle, then q.s. with water to the 60-mL mark. Shake well; label and dispense.

Quality Control

The preparation is a pink viscous suspension. There is no discernible settling of dispersed particles on standing when observed for at least 2 hours. The pH of the preparation is checked; pH = 7.

Labeling

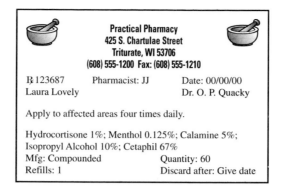

Practical Pharmacy
425 S. Chartulae Street
Triturate, WI 53706
(608) 555-1200 Fax: (608) 555-1210

℞ 123687   Pharmacist: JJ   Date: 00/00/00
Laura Lovely   Dr. O. P. Quacky

Apply to affected areas four times daily.

Hydrocortisone 1%; Menthol 0.125%; Calamine 5%;
Isopropyl Alcohol 10%; Cetaphil 67%
Mfg: Compounded   Quantity: 60
Refills: 1   Discard after: Give date

Auxiliary Labels: Shake well; For external use only

Patient Consultation

Hello, Ms. Lovely, I'm your pharmacist, Juliette Junco. Do you have any drug allergies? Are you currently taking any other medications? Do you know, or did your physician tell you, what this prescription is for and how to use it? This contains several ingredients that will stop inflammation and itching, act as an antiseptic, and protect, cleanse, and lubricate the skin. Shake this well before using it, and apply it to the affected area four times daily. Be careful not to get this in your eyes or mouth. If your condition gets worse, or you experience additional irritation, discontinue use and contact Dr. Quacky. This is in a childproof container, but it should be kept out of the reach of children. Store it at room temperature and keep the bottle tightly closed. Discard any unused portion after 2 weeks (give date). This may be refilled once. Do you have any questions?

➤ **Prescription 28.3**

Contemporary Physicians Group Practice
20 S. Park Street, Triturate, WI 53706
Tel: (608) 555-1333 Fax: (608) 555-1335

℞ # 633

Name *Prof. George Helmholtz*   Date *00/00/00*

Address *2160 Electron Circle*   *Age*   *Wt/Ht*

℞

Phenol   *1%*
White Lotion
~~*Methylcellulose 1500 cps 2%*~~   *aa qs ad 60 mL*
Na CMC med. viscosity 2%

J. Junco 00/00/00

Sig: *Apply to affected areas q am and hs*

Called Dr. Pasmak to change Methylcellulose to Na CMC due to compatibility concerns. JJ

Refills *3*   *R. Pasmak*   M.D.

DEA No. _____

Ingredients Used

Ingredient	Quantity Used	Manufacturer Lot #-Exp Date	Solubility	Dose Comparison		Use in the Prescription
				Given	Usual	
Phenol	0.6 g	JET Labs SS2831-mm/yy	1 g/15 mL water; v. sol in alcohol	1%	0.5–2%	antiseptic; local anesthetic;
Na CMC med visc. 2% soln	30 mL	Prac. Pharmacy XX2832-mm/yy	misc w/water and alcohol	—	—	viscosity inducer, vehicle
ZnSO₄ (to make 30 mL White Lotion)	1.2 g	JET Labs SS2833-mm/yy	sol in water	—	—	to make 30 mL White Lotion
Sulfurated Potash (to make 30 mL White Lotion)	1.2 g	JET Labs SS2834-mm/yy	sol in water	—	—	to make 30 mL White Lotion
White Lotion	30 mL	—	forms insol ZnS & S plus sol K₂SO₄	half-strength	full srength	antibacterial, antifungal, keratolytic
Purified Water	qs	Sweet Springs AL0529-mm/yy	—	—	—	solvent, vehicle

Compatibility–Stability/Beyond-Use Date

Stability–Compatibility: White Lotion is an official USP formulation. It is fairly stable, although the monograph states that it should be freshly made (10). Phenol is also fairly stable, but it is subject to oxidation.

It is necessary to change the Methylcellulose 1,500 cps to Sodium Carboxymethylcellulose (NaCMC) because Methylcellulose is reported to be incompatible with Phenol.

Preservative: This preparation contains Phenol and White Lotion; both have antimicrobial properties, so no additional preservative is needed.

Packaging and Storage and Beyond-use date: The *USP* monograph for White Lotion recommends that it be dispensed in tight containers (10). Pharmacist Junco will use the recommended maximum 14-day beyond-use date for compounded water-containing formulations prepared from ingredients in solid form when there is no stability information for the formulation (7). Because this is a topical product, controlled room temperature will be the recommended storage conditions.

Calculations

Dose/Concentration

All concentrations OK

Ingredient Amounts

Phenol in grams: *1% × 60 mL = 0.6 g*

Na CMC medium viscosity in grams: *2% × 30 mL = 0.6 g*

White Lotion:

The formula for 1,000 mL of White Lotion as given in the *USP* states that 40 g each of Sulfurated Potash and Zinc Sulfate are needed. Reducing this formula to make 30 mL:

$$\frac{40\ g}{1000\ mL\ White\ Lotion} = \frac{x\ g}{30\ mL\ White\ Lotion}; x = 1.2g\ of\ each$$

Compounding Procedure

Weigh 0.6 g each of Phenol and Na CMC med viscosity on a class 3 torsion or electronic balance. Place the Na CMC in a small beaker and add either hot or cold water to 30 mL, and allow it to stand until it clears (approximately 2 hours). Next make the White Lotion. Weigh 1.2 g each of $ZnSO_4$ and Sulfurated Potash, and dissolve each in 13.5 mL of water in separate beakers. Separately filter each of these two solutions; then add the Sulfurated Potash solution to the $ZnSO_4$ solution slowly with constant stirring. Pour this suspension into a 2-oz prescription bottle that has calibration marks, and use extra Purified Water to completely rinse the suspension into the bottle and q.s. to the 30-mL mark. Transfer the Phenol to this prescription bottle and agitate to dissolve the Phenol. Finally, q.s. with the Na CMC solution to the 60-mL mark. You may need to use extra Purified Water to rinse out the Na CMC solution and q.s. to the 60-mL mark. Shake the bottle well; label and dispense.

Quality Control

The preparation is a milky white suspension with very fine white particles. The suspension particles start to settle into a flocculated system in 20 to 30 minutes; at 2 hours the bottom 2/3 of the product shows a flocculated powder structure. The preparation is easily redispersed with shaking. The pH of the preparation is checked; pH = 7.5.

Labeling

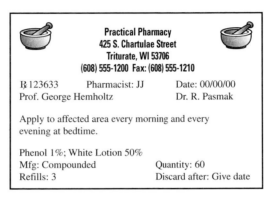

Auxiliary Labels: Shake well; For external use only

Patient Consultation

Hello, Prof. Helmholz, I'm your pharmacist, Justiens Junco. Do you have any drug allergies? Are you currently using any prescription or over-the-counter medication? What did your physician tell you about this prescription? This lotion contains several ingredients that are usually used to treat acne. Shake this well before using it, and apply it to the affected areas each morning and at bedtime daily. Be careful not to get this in your mouth or eyes. You may want to use a cotton ball to apply it. Be sure to wash the affected areas well before application, and wash your hands after applying the lotion. If your condition gets worse, or you experience additional irritation, discontinue use and contact Dr. Pasmak. This is in a childproof container, but it is still best to keep it out of the reach of children. It should be stored at room temperature. Discard any unused portion after 2 weeks (give date). This may be refilled 3 times. Do you have any questions?

➤ **Prescription 28.4**

Contemporary Physicians Group Practice
20 S. Park Street, Triturate, WI 53706
Tel: (608) 555-1333 Fax: (608) 555-1335

R # 632

Name *Dr. Kenneth Arrhenius*   Date *00/00/00*

Address *258 Kinetic Hill*   Age   Wt/Ht

℞

Sulfur	*9 g*
Resorcinol monoacetate	*3 mL*
LCD	*9 mL*
Dermabase	*qs*
Purified Water	*qs ad 90 mL*

Sig: *Apply to affected area bid*

B. Beastly 00/00/00

Refills *1*   *R. F. Gayle*   M.D.

DEA No. _____

Ingredients Used

Ingredient	Quantity Used	Manufacturer Lot #-Exp Date	Solubility	Dose Comparison Given	Dose Comparison Usual	Use in the Prescription
Sulfur Colloidal	9 g	JET Labs SS2841-mm/yy	prac. insol. in water; v. sl. sol in alcohol	10%	10%	antibacterial; antifungal; keratolytic
Resorcinol Monoacetate	3 mL	JET Labs SS2842-mm/yy	spar. sol. in water; sol. in alcohol	3.3%	1.5–3%	antibacterial; antifungal
LCD	9 mL	JET Labs SS2843-mm/yy	misc w/water and alcohol	10%	varies	antisebbhoraic; antipsoriatic
Dermabase	10 g	Paddock Labs UV5692-mm/yy	insol in water and alcohol	—	—	viscosity induction; emollient
Purified Water	qs ad 90 mL	Sweet Springs AL0529-mm/yy	—	—	—	vehicle

Compatibility–Stability/Beyond-Use Date

Stability–Compatibility: The Sulfur and tar ingredient (LCD) in this preparation are compatible and very stable when in a suspension. The Resorcinol Monoacetate is somewhat more difficult to assess. It is an ester that undergoes hydrolysis, but the result is the active principal Resorcinol. A lotion containing Sulfur and Resorcinol Monoacetate is described in the Resorcinol Monoacetate monograph in the 16th edition of *Remington's Pharmaceutical Sciences*, but no stability data are given.

Preservative: No extra preservative is needed because both Sulfur and Resorcinol Monoacetate have antimicrobial activity. In addition, the alcohol content is 8.4%.

Packaging and Storage and Beyond-use date: Pharmacist Beastly will use the recommended maximum 14-day beyond-use date for compounded water-containing formulations prepared from ingredients in solid form when there is no stability information for the formulation (7). Because this is a topical preparation, controlled room temperature will be the recommended storage conditions.

Calculations

Dose/Concentration

Sulfur:

$$\frac{9\ g\ Sulfur}{90\ mL\ lotion} = \frac{x\ g\ Sulfur}{100\ mL\ lotion}; x = 10g/100\ mL = 10\%$$

Resorcinol Monoacetate:

$$\frac{3\ mL\ R.M.}{90\ mL\ lotion} = \frac{x\ mL\ R.M.}{100\ mL\ lotion}; x = 3.3\ mL/100\ mL = 3.3\%$$

Coal Tar Topical Solution (LCD):

$$\frac{9\ mL\ LCD}{90\ mL\ lotion} = \frac{x\ mL\ LCD}{100\ mL\ lotion}; x = 10\ mL/100\ mL = 10\%$$

Alcohol Content:

We are adding 9 mL of LCD, which contains 84% alcohol. The content of C_2H_5OH in mL is: *84% × 9 mL = 7.56 mL.*

The final v/v% concentration of alcohol is calculated to be:

$$\frac{7.56\ mL\ C_2H_5OH}{90\ mL\ lotion} = \frac{x\ mL\ C_2H_5OH}{100\ mL\ lotion}; x = 8.4\ mL/100\ mL = 8.4\%$$

All concentrations are OK for the intended use.

Ingredient Amounts

All ingredient amounts are given in the prescription order except for the Dermabase. Pharmacist Beastly has decided to use 10 g of Dermabase. This amount is somewhat arbitrary and varies not only with the volume of the suspension, but also with the amount and type of solid ingredients. For this preparation, if you add 15 to 20 g of Dermabase for this volume of suspension, you will get a soft semisolid cream-type preparation that does not pour easily from a standard liquid prescription bottle.

Compounding Procedure

On a class 3 torsion or an electronic balance, weigh 9 g of Colloidal Sulfur and place the Sulfur in a mortar. Using a graduated cylinder or a syringe, measure 3 mL of Resorcinol Monoacetate. Add the Resorcinol Monoacetate to the Sulfur and triturate well to give a dry paste. Weigh 10 g of Dermabase and add with trituration to the Sulfur paste. Measure 20 mL of Purified Water in a 25-mL graduated cylinder and **very** gradually add to the Sulfur mixture with careful trituration. Measure 9 mL of Coal Tar Topical Solution (LCD) in a 10-mL graduated cylinder and gradually add the LCD in portions with trituration to Sulfur mixture. Add 15 mL of Purified Water with trituration, and then additional water until the preparation thins to a pourable suspension. Transfer to a 3-oz prescription bottle. Using successive water, rinse out the mortar and q.s. to the 90-mL mark on the bottle. Shake well; label and dispense. Note: Although the order of mixing may be varied, any change affects the viscosity and appearance (sometimes significantly) of the finished preparation.

Quality Control

When using Colloidal Sulfur, the resulting suspension is a beige-colored creamy base. The suspension is fairly thick but pours adequately after shaking. There is no significantly settling of solid particles on standing. The pH of the preparation is checked; pH = 5.

Labeling

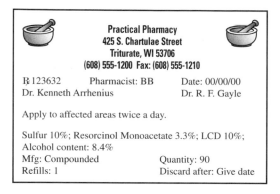

Auxiliary Labels: Shake well; For external use only

Patient Consultation

Hello, Dr. Arrhenius, I'm your pharmacist, Bing Beastly. Do you have any known drug allergies? Are you using any other medications, either over-the-counter or prescription? Do you know the purpose of this medicine? This is to treat the skin condition that your physician has diagnosed. You are to apply this to the affected area twice a day. Be sure to shake well before applying. You may want to place this on a cotton ball and use that to apply it, being careful not to get any in your eyes or mouth. Be sure to wash the areas well before application, and wash your hands after applying it. If this doesn't seem to be helping, if the condition gets worse, or if the area becomes irritated or inflamed, discontinue use and call your doctor. Be careful not to spill this or get any of the lotion on your clothes, because this suspension contains a tar-type ingredient that will stain. This is in a childproof bottle, but it's still a good idea to keep it out of reach of children. This may be stored at room temperature, and any unused portion should be discarded after 2 weeks (give date). You may have one refill if you need it. Do you have any questions?

➤ **Prescription 28.5**

Contemporary Physicians Group Practice
20 S. Park Street, Triturate, WI 53706
Tel: (608) 555-1333 Fax: (608) 555-1335

℞ # 667

Name *Joseph Wilding*	Date	*00/00/00*
Address *568 Mockingbird Lane*	Age	Wt/Ht

℞

Hydrochlorothiazide   *25 mg/5 mL*
Methylcellulose   *qs*

    M & Ft Suspension   *60 mL*

                                                      JET 00/00/00

Sig: 5 mL per NG tube bid

Refills   *11 X*   *Ozzie Wurtz*   M.D.

                           DEA No. _____

Ingredients Used

Ingredient	Quantity Used	Manufacturer Lot #-Exp Date	Solubility	Dose Comparison Given	Usual	Use in the Prescription
Hydrochloro-thiazide as 50 mg tablets	300 mg (6 × 50 mg tabs)	BJF Generics XY5739-mm/yy	sl sol in water, sol in alcohol	25 mg bid	25–200 mg/ day	antihypertensive; diuretic
Citrucel®	2 g	SK-Beecham XX2852-mm/yy	MC sol in water, insol in alcohol	3.33%	variable	viscosity induction
Sodium Benzoate	120 mg	JET Labs SS2851-mm/yy	1 g/1.8 mL water, 75 mL alcohol	0.2%	0.1–0.3%	preservative
Purified Water	q.s. 60 mL	Sweet Springs AL0529-mm/yy	—	—	—	vehicle

Compatibility–Stability/Beyond-Use Date

Stability–Compatibility: Pharmacist Thompson checked the stability of the Hydrochlorothiazide and found information in *The Chemical Stability of Pharmaceuticals* (11). The drug is most stable at pH 4, with a half-life of 720 days at 25°C.

Second, a methylcellulose suspending agent is needed, and Pharmacist Thompson selected Citrucel powder. This is an orange-flavored methylcellulose product marketed as an OTC bulk laxative. It is available sweetened with sucrose or as a sugar-free product sweetened with Aspartame. A flavored ingredient is not important for this preparation because this is for an NG tube, but Citrucel makes a convenient suspending medium for extemporaneous suspensions. It does not contain a preservative, so a preservative should be added to provide protection from growth of bacteria, yeasts, and molds. Either Potassium Sorbate or Sodium Benzoate would be effective because suspensions made with Citrucel have a pH of approximately 4. Pharmacist Thompson has chosen Sodium Benzoate 0.2%

Packaging and Storage and Beyond-use date: Because this is a formulation with some known stability information, Pharmacist Thompson has some flexibility in assigning a beyond-use date. Although the formulation is most likely stable for at least 6 months, the amount dispensed is only a 6-day supply, so a 14- to 30-day beyond-use date would be very adequate. Because this is an oral preparation, it should be stored in the refrigerator. This will enhance its stability, both chemical and microbiological, and also its taste.

Calculations

Dose/Concentration

Dose of 25 mg Hydrochlorothiazide two times daily is OK.

Ingredient Amounts

Hydrochlorothiazide: *25 mg/5 mL × 60 mL = 300 mg*

   Hydrochlorothiazide is available as 50-mg tablets. Exactly six tablets are needed for 300 mg.

Citrucel: Recommended amount is 2 g for 60 mL of suspension.

Preservative: Sodium Benzoate is selected. The amount in mg is calculated to be:

0.2% × 60 mL = 0.12 g = 120 mg

Compounding Procedure

Crush six 50-mg HCTZ tablets in a mortar, moistening tablets with a small amount of Purified Water to facilitate crushing. On a class 3 torsion or electronic balance, weigh 120 mg of Sodium Benzoate and 2 g of Citrucel powder. Combine them and either mix with about 40 mL of Purified Water in a small beaker and then slowly add this to the crushed tablets in the mortar with trituration, or add the Citrucel/Na Benzoate directly to the crushed tablets and gradually add the water in portions with trituration. Transfer to a 60-mL prescription bottle. Using more Purified Water, rinse out the mortar and transfer the rinsings to the prescription bottle. Add Purified Water to the calibration mark on bottle. Shake well; label and dispense.

Quality Control

The preparation is an orange suspension with white dispersed particles. The suspension is fairly viscous, and there is minimal settling on standing. Any settled particles redisperse with shaking. The pH of the preparation is checked; pH = 4.

Labeling

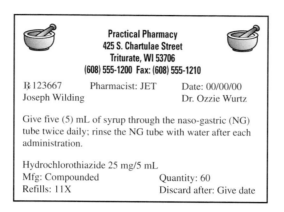

Practical Pharmacy
425 S. Chartulae Street
Triturate, WI 53706
(608) 555-1200 Fax: (608) 555-1210

℞ 123667   Pharmacist: JET   Date: 00/00/00
Joseph Wilding   Dr. Ozzie Wurtz

Give five (5) mL of syrup through the naso-gastric (NG)
tube twice daily; rinse the NG tube with water after each
administration.

Hydrochlorothiazide 25 mg/5 mL
Mfg: Compounded   Quantity: 60
Refills: 11X   Discard after: Give date

Auxiliary Labels: Shake well; Keep in the refrigerator

Patient Consultation

Hello, Mrs. Wilding, I'm your pharmacist, Judy Thompson. Here is the prescription for Mr. Wilding. How are things going at home with his care? What did Dr. Wurtz tell you about this drug? (Mrs. Wilding answers that he is taking it for water retention.) Has Mr. Wilding ever taken a medication like this before? If yes: Did he have any problems or adverse reaction to it? It is important to give 5 mL twice a day through his NG tube. If you forget to give a dose, give it as soon as you remember, but if it is close to the next dose, skip it. Mr. Wilding's potassium will need to be checked on a regular basis because this medicine can cause loss of potassium. This medication should cause increased urine output. Although uncommon, this medication may cause upset stomach, dizziness, lightheadedness, and loose stools. If side effects occur and become bothersome, contact Dr. Wurtz. Do you have something to measure 5 mL? (Provide dose syringe.) Rinse the NG tube with water after giving the dose. If the suspension seems to be too thick, you can measure the 5-mL dose and then dilute it with some water before putting it down the NG tube. Store this in the refrigerator for best stability. Shake well before giving. Discard any unused contents after 2 weeks. Keep out of reach of children. This may be refilled 11 times. Do you have any questions?

➤ **Prescription 28.6**

Contemporary Physicians Group Practice
20 S. Park Street, Triturate, WI 53706
Tel: (608) 555-1333 Fax: (608) 555-1335

R # 625

Name *Peter Childs*	Date *00/00/00*

Address *2530 Souffle Circle*	Age *10 yrs* Wt/Ht *68#*

R

    Captopril   *300 mcg/kg/dose*
    Flavored Syrup   *qs*
     Give enough for 10 days

             JR A 00/00/00

   Sig: Give one dose tid, one hr ac

Refills *1*   *Ozzie Wurtz*   M.D.

      DEA No. _____

Ingredients Used

Ingredient	Quantity Used	Manufacturer Lot #-Exp Date	Solubility	Dose Comparison Given	Dose Comparison Usual	Use in the Prescription
Captopril as 50 mg tablets	270 mg drug from 1156 mg crushed tablet powder	BJF Generics XY3692-mm/yy	1 g/6 mL water; fr sol in alcohol	300 mcg/kg t.i.d. or 9 mg t.i.d.	300 mcg/kg t.i.d. or 9 mg t.i.d.	antihypertensive
Cherry Flavor Concentrate	2 mL	JET Labs SS2861-mm/yy	mis w/water and alcohol	—	—	flavor
Disodium Edetate	150 mg	JET Labs SS2862-mm/yy	sol in water	0.1%	0.1%	chelating agent
Syrup NF	q.s. 150 mL	JET Labs SS2863-mm/yy	mis w/water and alcohol	—	—	sweet, viscous vehicle

Compatibility–Stability/Beyond-Use Date

Stability–Compatibility: Pharmacist Albers checked the stability of Captopril. The *USP/DI* states that this drug is unstable in liquid preparations, so when a liquid dosage form is needed, a solution of the drug should be made from crushed tablets that are dispersed in water, and the resulting solution should be used within a half-hour. However, research published in *AJHP* found that a suspension made with crushed tablets in undiluted Syrup or in 2% Methylcellulose with 0.1% Disodium Edetate was stable for 30 days at 5°C (12). Note that Captopril's stability in liquid preparations is very sensitive to conditions, because the same research found that if the Syrup was mixed 50:50 with water, the resulting preparation was chemically unstable. Pharmacist Albers has decided to use undiluted Syrup NF, which comes preserved with Sodium Benzoate 0.1%. To enhance the chemical stability of the Captopril, he will add 0.1% Disodium Edetate.

Packaging and Storage and Beyond-use date: Because this is a formulation with some known stability information, Pharmacist Albers has some flexibility in assigning a beyond-use date. Although the formulation is most likely stable for 1 month, the amount dispensed is only a 10-day supply, so a 14- to 30-day beyond-use date would be acceptable. Because this is an oral preparation, it should be stored in the refrigerator. Furthermore, the studies used in establishing the beyond-use date were conducted with storage at 5°C. Refrigeration will also enhance the taste of the preparation.

Calculations

Dose/Concentration

The 300 mcg/kg t.i.d. is OK (Checked in USP/DI)

$$Weight\ of\ child\ in\ kg: \frac{68\ lb}{2.2\ lb/kg} = 31\ kg$$

Dose in mg: 300 mcg/kg × 31 kg = 9,300 mcg = 9.3 mg ≈ 9 mg/dose

Amounts

Captopril:

Mg of drug for 10 days: *9 mg/dose × 3 doses/day × 10 days = 270 mg*

Captopril is available as 50-mg tablets. The number of tablets needed is calculated as:

$$\frac{270\ mg\ Captopril\ needed}{50\ mg\ Captopril\ /\ tablet} = 5.4\ or\ 6\ tablets$$

Six 50-mg Captopril tablets (300 mg of Captopril) are found to weigh 1,284 mg. The quantity of crushed tablet powder that will contain 270 mg of Captopril is calculated as:

$$\frac{300\ mg\ Captopril}{1284\ mg\ tablet\ powder} = \frac{270\ mg\ Captopril}{x\ mg\ tablet\ powder}; x = 1156\ mg\ crushed\ tablet\ powder\ needed$$

Disodium Edetate in g and mg: *0.1% × 150 mL = 0.15 g = 150 mg*

Volume of Suspension for 10 days using 5 mL/dose:

5 mL/dose × 3 doses/day × 10 days = 150 mL

Compounding Procedure

Weigh six tablets of Captopril 50 mg (total weight 1,284 mg, or 214 mg per tablet). Crush the six tablets in a mortar and weigh 1,156 mg of this crushed tablet powder. Place the weighed tablet powder in a clean mortar. On a digital balance, weigh 150 mg of Disodium Edetate and place in the mortar. Gradually with trituration add approximately 20–40 mL of Syrup NF to the mortar. Transfer to a 6-oz prescription bottle with calibration markings. Using more Syrup, rinse out the mortar and transfer the rinsings to the prescription bottle. Add 2 mL of Cherry Extract Flavoring and q.s. to the 150-mL calibration mark on the bottle with Syrup. Shake well; label and dispense.

Quality Control

The preparation is a colorless suspension with white dispersed particles. The suspension is fairly viscous, and there is minimal settling on standing. Any settled particles redisperse with vigorous shaking. The pH of the preparation is checked; pH = 5.

Labeling

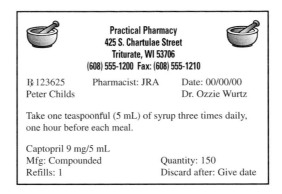

Practical Pharmacy
425 S. Chartulae Street
Triturate, WI 53706
(608) 555-1200 Fax: (608) 555-1210

R 123625   Pharmacist: JRA   Date: 00/00/00
Peter Childs   Dr. Ozzie Wurtz

Take one teaspoonful (5 mL) of syrup three times daily,
one hour before each meal.

Captopril 9 mg/5 mL
Mfg: Compounded   Quantity: 150
Refills: 1   Discard after: Give date

Auxiliary Labels: Shake well; Keep in the refrigerator

Patient Consultation

Hello, Mrs. Childs, I'm your pharmacist, John Albers. Here is the prescription for Peter. Is he allergic to any medications that you know of? Is he currently taking any other medications? What did Dr. Wurtz tell you about this drug and how to use it? Has Peter ever taken a medication like this before? It is important to give him one teaspoonful or 5 mL three times a day, approximately 1 hour before each meal. If you forget to give a dose, give it as soon as you remember, but if it is close to the next dose, skip it. Although uncommon, this medication may cause dizziness or lightheadedness, cough, and some skin reactions like rash or itching. If side effects occur and become bothersome, contact Dr. Wurtz. Do you have something to accurately measure the dose? Store this prescription in the refrigerator for best stability. Shake the bottle well before measuring the dose. Discard any unused contents after 14 days. Keep out of reach of children. This may be refilled one time. Do you have any questions?

References

1. The 2002 United States Pharmacopeia 25/National Formulary 20. Rockville, MD: The United States Pharmacopeial Convention, Inc., 2001;2222-2223.
2. Martin A, Bustamante P. Physical pharmacy, 4th ed. Philadelphia: Lea & Febiger, 1993;370.
3. Zografi G. Interfacial phenomena. In: Gennaro AR, ed. Remington: The science and practice of pharmacy, 19th ed. Easton, PA: Mack Publishing Co., 1995;247.
4. Martin A, Bustamante P. Physical pharmacy, 4th ed. Philadelphia: Lea & Febiger, 1993;384.
5. Martin A, Bustamante P. Physical pharmacy, 4th ed. Philadelphia: Lea & Febiger, 1993;477–479.
6. The 2002 United States Pharmacopeia 25/National Formulary 20. Rockville, MD: The United States Pharmacopeial Convention, Inc., 2001;977.
7. The 2002 United States Pharmacopeia 25/National Formulary 20. Rockville, MD: The United States Pharmacopeial Convention, Inc., 2001;2054.
8. The 2002 United States Pharmacopeia 25/National Formulary 20. Rockville, MD: The United States Pharmacopeial Convention, Inc., 2001;275-276.
9. Timmons P, Gray EA. Degradation of hydrocortisone in a zinc oxide lotion. J Clin Hosp Pharm 1983;8:79-85.
10. The 2002 United States Pharmacopeia 25/National Formulary 20. Rockville, MD: The United States Pharmacopeial Convention, Inc.; Official Monographs.
11. Connors KA, Amidon GL, Stella VJ. Chemical Stability of Pharmaceuticals, 2nd ed. New York: John Wiley and Sons, 1986;478-482.
12. Lye MYF, Yow KL, et al. Effects of ingredients on stability of captopril in extemporaneously prepared oral liquids. Am J Health-Syst Pharm 1997;54:2483–2487.

CHAPTER 29

Liquid Emulsions

I. DEFINITIONS

A. **Emulsions:** "Emulsions are two-phase systems in which one liquid is dispersed throughout another liquid in the form of small droplets." (1) —*USP*

B. **Emulsification:** Emulsification of two immiscible phases can be accomplished when energy is applied to the system (e.g., trituration or homogenization) to create small droplets and cause a physical and/or electrostatic barrier to form around the droplets to prevent them from coalescing. This is accomplished by the use of emulsifying agents. The dispersed droplets are collectively termed the internal phase, and the continuous liquid is called the external phase.

C. **Emulsifying Agents:** These are surfactants that concentrate at the interface of the two immiscible phases, reduce the interfacial tension between the immiscible phases, provide a barrier around the droplets as they form, and prevent coalescence of the droplets. Some emulsifying agents also increase the viscosity of the system, slowing aggregation of the droplets and decreasing the rate of creaming. Surfactants and emulsifying agents commonly used for compounding purposes are described and discussed in Chapter 19, Surfactants and Emulsifying Agents.

D. **Creaming:** This is the migration of the droplets of the internal phase to the top or bottom of the emulsion. The migration is caused by the difference in density between the two phases, and the direction of the movement depends on whether the internal phase is more or less dense than the continuous or external phase.

E. **Coalescence:** This is the merging of small droplets into larger droplets, with eventual complete separation of phases so that the droplets cannot be re-emulsified by simple shaking of the product. With coalescence, the barrier formed by the emulsifying agent(s) is broken or destroyed. This irreversible coalescence of the droplets is also called "cracking."

II. USES OF EMULSIONS

A. **Oral Products:** As discussed in the chapters on solutions and suspensions, there are times when oral liquid preparations are needed. Generally, oral liquid emulsions are less acceptable to patients than solutions or suspensions because of the objectionable oily feel of emulsions in the mouth. Therefore, an oral emulsion is formulated only when it is necessary to make a liquid product of an oil or when the solubility or bioavailability characteristics of a drug make this delivery system clearly superior.

B. **Topical Products:** Topical emulsions are more common. Emollient (soothing of the skin) or protective properties are often desired of topical preparations, and oils can serve these functions. When the oils are emulsified, they feel less greasy and are more esthetically appealing to patients.

III. EMULSION TYPE

A. **Oil-in-Water** (o/w): In this type, the oil is dispersed as droplets in an aqueous solution. This is the most common emulsion type. It is always preferred for oral products where an oily feel in the mouth is objectionable. It is also used for external products when ease of removal and/or a nongreasy-feeling preparation is desired.

B. **Water-in-Oil** (w/o): In this type, the water is dispersed as droplets in an oil or oleaginous material. This type is used for external products when emollient, lubricating, or protective properties are desired. Many ointments that are emulsion systems are w/o emulsions.

C. Factors That Determine Emulsion Type
1. Emulsifier
   As described in Chapter 19, Surfactants and Emulsifying Agents, some emulsifiers will form either w/o or o/w emulsions; others form only one type.
2. Phase ratio (that is, relative amounts of oil and water)
   All other things being equal, the phase that is present in the greater concentration tends to be the external phase, but an emulsifying agent that strongly favors a particular emulsion type and that forms a good barrier at the interface can overcome an unfavorable phase ratio.
3. Order of mixing
   Because the phase that is present in the greater concentration tends to be the external phase, the phase that is being added, usually by portions, tends to be the internal phase. The bulk external phase will continue to accommodate added internal phase as small droplets until either the bulk phase becomes completely packed or there is no longer sufficient emulsifying agent to serve as a barrier to coalescence. Then, if more internal phase is added, either it will fail to be emulsified and will remain as separate droplets, or the emulsion will coalesce; or, if the emulsifier will allow it, phase inversion will occur. The external phase, which was the continuous phase, now becomes the dispersed droplets, the internal phase.

IV. DESIRED PROPERTIES OF A LIQUID EMULSION

A. Fine Droplets
Emulsions with fine droplet size are desired. Many factors can contribute to small droplets.
1. One factor is the mechanical method used for mixing and shearing the two immiscible liquids. The pharmaceutical industry has specialized equipment for this task. For extemporaneous compounding, a rough-sided Wedgewood mortar is usually used for the emulsification process. Simple, relatively inexpensive hand-homogenizers and high-speed blenders are available, which may give finer, and more uniform, droplets.
2. Certain techniques, such as phase inversion, can be used to give fine, uniform-sized droplets.
3. Finally, some emulsifying agents give finer emulsions. For example, amino-soaps are better balanced emulsifiers than are the alkali soaps and give more stable emulsions of finer droplet size (2).

B. Slow Aggregation of the Droplets and Creaming of the Product
1. Although almost all emulsions eventually cream, the rate of creaming should be slow enough to ensure accurate measurement of a dose or application of a uniform product.

2. Aggregation and creaming can be slowed through proper emulsification and through the use of various additives, such as viscosity-increasing agents. To control the rate of creaming, you can adjust some of the parameters found in Stoke's Law. Although this equation was developed for particles settling in a suspension, many of the same factors affect the rate of creaming for droplets in an emulsion. These include droplet size, viscosity of the continuous phase, and relative density difference of the droplets and the continuous phase. For a more complete discussion of Stoke's Law, see Chapter 28, Suspensions.

C. Ease of Redispersion When Shaken
Although aggregation and creaming are usually unavoidable, the product should be formulated so that the internal phase readily redisperses to give a uniform emulsion when the product is shaken. Furthermore, coalescence should not occur.

V. COMPOUNDING BASIC EMULSION TYPES

A. Acacia emulsions: Acacia is unique among the polymer emulsifiers in its ability to form emulsions using only a Wedgewood mortar and pestle. It is therefore a useful ingredient for extemporaneous compounding of emulsions.
   1. The emulsification process for Acacia emulsions requires the formation of a primary emulsion. The term "primary emulsion" is used to describe the initial emulsion formed with a prescribed ratio of ingredients. This prescribed set of ingredients gives a system of optimal viscosity and consistency so that the shearing force exerted in the mortar is maximized to allow the formation of an emulsion.
   2. Ingredient ratio for primary Acacia emulsions
      a. For fixed oils, such as vegetable oils and mineral oil, the oil to water to Acacia ratio (o:w:a) is 4:2:1.
      b. The ratio for volatile and essential oils is 3:2:1 or 2:2:1.
      c. The amounts in the ratio are predicated on the total amount of oil in the formulation. Because Acacia forms o/w emulsions, the oil is the internal phase. Therefore, all of the oil must be emulsified when making the primary emulsion. After the primary emulsion is formed, the emulsion may be diluted with any extra water or water-miscible phase, as required.
   3. Methods of forming the primary emulsion
      a. **Dry gum method.** This usually is the preferred method. Its steps are as follows:
         (1) The calculated amount of Acacia and all the oil contained in the formulation are put in a Wedgewood mortar and triturated until a smooth slurry results and all the Acacia is properly wet by the oil.
         (2) The amount of the aqueous phase, which is calculated from the ratio given above, is measured in a **clean, dry** graduated cylinder and is added, all at once, with **hard and fast** trituration. Trituration is continued until the primary emulsion is formed. You know this has occurred when the system changes from a translucent, oily-appearing liquid into a thick, white liquid. The sound of trituration also changes to give a crackling sound.
         (3) Once the primary emulsion is formed, other ingredients may be added.
      b. **Wet gum method.** With this method, the order of mixing is as follows:
         (1) The appropriate amount of Acacia is put in a Wedgewood mortar, and a small amount of water-miscible wetting agent, such as glycerin, is added to wet the Acacia. This is necessary because powdered Acacia gets lumpy when water is added directly to it.
         (2) The calculated amount of water is then gradually added in portions with trituration.
         (3) The oil is then gradually added with trituration until all the oil has been added and the primary is formed.
         (4) As with the dry gum method, once the primary emulsion is formed, water or other ingredients may be added.

4. Order of mixing for Acacia emulsions

   a. Make the primary emulsion first using all the oil(s), the Acacia, and Purified Water, in the appropriate ratio.

   b. Additional water, water-miscible liquids, including flavored syrups, and water-soluble drugs or chemicals may then be added directly to the primary emulsion. Soluble ingredients that are in solid form may be dissolved first in water or another appropriate solvent before being added to the emulsion.

   c. Insoluble ingredients, such as Zinc Oxide and Calamine, should be put in a separate mortar, and the primary emulsion should be added to the powders in portions with trituration. This is done to wet the powders and reduce their particle size so that a smooth preparation results. This process is illustrated in Sample Prescription 29.1.

   d. In some cases, oil-soluble ingredients may be dissolved in the oil phase before the formation of the primary emulsion. This is illustrated with the active ingredients Dioxybenzone and Oxybenzone in Sample Prescription 29.1. If the primary emulsion fails to form with the extra ingredient(s) in the oil phase, the ingredients should be handled as described in c. above.

5. Preservation and Storage

   a. Preservatives are required by the *USP* for all emulsions. This is especially important with Acacia emulsions because they are very susceptible to microbial (especially mold) growth.

   b. Unless the formulation contains an additive that would alter the pH, Acacia emulsions have a pH in the range of 4.5–5.0. Therefore, preservatives that require a slightly acid pH, such as Benzoic Acid or Sorbic Acid, are effective preservatives for Acacia emulsions. For an official Acacia emulsion, Mineral Oil Emulsion USP, the use of either Benzoic Acid 0.2% or Alcohol 4–6% is recommended. The Benzoic Acid can be added as its sodium salt. Methylparaben 0.2% with Propylparaben 0.02% is also an acceptable preservative system. The quaternary ammonium preservatives, such as Benzalkonium Chloride, Benzethonium Chloride, and Cetylpyridinium Chloride, are not recommended because they are inactivated through binding with Acacia.

   c. For reasons of improved stability and taste, internal preparations should be stored in a refrigerator. External preparations are generally stored at controlled room temperature.

6. A complete description of Acacia, including its incompatibilities and limitations, is given in Chapter 18, Viscosity-inducing Agents.

B. Nascent Soap Emulsions: The term "nascent" means beginning to exist or to develop. As the name implies, the emulsifier is formed as these emulsions are made. These emulsifiers are the hard and soft soaps, which are discussed in Chapter 19, Surfactants and Emulsifying Agents. The current section concentrates on a prototype of this emulsion type, so-called Lime Water emulsions, in which the emulsifier, calcium oleate, is formed when Calcium Hydroxide Topical Solution (Lime Water) is added to a vegetable oil.

1. Oil phase

   a. Olive Oil was the original oil used in these emulsions because, of the vegetable oils, it has the largest amount of free fatty acid necessary for forming the soap emulsifying agent.

   b. Olive Oil may be replaced by other vegetable oils; however, in this case, extra free fatty acid in the form of Oleic Acid must be added.

   c. Depending on its source, Olive Oil may also need fortification with extra Oleic Acid. It may be advisable to add 3–5 drops of Oleic Acid/30 mL of Olive Oil and 1–1.5 mL Oleic Acid/30 mL of any other vegetable oil before the emulsification process is begun. Extra Oleic Acid can be added drop-wise during emulsification if necessary. This is illustrated in Sample Prescription 29.2.

2. Lime Water should be freshly prepared. The formula can be found in the *USP* under Calcium Hydroxide Topical Solution. It is reproduced below:

Calcium Hydroxide   3 g
Purified Water   1,000 mL

Add the Calcium Hydroxide to 1,000 mL of cool Purified Water, and agitate the mixture vigorously and repeatedly during 1 hour. Allow the excess calcium hydroxide to settle. Dispense only the clear, supernatant liquid (3).

3. Methods of preparation
   a. Bottle method: With this method, equal amounts of oil (containing adequate Oleic Acid) and Lime Water are placed in a bottle. The bottle is shaken vigorously to form the emulsion. The emulsion can then be used as a wetting agent for any solid insoluble ingredients.
   b. Mortar method: This method is often preferred when the formulation contains solid insoluble ingredients, such as Zinc Oxide or Calamine. These solids concentrate at the oil–water interface as the emulsion is being formed and enhance the interfacial barrier, which improves the stability of the system. With this method, the solids are placed in a mortar. The oil (containing Oleic Acid) is added in portions with trituration until all the oil has been added and a smooth slurry of oil-powders is obtained. The Lime Water is then added in portions with trituration to form the emulsion.

4. Order of mixing: This depends somewhat on the method of emulsification as described above.
   a. With either method, water-miscible liquids and water-soluble drugs or chemicals should be added to the Lime Water before it is added to the bottle or mortar for emulsification. This is because water is the internal phase.
   b. Because oil is the external phase, oil-soluble and oil-miscible ingredients can be added to the oil before emulsification or to the emulsion after the water phase is emulsified.
   c. Any insoluble ingredients should be placed in a mortar. If the bottle method is used, the formed emulsion can serve as a wetting agent in triturating and incorporating these solids. Insoluble solids should never be merely added to the bottle with shaking. As described previously, when the mortar method is used, insoluble ingredients may be placed in the mortar at the beginning of the compounding process. In all cases, the wetting liquid should be added in portions with trituration to ensure the formation of a smooth preparation.

5. Handling incompatibilities: As indicated in the section on soaps in Chapter 19, adding acidic ingredients to emulsions using soap emulsifiers shifts the equilibrium from the salt form of the soap, which is the surface active form, toward the undissociated acid form, which is oil-soluble. This destroys the barrier necessary for maintaining the emulsion.

Nascent soap emulsion using the bottle method—before (left) and after (right)

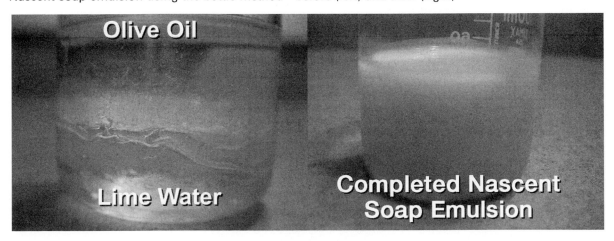

    a. Examples of acidic ingredients commonly used in topical products that may be prescribed in nascent soap emulsions include Phenol, Resorcinol, Menthol, Salicylic Acid, Lactic Acid, Acetic Acid, Aluminum Acetate Topical Solution (Burow's Solution), and Aluminum Subacetate Topical Solution.

    b. The soap emulsifier may be protected from these acid ingredients by incorporating the offending acid ingredient or ingredients in 2–4 grams of absorption base (e.g., Lanolin, Hydrophilic Petrolatum, Aquabase®) per 30 mL of oil phase before the acid ingredients are incorporated in the formulation. This procedure is illustrated in Sample Prescription 29.2.

6. Preservation and storage

    a. Preservatives are not usually required for Lime Water emulsions because the Calcium Hydroxide generates a high pH, which is not favorable for microbial or mold growth. Furthermore, these are external-use emulsions that often contain antiseptic or antimicrobial active ingredients.

    b. For other nascent soap emulsions, if a preservative is needed, Alcohol or the parabens are suitable agents. Benzoic Acid/Sodium Benzoate and Sorbic Acid/Potassium Sorbate are not effective because of the alkaline pH of these emulsions.

    c. As external use preparations, nascent soap emulsions are stored at controlled room temperature.

C. Non-ionic surfactant emulsions: The most common non-ionic emulsifying agents for liquid emulsions are combinations of polysorbates with sorbitan esters, the so-called Span-Tween surfactants.

1. Total amount of emulsifier needed

    a. A 2–5% w/v emulsifier combination has been recommended for liquid emulsions. Some sources report that using an amount in the upper range gives more stable preparations. This means that for 100 mL of a preparation, 5 g total of a polysorbate-sorbitan ester combination would be used.

    b. Other references recommend that the amount of emulsifier used should depend on the amount of internal phase to be emulsified. In this case, 10–20% w/v of the internal phase is a suggested guideline.

2. Relative amounts of emulsifier combinations

    a. A system was needed to aid formulators in making systematic decisions for amounts and types of surfactants to use in giving products of maximum stability. The HLB (Hydrophile-Lipophile-Balance) system was developed by Griffin (4). It is based on the fact that all surfactant molecules have both hydrophilic (water-loving) and lipophilic (oil-loving) portions. The balance between these two parts varies with the surfactant. Numbers from 1 to 20 were assigned to surfactants based on this balance, with the lower numbers given to lipophilic compounds and the higher numbers assigned to hydrophilic compounds. The former Atlas Powder Company, the firm that originally developed and marketed a number of non-ionic surfactants, including Span®, Tween®, Arlacel®, Brij®, and Myrj®, further developed and advocated this system.

    b. Span and Arlacel surfactants are considered lipophilic, with HLB numbers in the range of 1.8–8.6. They tend to form w/o emulsions. Tween emulsifiers have HLB numbers in the range of 9.6–16.7; they are more hydrophilic and favor o/w emulsions. Table 29.1 gives HLB values for some common non-ionic surfactants used in compounding.

    c. Experimental work was also done to determine "required HLB" values for various types of formulations and ingredients. Table 29.2 gives some of these "required" values for both o/w and w/o emulsions with common pharmaceutical ingredients. Some sample calculations using HLB values are given below, and Sample Prescription 29.3 gives an additional illustration.

    d. When a blend of oil/wax ingredients is used, the final "required HLB" is a total calculated from the sum of individual required HLBs of each ingredient times its weight fraction of all oil-type ingredients.

TABLE 29.1   HLB Values of Some Surfactants

Surfactant	HLB
Sorbitan trioleate (Span® 85)*	1.8
Sorbitan tristearate (Span® 65)*	2.1
Sorbitan sesquioleate (Arlacel 83)*	3.7
Glyceryl monostearate, N.F.	3.8
Sorbitan monooleate, N.F., (Span® 80)*	4.3
Sorbitan monostearate, N.F., (Span® 60)*	4.7
Sorbitan monopalmitate, N.F., (Span® 40)*	6.7
Sorbitan monolaurate, N.F., (Span® 20)*	8.6
Polyoxyethylene sorbitan tristearate (Tween® 65)*	10.5
Polyoxyethylene sorbitan trioleate (Tween® 85)*	11.0
Polyethylene glycol 400 monostearate	11.6
Polysorbate 60, N.F., (Tween® 60)*	14.9
Polyoxyethylene monostearate (Myrj 49)*	15.0
Polysorbate 80, N.F., (Tween® 80)*	15.0
Polysorbate 40, N.F., (Tween® 40)*	15.6
Polysorbate 20, N.F., (Tween® 20)*	16.7

*ICI Americas, Inc., Wilmington, Delaware.

e. Some formulators maintain that using a 50-50 blend of Span and Tween gives emulsions that are as satisfactory as those made using Span-Tween blends calculated from the HLB system. Although this is often true for o/w systems, it may fail for w/o emulsions. The reason for this is readily apparent if the HLB values of common Spans and Tweens are observed. A 50-50 blend of many polysorbate-sorbitan ester combinations gives a final HLB of 10 or greater; this is a desirable HLB for most o/w emulsions. Such a resultant HLB is, however, often too high for stable w/o systems.

f. Phase ratio also plays an important role in the type of emulsion formed using these emulsifiers.

3. Measurement of polysorbate-sorbitan ester emulsifiers: All are customarily measured by weight, not by volume. This is because, at room temperature, some of these emulsifiers are solids and others are thick liquids.

4. Order of mixing

a. Although some sources recommend dissolving the oil-soluble sorbitan ester portions (the Spans) in the oil, and the water-soluble polysorbate part (the Tweens)

TABLE 29.2   "Required HLB" Values of Some Ingredients

Ingredient	"Required HLB" for w/o emulsion	o/w emulsion
Acid, Lauric	–	15–16
Acid, Oleic	–	17
Acid, Stearic	6	15
Alcohol, Cetyl	–	15
Alcohol, Lauryl	–	14
Alcohol, Stearyl	–	14
Lanolin, Anhydrous	8	10
Oil, Castor	6	14
Oil, Cottonseed	5	10
Oil, Mineral	5	12
Oil, Olive	6	14
Petrolatum	5	12
Wax, Beeswax	4	12
Wax, Paraffin	4	11

in the water, many pharmacists find it much easier to dissolve or disperse both emulsifiers in the oil phase. Although the polysorbate compound eventually dissolves in water, it tends to "lump up" initially, making it difficult to work with.

b. If no solid ingredients are present in the formulation, the emulsion can easily be made directly in the dispensing bottle. Put all ingredients in the bottle and shake well. A more uniform preparation, with finer emulsion droplets, can be achieved by passing the emulsion through a hand-homogenizer or by processing the emulsion in a blender.

c. If solids are to be added, this must be done in a mortar. Either make the emulsion first using the bottle method and then add the emulsion, in portions with trituration, to the solids in the mortar, or put the solids in a Wedgewood mortar, add the oil-emulsifier with trituration, and then **gradually** add the water phase in portions with trituration.

5. Unlike gums, non-ionic surfactants are not viscosity-inducing agents. When using these emulsifiers, it may be necessary to add a viscosity-increasing agent or a viscous vehicle to retard the rate of creaming. This, of course, depends on the phase ratio of the ingredients; an emulsion with a high concentration of internal phase will be more viscous than a preparation with a small amount of dispersed phase. For an o/w oral preparation, a flavored syrup, such as orange or cherry syrup, may be substituted for all or part of the water because it will serve the dual functions of flavoring and increasing the viscosity and density of the external phase.

6. Sample calculations

Rx	Mineral Oil		50 mL
	Span 60	q.s.	
	Tween 40	q.s.	
	Cherry Syrup		40 mL
	Distilled Water	q.s. ad. 120 mL	

Total amount of emulsifier needed: *5% × 120 mL = 6 g*

This is a preparation for internal use, so an o/w emulsion is preferred. Mineral Oil has a "required HLB" of 12 (some sources give 10) for an o/w emulsion.

HLB of Span 60: 4.7   HLB of Tween 40: 15.6

If a 50-50 mixture is used, weigh 3 g each of Span 60 and Tween 40.
This combination has an HLB of:

50% × 4.7	*=*	*2.35*
50% × 15.6	*=*	*7.8*
Total HLB	*=*	*10.15*

This value is between the recommended HLBs of 10 and 12 and would give a perfectly satisfactory emulsion.
The amount of Span 60 and Tween 40 based on "required HLB" can be calculated using either alligation or algebra.

• By algebra:

$$HLB = f_T (HLB_T) + f_S (HLB_S)$$

where: HLB = Total desired HLB
HLB_T = HLB of the Tween
HLB_S = HLB of the Span
f_T & f_S = weight-fractions of Tween and Span

because $f_T + f_S = 1$, then $f_T = 1 - f_S$
$$\therefore 12 = (1 - f_S) (15.6) + f_S(4.7)$$
$$12 = 15.6 - (f_S)(15.6) + f_S(4.7)$$
$$10.9 f_S = 3.6$$

$f_S = 0.33$ This is the weight-fraction of Span.

The weight-fraction of Tween is:

$$f_T = 1 - f_S = 1 - 0.33 = 0.67$$

The weight in grams of Span 60 for 6 g of total emulsifier is:

0.33 × 6 g = 1.98 g

The weight in grams of Tween 40 for 6 g of total emulsifier is:

0.67 × 6 g = 4.02 g

- By alligation:

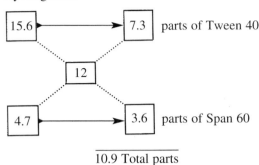

$$\frac{7.3\ g\ Tween\ 40}{10.9\ g\ total\ emulsifier} = \frac{x\ g\ Tween\ 40}{6\ g\ total\ emulsifier};\ x = 4.02\ g\ Tween\ 40$$

$$\frac{3.6\ g\ Span\ 60}{10.9\ g\ total\ emulsifier} = \frac{x\ g\ Span\ 60}{6\ g\ total\ emulsifier};\ x = 1.98\ g\ Span\ 60$$

VI. STABILITY

A. Physical stability of the system: Maintenance of small droplets and ease of redispersion are both essential to the physical stability of emulsion systems. Because emulsions are by nature physically unstable systems, beyond-use dates for these preparations should be conservative even with ingredients that are chemically stable.

B. Chemical stability of the ingredients: Because the preparation beyond-use date depends on the stability of the ingredients, check suitable references such as those listed in Chapter 34. The *USP* chapter on pharmacy compounding, Chapter ⟨795⟩, recommends a maximum 14-day dating for all water-containing preparations, such as emulsions, made with ingredients in solid form when the stability of the ingredients in the formulation is unknown (5). When ingredients of questionable stability are present, more conservative datings should be considered. Many external-use preparations are formulated from ingredients, such as Zinc Oxide and Calamine, that are known to be very stable. For these preparations, a 1-month dating would be satisfactory.

C. Microbiologic stability: The *USP* states that all emulsions require an antimicrobial agent because the aqueous phase is favorable to the growth of microorganisms. This is especially true of o/w emulsions and emulsions made with natural gums. Growth of fungi (molds) and yeasts is especially problematic, so the preservative chosen should have fungistatic as well as bacteriostatic properties. Bacteria have been shown to degrade non-ionic and anionic surfactants, as well as natural gums (1). If antimicrobial ingredients are present in the formulation, extra preservatives may not be needed. For acceptable preservatives, see the previous discussion of individual emulsion types and see Chapter 15, Preservatives.

VII. SPECIAL LABELING REQUIREMENTS FOR EMULSIONS

A. All emulsions are disperse systems and need a "Shake Well" auxiliary label.

B. External use emulsions should be labeled "For External Use Only."

SAMPLE PRESCRIPTIONS

➤ Prescription 29.1

Contemporary Physicians Group Practice
20 S. Park Street, Triturate, WI 53706
Tel: (608) 555-1333 Fax: (608) 555-1335

R # 466

Name *Laurie Mower*   Date *00/00/00*

Address *905 Chickadee Lane*   Age   Wt/Ht

Rx

Calamine	5%
Zinc Oxide	5%
Dioxybenzone	3%
Oxybenzone	3%
Almond Oil	45 mL
Acacia	qs
Rose Water	qs ad 90 mL

Ted Fence   00/00/00

Sig: *Apply to exposed areas of skin prior to sun exposure*

Refills   5   *Jackson Parker*   M.D.

DEA No. _____

Ingredients Used

Ingredient	Quantity Used	Manufacturer Lot #-Exp Date	Solubility	Dose Comparison Given	Dose Comparison Usual	Use in the Prescription
Almond Oil	45 mL	JET Labs EM2911-mm/yy	immisc w/water, alcohol	—	—	part of emulsion vehicle system
Zinc Oxide	4.5 g	JET Labs SS2812-mm/yy	insol. in water and alcohol	4.4%	5–20%	astringent, protective, antiseptic
Calamine	4.5 g	JET Labs SS2811-mm/yy	insol. in water and alcohol	4.4%	5–20%	astringent, protective, antiseptic
Dioxybenzone	2.7 g	JET Labs EM2912-mm/yy	pr. insol in water; fr sol. in alcohol	3%	3%	sunscreen
Oxybenzone	2.7 g	JET Labs EM2913-mm/yy	pr. insol in water; fr sol. in alcohol	3%	3%	sunscreen
Acacia	11.25 g	JET Labs EM2914-mm/yy	1 g/2 mL water insol. alcohol	—	—	emulsifying agent
Rose Water	qs ad 90 mL	JET Labs EM2915-mm/yy	—	—	—	part of emulsion vehicle system
Alcohol USP	5.7 mL	JET Labs EM2916-mm/yy	miscible w/water	6%	6%	preservative

Compatibility–Stability/Beyond-Use Date

Stability–Compatibility: The Calamine and Zinc Oxide in this preparation are compatible and very stable when in an Acacia emulsion. The stability of the Oxybenzone and the Dioxybenzone is more difficult to assess. There is a manufactured sunscreen lotion that contains these two ingredients, but that product is a suspension and the current formulation is an emulsion. Also, the prescribed preparation contains extra ingredients that could affect the stability of these compounds.

Preservative: Although the Zinc Oxide and Calamine have antimicrobial properties, Pharmacist Fence wants to be on the safe side and add a preservative because of the susceptibility to microbial growth of Acacia emulsions. One traditional preservative for Acacia emulsions is Sodium Benzoate, which works well in the usual pH of 4.5 to 5 for these emulsions. Pharmacist Fence wisely checked the pH of the final preparation because he was concerned that the Zinc Oxide might impart a higher pH to the emulsion. The pH was found to be 7, too high for use of Sodium Benzoate. He therefore selected Alcohol 6% as the preservative.

Packaging and Storage and Beyond-use date: Pharmacist Fence will use the *USP* recommended maximum 14-day beyond-use date for compounded water-containing formulations prepared from ingredients in solid form when there is no stability information for the formulation (5). The *USP* monographs for Oxybenzone and Dioxybenzone recommend storage in tight, light-resistant containers (6). Because this is a topical preparation, controlled room temperature will be the recommended storage conditions.

Calculations

Dose/Concentration

All concentrations OK

Ingredient Amounts

Zinc Oxide and Calamine in g: *5% × 90 mL = 4.5 g*

Dioxybenzone and Oxybenzone in g: *3% × 90 mL = 2.7 g*

Calculation of oil:water:Acacia content for primary emulsion:

Oil:Water:Acacia = 4:2:1 = 45 mL:22.5 mL:11.25 g

Preservative: Alcohol 6% is used. The volume of pure ethyl alcohol is calculated here.

6% × 90 mL = 5.4 mL ethyl alcohol

Ethyl Alcohol is available as Alcohol USP, which is 95% ethyl alcohol. The volume of Alcohol USP that contains 5.4 mL of ethyl alcohol is calculated to be:

95% × x mL Alcohol = 5.4 mL ethyl alcohol; x = 5.7 mL Alcohol USP

Compounding Procedure

All weighing is done on a class 3 torsion or an electronic balance. Weigh 11.25 g of Acacia and put in a dry Wedgewood mortar. Gradually add 45 mL of Almond Oil and triturate well. Weigh 2.7 g each of Dioxybenzone and Oxybenzone and add these to the Almond Oil–Acacia mixture and triturate to disperse and dissolve the drugs. In a clean 25-mL graduated cylinder, measure 22.5 mL of Rose Water. Add this all at once to the oil–drug–Acacia mixture in the mortar and triturate rapidly to form the primary emulsion. Add some extra Rose Water to reduce the viscosity of the emulsion. Weigh 4.5 g each of Zinc Oxide and Calamine and place in a mortar. Wet the powders by adding the previously formed emulsion to them with trituration. If it gets too thick, small amounts of additional Rose Water may be added. To preserve, add 5.7 mL of Alcohol USP to the emulsion. Pour the emulsion into a 3-oz prescription bottle with a child-resistant closure. Use successive rinses of the mortar with the Rose Water to q.s. to the 90-mL mark. Cap tightly. Shake the bottle well; label and dispense.

Quality Control

This preparation is a pink oil-in-water emulsion. It is fairly viscous, and no creaming or settling occurs in 2 hours. The preparation pours easily after shaking. The pH of the preparation is checked and recorded; pH = 7.

Labeling

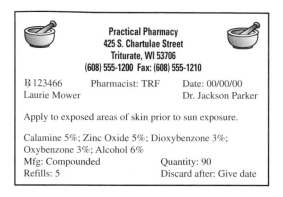

Practical Pharmacy
425 S. Chartulae Street
Triturate, WI 53706
(608) 555-1200 Fax: (608) 555-1210

R 123466   Pharmacist: TRF   Date: 00/00/00
Laurie Mower   Dr. Jackson Parker

Apply to exposed areas of skin prior to sun exposure.

Calamine 5%; Zinc Oxide 5%; Dioxybenzone 3%;
Oxybenzone 3%; Alcohol 6%
Mfg: Compounded   Quantity: 90
Refills: 5   Discard after: Give date

Auxiliary Labels: Shake well; For external use only

Patient Consultation

Hello, Ms. Mower, I'm your pharmacist, Ted Fence. Do you have any drug allergies? Are you taking any other medications? What did your doctor tell you about this lotion? This is a specially formulated sunscreen. Prior to sun exposure, you are to apply this to areas of your skin that are not covered with clothing and that therefore will be exposed to the sun's rays. This lotion will also lubricate and protect the area. If you experience any type of skin reaction or allergy, or if this does not seem to be working, discontinue use and contact Dr. Parker. Be sure to shake this up well before applying. This is for external use only. Store it at room temperature and out of the reach of children. Discard any unused portion after 2 weeks (give date). This may be refilled five times.

➤ Prescription 29.2

Contemporary Physicians Group Practice
20 S. Park Street, Triturate, WI 53706
Tel: (608) 555-1333 Fax: (608) 555-1335

R # 462

Name *Fr. Paul Saint*	Date *00/00/00*

Address *926 Holy Lane*	Age	Wt/Ht

R

Phenol	1.2 g
Menthol	0.3 g
Zinc Oxide	8 g
Lime water	60 mL
Cottonseed Oil	q s ad 120 mL

B. Bellfree 00/00/00

Sig: *Apply to affected areas prn ut dict*

Refills   1   *J. T. Largay*   M.D.

DEA No. _____

Ingredients Used

Ingredient	Quantity Used	Manufacturer Lot #-Exp Date	Solubility	Dose Comparison Given	Dose Comparison Usual	Use in the Prescription
Menthol	300 mg	JET Labs SS2822-mm/yy	sl. sol. water; v. sol. alcohol	0.25%	1–3%	antipyretic, counterirritant
Phenol	1.2 g	JET Labs SS2831-mm/yy	1 g/15 mL water; v. sol. alcohol, glycerin	1.0%	0.5–2.0%	antiseptic, topical anesthetic
Zinc Oxide	8 g	JET Labs SS2812-mm/yy	insol in water and alcohol	6.7%	5–20%	astringent, protective, antiseptic
Lime Water (Contents in Calculations)	60 mL	Prac. Pharmacy JT1143-mm/yy	misc w/water and alcohol	—	—	part of emulsion vehicle system
Cottonseed Oil	qs ad 120 mL	JET Labs EM2921-mm/yy	immisc w/water and alcohol	—	—	emollient, part of emulsion system
Oleic Acid	1.8 mL	JET Labs EM2922-mm/yy	prac insol in water; misc w/alcohol & oils	—	—	part of emulsifier
Aquabase®	4 g	Paddock Labs RA012-mm/yy	insol in water and alcohol	—	—	auxiliary emulsifier

Compatibility–Stability/Beyond-Use Date

Stability–Compatibility: The ingredients in this preparation are compatible and most likely quite stable when in this emulsion. The content of this preparation is similar to the official product Phenolated Calamine Lotion (5), although the official product is a suspension and the prescribed formulation is an emulsion. This preparation also contains Menthol, which is also probably quite stable in this formulation.

Preservative: No extra preservative is needed because of the alkaline pH and because Phenol is an excellent antimicrobial agent.

Packaging and Storage and Beyond-use date: Although this is probably a fairly stable preparation, Pharmacist Bellfree will use the *USP* recommended maximum 14-day beyond-use date for compounded water-containing formulations prepared from ingredients in solid form when there is no stability information for the formulation (5). Because this is a topical preparation, storage should be in controlled room temperature, and the preparation should be packaged in a tight container.

Calculations

Dose/Concentration

Phenol in %:

$$\frac{1.2 \ g \ Phenol}{120 \ mL \ lotion} = \frac{x \ g \ Phenol}{100 \ mL \ lotion}; \ x = 1 \ g \ Phenol \, / \, 100 \ mL = 1\%$$

Menthol in %:

$$\frac{0.3 \ g \ Menthol}{120 \ mL \ lotion} = \frac{x \ g \ Menthol}{100 \ mL \ lotion}; \ x = 0.25 \ g \ Menthol \, / \, 100 \ mL = 0.25\%$$

Zinc Oxide in %:

$$\frac{8 \ g \ Zinc \ Oxide}{120 \ mL \ lotion} = \frac{x \ g \ Zinc \ Oxide}{100 \ mL \ lotion}; \ x = 6.7 \ g \ Zinc \ Oxide \, / \, 100 \ mL = 6.7\%$$

All concentrations are OK for the intended use.

Ingredient Amounts

Calculation of Calcium Hydroxide amount to make Lime Water: Make any reasonable amount greater than or equal to 60 mL; 150 mL is a suggested amount so you will have a sufficient amount to make the product twice in case of problems.

$$\frac{3\,g\,Calcium\,Hydroxide}{1000\,mL\,water} = \frac{x\,g\,Calcium\,Hydroxide}{150\,mL\,water};\ x = 0.45\,g\,Calcium\,Hydroxide$$

Compounding Procedure

On a class 3 or an electronic digital balance, weigh 450 mg of Calcium Hydroxide, 300 mg of Menthol, 1.2 g of Phenol, and 8 g of Zinc Oxide. Place the Calcium Hydroxide in a graduate and q.s. to 150 mL with Purified Water; stir occasionally over 1 hour and then allow any solid to settle. Place Menthol and Phenol in a Wedge-wood mortar and triturate to force liquification of the eutectic mixture. Weigh 4 g of Aquabase® and add to the eutectic mixture with trituration. Measure 45–50 mL of Cottonseed Oil in a graduated cylinder and draw 3 mL of Oleic Acid into a syringe. Add 1.5 mL of the Oleic Acid to the Cottonseed Oil. Add alternating portions of the Zinc Oxide and Cottonseed Oil to the Phenol mixture with trituration. Continue adding these alternately to maintain a proper consistency for making a smooth product until all the Zinc Oxide and Cottonseed Oil are added. Decant 60 mL of the Lime Water from the graduate and add it in portions with trituration to the Wedge-wood mortar. If emulsion appears to be coalescing, add several more drops of Oleic Acid, keeping track of the total amount of Oleic Acid added. Transfer the product to a 4-oz prescription bottle with child-resistant closure. Use some Cottonseed Oil to rinse the mortar and to q.s. to the 120-mL mark on the prescription bottle. Label and dispense.

Quality Control

This preparation is a white water-in-oil emulsion. It is fairly viscous, and there is no apparent creaming or settling in 2 hours. Although viscous, the preparation pours smoothly after shaking. The pH of the preparation is checked with pH paper and recorded; pH = 12.

Labeling

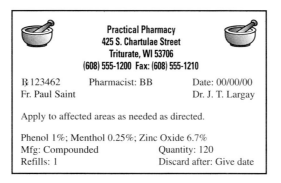

Practical Pharmacy
425 S. Chartulae Street
Triturate, WI 53706
(608) 555-1200 Fax: (608) 555-1210

℞ 123462   Pharmacist: BB   Date: 00/00/00
Fr. Paul Saint   Dr. J. T. Largay

Apply to affected areas as needed as directed.

Phenol 1%; Menthol 0.25%; Zinc Oxide 6.7%
Mfg: Compounded   Quantity: 120
Refills: 1   Discard after: Give date

Auxiliary Labels: Shake well; For external use only

Patient Consultation

Hello, Father Saint, I'm your pharmacist, Batziner Bellfree. Do you have any drug allergies? Are you using any other medication products? What did your doctor tell you about this lotion? This is to treat the skin condition that Dr. Largay diagnosed. The directions say to apply to affected areas as needed as directed. Did Dr. Largay explain how you were to use it? Don't use any other topical medication on the area unless you were advised to do so by Dr. Largay. Shake the bottle well before using. Remember, this is for external use only. If the condition doesn't improve, or gets worse, contact Dr. Largay. This should be stored at room temperature away from heat and light, and out of the reach of children. Discard any unused portion after 2 weeks (give date). You may have one refill. Do you have any questions?

➤ **Prescription 29.3**

Contemporary Physicians Group Practice
20 S. Park Street, Triturate, WI 53706
Tel: (608) 555-1333 Fax: (608) 555-1335

R # 465

Name *Mildred Stauffacher*   Date *00/00/00*

Address *88 1/3 Third Avenue*   *Age*   *Wt/Ht*

℞

Castor Oil	45 mL
Tween 80	qs
Span 20	qs
Orange Syrup	q s ad 90 mL

J. Jupiter 00/00/00

Sig: *Take entire contents of bottle at 4 PM on afternoon*
before procedure. Follow in 4 hours with X-Prep

Refills   *0*   *Olive Quacky*   M.D.

DEA No. _____

Ingredients Used

Ingredient	Quantity Used	Manufacturer Lot #-Exp Date	Solubility	Dose Comparison Given	Dose Comparison Usual	Use in the Prescription
Castor Oil	45 mL	JET Labs EM2931-mm/yy	immis with water; misc with alcohol	45 mL	15–60 mL	laxative
Tween 80	3.8 g	JET Labs EM2932-mm/yy	misc with water, alcohol, oils	—	—	emulsifying agent
Span 20	0.7 g	JET Labs EM2933-mm/yy	insol in water, misc w/oils	—	—	emulsifying agent
Orange Syrup	qs ad 90 mL	JET Labs EM2934-mm/yy	miscible with water	—	—	flavored vehicle

Compatibility–Stability/Beyond-Use Date

Stability–Compatibility: This is a very simple preparation containing just Castor Oil in an emulsion, and it should be very stable. There is an official *USP* Castor Oil Emulsion, but no formulation information is given (6).

Preservative: No extra preservative is needed because the Orange Syrup comes preserved with Sodium Benzoate.

Packaging and Storage and Beyond-use date: The *USP* monograph for Castor Oil Emulsion recommends storage in tight containers (6). Although there are manufactured versions of this formulation with expiration dates of several years, Pharmacist Jupiter will use a more conservative 1-month beyond-use date for this compounded preparation. Because it is an oral emulsion, it should be stored in the refrigerator; this will enhance the taste and improve microbiological stability.

Calculations

Dose/Concentration

Dose of Castor Oil OK

Ingredient Amounts

Total emulsifier concentration is 5%. This amount in g is: *5% × 90 mL = 4.5 g*

Span 20 and Tween 80 are the emulsifiers. The amount of each in g is calculated using the HLB system and either algebra or alligation. The alligation method is shown here. See the chapter text for an example using algebra.

Because this is an oral emulsion, an o/w system is desired. The required HLB for Castor Oil o/w emulsions is 14.

Using Span 20 and Tween 80 for emulsifiers, calculate the number of grams of each necessary to compound this prescription. Span 20 has an HLB of 8.6 and Tween 80 has an HLB of 15.

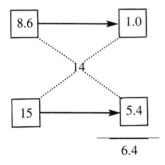

Span 20 in g:

$$\frac{5.4}{6.4} \times 4.5\,g = 3.8\,g\ Tween\ 80$$

Tween 80 in g:

$$\frac{1}{6.4} \times 4.5\,g = 0.7\,g\ Span\ 20$$

Compounding Procedure

On a class 3 torsion or electronic balance, weigh 3.8 g of Tween 80 and 0.7 g of Span 20. Using a 3-oz prescription bottle that has calibration marks at 45 mL and at 90 mL, pour Castor Oil into the bottle to the 45-mL mark. Transfer the Tween and the Span into the bottle and agitate to mix. Add Orange Syrup to the 90-mL mark, and shake well to form the emulsion. Label and dispense.

Quality Control

This preparation is an orange oil-in-water emulsion. It has moderate viscosity; after 2 hours there appears a slightly transparent zone of orange syrup at the bottom of the bottle, indicating some creaming. The preparation is very easily redispersed with shaking. The pH of the preparation is checked with pH paper and recorded; pH = 3.

Labeling

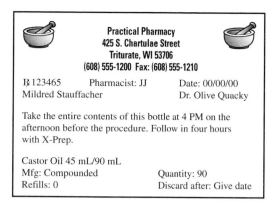

> **Practical Pharmacy**
> **425 S. Chartulae Street**
> **Triturate, WI 53706**
> **(608) 555-1200 Fax: (608) 555-1210**
>
> ℞ 123465   Pharmacist: JJ   Date: 00/00/00
> Mildred Stauffacher   Dr. Olive Quacky
>
> Take the entire contents of this bottle at 4 PM on the afternoon before the procedure. Follow in four hours with X-Prep.
>
> Castor Oil 45 mL/90 mL
> Mfg: Compounded   Quantity: 90
> Refills: 0   Discard after: Give date

Auxiliary Labels: Shake well; Keep in the Refrigerator

Patient Consultation

Hello, Ms. Stauffacher, I'm your pharmacist, Jor-el Jupiter. Do you have any drug allergies? Are you currently using any other prescription or over-the-counter drug products? What has your physician told you about using the medication? This is a laxative/purgative to prepare your gastrointestinal tract for your scheduled examination. Have you ever used anything like this before? This is rather fast-acting and may cause stomach cramps and diarrhea. I recommend that you don't wander too far from a restroom after you have taken this medication. You should take the entire contents of this bottle at 4 p.m. on the afternoon before your test; then 4 hours after taking this, take a full dose of X-Prep. Shake this bottle well before taking the contents. Keep it in the refrigerator until the day you have to take it—it will taste somewhat better if it is cold. You might want to have a little something like soda or juice to rinse your mouth and wash this down. This expires in 1 month (give date), so if your appointment gets changed to a date beyond the expiration date of this preparation, contact Dr. Quacky for a new prescription order. Do you have any questions?

References

1. The 2002 United States Pharmacopeia 25/National Formulary 20. Rockville, MD: The United States Pharmacopeial Convention, Inc., 2001;2217.
2. Spalton LM. Pharmaceutical emulsions and emulsifying agents. Brooklyn, NY: Chemical Publishing, Inc., 1950;10.
3. The 2002 United States Pharmacopeia 25/National Formulary 20. Rockville, MD: The United States Pharmacopeial Convention, Inc., 2001;289.
4. Griffin WC. J Soc Cos Chem 1954;5:249.
5. The 2002 United States Pharmacopeia 25/National Formulary 20. Rockville, MD: The United States Pharmacopeial Convention, Inc., 2001;2054.
6. The 2002 United States Pharmacopeia 25/National Formulary 20. Rockville, MD: The United States Pharmacopeial Convention, Inc., 2001; Official Monographs.

CHAPTER 30

Ointments, Creams, Gels, and Pastes

I. DEFINITIONS

A. Ointments
"Ointments are semisolid preparations intended for external application to the skin or mucous membranes." (1)—*USP*

B. According to the *USP*, there are four general classes of ointment bases: hydrocarbon, absorption, water-removable, and water-soluble. Pastes and gels met the general classification of an ointment, but they are defined separately by the *USP*. Although creams have also been given a separate class by the *USP*, the term is now commonly reserved for ointment bases of the water-removable class. Creams, pastes, and gels are defined and described in Chapter 22, and the four classes of ointment bases, their composition, and characteristics are also discussed. For the purpose of this chapter, the word *ointment* is used in its most general sense, encompassing all semisolid dosage forms intended for external application.

II. USES OF OINTMENTS, CREAMS, GELS, AND PASTES

A. To protect skin or mucous membrane from chemical or physical irritants in the environment and to permit rejuvenation of the tissue

B. To provide hydration of the skin or an emollient effect

C. To provide a vehicle for applying a medication either for local or systemic effect (e.g., local—a topical antibiotic; systemic—a nitroglycerin ointment for treating angina)

III. CHOICE OF A BASE

A. The choice of a base depends on:
1. The action or effect desired (see item II above)
2. The nature of the incorporated medication
    a. Bioavailability
    b. Stability
    c. Compatibility
3. The area of application

B. If a prescription order specifies a particular ointment base and a change of base is necessary for compatibility or stability reasons, the prescriber should be consulted.

IV. PRINCIPLES OF COMPOUNDING OINTMENTS

A. Compounding Equipment

1. **Ointment slabs or pads**

   a. In the United States, ointments are commonly made using a spatula and an ointment slab or pad. In some other countries, mortars and pestles are the preferred compounding equipment.

   b. Although ointment pads are nice because they minimize cleanup, they do have some limitations. Ointment slabs are preferred when a liquid ingredient must be incorporated into the ointment, especially if the liquid is an aqueous solution. Liquids soak into the parchment paper of ointment pads, and excess weight can be lost. Very sticky or thick ointments are often more easily made on a slab. Loss is usually less when an ointment is compounded on an ointment slab than on a pad.

2. **Spatulas**

   a. Generally, large metal spatulas are used for levigation, spatulation, and incorporation of solid and liquid ingredients. Smaller metal spatulas are useful for removing product from the large spatula and for transferring product from the ointment slab or pad to the ointment jar.

   b. Black rubber or plastic spatulas are special-purpose spatulas that are used when an ingredient (e.g., iodine) reacts with a metal spatula. They are not for general use in compounding ointments because they do not have the proper combination of flexibility and strength to give adequate shear and mixing.

3. For pharmacies that do significant compounding of customized ointments and creams, small-scale ointment mills and specialized electric ointment mixers are available. This sort of equipment can produce smooth, elegant preparations with minimal effort.

B. Amount of excess product to make to compensate for loss during compounding

1. Depending on factors such as compounding technique, number and type of ointment ingredients, and difficulty of the compounding process, between 2 and 4 g of an ointment may be lost in the compounding process when preparing a moderate amount of ointment (e.g., 15–120 g).

2. Either a percentage of excess (e.g., 10%) or a given amount of excess product (e.g., 3 g) is usually made to compensate for this loss. The amount of excess made is based on the pharmacist's own experience and professional judgment.

C. Incorporation of Solid Drugs and Chemicals

1. **General Principles**

   a. Because a smooth, nongritty product is desired, any solids incorporated into an ointment base should be either solubilized or in the finest state of subdivision possible.

   b. Auxiliary agents, such as levigating agents and solvents, are sometimes added during the formulation of an ointment to facilitate making a smooth, elegant product. Auxiliary agents that make a substantive change in the product's properties should be avoided. For example, if a stiff, paste-like ointment is desired, avoid adding an auxiliary agent that would significantly decrease the viscosity of the formulation.

2. **Choice of drug form**

   a. If possible, pick a form of the drug that is a fine powder (for example, Boric Acid powder rather than Boric Acid crystals, or colloidal sulfur rather than Precipitated Sulfur).

   b. If the prescription order specifies a certain form, that form should be used unless the prescriber is consulted.

    c. If a drug or chemical is available in more than one form, the selected form should be specified on the face of the prescription document or in the compounding log.

3. Levigation

    a. Levigation is the process of reducing the particle size of a solid by triturating it in a mortar or spatulating it on an ointment slab or pad with a small amount of a liquid or melted base in which the solid is not soluble.

    b. Optimally the liquid, called a **levigating agent**, is somewhat viscous and has a low surface tension to improve ease of wetting the solid. When solids are added directly to an ointment base, a certain amount of energy is required just to overcome the high resistance to flow of the semisolid ointment base. This resistance to flow makes it difficult to provide adequate shear to reduce the particle size of a solid when the manual techniques used in compounding are employed. Levigating agents act as lubricating agents. They make incorporating solids easier, and they usually give smoother products.

    c. Often the ointment formulation contains an ingredient that can be used as a levigating agent. This is the preferred situation. If the prescribed formula does not contain an ingredient that may be used for this purpose, it is generally acceptable to add an auxiliary agent, provided it is bland and nontoxic and does not make a substantive change in the product's physical or therapeutic properties.

    d. It is important to remember that auxiliary levigating agents are added to facilitate making a smooth, elegant preparation. An added levigating agent is not needed when:

        (1) The solid being incorporated has a very fine particle size

        (2) The quantity of solid to incorporate is small

        (3) The ointment base is soft

        (4) The final product is to be a stiff ointment or paste

    e. Types of levigating agents

        (1) Commonly used levigating agents are listed in Table 30.1; their specific gravities, miscibilities, and general uses are given. More complete descriptions of the oils and solvents can be found in Chapter 14, Pharmaceutical Solvents, and Polysorbate 80 is described in Chapter 19, Surfactants and Emulsifying Agents.

        (2) Melted ointment base may also be used.

        (3) Special levigating agents are sometimes required for compatibility or stability reasons.

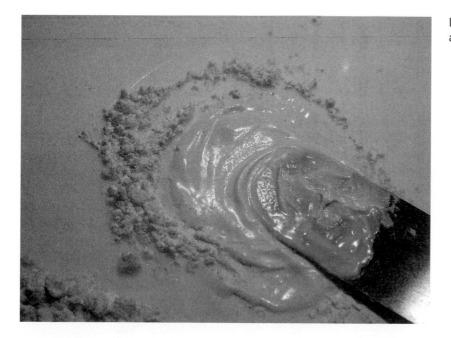

Levigation of a powder on an ointment slab

TABLE 30.1 Levigating Agents

Levigating Agents	Specific Gravity	Miscibility	Uses
Mineral Oil (Also known as Heavy Mineral Oil)	0.88 Light: 0.85	Miscible with fixed oils* except castor oil Immiscible with water, alcohol, glycerin, propylene glycol, PEG 400, and castor oil	– Oleaginous Bases – Absorption Bases – Water-in-Oil Emulsion Bases
Glycerin	1.26	Miscible with water, alcohol, propylene glycol, and PEG 400 Immiscible with mineral oil, and fixed oils*	– Oil-in-Water Emulsion Bases – Water Soluble Bases – Ichthammol
Propylene Glycol	1.04	Miscible with water, alcohol, glycerin, and PEG 400 Immiscible with mineral oil and fixed oils*	– Oil-in-Water Emulsion Bases – Water Soluble Bases
PEG 400	1.13	Miscible with water, alcohol, glycerin, and propylene glycol Immiscible with mineral oil and fixed oils*	– Oil-in-Water Emulsion Bases – Water Soluble Bases
Cottonseed Oil	0.92	Miscible with mineral oil and other fixed oils,* including castor oil Immiscible with water, alcohol, glycerin, propylene glycol, and PEG 400	– Cottonseed or any other vegetable oil can be used as a substitute for mineral oil when a vegetable oil is preferred or when the solid to be incorporated is more soluble or mixes more smoothly with a vegetable oil than with mineral oil
Castor Oil	0.96	Miscible with alcohol and other fixed oils* Immiscible with water, glycerin, propylene glycol, PEG 400, and mineral oil	–Ichthammol or Balsam of Peru – Same uses as described above with cottonseed oil
Polysorbate 80 (Tween® 80)	1.06–1.09 (Usually Weighed)	Miscible with water, alcohol, glycerin, propylene glycol, PEG 400, mineral oil, and fixed oils*	– Coal Tar – Other instances when a surfactant is desired – May be incompatible with some water-in oil emulsion bases

*Fixed oils consist of glyceryl esters of fatty acids that are liquids at room temperature and nonvolatile under ordinary conditions. Examples of fixed oils are cottonseed oil, castor oil, olive oil, sesame oil and corn oil.

    f. Choosing a levigating agent

        (1) If the formulation already contains an ingredient that is a suitable levigating agent, that liquid should be used.

        (2) For an added levigating agent, check for compatibility with the other ointment ingredients and with the ointment base. Fortunately, most levigating agents are fairly unreactive and cause few compatibility problems.

        (3) **General rule:** Assuming that there are no compatibility problems with other ointment ingredients, levigating agents are usually chosen to be chemically similar to the ointment base. For example, Mineral Oil is the levigating agent of choice for oily bases, such as hydrocarbon, absorption, and water-in-oil emulsion bases (See Sample Prescription 30.1). Glycerin, which is miscible with water, is usually used for water-removable and water-soluble bases.

(4) Some active ingredients require special levigating agents. Several of these are listed below.

  (a) Polysorbate 80 (Tween 80) is used as the levigating agent for Coal Tar. Coal Tar Ointment USP contains an amount of Polysorbate 80 equal to half the weight of Coal Tar (see Sample Prescription 30.3). Coal Tar will not mix with Mineral Oil or Glycerin, but it can be directly incorporated into some ointment bases.

  (b) Castor Oil is recommended for levigating Peruvian Balsam. *Remington: The Science and Practice of Pharmacy* states that the resinous part of Peruvian Balsam separates out from ointments that also contain Sulfur unless an equal quantity of Castor Oil is used as the levigating agent for the Balsam of Peru. Sample Prescription 30.6 illustrates this use.

  (c) Although Ichthammol is a black, tarry substance, it is water-washable. Because it mixes with Glycerin and fixed oils, these are suitable levigating agents. Some pharmacists think they get a better product by levigating Ichthammol with an absorption base such as Hydrophilic Petrolatum or Aquabase®. In this case, the amount of absorption base used is equal to the amount of Ichthammol in the prescription order.

(5) Some levigating agents have compatibility problems with certain ointment bases or additives. Some examples are listed below.

  (a) Some nonionic surfactants may be incompatible with certain emulsion ointment bases if the surfactant favors the opposite emulsion type. For example, Polysorbate 80, which forms o/w emulsions, can cause a phase inversion and breakdown when mixed with some w/o emulsion ointment bases.

  (b) Depending on the relative amounts, Castor Oil can be incompatible with ointment bases or formulations that contain a significant amount of Mineral Oil. This is because Castor Oil is immiscible with Mineral Oil.

(6) Levigating agents should be nonsensitizing and nonallergenic. Because some patients are allergic to lanolin-type compounds (a much smaller percentage are allergic to purified derivatives, such as those present in Hydrophilic Petrolatum or Aquabase®), the prescriber and patient should be consulted before these are added to a prescription product.

g. Amount of levigating agent to use

(1) Factors that determine the amount of levigating agent needed include:

  (a) The quantity and properties of the solids to be incorporated

  (b) The levigating agent selected

  (c) The properties of the ointment base

  (d) The desired spreading consistency of the ointment

(2) Amounts of levigating agents used in official products can serve as a guide, but these vary considerably. Several examples illustrate this point.

  (a) Zinc Oxide Ointment USP calls for 15% Mineral Oil to be used for 20% Zinc Oxide in a White Ointment base (White Ointment contains the stiffening agent White Wax 5% in the ointment base White Petrolatum).

  (b) Zinc Oxide Paste USP uses no levigating agent for 50% solids (25% Zinc Oxide and 25% Starch) in White Petrolatum.

  (c) Sulfur Ointment USP uses 10% Mineral Oil for 10% Sulfur in White Petrolatum.

(3) **General rule:** Unless a prescription order specifically calls for a given amount of levigating agent, the **minimum amount** of levigating agent necessary to lubricate the powders is generally recommended.

  (a) To give you some idea of how much this is, 3 g of Zinc Oxide (10% Zinc Oxide for a 30-g ointment) requires approximately 1.5–2 mL of Mineral Oil or 1–1.25 mL of Glycerin to get adequate lubrication of the powder for levigation.

(b) In both of these cases, the percent w/w concentration of levigating agent for a 30-g ointment is 4–6%. This is the rationale for the recommendation of a maximum of 5% levigating agent that is found in some compounding references. You can easily see, however, that the amount really depends on the amount of powder to be levigated.

(4) The amount of levigating agent used should be measured in a syringe or graduate. The weight of the levigating agent that is used should be calculated from the volume incorporated using the agent's specific gravity. There should be a corresponding decrease in the weight of the ointment base to bring the product to the desired final weight. This is illustrated with Sample Prescription 30.6. Specific gravities of various levigating agents are given in Table 30.1.

h. Documentation: The name of the levigating agent and the quantity used should be noted on the face of the prescription order or the compounding log.

4. Dissolution

a. Under certain circumstances, dissolving a solid ingredient in a solvent or oil and subsequent incorporation of the solution into the ointment base is the preferred treatment. Certain crystalline ingredients such as Urea and Camphor are difficult or impossible to levigate to a fine powder and should be dissolved in a suitable solvent before incorporation in the ointment base. Testosterone is an example of a compound that gives gritty ointments unless it is first dissolved in an appropriate vegetable oil. It is not soluble in Mineral Oil.

b. Types of solvents

(1) Water-miscible solvents include Water, Alcohol, Isopropyl Alcohol, Glycerin, Propylene Glycol, and Polyethylene Glycol 400. Descriptions of these solvents can be found in Chapter 14.

(2) Lipophilic solvents include Mineral Oil and the various fixed oils, including Castor Oil, Cottonseed Oil, Olive Oil, and Corn Oil. Descriptions of these oils can also be found in Chapter 14.

c. Choosing a solvent

(1) Check a reference such as *Remington: The Science and Practice of Pharmacy, The Merck Index,* or *Martindale—The Complete Drug Reference* (formerly *The Extra Pharmacopoeia*) for solubility information on the ointment ingredient(s) to be dissolved.

(2) If the formulation already contains an ingredient that would be a suitable solvent, that liquid should be used to dissolve the solid.

(3) Check for compatibility of the solvent with the ointment base and other ointment ingredients.

d. Capacity of various ointment bases to absorb solvents

Based on their make-up, ointment bases have varying capacities to absorb liquids.

(1) Hydrocarbon bases absorb no water and only very limited amounts of alcoholic solutions. Most oil solvents mix easily with hydrocarbon bases, but they reduce the viscosity of the ointment.

(2) Anhydrous absorption bases can absorb large quantities of aqueous solutions and lesser amounts of alcoholic solutions.

(a) Hydrophilic Petrolatum and its branded commercial counterparts such as Aquabase® and Aquaphor® absorb an equal weight of water with relative ease, and up to several times their weight of water with adequate spatulation and patience.

(b) These bases absorb less alcohol, possibly up to an equal weight, because the alcohol eventually dissolves the emulsifiers in these absorption bases and destroys their ability to emulsify extra hydroalcoholic liquid.

(c) As with hydrocarbon bases, absorption bases easily incorporate most oils, with a corresponding decrease in the viscosity of the system.

(3) **Water-in-oil emulsion bases** accept varied amounts of water and alcoholic solutions.

- **(a)** Cold Cream and Rose Water Ointment are w/o emulsion bases that can absorb very little water.
- **(b)** Hydrocream® and Eucerin®, also w/o emulsion bases, absorb much more water than these but much less than their counterpart anhydrous absorption base Hydrophilic Petrolatum.
- **(c)** Although w/o emulsion bases easily accept most oils, as with hydrocarbon and absorption bases, their consistency may be decreased, depending on the amount of oil added.

(4) **Water-removable oil-in-water emulsion bases** accept water or water-miscible liquids in their external phase but eventually thin out to a fluid lotion with the addition of significant amounts of water.

- **(a)** The o/w emulsion base Hydrophilic Ointment USP and its commercial counterparts such as Dermabase®, and Aquaphilic® Ointment take up about 30% of their weight of water without thinning. They will accept a somewhat lesser amount of alcohol and will eventually break down if too much alcohol is added.
- **(b)** These ointment bases emulsify some amount of added oil because there is usually some excess emulsifying agent in the formulation. Larger quantities of oil may require the addition of a small amount of an o/w emulsifier, such as Polysorbate 80 (Tween 80).

(5) As their name indicates, **water-soluble bases** are soluble in water. They are also soluble in alcohol.

- **(a)** They accept a very limited amount of water or alcohol without loss of viscosity.
- **(b)** Addition of an oil may require prior levigation with a liquid of intermediate chemical properties, such as Glycerin or Propylene Glycol.

e. Strategies for adding solvents to nonabsorbing bases

If an aqueous or alcoholic solution must be added to a base that will not absorb it, the pharmacist may use one of the following strategies:

(1) Change the ointment base, in part or whole, to an absorption base or other base that will take up the liquid. If it is possible, stay within the same base class. For example, change from Cold Cream to Hydrocream®, both w/o emulsion bases, rather than to Aquabase®, an anhydrous absorption base. The prescriber should be consulted about base changes. This is illustrated with Sample Prescription 30.5.

(2) Add a nonionic auxiliary emulsifier or emulsifier combination.

- **(a)** Fatty alcohols such as Cetyl or Stearyl Alcohol can be added to hydrocarbon bases for this purpose. For example, when 5% Cetyl Alcohol is added to White Petrolatum, the combination will absorb 40–50% of its weight in water. Because these fatty alcohols are waxy substances, the combination must be melted and then allowed to congeal so that a smooth base results.
- **(b)** Span non-ionic surfactants are very useful for this purpose. For example, 2–5% Span 80, when directly incorporated into a hydrocarbon base, will enable the ointment to take up a significant amount of aqueous solution. This is illustrated with Sample Prescription 30.4.
- **(c)** Stearyl or Cetyl Alcohol can also be added to water-soluble Polyethylene Glycol bases to improve their water or alcohol absorption properties. The Polyethylene Glycol Ointment monograph in the *National Formulary* notes that 6–25% of an aqueous solution can be incorporated in Polyethylene Glycol Ointment if 5% of the PEG 3350 is replaced with an equal quantity of Stearyl Alcohol (2).

(3) Spatulate the solution and ointment base until a sufficient amount of the solvent evaporates.

    f. Be cautious when adding water to formulations containing drugs that are subject to hydrolysis. It may affect the stability of the preparation.

    g. Amount of solvent to add

      (1) General rule: Unless a prescription order specifically calls for a given amount of the solvent, use the **minimum amount** necessary to dissolve the powders.

      (2) The amount of solvent used should be measured in a syringe or graduate. The weight of the solvent that is used should be calculated from the volume incorporated using the solvent's specific gravity. There should be a corresponding decrease in the weight of the ointment base to bring the product to the desired final weight. This is illustrated with Sample Prescriptions 30.4 and 30.5. Specific gravities of some solvents are given in Table 30.2 and in the solvent descriptions in Chapter 14.

    h. Documentation: The name of the solvent and the quantity used should be noted on the face of the prescription order or in the compounding log.

D. Incorporation of Liquids

    1. Formulations that include liquids require ointment bases that will absorb the liquid. If a liquid must be added to a base that will not absorb it, one of the strategies given above for incorporating solutions may be used.

    2. When adding a nonviscous liquid such as an aqueous or hydroalcoholic solution, good technique and care must be used during incorporation. Ointment bases are by definition semisolids, and even those bases that can take up a significant amount of liquid do not just absorb the liquid; the liquid must be carefully spatulated into the base. Some pharmacists find it works best to create a depression in the ointment base mass; they then put the liquid to be incorporated in that depression to keep the liquid contained during the process. The liquid is then carefully spatulated in small portions into the base.

    3. Certain thick liquids are measured by weight rather than by volume. Examples include Coal Tar, Peru Balsam, Ichthammol, and the polysorbate-sorbitan type emulsifiers. For the thick and sticky liquids, it works well to wipe the weighing paper first with

TABLE 30.2   Densities of Selected Liquids

Liquid	Density
Acetic Acid, Glacial	1.05
Acetone	0.79
Alcohol	0.82
Benzoin Tincture	0.85
Castor Oil	0.96
Chloroform	1.48
Coal Tar Solution (LCD)	0.87
Compound Benzoin Tincture	0.91
Cottonseed Oil	0.92
Glycerin	1.26
Hydrochloric Acid	1.18
Isopropyl Alcohol	0.78
Lactic Acid	1.20
Liquefied Phenol	1.06
Methyl Salicylate (Oil of Wintergreen)	1.18
Mineral Oil, Heavy	0.88
Mineral Oil, Light	0.85
Peppermint Oil	0.91
Phosphoric Acid	1.71
Polyethylene Glycol 400	1.13
Propylene Glycol	1.04
Resorcinol Monoacetate	1.20
Soluble Rose	1.16
Witch Hazel	0.98

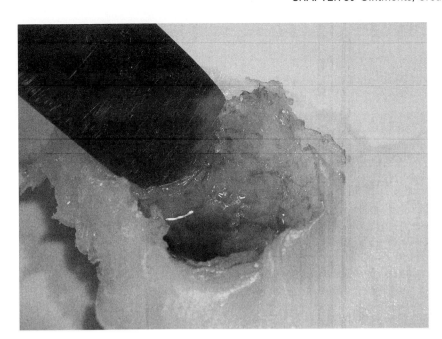

Using a depression in Hydrophilic Petrolatum to incorporate Coal Tar Solution

the chosen levigating agent before taring out the weight of the paper and adding the sticky liquid. The thick liquid is then easier to transfer completely from the weighing paper onto the ointment slab because the thick liquid slides more readily off the slippery surface of the weighing paper.

4. Some liquids require special levigating agents. Several of these are listed above in the section on levigating agents.

5. Some liquids, especially aqueous and alcoholic solutions, soak into the paper of ointment pads. Ointment slabs are the preferred equipment for these products.

V. COMPATIBILITY AND STABILITY

A. Physical Stability of the System

1. Ointments are semisolid dosage forms and are therefore naturally more physically stable than are liquid preparations such as solutions, suspensions, or emulsions; sedimentation, caking, creaming, and precipitation of solids are not problems we encounter with ointments. This allows more flexibility with assigning beyond-use dates.

2. The strategies for achieving uniform, smooth, nongritty ointments and of incorporating liquid ingredients in ointment bases have been discussed previously in this chapter.

3. "Bleeding" of liquid ingredients and phase separation can occur. Special levigating agents, as outlined previously, may be helpful.

4. Glycerin or Propylene Glycol may be added as humectants to ointment bases containing water to retard evaporation of the water and prevent drying out of the ointment base.

B. Chemical Stability

1. Ingredients

a. Check suitable references for information on chemical stability of the active ingredients and other formulation components. Issues of chemical stability in general are discussed in Chapter 34, and specific illustrations are given with sample prescriptions in this chapter and in previous dosage-form chapters.

b. When stability information is not known for a specific formulation that contains water and ingredients in solid form, the *USP* chapter on pharmacy compounding,

Chapter ⟨795⟩, allows a beyond-use dating of 14 days. For nonaqueous formulations of unknown stability (3), the limit varies from 30 days to 6 months, depending on the source of ingredients. Concerns for chemical stability of known labile active ingredient(s) may further limit beyond-use dates. Beyond-use dating is discussed in Chapter 4.

2. Emulsifiers: For general compatibility information on emulsifiers, see Chapter 19, Surfactants and Emulsifying Agents. Soap-type emulsifiers cause most of the compatibility problems. Some specific ointment base examples include:

   a. Oil-in-water emulsions: Traditional vanishing creams used stearate soap-type emulsifiers, which are sensitive to pH and multivalent ions. Some manufacturers have reformulated vanishing creams to use non-ionic surfactants. The formula of a cream should be checked if compatibility problems are suspected. Some o/w emulsions, such as Hydrophilic Ointment USP, do not have these compatibility problems because the emulsifying agent is a detergent, Sodium Lauryl Sulfate in this case, plus the nonionic emulsifiers Stearyl and Cetyl Alcohol.

   b. Water-in-oil emulsions: Again, emulsion ointments that have soap-type emulsifiers may have problems. Two examples are Cold Cream and Rose Water Ointment. Both have emulsifiers formed by the reaction of Sodium Borate with the fatty acids in Cetyl Esters Wax. This emulsion is sensitive to acid ingredients such as Salicylic Acid or phenolic compounds. Eucerin® and Hydrocream® are w/o emulsion bases that contain nonionic emulsifiers. These bases are stable to acid ingredients.

C. Microbiological Stability

1. Ointments that contain water are subject to microbial growth. The *USP* specifically states that **all emulsions** require an antimicrobial agent because the aqueous phase is favorable to the growth of microorganisms (1). This is especially true of ointments in which water is the external phase. For information on acceptable preservatives, see Chapter 15, Preservatives.

2. If antimicrobial ingredients are present in the formulation, either for therapeutic purposes or as part of the preservative system of an ingredient, extra preservatives may not be needed. For example, Hydrophilic Ointment USP and manufactured emulsion ointment bases such as Dermabase®, Acid Mantle Cream®, Aquaphilic Ointment®, Velvachol®, and Dermovan® contain preservatives.

3. It is important to remember that some preservatives, such as parabens and Benzoic Acid, are highly lipophilic; a significant portion of these may partition into the oil phase of the ointment and leave the water phase with an insufficient preservative concentration. Extra preservative may be needed.

VI. LABELING

A. "External Use Only" labels are customarily used on ointments.

SAMPLE PRESCRIPTIONS

➤ Prescription 30-1

Note: The following prescription order is for a USP formulation that is available as a manufactured product from various sources. It would, therefore, not normally be compounded in the pharmacy. It is given here as an example of a basic ointment preparation that uses a levigating agent for incorporation of insoluble powder.

Contemporary Physicians Group Practice
20 S. Park Street, Triturate, WI 53706
Tel: (608) 555-1333 Fax: (608) 555-1335

℞ # 310

Name *Basil Hoepe*   Date *00/00/00*

Address *612 Companion Lane*   Age   Wt/Ht

℞

Zinc Oxide Ointment USP

Disp 30 g

J. Jensen 00/00/00

Sig: Apply to affected areas qid ut dict

Refills *1*   *Linus Ashman*   M.D.

DEA No. _____

Ingredients Used (Amounts given are for 33 g, 3 g excess)

Ingredient	Quantity Used	Manufacturer Lot #-Exp Date	Solubility	Dose Comparison		Use in the Prescription
				Given	Usual	
Zinc Oxide	6.6 g	JET Labs SS2812-mm/yy	insol in water and alcohol	20%	varies from 1–25%	astringent, protective, antiseptic
Mineral Oil	5.6 mL	JET Labs EM2912-mm/yy	immisc w/water and alcohol	—	—	levigating agent
White Ointment	21.45 g	JET Labs ON3011-mm/yy	immisc with water & alcohol	—	—	base

Compatibility–Stability/Beyond-Use Date

Stability–Compatibility: The is an official USP formulation that is known to be very stable.
Preservative: No preservative is needed; Zinc Oxide is an antiseptic and there is no water present in this formula.
Packaging and Storage and Beyond-use date: The *USP* monograph for this preparation recommends storage in well-closed containers (2). Although manufactured versions of this formulation are given expiration dates of several years, Pharmacist Jensen will use a more conservative 6-month beyond-use date for this compounded preparation.

Calculations

Dose/Concentration

This is a USP formulation; the concentration of Zinc Oxide is OK (See below).

Zinc Oxide is often used as a protectant, which is defined as a substance that protects injured or exposed skin surfaces from harmful or annoying stimuli. The concentration range specified by the FDA for Zinc Oxide as a protectant is 1–25%. Using the USP formula given below, the concentration of Zinc Oxide in this preparation can be calculated as:

$$\frac{200 \text{ g } ZnO}{1000 \text{ g } ointment} = \frac{x \text{ g } ZnO}{100 \text{ g } ointment}; x = 20 \text{ g}/100 \text{ g} = 20\%$$

Ingredient Amounts

Zinc Oxide Ointment USP has the following formula (2):

Zinc Oxide	200 g
Mineral Oil	150 g
White Ointment	650 g
To make	1,000 g

Amounts of each ingredient in g to make 33 g of ointment (3 g excess):

Zinc Oxide:
$$\left(\frac{200 \text{ g } ZnO}{1000 \text{ g } ointment}\right)\left(\frac{33 \text{ g } ointment}{}\right) = 6.6 \text{ g } ZnO$$

Mineral Oil:
$$\left(\frac{150 \text{ g } Min. Oil}{1000 \text{ g } ointment}\right)\left(\frac{33 \text{ g } ointment}{}\right) = 4.95 \text{ g } Mineral Oil$$

White Ointment:
$$\left(\frac{650 \text{ g } White Ointment}{1000 \text{ g } ointment}\right)\left(\frac{33 \text{ g } ointment}{}\right) = 21.45 \text{ g } White Ointment$$

The quantity of Mineral Oil is given in grams, but in small-scale compounding, it is usually measured volumetrically. Using the specific gravity of Mineral Oil, the number of milliliters needed for this prescription is calculated:

s. g. = 0.860–0.905   avg. s.g. = 0.88

$$\left(\frac{mL \text{ } Mineral Oil}{0.88 \text{ g } Mineral Oil}\right)\left(\frac{4.95 \text{ g } Mineral Oil}{}\right) = 5.6 \text{ } mL$$

Compounding Procedure

On a class 3 torsion or electronic balance, weigh 6.6 g of Zinc Oxide (ZnO). Levigate it with 5.6 mL Mineral Oil on an ointment pad or slab, forming a smooth paste. Weigh 21.45 g of White Ointment, and incorporate the ZnO-Mineral Oil paste into the White Ointment and spatulate well to achieve a smooth, uniform ointment. Transfer to an ointment jar; label and dispense.

Quality Control

Preparation is a smooth, white opaque ointment of moderate consistency and with a slight sheen. The actual weight is checked and is 30.6 g, within the range of 30–33 g, which matches the theoretical weight.

Labeling

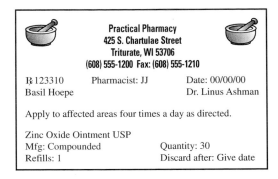

> **Practical Pharmacy**
> **425 S. Chartulae Street**
> **Triturate, WI 53706**
> **(608) 555-1200 Fax: (608) 555-1210**
>
> ℞ 123310   Pharmacist: JJ   Date: 00/00/00
> Basil Hoepe   Dr. Linus Ashman
>
> Apply to affected areas four times a day as directed.
>
> Zinc Oxide Ointment USP
> Mfg: Compounded   Quantity: 30
> Refills: 1   Discard after: Give date

Auxiliary Labels: For External Use only;

Patient Consultation

Hello, Mr. Hoepe, I'm your pharmacist, Julia Jensen. Do you have any drug allergies? Are you taking or using any other medication products? What has your physician told you about this medication and how to use it? This ointment contains Zinc Oxide and is used to treat the skin condition that your physician has diagnosed. Apply a thin coat to the affected areas four times daily as directed. Be careful not to get this near your eyes or mouth. This is a somewhat greasy ointment that is intended to afford better protectant action, but it may soil clothing or sheets, so take precautions. If your condition doesn't improve or gets worse, contact Dr. Ashman and discontinue use until you talk with him. You may store this at room temperature, away from the reach of children. Discard any unused portion after 6 months (give date). This may be refilled one time. Do you have any questions?

➤ Prescription 30-2

> **Contemporary Physicians Group Practice**
> **20 S. Park Street, Triturate, WI 53706**
> **Tel: (608) 555-1333 Fax: (608) 555-1335**
>
> ℞ # 311
>
> Name *Justiens Case*   Date *00/00/00*
>
> Address *532 Lazy Acres Road*   Age   Wt/Ht
>
> ℞
>
>   Zinc Oxide
>   Calamine   │ aa   7.5 g
>   Starch   15 g
>   White Petrolatum   q s ad   60 g
>   *G. Giles 00/00/00*
>
>   Sig: *Apply after each diaper change prn*
>
> Refills   *Ozzie Wurtz*   M.D.
>
>   DEA No. _____

Ingredients Used

(No excess is calculated here; may calculate for excess if desired)

Ingredient	Quantity Used	Manufacturer Lot #-Exp Date	Solubility	Dose Comparison Given	Dose Comparison Usual	Use in the Prescription
Zinc Oxide	7.5 g	JET Labs SS2812-mm/yy	insol in water and alcohol	12.5%	1–25%	protective astringent antiseptic
Calamine	7.5 g	JET Labs SS2811-mm/yy	insol in water and alcohol	12.5%	1–25%	protective astringent antiseptic
Starch	15 g	JET Labs ON3021-mm/yy	insol cold water and alcohol	25%	varies	absorbent protective demulcent
White Petrolatum	30 g	JET Labs ON3022-mm/yy	immisc with water and alcohol	—	—	base

Compatibility–Stability/Beyond-Use Date

Stability–Compatibility: The preparation is very similar to the official USP formulation Zinc Oxide Paste, which is known to be very stable.

Preservative: No preservative is needed; Zinc Oxide and Calamine are antiseptics and there is no water present in this formula.

Packaging and Storage and Beyond-use date: The *USP* monograph for Zinc Oxide Paste recommends storage in well-closed containers (2). Although manufactured versions of this formulation are given expiration dates of several years, Pharmacist Giles will use a more conservative 6-month beyond-use date for this compounded preparation.

Calculations

Dose/Concentration

Percent concentration of ZnO and Calamine:

$$\frac{7.5\ g\ ZnO/Cal.}{60\ g\ ointment} = \frac{x\ g\ ZnO/Cal.}{100\ g}; x = 12.5\ g/100\ g = 12.5\%$$

Percent concentration of Starch:

$$\frac{15\ g\ Starch}{60\ g\ ointment} = \frac{x\ g\ Starch}{100\ g}; x = 25\ g/100\ g = 25\%$$

This formulation is very similar to Zinc Oxide Paste USP. All concentrations are OK for the intended use. Because this product is for treatment of diaper rash, a very thick, stiff formulation (such as a paste) is desired. For this reason, no levigating agent was added. Making such a product with a smooth, non-gritty texture requires extra time and skill. It is best done by incorporating a small amount of powder at a time in a small amount of base until all the powder has been added and a smooth paste is obtained.

Ingredient Amounts

The weights in g of all ingredients except the ointment base are given in the prescription order. The amount of White Petrolatum is calculated by subtracting the weights of all the other ingredients from the total weight desired.

Weight of Zinc Oxide:	7.5 g
Weight of Calamine:	7.5 g
Weight of Starch:	15 g
Total weight of ingredients:	30 g

Weight of White Petrolatum: *60 g − 30 g = 30 g*

Compounding Procedure

On a class 3 torsion or electronic balance, weigh 7.5 g each of Calamine and Zinc Oxide, 15 g of Starch, and 30 g of White Petrolatum. Spatulate the Calamine and Zinc Oxide together on an ointment slab, and then spatulate the Starch into the powders until the combined powders are thoroughly mixed. Incorporate the powders directly into the White Petrolatum in small portions with careful spatulation until a smooth paste is produced. Transfer to a 2-oz ointment jar; label and dispense.

Quality Control

Preparation is a smooth, pink opaque ointment of very stiff consistency and with a "dry" matte appearance. The actual weight is checked and is 58.3 g, which is within the range of ±5% of the theoretical weight of 60 g.

Labeling

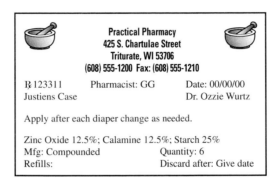

Auxiliary Labels: External Use only

Patient Consultation

Hello, Mr. Case, I'm pharmacist, Georgette Giles, and I have prepared this prescription for Justiens. Is he allergic to any medication? Is he using or taking any other medications? What has Dr. Wurtz told you about this ointment? This is used to treat diaper rash. It will protect the affected area from irritation caused by urine and feces. At each diaper change, wash and rinse the area thoroughly but gently, then apply this ointment as needed. Because the area is already irritated and raw, it is most important to change Justiens' diaper as soon as possible after he wets or has a bowel movement. If the condition doesn't improve, or gets worse, call Dr. Wurtz. This is for external use only and should be stored at room temperature, out of the reach of children. Discard any unused portion after 6 months (give date). Dr. Wurtz has not indicated any refills on this prescription, but if you find this product useful, I am sure that he would authorize refills. Just give me a call. You can also buy a similar product, Zinc Oxide Paste, without a prescription. I would be happy to assist you if you need advice. Do you have any questions?

➤ **Prescription 30-3**

Note: The following prescription order is for a USP formulation that may be available as a manufactured product. If available, it would not normally be compounded in the pharmacy. It is given here as an example of an ointment preparation containing a tar ingredient that uses a special levigating agent for incorporation of the tar.

Contemporary Physicians Group Practice
20 S. Park Street, Triturate, WI 53706
Tel: (608) 555-1333 Fax: (608) 555-1335

℞ # 312

Name *P. Sandra Smith*   Date *00/00/00*

Address *2530 Hosta Haven*   Age   Wt/Ht

℞

Coal Tar Ointment USP

Dispense 1 oz

Sig: Apply to affected areas at bedtime for psoriasis

J. Jolson 00/00/00

Refills *3*   *Penelope Pixce*   M.D.

DEA No. _____

Ingredients Used

(No excess is calculated here; may calculate for excess if desired)

Ingredient	Quantity Used	Manufacturer Lot #-Exp Date	Solubility	Dose Comparison Given	Usual	Use in the Prescription
Coal Tar	300 mg	JET Labs ON3031-mm/yy	sl sol in water; part sol in alcohol	1%	varies	antipruritic anti-eczema keratoplastic
Polysorbate 80	150 mg	JET Labs ON3032-mm/yy	misc with water, oils	0.5%	$^1/_2$–1 times the amount of Coal Tar	dispersing, emulsifying agent
Zinc Oxide Paste	29.55 g	JET Labs ON3033-mm/yy	immisc with water	—	—	protective, vehicle

Compatibility–Stability/Beyond-Use Date

Stability–Compatibility: The is an official USP formulation that is known to be very stable.
Preservative: No preservative is needed; Zinc Oxide in the Zinc Oxide Paste is an antiseptic and there is no water present in this formula.
Packaging and Storage and Beyond-use date: The *USP* monograph for this preparation recommends storage in tight containers (2). Although manufactured versions of this formulation are given expiration dates of several years, Pharmacist Jolson will use a more conservative 6-month beyond-use date for this compounded preparation.

Calculations

Dose/Concentration

This is a USP formulation; all concentrations are OK.

Ingredient Amounts

Coal Tar Ointment USP has the following formula (2):

Coal Tar	10 g
Polysorbate 80	5 g
Zinc Oxide Paste	985 g
To make	1,000 g

Amounts of each ingredient in g to make 30 g of ointment:

Coal Tar: $\left(\dfrac{10\ g\ Coal\ Tar}{1000\ g}\right)\left(\dfrac{30\ g}{}\right) = 0.3\ g\ Coal\ Tar$

Polysorbate 80: $\left(\dfrac{5\ g\ Polysorbate\ 80}{1000\ g}\right)\left(\dfrac{30\ g}{}\right) = 0.15\ g\ Polysorbate\ 80$

Zinc Oxide Paste: $\left(\dfrac{985\ g\ ZnO\ Paste}{1000\ g}\right)\left(\dfrac{30\ g}{}\right) = 29.55\ g\ ZnO\ Paste$

Compounding Procedure

On a class 3 torsion or electronic balance, weigh 300 mg of Coal Tar, 150 mg of Polysorbate 80, and 29.55 g of ZnO Paste. Because the Coal Tar is thick and sticky, it works well to wipe the weighing paper first with Mineral Oil or Polysorbate 80 before taring out the weight of the paper and adding the Coal Tar. The Coal Tar is then easier to transfer completely onto the ointment slab with a metal spatula. Levigate the Polysorbate 80 and Coal Tar together on an ointment slab, then incorporate this mixture into the ZnO Paste by spatulation using geometric dilution. Transfer completely to a 1-oz ointment jar or tube; label and dispense.

Quality Control

Preparation is a smooth, grayish-black opaque ointment with a moderately stiff consistency and with a slight sheen. There should be no apparent white particles in the ointment. It has the characteristic odor of Coal Tar. The actual weight is checked and is 29.1 g, which is within the range of ±5% of the theoretical weight of 30 g.

Labeling

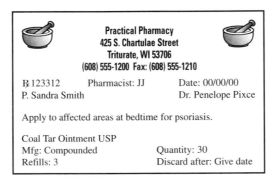

Practical Pharmacy
425 S. Chartulae Street
Triturate, WI 53706
(608) 555-1200 Fax: (608) 555-1210

℞ 123312	Pharmacist: JJ	Date: 00/00/00
P. Sandra Smith		Dr. Penelope Pixce

Apply to affected areas at bedtime for psoriasis.

Coal Tar Ointment USP	
Mfg: Compounded	Quantity: 30
Refills: 3	Discard after: Give date

Auxiliary Labels: For External Use only; Photosensitivity Warning

Patient Consultation

Hello, Ms. Smith, I'm your pharmacist, Jennifer Jolson. Are you allergic to any drugs? Are you currently using (orally or topically) any other medications? What did Dr. Pixce tell you about this medication? This ointment is to treat your psoriasis. Apply it to the affected areas each night at bedtime. This will stain fabrics, so cover areas with some clean, disposable material (some dermatologists recommend using a plastic food wrap). This product might make the affected areas more sensitive to sunlight, causing redness of the skin or dermatitis. Avoid using in ano-genital areas, and don't get this in or near your eyes. If your condition seems to be getting worse, or if other types of irritation occur, discontinue use and contact Dr. Pixce. This should be kept at room temperature, out of the reach of children. Discard any unused contents after 6 months. Dr. Pixce has authorized three refills. Do you have any questions?

➤ **Prescription 30-4**

Contemporary Physicians Group Practice
20 S. Park Street, Triturate, WI 53706
Tel: (608) 555-1333 Fax: (608) 555-1335

R # 365

Name *Chevy Hunt*   Date *00/00/00*

Address *95 Lampoon Drive*   Age   Wt/Ht

R

        Hydrocortisone   *0.6 g*
        Urea   *6 g*
        ~~*White Petrolatum*~~ *q s ad 60 g*

Per telephone consult with Dr. Stark, changed White
     Petrolatum to Hydrophilic Petrolatum   **Bill Bailey 00/00/00**

Sig: Apply to affected area up to qid

Refills *4*   *Art Stark*   M.D.

               DEA No. _____

Ingredients Used (No excess is calculated here; may calculate for excess if desired)

Ingredient	Quantity Used	Manufacturer Lot #-Exp Date	Solubility	Dose Comparison		Use in the Prescription
				Given	Usual	
Hydrocortisone	0.6 g	JET Labs SS2821-mm/yy	v sl sol in water; 1 g/40 mL alcohol	1.0%	0.25–2.5%	anti-inflammatory antipruritic
Paraben-Propylene Glycol Stock	3 g	Prac. Pharm. JT4872-mm/yy	misc w/water, alcohol	0.2% MP 0.02% PP	0.2% MP 0.02% PP	preservative
Urea	6 g	JET Labs ON3041-mm/yy	1 g/1.5 mL water; 10 mL alcohol	10%	5–30%	mild keratolytic; hydrates skin; removes scales
Purified Water	9 mL	Sweet Springs ALO529-mm/yy	—	—	—	solvent
Hydrophilic Petrolatum	41.4 g	JET Labs ON3042-mm/yy	insol in water and alcohol	—	—	vehicle; emollient

MP = Methylparaben PP = Propylparaben

Compatibility–Stability/Beyond-Use Date

Stability–Compatibility: Because of the multiple ingredients in this formulation, this is somewhat difficult to evaluate. Urea creams, alone and with Hydrocortisone, are available from various manufacturers.

Compounded Urea topical preparations have been evaluated and reported in the literature, but with mixed results. A good review of the subject can be found in *Trissel's Stability of Compounded Formulations* (4). *The Merck Index* reports that 10% solutions of Urea in water have a pH of 7.2.

The stability of Hydrocortisone in this preparation is also difficult to assess. It undergoes oxidation and other complex degradation reactions. It is most stable at pH 3.5-4.5, and its stability is quite dependent on pH, with steep slopes for its pH profile in both the acidic and basic regions (5). No stability data for this specific formulation are available.

Because Urea is a hard crystalline substance that is difficult to levigate to a fine powder, it is usually first dissolved in water before incorporation into the ointment base. Therefore, Pharmacist Bailey has called the prescriber to discuss a change in the ointment base, because the White Petrolatum will not absorb the water needed to make this prescription. The White Petrolatum may be replaced in whole or part with an absorption base such as Hydrophilic Petrolatum or a similar branded absorption base. Another alternative would be to add 2–5% of Span 80 to emulsify the Urea solution. For the purpose of this prescription, it was decided to change the base to Hydrophilic Petrolatum.

Preservative: Because of the addition of water, a preservative must be added. Pharmacist Bailey has selected the combination 0.2% Methylparaben and 0.02% Propylparaben in Propylene Glycol.

Packaging and Storage and Beyond-use date: Pharmacist Bailey will use the *USP* recommended maximum 14-day beyond-use date for compounded water-containing formulations prepared from ingredients in solid form when there is no stability information for the formulation (3). Packaging should be in a tight, light-resistant container, with recommended storage at controlled room temperature.

Calculations

Dose/Concentration

Concentration in percent for each active ingredient is calculated here.

Hydrocortisone:
$$\frac{0.6\ g\ Hydrocortisone}{60\ g\ ointment} = \frac{x\ g\ Hydrocortisone}{100\ g}; x = 1\ g/100\ g = 1\%$$

Urea:
$$\frac{6\ g\ Urea}{60\ g\ ointment} = \frac{x\ g\ Urea}{100\ g}; x = 10\ g/100\ g = 10\%$$

All concentrations are OK.

Ingredient Amounts

The Hydrocortisone and the Urea are solids and the prescription order gives the amounts of each in g.

The Urea has a hard crystalline structure that requires dissolution in water for a smooth ointment preparation. The solubility of Urea in water is 1 g/1.5 mL. The amount of water required to dissolve the Urea can be calculated:

$$\left(\frac{1.5\ mL\ water}{1\ g\ Urea}\right)\left(\frac{6\ g\ Urea}{}\right) = 9\ mL\ water$$

This addition of water means that a preservative must be added. Pharmacist Bailey has the following stock solution of Methylparaben and Propylparaben in Propylene Glycol:

Methylparaben	1.2 g
Propylparaben	0.12 g
Propylene Glycol	28.68 g
Total weight:	30.00 g

By taking 3 g of this stock solution, Pharmacist Bailey will have 120 mg of Methylparaben (0.2% w/w of the ointment) and 12 mg of Propylparaben (0.02% w/w of the ointment), which is the recommended - concentration for these preservatives. The 3 g of solution could be weighed in a tared graduate, but a close estimate can be made by measuring this amount volumetrically. Propylene Glycol has a specific gravity of 1.036. If you ignore the powder volume of the parabens and use this as the specific gravity of the stock solution, a weight of 3 g would correspond to a volume of 2.9 mL or approximately 3 mL.

As discussed above, the base had to be changed from White Petrolatum to the absorption base Hydrophilic Petrolatum. The amount of base is calculated by subtracting the weights of all the other ingredients from the total weight desired. The first step is to determine the actual weights of all the ingredients. The weights for Hydrocortisone and Urea are given. The weight in g of the paraben-Propylene Glycol is 3 g. The weight of 9 mL of Purified Water with a density of 1 g/mL is 9 g.

Weight of all ingredients:

Weight of Hydrocortisone:	0.6 g
Weight of paraben-PG	3. g
Weight of Urea:	6. g
Weight of Water:	9. g
Total weight of ingredients:	18.6 g

Weight of Hydrophilic Petrolatum: $60\ g\ -\ 18.6\ g = 41.4\ g$

Compounding Procedure

All weighings are done on a class 3 torsion or an electronic balance. Weigh 6 g of Urea and dissolve in 9 mL Purified Water. Measure and add 3 mL of paraben–Propylene Glycol stock solution. Subtract the weights of all ingredients from 60 g to determine the weight of ointment base (e.g., 41.4 g). Weigh 41.4 g of Hydrophilic Petrolatum. Weigh 0.6 g of Hydrocortisone powder. Levigate this on ointment slab with a small amount of Hydrophilic Petrolatum, then geometrically incorporate the rest of the Hydrophilic Petrolatum. Incorporate the Urea/paraben–PG solution into the ointment very gradually, using a spatula and being careful not to lose any of the solution. Transfer to a 2-oz. ointment jar; label and dispense.

Quality Control

Preparation is a smooth, white, slightly translucent ointment of moderate consistency and with a slight sheen. The actual weight is checked and is 57.9 g, which is within the range of ±5% of the theoretical weight of 60 g.

Labeling

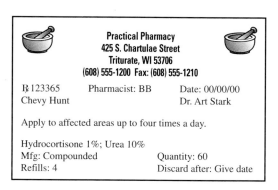

Auxiliary Labels: For External Use only

Patient Consultation

Hello, Mr. Hunt, I'm your pharmacist, Bill Bailey. Are you allergic to any drugs? Are you currently using or taking any other medications? What has Dr. Stark told you, or what do you know about, this ointment? This ointment contains anti-itch and anti-inflammatory drugs, as well as a skin softening agent. This may be applied up to four times daily. Use it sparingly and rub in well. If the condition doesn't seem to respond to the treatment or if the condition gets worse, discontinue use and contact your physician. This is for external use only and should be stored at room temperature, away from light and heat, and out of the reach of children. Discard any unused portion after 2 weeks (give date). This may be refilled four times. Do you have any questions?

➤ **Prescription 30-5**

Contemporary Physicians Group Practice
20 S. Park Street, Triturate, WI 53706
Tel: (608) 555-1333 Fax: (608) 555-1335

R # 354

Name *Bobby Armstrong*   *Date   00/00/00*

Address *8573 High Point Place*   *Age*   Wt/Ht

R

      Peru Balsam
      Sulfur | aa   5 g
      Salicylic Acid   3 g
      Lanolin   q s ad   30 g
                                    Hank Bassettlab 00/00/00

          Sig: *Apply locally ut dict*

Refills   2   *E. S. Clyde*   M.D.

                    DEA No. _____

Ingredients Used (No excess is calculated here; may calculate for excess if desired)

Ingredient	Quantity Used	Manufacturer Lot #-Exp Date	Solubility	Dose Comparison		Use in the Prescription
				Given	Usual	
Peru Balsam	5 g	JET Labs ON3061-mm/yy	nearly insol in water; sol in alcohol	17%	varies-prn	healing-promotes growth of epithelial cells
Colloidal Sulfur	5 g	JET Labs SS2841-mm/yy	prac insol in water; v sl sol. in alcohol	17%	10% (varies)	antibacterial, antifungal, keratolytic
Salicylic Acid	3 g	JET Labs XY1148-mm/yy	1 g/460 mL water, 3 mL alcohol	10%	2–60%	keratolytic
Lanolin	12 g	JET Labs ON3062-mm/yy	insol in water; but takes up water	—	—	base
Castor Oil	5 g (5.2 mL)	JET Labs EM2932-mm/yy	immisc w/water; misc w/alcohol	16.7%	—	levigating agent; stabilizer

Compatibility–Stability/Beyond-Use Date

Stability–Compatibility: The Sulfur and Salicylic Acid in this preparation are compatible and very stable when in an ointment. The Peru Balsam is a natural product that has been formulated in ointments and suppositories for many years. The Peru Balsam monograph in *Remington's Pharmaceutical Sciences* states that the resinous part of Peruvian Balsam separates out from ointments that also contain Sulfur unless an equal quantity of Castor Oil is used as the levigating agent (6), so Castor Oil is used in this preparation as the levigating agent.
Preservative: No extra preservative is needed because both Sulfur and Peru Balsam have antimicrobial activity. Lanolin, as currently described in the *USP*, is anhydrous, so no water is present in this preparation.
Packaging and Storage and Beyond-use date: Although the *USP* allows a 6-month beyond-use date for compounded nonaqueous solid preparations that are made from official substances, Pharmacist Bassettlab will use

a more conservative 30-day beyond-use date because of the propensity of Peruvian Balsam preparations to separate (3). The ointment should be packaged in a tight, light-resistant container. Controlled room temperature will be the recommended storage conditions.

Calculations

Dose/Concentration

Concentration in percent for each active ingredient is calculated here.

Peru Balsam and Sulfur: $\dfrac{5\,g\,Sulfur\,/\,P.B.}{30\,g\,ointment} = \dfrac{x\,g\,Sulfur\,/\,P.B.}{100\,g}; x = 16.7\,g/100\,g = 16.7\% \approx 17\%$

Salicylic Acid: $\dfrac{3\,g\,Sal.\,Acid}{30\,g\,ointment} = \dfrac{x\,g\,Sal.\,Acid}{100\,g}; x = 10\,g/100\,g = 10\%$

All concentrations are OK.

Ingredient Amounts

The Sulfur and the Salicylic Acid are solids and the prescription order gives the amounts of each in g. Peru Balsam is a viscous liquid that is also measured in g.

An amount of Castor Oil equal in quantity to the amount of Peru Balsam is recommended for levigating Peru Balsam, especially in ointments that also contain Sulfur. Therefore, 5 g of Castor Oil should be added. Castor Oil is usually measured by volume. The volume equivalent to 5 g can be calculated using the specific gravity or density of Castor Oil.

Castor Oil: s.g. = 0.96

$$\left(\frac{mL\,Castor\,Oil}{0.96\,g\,Castor\,Oil}\right)\left(\frac{5\,g\,Castor\,Oil}{}\right) = 5.2\,mL\,Castor\,Oil$$

The amount of Lanolin is calculated by subtracting the weights of all the other ingredients from the total weight desired.

Weight of Peru Balsam	5 g
Weight of Sulfur:	5 g
Weight of Salicylic Acid:	3 g
Weight of Castor Oil:	5 g
Total weight of ingredients:	18 g

Weight of Lanolin: *30 g − 18 g = 12 g*

Compounding Procedure

On a class 3 torsion or an electronic balance, weigh 5 g of Peru Balsam and place on one corner of an ointment slab. As with Coal Tar, Peru Balsam is thick and sticky, and it works well to wipe the weighing paper first with Castor Oil before taring out the weight of the paper and adding the Peru Balsam. The Peru Balsam is then easier to transfer completely from the slick weighing paper onto the ointment slab using a metal spatula. Measure 5.2 mL (5 g) Castor Oil in a graduated cylinder or a disposable syringe. Add part of it to the Peru Balsam and levigate. Weigh 5 g of Colloidal Sulfur (may also use Precipitated Sulfur, but must specify the type used on the prescription order or compounding record) and 3 g of Salicylic Acid and levigate these powders with the rest of the Castor Oil on another part of ointment slab. Weigh 12 g of Lanolin and divide into two portions. Incorporate the Peru Balsam into one portion and the Sulfur/Salicylic Acid into the other portion with spatulation. Combine the two portions with spatulation and transfer to a 1-oz ointment jar; label and dispense.

Quality Control

Preparation is a smooth, yellowish-brown opaque ointment of moderate consistency and with a slight sheen. It has the characteristic odor of Peruvian Balsam. The actual weight is checked and is 29.2 g, which is within the range of ±5% of the theoretical weight of 30 g.

Labeling

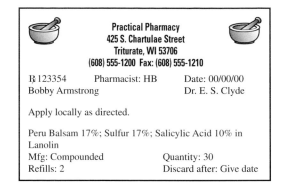

Practical Pharmacy
425 S. Chartulae Street
Triturate, WI 53706
(608) 555-1200 Fax: (608) 555-1210

℞ 123354   Pharmacist: HB   Date: 00/00/00
Bobby Armstrong   Dr. E. S. Clyde

Apply locally as directed.

Peru Balsam 17%; Sulfur 17%; Salicylic Acid 10% in
Lanolin
Mfg: Compounded   Quantity: 30
Refills: 2   Discard after: Give date

Auxiliary Labels: For external use only

Patient Consultation

Hello, Mr. Armstrong, I'm your pharmacist, Hank Bassettlab. Do you have any drug allergies? Are you allergic to Lanolin or wool? Are you using any other medications at the present time? Do you know, or has Dr. Clyde discussed with you. what we are treating with this ointment? It will soften and remove dead skin, promote new skin growth, and act as an anti-infective. You are to apply it locally as directed. Did Dr. Clyde tell you how often to apply it? Use a small amount and spread it thinly and evenly over the affected area(s), being careful not to get too close to your eyes or mouth. This may stain your clothing, so it may be a good idea to cover the area with gauze, a bandage, plastic wrap, or something similar. If the condition gets worse or you develop severe irritation and/or inflammation, contact Dr. Clyde. This may be stored at room temperature, out of reach of children. Any unused portion should be discarded after 1 month (give date). You may have two refills. Do you have any questions?

➤ **Prescription 30-6**

Contemporary Physicians Group Practice
20 S. Park Street, Triturate, WI 53706
Tel: (608) 555-1333 Fax: (608) 555-1335

℞ # 321

Name *Millie Butler*   Date *00/00/00*

Address *624 Cottage Grove Rd.*   Age   Wt/Ht

℞

Urea	*10%*
Neomycin Sulfate	*0.5%*
Lactic Acid	*5%*
Triamcinolone Acetonide	
Ointment 0.1%	*q s ad 15 g*

Sig: Apply to affected area tid

J. Jacquisch 00/00/00

Refills *1*   *Conway Sprague*   M.D.

DEA No. _____

Ingredients Used (The quantities below represent amounts for 10% excess, or 16.5 g)

Ingredient	Quantity Used	Manufacturer Lot #-Exp Date	Solubility	Dose Comparison Given	Dose Comparison Usual	Use in the Prescription
Urea	1.65 g	JET Labs ON3041-mm/yy	1 g/1.5 mL water, 10 mL alcohol	10%	5 to 30%	keratolytic; humectant
Neomycin Sulfate	165 mg weighed 82.5 mg used	JET Labs SN2693-mm/yy	1 g/1 mL water; v sl sol in alcohol	0.5%	0.5%	antimicrobial
Lactic Acid USP	0.76 mL (0.92 g)	JET Labs SN2672-mm/yy	misc w/water, alcohol	5%	1–10%	increases hydration of skin
Purified Water	1 mL for Neomycin; 2.5 mL for Urea	Sweet Springs AL0529-mm/yy	—	—	—	solvent
Paraben- Propylene Glycol Stock	0.82 g (0.8 mL)	Prac. Pharm. JT4872-mm/yy	miscible w/water and alcohol	0.2% MP 0.02% PP	0.2% MP 0.02% PP	preservative
Sorbitan Monooleate (Span 80)	330 mg	JET Labs ON3042-mm/yy	miscible w/water and oil	2%	—	emulsifying agent
TCNL oint 0.1%	9.28 g	BJF Generics JF4985-mm/yy	immisc w/water, alcohol	0.05%	0.025–0.5%	topical steroid

Compatibility–Stability/Beyond-Use Date

Stability–Compatibility: No stability data for this specific formulation are available. Because of the multiple ingredients in this formulation, this is a difficult order to evaluate.

Making a smooth ointment with Urea requires the addition of water, but the ointment base in this case will not absorb water. Sample Prescription 30.4 is similar, but the base ointment in that preparation did not contain any active ingredient, so the hydrocarbon base could be changed to an absorption base. In this prescription order, the base ointment is a hydrocarbon type, but it contains the active ingredient Triamcinolone Acetonide, so a change like that cannot be made. Therefore, an emulsifying system must be added to the formulation to enable the aqueous solution to be incorporated into the Triamcinolone Ointment. Span 80 in a concentration of 2% w/w works well for this.

Urea creams, alone and with Lactic Acid, are available from various manufacturers. Compounded Urea topical preparations have also been evaluated and reported in the literature, but with mixed results. A good review of the subject can be found in *Trissel's Stability of Compounded Formulations* (4). *The Merck Index* reports that 10% solutions of Urea in water have a pH of 7.2. The addition of Lactic Acid to the Urea solution will lower the pH. The Lactic Acid itself is a rather stable chemical in solution.

Aqueous solutions of Neomycin Sulfate are reported to be stable over a fairly wide pH range, pH 2 to 9, but the drug is subject to oxidation, and tight, light-resistant containers should be used (7).

The stability of the Triamcinolone Acetonide in this complex preparation is difficult to assess. According to the review of Triamcinolone in *Analytical Profiles of Drug Substances*, this drug is very stable as a solid, but in aqueous or alcoholic solutions, it is similar to Hydrocortisone and other corticosteroids in that it undergoes complex oxidative rearrangements with decomposition at alkaline pH's (8). Although in this preparation the Triamcinolone Acetonide is not in a water or alcohol environment, it will be in contact with the emulsified droplets of the Urea–Lactic Acid solution. This should have a limited effect, and the Triamcinolone should be relatively stable in this product.

Preservative: Because of the addition of water to this ointment, a preservative must be added. Pharmacist Jacquisch has selected the combination 0.2% Methylparaben and 0.02% Propylparaben in Propylene Glycol. Packaging and Storage and Beyond-use date: Pharmacist Jacquisch will use the *USP* recommended maximum 14-day beyond-use date for compounded water-containing formulations prepared from ingredients in solid form when there is no stability information for the formulation (3). Packaging should be in a tight, light-resistant container, with recommended storage at controlled room temperature.

Calculations

Dose/Concentration

All concentrations OK for expected use.

Ingredient Amounts

Because this is a rather complex ointment, there is a good chance of material loss in the compounding process. Furthermore, the amount prescribed is relatively small, so that even a small loss would mean a significant percent decrease in the amount dispensed. Therefore, Pharmacist Jacquisch has decided to prepare a 10% excess. The following calculations are for 16.5 g of ointment, a 10% excess.

Urea: $10\% \times 16.5\ g = 1.65\ g$

Neomycin SO$_4$: $0.5\% \times 16.5\ g = 0.0825\ g = 82.5\ mg$

This amount is below the MWQ, so an aliquot is needed. A solid-liquid aliquot, using water as the diluent, would be the most convenient. Neomycin SO$_4$ has a water solubility of 1 g/mL. Because this is an ointment, we want to use a minimal amount of water. If we weigh two times the amount of Neomycin needed ($2 \times 82.5\ mg = 165\ mg$) and dissolve it in 2 mL of water, and then take half of this volume or 1 mL (measured in a 1- or 3- mL syringe or a pipette), we will have the 82.5 mg needed. This 1 mL of solution weighs ~1 g because it is mostly water (s.g. of water = 1.0).

Lactic Acid: $5\% \times 16.5\ g = 0.825\ g$

This amount of Lactic Acid is subject to interpretation. Lactic Acid is available as the USP liquid, which is 90% w/w with respect to the chemical lactic acid, and it has a density of 1.2 g/mL. The 0.825 g in this prescription could be interpreted as 0.825 g Lactic Acid USP, or 0.825 g of lactic acid, the pure chemical. In either case, it would usually be measured volumetrically, so the 0.825 g should be converted to a volume.

For example:
1) For the 0.825 g of Lactic Acid USP interpretation, calculate the volume to measure as follows:

$$\left(\frac{mL\ L.A.\ USP}{1.2\ g\ L.A.\ USP}\right)\left(\frac{0.825\ g\ L.A.\ USP}{}\right) = 0.69\ mL\ Lactic\ Acid\ USP$$

2) For the 0.825 g of the pure chemical interpretation, calculate the volume to measure as follows:

$$\left(\frac{mL\ L.A.\ USP}{1.2\ g\ L.A.\ USP}\right)\left(\frac{100\ g\ L.A.\ USP}{90\ g\ lactic\ acid}\right)\left(\frac{0.825\ g\ lactic\ acid}{}\right) = 0.76\ mL\ Lactic\ Acid\ USP$$

Note: Another interpretation is also possible. Since Lactic Acid USP is a liquid, the original calculation could also be: $5\% \times 16.5\ g = 0.825\ mL$, in which case 0.825 mL of Lactic Acid USP would be measured. Fortunately for this situation, the amounts are all close and this is not a potent drug that requires a precise quantity. Pharmacist Jacquisch consulted with Dr. Sprague, and it was decided that interpretation #2, 0.825 g of the pure lactic acid chemical, would be used with a volume of 0.76 mL of Lactic Acid USP.

This volume can be measured in a 1-mL syringe.

The weight of this volume of Lactic Acid USP is:

$$1.2\ g/mL \times 0.76\ mL = 0.92\ g$$

As stated in sample Prescription 30.4, because Urea is difficult to pulverize, it is usually dissolved first in water and the solution is incorporated. The solubility of Urea is 1 g/1.5 mL. The amount of water required to dissolve the Urea can be calculated:

$$\left(\frac{1.5\,mL\,water}{1\,g\,Urea}\right)\left(\frac{1.65\,g\,Urea}{}\right)=2.5\,mL\,water$$

This addition of water means that a preservative must be added. Pharmacist Jacquisch has the following stock solution of Methylparaben and Propylparaben in Propylene Glycol:

Methylparaben	1.2 g
Propylparaben	0.12 g
Propylene Glycol	28.68 g
Total weight:	30.00 g

By taking 0.825 g of this stock solution, Pharmacist Jacquisch will have 33 mg of Methylparaben (0.2% w/w of the 16.5 g ointment) and 3.3 mg of Propylparaben (0.02% w/w of the 16.5 g ointment), which is the recommended concentration for these preservatives. This can be verified with the following calculation:

$$\frac{1.2\,g\,MP}{30\,g\,solution}=\frac{0.033\,g\,MP}{x\,g\,solution};x=0.825\,g\,solution$$

The amount could be weighed in a tared graduate, but a close estimate can be made by measuring this amount volumetrically. Propylene Glycol has a specific gravity of 1.036. If you ignore the powder volume of the parabens and use this as the specific gravity of the stock solution, a weight of 0.825 g would correspond to a volume of approximately 0.8 mL.

As discussed above, an emulsifying system must be added to enable the aqueous solutions to be incorporated into the Triamcinolone Ointment. Span 80 in a concentration of 2% w/w will be used. The weight in g of Span 80 needed is calculated:

$$2\%\times16.5\,g=0.33\,g$$

To determine the amount of Triamcinolone Ointment needed, add the weights of all ingredients (including the water and emulsifying agent) and subtract this from the final desired ointment weight.

Urea	1.65 g
Water to dissolve the Urea	2.5 g
Lactic Acid USP	0.92 g
Neomycin SO$_4$ solution	1.0 g
PG–paraben solution	0.82 g
Span 80	0.33 g
Total ingredient weight:	7.22 g

Weight of Triamcinolone Acetonide 0.1% Ointment: $16.5\,g-7.22\,g=9.28\,g$

Weight in g of Triamcinolone Acetonide (TA) in final ointment:

$$0.1\%\,TA\times9.28\,g=0.009\,g\,TA$$

Final percent w/w of TA in the final product:

$$\frac{0.009\,g\,T.A.}{16.5\,g\,ointment}=\frac{x\,g\,T.A.}{100\,g};x=0.05\,g/100\,g=0.05\%$$

Compounding Procedure

On a class 3 torsion or electronic balance, weigh 1.65 g of Urea and dissolve it in 2.5 mL of Purified Water in a beaker. Dissolve 165 mg of Neomycin Sulfate in 2 mL Purified Water and, using a 3-mL syringe, measure 1 mL of solution. Using 1-mL syringes, measure 0.76 mL of Lactic Acid USP and 0.82 mL of the Propylene Glycol–paraben stock solution. Weigh 330 mg of Span 80 and 9.28 g of Triamcinolone 0.1% Ointment. On an ointment slab, first incorporate the Span into the Triamcinolone Ointment, then incorporate the rest of the liquids, levigating well with each addition to ensure uniform mixing and absorption of the solutions by the base. Transfer the preparation to a ½-oz ointment jar; label and dispense.

Quality Control

Preparation is a smooth, whitish, slightly translucent ointment with a soft consistency and with moderate sheen. The actual weight is checked and is 14.9 g, which is an expected loss of material from the theoretical weight of 16.5 g. It is within the range of ±5% of the prescribed weight of 15 g.

Labeling

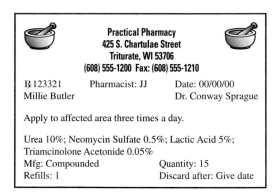

Practical Pharmacy
425 S. Chartulae Street
Triturate, WI 53706
(608) 555-1200 Fax: (608) 555-1210

℞ 123321   Pharmacist: JJ   Date: 00/00/00
Millie Butler   Dr. Conway Sprague

Apply to affected area three times a day.

Urea 10%; Neomycin Sulfate 0.5%; Lactic Acid 5%;
Triamcinolone Acetonide 0.05%
Mfg: Compounded   Quantity: 15
Refills: 1   Discard after: Give date

Auxiliary Labels: For external use only

Patient Consultation

Hello, Ms. Butler, I'm Jordan Jacquisch, your pharmacist. Do you have any drug allergies? Are you taking or using any nonprescription or prescription medications? What has Dr. Sprague told you about this prescription? Have you ever used anything like it before? This medication contains agents to help with dry, cracked, irritated, inflamed, or infected skin. It also has an antibiotic to cure any infection and speed healing. You are to apply it in a thin layer to the affected area three times a day. If the irritation or condition gets worse, or if you don't seem to be getting any relief, contact Dr. Sprague. You should store this at room temperature, out of the reach of children. This may be refilled one time. Discard any unused portion after 2 weeks (give date). Do you have any questions?

➤ Prescription 30-7

Contemporary Physicians Group Practice
20 S. Park Street, Triturate, WI 53706
Tel: (608) 555-1333 Fax: (608) 555-1335

℞ # 712

Name _Jeff Diaz_   Date _00/00/00_

Address _2396 Rosario Lane_   Age   Wt/Ht

℞

Hydrocortisone   2%
Hydroxypropylcellulose   1.05 g
Propylene Glycol   2.5 g
Polysorbate 80   1.3 g
Isopropyl Alcohol 70% q s ad   60 g

Juan Valdez 00/00/00

Sig: _Apply to affected areas on scalp 2 x daily ut dict_

Refills   1   _Marcy Dacy_   M.D.

DEA No. _____

Ingredients Used   (No excess is calculated here; may calculate for excess if desired)

Ingredient	Quantity Used	Manufacturer Lot #-Exp Date	Solubility	Dose Comparison Given	Dose Comparison Usual	Use in the Prescription
Hydrocortisone	1.2 g	JET Labs SS2821-mm/yy	v sl sol in water; 1 g/40 mL alcohol	2%	0.5–2.5%	anti-inflammatory, antipruritic
Hydroxyproyl-cellulose	1.05 g	JET Labs ON3071-mm/yy	sol in water and alcohol	—	—	suspending agent
Propylene Glycol	2.5 g (2.4 mL)	JET Labs SN2662-mm/yy	misc with water and alcohol	—	—	solvent, preservative, humectant
Polysorbate 80	1.3 g	JET Labs ON3032-mm/yy	v sol in water and alcohol	—	—	wetting and dispersing agent
Isopropyl Alcohol 70%	61.3 mL	JET Labs SS2824-mm/yy	miscible with water	56 % w/w IPA	—	antiseptic and vehicle

Compatibility–Stability/Beyond-Use Date

Stability–Compatibility: No stability data for this specific formulation are available. The formulation was patterned after a Piroxicam gel formulation in the *International Journal of Pharmaceutical Compounding* (9), but that article states that no stability studies have been performed. Furthermore, this contains a different active ingredient, Hydrocortisone. As described in sample Prescription 30.4, the stability of Hydrocortisone in preparations such as these is difficult to assess. Hydrocortisone undergoes oxidation and other complex degradation reactions. It is most stable at pH 3.5-4.5, and its stability is quite dependent on pH, with steep slopes for its pH profile in both the acidic and basic regions (5).

Preservative: No additional preservative is needed because of the high content of Isopropyl Alcohol in the formula.

Packaging and Storage and Beyond-use date: Pharmacist Valdez will use the *USP* recommended maximum 14-day beyond-use date for compounded water-containing formulations prepared from ingredients in solid form when there is no stability information for the formulation (3). Packaging should be in a tight, light-resistant container, with recommended storage at controlled room temperature.

Calculations

Dose/Concentration

Hydrocortisone: The 2% concentration is OK.

Isopropyl Alcohol: Any preparation containing either ethyl or isopropyl alcohol should have the final percent concentration of the alcohol specified on the prescription label. Although this would seem to be simple enough, when a semisolid dosage form is involved, we are dealing with conflicting formats for expressing concentration. The prototype for expressing alcohol concentration in liquid preparations is given for ethyl alcohol in the General Notices of the *USP*. This is discussed in detail with numerous examples in Chapter 7. Basically, the standard for alcohol in liquid preparations is a v/v percent of the pure alcohol in the preparation. Juxtaposed with this standard is the General Notices standard for expressing percent concentrations, which gives w/w percent for mixtures of solids and semisolids, w/v percent for solids in liquids, and v/v percent for liquids in liquids. Unfortunately, we have no direction for percent concentration of liquids in semisolids. Obviously, we would want to select a format that would be most meaningful.

According to the USP monographs, pure IPA has a s.g. of 0.78; 70% IPA is a 70% v/v solution of IPA in water with a s.g. of 0.88. As can be seen from the calculations below, the 60-g preparation contains 53.95 g or 61.3 mL of 70% Isopropyl Alcohol (IPA):

$$60 \ g - (1.2 \ g \ HC + 1.05 \ g \ HPC + 2.5 \ g \ PG + 1.3 \ g \ Tween \ 80) = 53.95 \ g \ 70\% \ IPA$$

$$\left(\frac{mL \ 70\% \ IPA}{0.88 \ g \ 70\% \ IPA} \right) \left(\frac{53.95 \ g \ 70\% \ IPA}{} \right) = 61.3 \ mL \ 70\% \ IPA$$

Using these numbers, we can calculate a final percent concentration in one of the following ways:

1) w/w percent of the 70% IPA solution in the preparation:

$$\frac{53.9\ g\ 70\%\ IPA}{60\ g\ ointment} = \frac{x\ g\ 70\%\ IPA}{100\ g}; x = 89.8\% \approx 90\%$$

2) v/w percent of the 70% IPA solution in the preparation:

$$\frac{61.3\ mL\ 70\%\ IPA}{60\ g\ ointment} = \frac{x\ mL\ 70\%\ IPA}{100\ g}; x = 102\%$$

Note that a percent greater than 100% is an anomaly that results from using a v/w percent and the fact that 70% IPA has a density less than 1.0.

3) w/w percent of pure IPA in the preparation:

$$\left(\frac{70\ mL\ IPA}{100\ mL\ 70\%\ IPA}\right)\left(\frac{61.3\ mL\ 70\%\ IPA}{}\right) = 42.9\ mL\ pure\ IPA$$

$$\left(\frac{0.78\ g\ IPA}{mL\ IPA}\right)\left(\frac{42.9\ mL\ IPA}{}\right) = 33.5\ g\ IPA$$

$$\frac{33.5\ g\ IPA}{60\ g\ ointment} = \frac{x\ g\ IPA}{100\ g}; x = 55.8\%$$

4) v/w percent of pure IPA in the preparation:

$$\left(\frac{70\ mL\ IPA}{100\ mL\ 70\%\ IPA}\right)\left(\frac{61.3\ mL\ 70\%\ IPA}{}\right) = 42.9\ mL\ pure\ IPA$$

$$\frac{42.9\ mL\ IPA}{60\ g\ ointment} = \frac{x\ mL\ IPA}{100\ g}; x = 71.5\%$$

It is apparent that the numbers vary considerably from approximately 56% to 102%, and while method #3 is probably the most correct method, it is also the most laborious to calculate. Methods #1 and #4 (although by definition there is no such thing as a v/w percent) are probably most commonly used by pharmacists. In this case, because the 70% IPA is not just one of the listed ingredients, but is used to q.s. to a final weight, a final method could be used: label the various ingredients "in 70% Isopropyl Alcohol." This method has the advantage of simplicity (no calculations are needed) and it accurately describes the product. Whichever method is used, the label should make it clear what is being reported.

Ingredient Amounts

No excess was calculated for this product, but excess could be made if desired.

Hydrocortisone: $2\% \times 60\ g = 1.2\ g$

Propylene Glycol: The amount given in the prescription order is in grams, but this is usually measured in volume. The volume can be calculated using the specific gravity or density of the Propylene Glycol (s.g. = 1.04).

$$\left(\frac{mL\ P.G.}{1.04\ g\ P.G.}\right)\left(\frac{2.5\ g\ P.G.}{}\right) = 2.4\ mL\ Propylene\ Glycol$$

The Hydroxypropyl Cellulose and the Polysorbate 80 are given in grams and are weighed.

To determine the amount of Isopropyl Alcohol 70% needed, add the weights of all ingredients and subtract this from the final desired ointment weight (this is also briefly shown above):

Hydrocortisone	1.2 g
Propylene Glycol	2.5 g
Hydroxypropyl Cellulose	1.05 g
Polysorbate 80 (Tween 80)	1.3 g
Total ingredient weight	6.05 g

Weight of Isopropyl Alcohol 70%:   *60 g − 6.05 = 53.95 g*

Isopropyl Alcohol 70% has a specific gravity = 0.88. The volume of 70% Isopropyl Alcohol to measure can be calculated:

$$\left(\frac{mL\ 70\%\ IPA}{0.88\ g\ 70\%\ IPA} \right)\left(\frac{53.95\ g\ 70\%\ IPA}{} \right) = 61.3\ mL\ 70\%\ IPA$$

Compounding Procedure

Weigh 1.05 g of Hydroxypropylcellulose and sprinkle in portions over 61.3 mL of Isopropyl Alcohol 70%, allowing each portion to become thoroughly wetted without stirring. Once the powder is wetted, stir gently. Allow this to sit overnight (at least 8–10 hours), stirring occasionally. Weigh 1.2 g of Hydrocortisone and place in a glass mortar. Measure 2.4 mL of Propylene Glycol and weigh 1.3 g of Polysorbate 80. Add these with trituration to the Hydrocortisone. Slowly with trituration add the Hydroxypropylcellulose gel to the mortar. Triturate well to a uniform consistency. Place in a 2-oz ointment jar; label and dispense.

Quality Control

Preparation is a colorless to slightly whitish transparent gel with a soft consistency. The actual weight is checked and is 59.1 g. which is an expected loss of material from the theoretical weight 60 g and is within the range of ±5% of the prescribed weight of 60 g.

Labeling

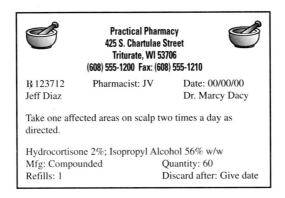

Practical Pharmacy
425 S. Chartulae Street
Triturate, WI 53706
(608) 555-1200 Fax: (608) 555-1210

℞ 123712   Pharmacist: JV   Date: 00/00/00
Jeff Diaz   Dr. Marcy Dacy

Take one affected areas on scalp two times a day as directed.

Hydrocortisone 2%; Isopropyl Alcohol 56% w/w
Mfg: Compounded   Quantity: 60
Refills: 1   Discard after: Give date

Auxiliary Labels: Caution: Flammable; For External Use Only
Keep out of the reach of children

Patient Consultation

Hello, Mr. Diaz, I'm your pharmacist, Juan Valdez. Are you currently using any other medications? Are you allergic to any drugs? What has your doctor told you about this medication? This is used to treat the seborrhea on your scalp. Apply it to your scalp two times daily as directed by your physician. It is a clear gel and is not greasy, so you should be able to use it during the day without it being noticeable. Because it contains Isopropyl Alcohol, it may sting. If your condition seems to be showing no improvement or seems to be getting worse, contact your doctor. If any intense reaction should occur in the application area, discontinue use and contact your doctor. Keep the container tightly closed, in a cool dry place. This is in a non-safety container, so be sure to keep it out of the reach of children. Because of the high alcohol content, it is flammable, so do not use it around any flame or lighted smoking material. Discard any unused portion after 2 weeks. This prescription has one refill. Do you have any questions?

➤ **Prescription 30-8**

Contemporary Physicians Group Practice
20 S. Park Street, Triturate, WI 53706
Tel: (608) 555-1333 Fax: (608) 555-1335

R # 383

Name *Lacey Bindl*	Date *00/00/00*	
Address *256 River Valley Lane*	Age	Wt/Ht

℞

Lidocaine HCl	*600 mg*
Diphenhydramine HCl	*300 mg*
Polyoxamer Lecithin Organogel q s ad	*30 g*

C. Kraemer 00/00/00

Sig: Apply to affected areas tid prn pain and itching

Refills   4   *Louis Tacky*   M.D.

DEA No. _____

Ingredients Used   (Amounts are for 33 g, 3 g excess)

Ingredient	Quantity Used	Manufacturer Lot #-Exp Date	Solubility	Dose Comparison Given	Dose Comparison Usual	Use in the Prescription
Lidocaine HCl	660 mg	JET Labs ON3081-mm/yy	v sol in water and alcohol	2%	1–5%	local anesthetic
Diphenhydramine HCL	330 mg	JET Labs ON3082-mm/yy	1g/mL water or 2 mL alcohol	1%	1–2%	anthihistamine
Lecithin/Iso-propyl palmitate	6.4 g	JET Labs ON3083-mm/yy	dispersible in water	—	—	vehicle
Polyoxamer Gel 20%	25.6 g	JET Labs ON3084-mm/yy	misc with water and alcohol	—	—	vehicle

Compatibility–Stability/Beyond-Use Date

Stability–Compatibility: No stability data for this specific formulation are available. The formulation was patterned after a similar gel formulation in the *International Journal of Pharmaceutical Compounding* (10), but that article states that no stability studies have been performed. Furthermore, while both formulations contain Lidocaine, this preparation contains Diphenhydramine HCl and it does not include Ketoprofen and Cyclobenzaprine. Both Diphenhydramine HCl and Lidocaine HCl are available in manufactured aqueous and alcoholic solutions and are reported to be quite stable (11,12).

Preservative: No additional preservative is needed because Pharmacist Kraemer has decided to use commercial brands of lecithin-isopropyl palmitate and poloxamer 20% gel. Both are preserved with Sorbic Acid and the parabens. (See Chapter 18 for a more complete description.)

Packaging and Storage and Beyond-use date: Pharmacist Kraemer will use the *USP* recommended maximum 14-day beyond-use date for compounded water-containing formulations prepared from ingredients in solid form when there is no stability information for the formulation (3). Packaging should be in a tight, light-resistant container, with recommended storage at controlled room temperature.

Calculations

Dose/Concentration

Lidocaine HCl: w/w % is calculated to be:

$$\frac{0.6 \text{ g Lidocaine}}{30 \text{ g gel}} = \frac{x \text{ g Lidocaine}}{100 \text{ g gel}}; x = 2 \text{ g} / 100 \text{ g} = 2\%$$

Diphenhydramine HCl (DPH): w/w % is calculated to be:

$$\frac{0.3 \text{ g DPH}}{30 \text{ g gel}} = \frac{x \text{ g DPH}}{100 \text{ g gel}}; x = 1 \text{ g} / 100 \text{ g} = 1\%$$

These concentrations are OK.

Ingredient Amounts

Pharmacist Kraemer has decided to make 3 g excess to compensate for loss on compounding.

Lidocaine HCl in g for 33 g of gel is calculated to be:

$$\frac{0.6 \text{ g Lidocaine}}{30 \text{ g gel}} = \frac{x \text{ g Lidocaine}}{33 \text{ g gel}}; x = 0.66 \text{ g Lidocaine}$$

Diphenhydramine HCl (DPH) in g for 33 g of gel is calculated to be:

$$\frac{0.3 \text{ g DPH}}{30 \text{ g gel}} = \frac{x \text{ g DPH}}{33 \text{ g gel}}; x = 0.33 \text{ g DPH}$$

Poloxamer Lecithin Organogel (PLO) can be made from the individual ingredients, or the 20% Poloxamer Gel and the combined isopropyl palmitate and lecithin (IPP-Lecithin) solution may be purchased. These two liquids are then mixed together in a ratio of 4 parts of the Poloxamer Gel with 1 part of the IPP-Lecithin solution. For this prescription, Pharmacist Kraemer purchased the prepared gel and IPP-Lecithin solution.

First, the weight in g of the Poloxamer Lecithin Organogel is calculated by subtracting the weight of all the other ingredients from total preparation weight of 33 g:

$$33 \text{ g} - (0.33 \text{ g DPH} + 0.66 \text{ g Lidocaine}) = 33 \text{ g} - 0.99 \text{ g} = 32.01 \text{ g} \approx 32 \text{ g}$$

Second, using the ratio of 4 parts to 1 part for a total of 5 parts, calculate the weight in g of Poloxamer Gel 20% and of IPP-Lecithin solution:

$$\frac{1 \text{ part IPP} - Lec.}{5 \text{ parts organogel}} = \frac{x \text{ g IPP} - Lec.}{32 \text{ g organogel}}; x = 6.4 \text{ g IPP} - Lec.$$

$$\frac{4 \text{ part Pol 20\% Gel}}{5 \text{ parts organogel}} = \frac{x \text{ g Pol 20\% Gel}}{32 \text{ g organogel}}; x = 25.6 \text{ g Pol 20\% Gel}$$

If made from the individual ingredients, the 20% w/v Poloxamer Gel is made from poloxamer 407 (Pluronic® F 127), as described in Chapter 18. This requires overnight storage in a refrigerator for the clear gel to form. The IPP-Lecithin solution is made by adding 10 g of soya lecithin to 10 g of isopropyl palmitate and allowing the mixture to set overnight. Neither preparation is difficult to make, but both have to be made ahead of time because they require setting overnight. Furthermore, the manufactured solutions come already buffered and preserved, but if the solutions are made in the pharmacy, a preservative system and possibly a buffer must be added.

Compounding Procedure

On a digital balance weigh 660 mg of Lidocaine HCl and 330 mg of Diphenhydramine HCl and place in a glass mortar. Tare a small beaker and weigh 6.4 g of the IPP-Lecithin, and in another tared beaker weigh 25.6 g of Poloxamer Gel 20%, and combine the two in one beaker. Slowly add a small portion of this to the powders in the mortar to make a smooth paste. Using trituration, continue to slowly add the PLO mixture until it is all blended together and you have obtained a uniform gel. Transfer this to a 1-oz ointment jar; label and dispense.

Quality Control

Preparation is a pale yellowish-white opaque gel. It is a viscous liquid when refrigerated but is more gel-like in consistency when at room temperature. The actual weight is checked and is 30.9 g, which is an expected loss of material from the theoretical weight 33 g and is within the range of ±5% of the prescribed weight of 30 g.

Labeling

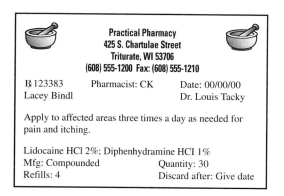

Practical Pharmacy
425 S. Chartulae Street
Triturate, WI 53706
(608) 555-1200 Fax: (608) 555-1210

℞ 123383   Pharmacist: CK   Date: 00/00/00
Lacey Bindl   Dr. Louis Tacky

Apply to affected areas three times a day as needed for pain and itching.

Lidocaine HCl 2%; Diphenhydramine HCl 1%
Mfg: Compounded   Quantity: 30
Refills: 4   Discard after: Give date

Auxiliary Labels: For External Use Only; Keep in the Refrigerator

Patient Consultation

Hello, Lacey, I'm Chelsey Kraemer, your pharmacist. Do you have any drug allergies? Are you using any OTC or prescription medications? What has your physician told you about the use of this gel? It should give you some relief from your pain and itching. You are to apply the gel three times daily as needed to the affected areas. If the itching or pain gets worse, or if you don't seem to be getting any relief, contact Dr. Tacky. This is for external use only. You may store this at room temperature but it does apply better if it has been refrigerated. This gel has the unique property of being a liquid when at cool temperature, but it firms up when it is applied to a warm skin surface. This means that if cool, it is easy to apply but it stays in place on the applied skin area. Keep this out of the reach of children. This may be refilled four times. You should discard any unused portion after 2 weeks. Do you have any questions?

➤ **Prescription 30-9**

Contemporary Physicians Group Practice
20 S. Park Street, Triturate, WI 53706
Tel: (608) 555-1333 Fax: (608) 555-1335

R # 950

Name *Addie McPeel*   Date *00/00/00*

Address *202 Council Bluff Circle*   Age   Wt/Ht

R

Methyl Salicylate	*3.5 g*	
Menthol	*1.5 g*	
Sodium Stearate	*1.3 g*	
Propylene Glycol	*2.5 g*	
Purified Water	*1.2 g*	

Disp 5 g Medication Stick

J. Jetson 00/00/00

Sig: Apply to affected areas tid prn pain

Refills *prn*

Emil Clyde   M.D.

DEA No. _____

Ingredients Used   (Amounts are for 10 g, 5 g excess)

Ingredient	Quantity Used	Manufacturer Lot#–Exp Date	Solubility	Dose Comparison Given	Dose Comparison Usual	Use in the Prescription
Methyl Salicylate	3.5 g (3 mL)	JET Labs ON3091–mm/yy	1 g/1500 mL water, misc w/ alcohol	35%	varies 10–35%	counterirritant, local analgesic
Propylene Glycol	2.5 g (2.4 mL)	JET Labs SN2662–mm/yy	misc w/ water, alcohol	____	____	solvent, preservative, humectant
Menthol	1.5 g	JET Labs ON3092–mm/yy	sl sol water, v sol alcohol	15%	0.5–20%	counterirritant, local analgesic
Purified Water	1.2 g (1 mL)	Sweet Springs AL0529–mm/yy	misc w/ alcohol	____	____	solvent
Sodium Stearate	1.3 g	JET Labs ON3093–mm/yy	readily sol in hot water and alcohol	____	____	emulsifier, stiffening agent

Compatibility–Stability/Beyond-Use Date

Stability–Compatibility: No stability data for this specific formulation is available, but the methyl salicylate and Menthol should be quite stable in this formulation. There are numerous commercial nonprescription products with similar formulations. This formulation was patterned after a similar medication stick formulation given on the Internet site for Paddock Labs (www.paddocklabs.com), under Publications, Secundum Artem, Vol. 5, No. 3, Compounding Medication Sticks. Another source of information is the January/February 2000 issue of the *International Journal of Pharmaceutical Compounding*.

Preservative: No additional preservative is needed because of the presence of Propylene Glycol (25%), Menthol, and methyl salicylate, all of which have preserving properties.

Packaging and Storage and Beyond-use date: Pharmacist Jetson will use the *USP* recommended maximum 30-day beyond-use date for compounded formulations prepared from ingredients in solid form when there is no stability information for the formulation (3). Packaging will be in a special medication stick tube container, with recommended storage at controlled room temperature.

Calculations

Dose/Concentration

The active ingredients in this formulation are methyl salicylate and menthol. For this topical preparation, a w/w % concentration is calculated for these ingredients.

Methyl salicylate: w/w % is calculated to be:

$$\frac{3.5\ g\ Methyl\ Sal.}{10\ g\ preparation} = \frac{x\ g\ Methyl\ Sal.}{100\ g\ preparation}; x = 35\ g/100\ g = 35\%$$

Menthol: w/w % is calculated to be:

$$\frac{1.5\ g\ Menthol}{10\ g\ preparation} = \frac{x\ g\ Menthol}{100\ g\ preparation}; x = 15\ g/100\ g = 15\%$$

These concentrations are OK.

Ingredient Amounts

Pharmacist Jetson will make 5 g excess to compensate for loss on compounding. The weights of all the ingredients are given for the 10-g formula. The methyl salicylate and the propylene glycol are liquids that would more conveniently be measured by volume. The volumes can be calculated using the specific gravity of each of these ingredients.

Methyl salicylate has a s.g. of 1.18; the volume of 3.5 g is calculated to be:

$$\left(\frac{mL\ Methyl\ Sal.}{1.18\ g\ Methyl\ Sal.}\right)\left(\frac{3.5\ g\ Methyl\ Sal.}{}\right) = 3.0\ mL\ Methyl\ Sal.$$

Propylene Glycol has a s.g. of 1.04; the volume of 2.5 g is calculated to be:

$$\left(\frac{mL\ P.G.}{1.04\ g\ P.G.}\right)\left(\frac{2.5\ g\ P.G.}{}\right) = 2.4\ mL\ Propylene\ Glycol$$

Compounding Procedure

On a class 3 torsion balance or a digital balance, weigh 1.5 g of Menthol and 1.3 g of Sodium Stearate. Place the Sodium Stearate in a small beaker. Measure 1.2 mL of Purified Water and 2.4 mL Propylene Glycol using a 3-mL syringe and add to the beaker containing the Sodium Stearate. Heat this mixture in a microwave oven for about 10 seconds. Place the Menthol in another small beaker. Measure 3 mL of methyl salicylate in a 10-mL graduated cylinder or a 3-mL syringe and add it to the beaker containing the Menthol; stir to mix until the Menthol is dissolved. Add this to the melted base in the other beaker and stir thoroughly. Allow this to cool further until it begins to become more viscous, then pour this into a medication tube and allow it to solidify. Label and dispense.

Quality Control

Preparation is a colorless to slightly whitish transparent soft solid stick. The actual weight of the stick is checked by weighing the medication stick tube before and after the preparation is added to the tube; the weight of the preparation is 5.4 g, which is an expected loss of material from the theoretical weight of 10 g and is within the range of ±5% of the prescribed weight of 5 g.

Labeling

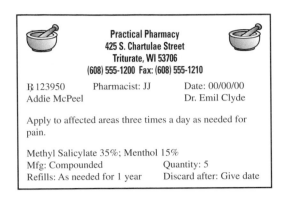

Practical Pharmacy
425 S. Chartulae Street
Triturate, WI 53706
(608) 555-1200 Fax: (608) 555-1210

℞ 123950   Pharmacist: JJ   Date: 00/00/00
Addie McPeel   Dr. Emil Clyde

Apply to affected areas three times a day as needed for pain.

Methyl Salicylate 35%; Menthol 15%
Mfg: Compounded   Quantity: 5
Refills: As needed for 1 year   Discard after: Give date

Auxiliary Labels: For External Use Only; Keep out of reach of children

Patient Consultation

Hi, Ms. McPeel, I'm your pharmacist, Judy Jetson. Do you have any drug allergies? Are you using any OTC or prescription medications? What has Dr. Clyde told you about the use of this medication stick? This is a preparation to treat your muscle pain. You are to apply this three times daily as needed to the affected areas as directed by Dr. Clyde. To use this, remove the cap and turn the bottom of the tube counter-clockwise and then rub the medication stick over the area. If you develop a rash or hives after you start using this medication, or if the pain does not improve or gets worse, stop using this preparation and contact Dr. Clyde. This is for external use only. You should store this in a cool, dry place. It is especially important to keep this out of the reach of children; it contains methyl salicylate, which smells like wintergreen, and some children may mistake it for candy. This may be refilled as needed for a year, but I would suggest that you call ahead when you need a new tube, since this is a custom-made preparation and it take a little while to make it. You should discard any unused portion after a month. Do you have any questions?

References

1. The 2002 United States Pharmacopeia 25/National Formulary 20. Rockville, MD: The United States Pharmacopeial Convention, Inc., 2001;2217-2219.
2. The 2002 United States Pharmacopeia 25/National Formulary 20. Rockville, MD: The United States Pharmacopeial Convention, Inc., 2001; Official Monographs.
3. The 2002 United States Pharmacopeia 25/National Formulary 20. Rockville, MD: The United States Pharmacopeial Convention, Inc., 2001;2054.
4. Trissel LA. Trissel's Stability of Compounded Formulations, 2nd ed. Washington, DC: American Pharmaceutical Association, 2001;385-386.
5. Connors KA, Amidon GL, Stella VJ. Chemical Stability of Pharmaceuticals, 2nd ed. New York: John Wiley & Sons, 1986;483-490.
6. Gennaro AR, ed. Remington: The Science and Practice of Pharmacy, 20th ed. Philadelphia: Lippincott Williams & Wilkins, 2000;1208.
7. Trissel LA. Trissel's Stability of Compounded Formulations, 2nd ed. Washington, DC: American Pharmaceutical Association, 2001;268-270.
8. Florey K, ed. Analytical Profiles of Drug Substances, Vol. 1. New York: Academic Press, 1972;383.
9. Allen Jr LV, ed. Piroxicam 0.5% in an Alcoholic Gel. IJPC 1997;1:181.
10. Allen Jr LV, ed. Ketoprofen 10%, Cyclobenzaprine 1% and Lidocaine 5% in Poloxamer Lecithin Organogel. IJPC 1998;2:154.
11. Trissel LA. Trissel's Stability of Compounded Formulations, 2nd ed. Washington, DC: American Pharmaceutical Association, 2001;130–131.
12. Trissel LA. Trissel's Stability of Compounded Formulations, 2nd ed. Washington, DC: American Pharmaceutical Association, 2001;218-220.

CHAPTER 31

Suppositories

I. GENERAL DEFINITION

"Suppositories are solid bodies of various weights and shapes, adapted for introduction into the rectal, vaginal, or urethral orifice of the human body. They usually melt, soften, or dissolve at body temperature. A suppository may act as a protectant or palliative to the local tissues at the point of introduction or as a carrier of therapeutic agents for systemic or local action." (1)—*USP*

II. USES

A. Suppositories are used when a local effect is needed in the rectum, vagina, or urethra.

B. Rectal and vaginal suppositories may also be used as carriers of drugs for systemic use.
   1. Rectal suppositories offer an alternative for the systemic delivery of drugs in patients who cannot take drugs orally. Examples include patients who are unconscious, those who are vomiting or having seizures, and those who have obstructions in the upper gastrointestinal tract.
   2. Some drugs that are ineffective orally may be successfully administered rectally or vaginally. Examples include drugs that are extensively metabolized by first-pass effect and drugs that are destroyed in the stomach or intestine. An example of a drug that is administered either rectally or vaginally for systemic effect is Progesterone.

C. Compounding suppositories is usually done as a last resort. This is because suppositories are, in general, more difficult to prepare than other dosage forms and because absorption of therapeutic agents from suppositories is relatively unpredictable.

D. As with other dosage forms, suppositories should be compounded extemporaneously only when a manufactured product is not available. This principle is especially true with suppositories containing drugs needed for a systemic effect because of the unpredictable absorption from suppositories.

III. SELECTING THE SUPPOSITORY BASE MATERIAL

A. To release drug for systemic action or to make drug available for local effect, the suppository base must melt, soften, or dissolve in the body orifice. Of the two most common suppository base materials, polyethylene glycol (PEG) dissolves, while fatty bases, like Cocoa Butter and its synthetic substitutes, melt at body temperature. A detailed description of suppository bases and their properties is given in Chapter 23. Consult this chapter when selecting a suppository base for a compounded drug preparation.

B. The selection of suppository base material depends both on the intended use (systemic versus local effect) and the route of administration (rectal, vaginal, or urethral). Other factors to consider include patient comfort and compatibility and stability of components in the base.

1. Patient comfort

a. In general, fatty-type bases are more comfortable for patients than are PEG bases.

b. Fatty bases are bland and nonirritating to the sensitive tissues of the rectum, vagina, and urethra, whereas PEG bases can give a stinging or burning sensation. PEG bases also can cause a defecating reflex when used rectally. These effects can be minimized by adding 10% water to the PEG base and by moistening the suppository with water before insertion (2).

2. Compatibility and stability

a. In most cases, fatty bases are less reactive than PEG bases, so they have fewer compatibility and stability problems with incorporated therapeutic agents.

b. One compatibility problem of fatty bases is the lowering of their melting point with the addition of drugs or other components that form lower melting eutectic mixtures. Chloral Hydrate in Cocoa Butter is the classic example of this effect. A small amount of white wax or of cetyl esters wax can be added to overcome this problem; however, adding too much wax may give a suppository that does not melt at body temperature.

c. Because PEG bases are designed to dissolve rather than melt at the site of action, they can be formulated so that they will not melt on storage, even at fairly warm temperatures. In contrast, fatty bases are formulated to melt at body temperature and are therefore much more sensitive to warm temperatures; they must be stored at controlled room temperature or in the refrigerator.

3. Route of administration

a. Fatty bases are preferred for rectal suppositories because rectal tissues are especially sensitive to the irritating effects of PEG bases. As stated previously, PEG suppositories may also cause a defecating reflex.

b. PEG bases are often preferred over fatty bases for vaginal and urethral suppositories; the vagina and urethra do not have sphincter muscles to prevent leakage from these body orifices, and the oily material of fatty bases is more undesirable in this regard.

c. Soft, rubbery suppository bases, such as glycerinated gelatin, are suitable for vaginal administration but are not firm enough for rectal or urethral use.

4. Systemic effects

a. In general, systemic absorption of drugs from suppositories is unpredictable. This is due to both the poor environment for absorption in the rectum and vagina (urethral inserts are used solely for local effect) and to the physical-chemical nature of the suppository base material coupled with the properties of the active ingredient(s).

(1) The amount of aqueous fluid in the rectum and vagina is variable but small. This affects the release of drug from the base. Although this influences both local action and systemic absorption, its major impact is upon systemic absorption.

(a) Because PEG bases require dissolution for release of the drug from the dosage form, systemic effect depends on the amount of dissolving fluid present in the rectum or vagina. This is part of the rationale for recommending that patients moisten PEG suppositories before insertion; this puts a layer of water in contact with the suppository to help hasten dissolution upon insertion. Even in excess water, PEG bases dissolve slowly, taking up to 1 hour (2).

(b) Although fatty bases melt rather than dissolve, the incorporated drug must partition out of the base into the aqueous medium at the site of action before absorption can occur. This too requires a sufficient amount of aqueous media at the administration site.

    (2) As discussed in Chapter 23, fatty bases give poor release of hydrophobic drugs. Because many organic drug molecules are water-insoluble and hydrophobic except when present in their ionized salt or water-soluble complex form, this must be considered when choosing both the drug form and the suppository base.

        (a) The release of a drug from a fatty, lipophilic suppository base to the aqueous medium in the rectum or vagina depends on the water/base partition coefficient of the drug.

        (b) For this reason, from a bioavailability point of view, water-soluble ionized (salt) forms of drugs (these have high water/base partition coefficients) should be used when possible with fatty bases. For example, Codeine Phosphate or Sulfate is preferred over Codeine base for systemic absorption when a fatty suppository base is being used. Some drugs like Acetaminophen and Diazepam do not have water-soluble forms and give slow and unpredictable release from fatty bases. These drugs are not good candidates for incorporation into fatty bases.

    (3) When formulated with an appropriate blend of polymers, PEG suppositories dissolve in body cavity fluids and release the active ingredient(s), both hydrophilic and hydrophobic drugs. Provided there are sufficient aqueous secretions in the body cavity, they provide more reliable release of hydrophobic drugs from the dosage form than do fatty bases.

  b. Suppositories made with bases that contain a dispersing agent, such as Silicon Dioxide or Bentonite, and/or a surfactant may break apart more easily and spread more effectively over the target tissue or absorbing surfaces.

  c. Because of the unpredictability of release of drug from suppository bases, it is important to monitor the effectiveness of the drug delivery system by frequent monitoring of therapeutic results. Drugs with narrow therapeutic windows should be administered in compounded suppositories only with the greatest of caution.

5. Local action

  a. Choice of a base is not as critical when local action is desired because nearly any base holds the active ingredient in contact with the affected tissue.

  b. Suppositories made with bases that contain a dispersing agent and/or a surfactant may break apart more easily and the active ingredients may be spread more effectively on the target tissue.

  c. When an emollient local effect is desired, a fatty base is preferred.

IV. SELECTING A METHOD OF COMPOUNDING

A. Suppositories can be made by hand-rolling or by fusion. At one time they were also made by compression, but this method is now rarely used in extemporaneous compounding.

B. Depending on the compounding method selected, special calculations, compounding techniques, and equipment may be required to give accurate doses of suppositories.

C. Hand-rolling suppositories

  1. Advantages

    a. Hand-rolled suppositories do not require special calculations.

    b. Special equipment is not required for this method. A pill roller is useful, but a broad-bladed spatula or any stiff, flat piece of nonreactive material can be used for this purpose.

    c. Cocoa Butter is the base used for hand-rolled suppositories. It is readily available in bars or push-up tubes from any drug wholesaler; it is also available in grated form from suppliers of compounding ingredients and equipment.

    2. Disadvantages
       a. Preparing and forming hand-rolled suppositories requires experience and good technique.
       b. Even when well-made, hand-rolled suppositories do not have the elegant appearance of suppositories made by fusion.

D. Fusion
    1. Advantages
       a. This method does not require well-developed manual compounding technique.
       b. Suppositories made by fusion have an elegant, professional appearance.

    2. Disadvantages
       a. Special suppository molds are required to make suppositories by fusion.
       b. Caution must be used when incorporating drugs sensitive to heat.
       c. Because the components are dosed and measured by weight but compounded by volume, density calculations, mold calibrations, or double-casting procedures are required to give accurate doses.
          (1) Because suppositories are semisolid at room temperature, most of the base components and active ingredients are solids and are measured by weight.
          (2) The components are then combined, melted, and poured into suppository mold cavities. This means that the dosage unit is measured by volume—the volume of the mold cavity. The final amount of drug in a dosage unit therefore depends on two factors: the w/w concentration of active ingredient in the base material and the weight of the mixture contained in each mold cavity. The weight of mixture in the mold cavity depends on the volume of the cavity and the density (ρ) of the molten mixture.
          (3) Consider the following example. The usual volume of a suppository mold cavity is 2 mL. Depending on the density of the melted mixture of ingredients, the weight of a 2-mL suppository can vary considerably. To calculate the weight per suppository, multiply the density of the mixture times the volume of the mold cavity.
          For example:

          Water, $\rho = 1$ g/mL: *1 g/mL $\times$ 2 mL = 2 g*

          Cocoa Butter, $\rho = 0.86$ g/mL: *0.86 g/mL $\times$ 2 mL = 1.72 g*

          PEG 400, $\rho = 1.125$ g/mL: *1.125 g/mL $\times$ 2 mL = 2.26 g*
          (4) Obviously, the density of the material has a significant effect on the final weight of the dosage unit. To determine the quantity of base and active ingredients(s) to weigh when compounding suppositories by fusion, it is necessary to either calibrate the mold cavities for the desired base or use a double-casting procedure. There are other factors to consider as well. Examples are given and discussed in the section of this chapter on fusion compounding methods.

V. COMPOUNDING METHODS FOR SUPPOSITORIES

A. Hand-Rolling Suppositories
This method is limited to suppositories made using Cocoa Butter as the base material because Cocoa Butter is the only suppository base that can be molded without the use of heat. Follow the steps given below.
    1. Check the doses of the active ingredients.
    2. Check the compatibility and stability of the active ingredients and the formulation.
    3. Decide on the desired finished weight per suppository. The usual weight per unit for various suppository types is as follows:

- **a.** Adult rectal: 2 g
- **b.** Vaginal: 2–5 g
- **c.** Pediatric rectal: 1 g
- **d.** Male urethral: 4 g
- **e.** Female urethral: 2 g

4. Calculate the quantity of each ingredient needed for compounding the preparation. Make enough material for two extra suppositories.
   - **a.** Multiply the dose per unit times the number of units to determine the amount of each active ingredient.
   - **b.** Multiply the finished weight per unit times the number of units.
   - **c.** Subtract the total weight of active ingredients from the total weight of the suppositories to determine the amount of base (Cocoa Butter) needed.
5. If the Cocoa Butter is in a bar or in large pieces, grate or reduce the Cocoa Butter to very small pieces.
6. Weigh the calculated amount of active ingredient(s) and Cocoa Butter.
7. Place the active ingredients(s) in a **glass** mortar and triturate to a fine powder.
8. Add a small amount of Cocoa Butter and triturate, using pressure to soften and/or liquefy the Cocoa Butter so that it acts as a levigating agent for the active ingredient(s).
9. Add the rest of the Cocoa Butter by geometric dilution, triturating and scraping down the sides of the mortar regularly.
10. Using a metal spatula, remove the mass from the mortar and place the material in a clean piece of white filter paper. Wash your hands carefully and put on plastic disposable gloves. Knead the mass in the filter paper until it is pliable but not soft and sticky.
11. While it is still in the filter paper, start to shape the mass into a cylindrical pipe by rolling it in the filter paper between your hands (in the same manner as you made "snakes" out of modeling clay when you were in preschool).
12. Put the cylindrical mass on an ointment slab and, using a **clean** pill roller or a broad-bladed spatula, roll the mass into a smooth cylindrical pipe. Use the gauge on the ointment slab or a ruler to determine the proper length of the pipe so that equal pieces of appropriate length can be cut. The approximate dimensions per suppository are as follows:
    - **a.** 1–1½ inch in length with a diameter of about 3/8 inch for adult rectal and vaginal suppositories
    - **b.** Proportionate, but smaller in size for pediatric rectal suppositories
    - **c.** 4 inches in length by 3/16 inch in diameter for male urethral inserts
    - **d.** 2–3 inches in length by 3/16 inches in diameter for female urethral inserts
13. As you roll the mass, use the pill roller or spatula to keep the ends of the pipe as blunt and square as possible; you may wish to roll the pipe slightly longer than necessary and cut off the irregular ends of the pipe before cutting it into equal pieces.
14. Using a razor blade, cut the pipe into equal-length pieces.
15. Form a point on one end of each suppository. Suppositories should be bullet-shaped for ease of insertion.
16. Weigh each suppository; if necessary, adjust each to the proper weight by slicing thin pieces from the blunt end.
17. Wrap each suppository in foil or seal in individual plastic bags.

B. Fusion

1. Suppository molds
   - **a.** A wide assortment of suppository molds are available from vendors of compounding supplies. Depending on the company, aluminum molds for rectal-vaginal suppositories are available with either 1- or 2-mL capacity cavities and with 10 to 1,000 cavities per mold. Urethral molds, both male and female, are also available. A wide variety of disposable molds can also be purchased.
   - **b.** Although preference for disposable versus aluminum molds depends on the individual using them, the type of suppository base being used, and the intended use

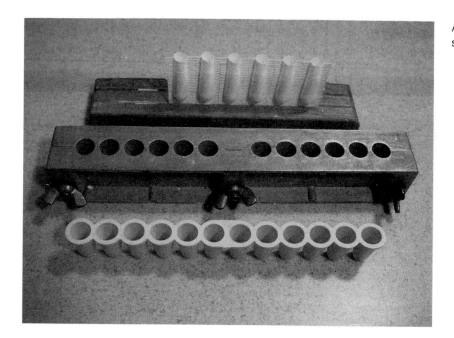

Aluminum and disposable suppository molds.

of the suppository, in general, aluminum molds give more uniform, accurate dosage units.

  c. Mold lubrication

    (1) Disposable molds have the advantage of not requiring any prior lubrication because the suppositories are just popped out or the plastic material peeled off at the time of use.

    (2) Although aluminum molds usually require lubrication before use, this is relatively easy with the use of spray vegetable oils. Just a light coating is needed; any excess should be wiped off with a tissue.

  d. Suppository wrappers

    (1) Disposable molds also have the advantage of providing the wrapping material for the suppositories—the suppositories are dispensed in the plastic shell that is used as the mold.

    (2) Suppositories that have been made in a nondisposable mold should have a protective covering applied before being placed in the dispensing container. They should either be wrapped individually in aluminum foil or sealed in small polyethylene plastic bags. The foil can be purchased precut in small squares (it even comes in colors), or the 3" × 3" squares can be cut from a sheet of aluminum foil. Alternatively, small polyethylene bags, zipper-lock or plain, can be purchased for a nominal price.

  e. Although aluminum molds have a greater initial investment cost, in the long term they may be less expensive to use than disposable molds.

2. Suppository base materials for the fusion method

  a. All four suppository base types that are recognized in the *USP* may be used with the fusion method. These bases and their properties are discussed in Chapter 23.

  b. Melting fatty bases

    (1) Microwave ovens are not recommended for melting fatty bases because these heating devices do not provide the carefully controlled temperature required. Similarly, although these bases could be carefully melted by direct heat on a hot plate, the more controlled temperature provided by a warm water bath is preferred. This is especially true when melting Cocoa Butter.

    (2) If the base is in a bar or in large solid blocks, grate or shred it into very small pieces.

    (3) Place the base in a beaker or crucible and carefully heat this on a warm water bath until the base has just turned to a fluid. If a warm water bath with a thermostat such as the one pictured in Chapter 12 is available, this would be preferred.

(4) If the base is Cocoa Butter, have the water bath temperature at approximately 55°C and melt the base carefully. Melted Cocoa Butter should maintain an opalescent, creamy appearance with a temperature of approximately 34°C. You can tell visually if the critical temperature has been exceeded for Cocoa Butter because the fluid changes to a clear, golden color. One recommendation to avoid overheating Cocoa Butter is to add it in portions to the heating vessel. Then, if the critical temperature is exceeded and the fluid becomes clear, the vessel can be removed from the heat source and extra grated Cocoa Butter can be added to reduce the temperature of the melt and provide new β-crystals for the desired polymorph.

(5) If a Cocoa Butter Substitute base such as Fattibase® is used, follow the manufacturer's instructions for the heating temperature. For example, the recommended melting temperature for Fattibase® is approximately 50°C, and this base should not be heated above 60°C.

c. Preparing and melting PEG and glycerinated gelatin bases

(1) Both PEG and glycerinated gelatin bases can be made using either a microwave oven or a hot plate. In either case, care must be exercised so that the material is not overheated.

(2) Preformulated blends of PEG, such as Polybase®, and typical solid PEG base components melt between 37° and 63°C, but they may be heated up to 100°C without danger of decomposition. The melting points of commonly used PEGs are given in Table 23.1 of Chapter 23.

(3) The formula and method of preparation for glycerinated gelatin suppository base are the same as the pediatric chewable gummy gel base given in Table 25.3 of Chapter 25.

3. Compounding procedures

These are discussed in the examples that follow.

➤ *EXAMPLE* Method using precalibration of the suppository mold

➤ **Prescription 31.1**

Contemporary Physicians Group Practice
20 S. Park Street, Triturate, WI 53706
Tel: (608) 555-1333 Fax: (608) 555-1335

R # 910

Name *Ellie Mae Clampett*   Date *00/00/00*

Address *598 Beverly Hills Court*   Age *1 y.o.*   Wt/Ht *22 lbs*

R

Aspirin   100 mg
Cocoa Butter   q s

M. & ft. Suppositories #6

R.Harrington 00/00/00

Sig: Insert 1 suppository pr q 4-6 hr prn pain

Refills *NR*   *Olive Quacky*   M.D.

DEA No. _____

---

1. Check the dose.

   Usual: A reference gives a pediatric dose of Aspirin of 10–15 mg/kg of body weight every 4 hours up to 60–80 mg/kg/day. Pharmacist Harrington should check with Dr. Quacky to be certain that patient Ellie Mae does not have an acute illness that predisposes to Reye's syndrome with Aspirin therapy.

   This prescription: Our patient weighs 22 lbs or 10 kg. The dose, as written, is 100 mg every 4–6 hours. For our patient, this is 10 mg/kg every 4–6 hours, a dose within the reference range.

2. Check compatibility–stability: Aspirin suppositories are an official USP product, and the monograph recommends storage in well-closed containers in a cool place (3). Although Aspirin is subject to hydrolysis in the presence of water, this preparation does not include any water.

3. Procedure

   a. Calibrate the suppository mold for the suppository base being used for this preparation by melting the base, pouring five suppositories, trimming and removing each suppository from its mold cavity, and weighing each. When melting the base, note and record the temperature of the melt so that this fusion temperature can be used each time for this calibration weight. The density of some bases will vary depending on temperature of the melt. In this example, the base is Cocoa Butter, the temperature of the melt is 34°C, and the average weight per suppository is 1.720 grams.

   b. Calculate the amount of active ingredient(s) for the prescription order plus two extras:

   $$8 \times 100 \ mg = 800 \ mg \ Aspirin$$

   c. Calculate the final weight of base and active ingredient(s) for all suppositories:

   $$8 \times 1.720 = 13.760 \ g \ total \ weight \ for \ 8 \ suppositories$$

   d. Calculate the amount of Cocoa Butter needed:

   $$Amount \ of \ Cocoa \ Butter = 13.760 \ g - 0.8 \ g = 12.960 \ g \ Cocoa \ Butter$$

   (but see the next example)

   e. Prepare the powdered active ingredient(s). Weigh a small excess of the amount of the active ingredient needed, and reduce this to a fine powder by trituration in a mortar. The excess is to allow for any loss in trituration and transfer of the active ingredient(s) from the mortar to the vessel used for heating the formulation. Weigh the calculated amount of active ingredient needed, in this case 800 mg of Aspirin.

   f. Prepare the suppository base material. If the suppository base material is in a bar or in large pieces, grate or reduce it to small pieces. Weigh the calculated amount of suppository base, in this case 12.96 g of Cocoa Butter.

   g. Before melting the base and combining the ingredients, prepare the suppository mold. Make certain it is clean. Apply a lubricant to the mold if needed. A thin film of vegetable oil spray usually works well.

   h. Put a small portion of the base in a beaker or crucible and carefully heat this on a warm water bath until the base has just turned to a fluid. If the base is Cocoa Butter, melt it carefully on a warm (approximately 55°C) water bath. The Cocoa Butter should have an opalescent appearance (approximately 34°C). If another base is used, follow the manufacturer's instructions for heating temperature.

   i. Add the powdered drug to the melted base and stir well to mix.

   j. Add the remainder of the grated base in portions with stirring, being careful not to overheat. Stir to ensure a uniform mixture. The temperature of the melt should be the same as the temperature for the base when the calibration was done.

   k. Pour the molten mixture into six or seven suppository mold cavities. Overfill the cavities slightly, as the base will contract somewhat as it cools.

   l. Allow the suppositories to solidify at room temperature, then place the mold in the refrigerator for about 30 minutes to allow the suppositories to harden. Do not put the mold in the refrigerator until the suppositories have congealed, or the base will contract too rapidly and thin cavities will form down the center of each suppository.

   m. Trim any excess material from the top of the mold using a warm spatula or a razor blade.

   n. Perform a quality control check on the suppositories by weighing a finished suppository. If many suppositories are molded at one time, a random sample of suppositories should be weighed.

o. If you are using a disposable mold as a dispensing wrapper, place the suppositories in a dispensing container. If a reusable mold is used, carefully remove the suppositories from the mold cavities. Wrap each suppository in foil or put in individual small plastic bags and place the suppositories in a dispensing container.

➤ *EXAMPLE* Determination and use of density displacement factors

1. The above procedure supposes that 800 mg of Aspirin occupies the same volume as 800 mg of Cocoa Butter. This is not exactly accurate. In Table 31.1, check the density factor for Aspirin with Cocoa But-

TABLE 31.1 Density Factors for Cocoa Butter Suppositories[a]

Medication	Factor
Aloin[c]	1.3
Alum	1.7
Aminophylline	1.1
Aminopyrine	1.3
Aspirin	1.3
Aspirin[c]	1.1
Barbital	1.2
Belladonna extract	1.3
Benzoic acid	1.5
Bismuth carbonate	4.5
Bismuth salicylate	4.5
Bismuth subgallate	2.7
Bismuth subnitrate	6.0
Boric acid	1.5
Castor oil	1.0
Chloral hydrate	1.3
Cocaine hydrochloride	1.3
Codeine phosphate[c]	1.1
Digitalis leaf	1.6
Dimenhydrinate[c]	1.3
Diphenhydramine hydrochloride[c]	1.3
Gallic acid	2.0
Glycerin	1.6
Ichthammol	1.1
Iodoform	4.0
Menthol	0.7
Morphine hydrochloride	1.6
Opium	1.4
Paraffin	1.0
Pentobarbital[c]	1.2
Peruvian Balsam[b]	1.1
Phenobarbital	1.2
Phenol[b]	0.9
Potassium bromide	2.2
Potassium iodide	4.5
Procaine	1.2
Quinine hydrochloride	1.2
Resorcinol	1.4
Salicylic acid	1.3
Secobarbital sodium[c]	1.2
Sodium bromide	2.3
Spermaceti	1.0
Sulfathiazole	1.6
Tannic acid	1.6
White wax	1.0
Witch hazel fluidextract	1.1
Zinc oxide	4.0
Zinc sulfate	2.8

[a] Davis H: *Bentley's Textbook of Pharmaceutics*, 5th ed., Williams & Wilkins, Baltimore, 1949; Büchi J. *Pharm Acta Helv 20:* 403, 1940.
[b] Density adjusted taking into account white wax in mass.
[c] King RE: In *Dispensing of Medication*, 9th ed, Mack Publishing Co., Easton, PA, 1984, p. 96.

ter. Notice that Aspirin has a density factor of 1.1 (or 1.3, depending on the reference) with Cocoa Butter; that is, 1.1 grams of Aspirin will displace 1 g of Cocoa Butter. This should be taken into account in calculating the amount of Cocoa Butter needed for these suppositories.

a. Using the density displacement factor for the drug, calculate the amount of base (e.g., Cocoa Butter) that is displaced by the amount of drug used (e.g., 800 mg Aspirin):

$$\frac{1.1\,g\,Aspirin}{1\,g\,Cocoa\,Butter} = \frac{0.8\,g\,Aspirin}{x\,g\,Cocoa\,Butter} ; x = 0.727\,g\,Cocoa\,Butter\,displaced\,by\,0.8\,g\,Aspirin$$

b. Based on this amount, calculate the weight of Cocoa Butter needed for the prescription order:

$$13.76\,g - 0.727\,g = 13.032\,g\,Cocoa\,Butter$$

Therefore, the amount of Cocoa Butter to weigh in the procedure given above is 13.032 g rather than 12.96 g.

2. When should you be concerned with compensating for differences in volume displacement? Density factors are important when the following conditions are met:

a. The drug has a quantity dose and is being used for systemic effect. If the drug is being used topically, we just want it in contact with the tissue in the body cavity, and precise quantities per dosage unit are not significant.

b. The drug makes up a significant portion of the dosage form. For example, if the drug is 5 mg in a 2-g (2,000 mg) dosage form, any difference in displacement volume is insignificant.

c. A density difference exists between the base and the drug. If the density factor for a drug in a base is 1.0, a density displacement calculation is not needed.

d. Because we often do not have a density factor for the drug and base in question, it is helpful to analyze the possibilities mathematically so that we can make informed judgments about when to compensate for displacement differences. For example, take the case of Cocoa Butter, and look at the density factors for various drugs with Cocoa Butter in Table 31.1.

   1. Notice that for inorganic substances like Zinc Oxide and salts like Sodium Bromide, the density factors are all at least 2.0, and many are in 4.0 or more. For a drug like this, unless it is being used topically, the displacement factor should probably be considered.

   2. Now notice the organic drugs like Diphenhydramine HCl and Codeine Phosphate; these density factors are lower, in the range of 0.7 to 2.0, with a mean value of 1.3, much closer to the neutral value of 1.0. Now pick a dosage amount per suppository and a reasonable density factor and calculate the difference in amount of Cocoa Butter base per suppository.

   Drug amount/suppository = 100 mg   D.F. = 1.3

   Calibrated weight of base/suppository = 2.000 g

   Calculate the weight of Cocoa Butter displaced by 100 mg of drug if the D. F. of the drug with Cocoa Butter is 1.3:

$$\frac{1.3\,g\,Drug}{1\,g\,Cocoa\,Butter} = \frac{0.1\,g\,Drug}{x\,g\,Cocoa\,Butter} ; x = 0.077\,g\,Cocoa\,Butter\,displaced\,by\,0.1\,g\,Drug$$

   Weight of Cocoa Butter/suppository if not compensating for D.F.:

   $\quad$ 2.000 g weight of suppository
   $\underline{-\ 0.100\ g\ drug}$
   $\quad$ 1.900 g Cocoa Butter needed/suppository

   Weight of Cocoa Butter/suppository when considering D.F.:

   $\quad$ 2.000 g weight of suppository
   $\underline{-\ 0.077\ g\ drug\ displacement}$
   $\quad$ 1.923 g Cocoa Butter needed/suppository

   The difference in weight of Cocoa Butter per suppository is 23 mg. To put this in perspective, the standard deviation found for Cocoa Butter suppository weights made in an aluminum mold was determined by a group of laboratory students to be ±22 mg. In other words, there is about as much chance for there to be this amount of difference in any 68% (the percent amount for ±1 standard deviation from the mean in a normally distributed population) of the Cocoa Butter suppositories we make.

The same exercise can be repeated for a density factor of 2.0; the result is about the same, 23 mg, for a drug content per unit of 50 mg.

These values should give you some idea of the point at which it is prudent to consider density displacement. What can be done when you have a drug for systemic use that has a dose of 100 mg or greater and you do not have a density factor? The double casting method shown below can be used in these circumstances.

➤ **EXAMPLE** Double casting method

The following is an example of a suppository prescription in which the drug makes up a considerable amount of the dosage unit, but there is no reported density factor for the drug in this base. In cases like this, a double casting procedure may be used.

➤ **Prescription 31.2**

Contemporary Physicians Group Practice
20 S. Park Street, Triturate, WI 53706
Tel: (608) 555-1333 Fax: (608) 555-1335

R # 911

Name *Granny Clampett*   Date *00/00/00*

Address *7486 Critter Lane*   Age *38*   Wt/Ht

R

Progesterone   100 mg
PEG Base   qs

M & ft. Suppositories #6

G. Giles 00/00/00

Sig: Insert 1 supp vaginally ut dict for PMS

Refills   *Ima Hack*   M.D.

DEA No. _____

---

1. Check the dose.
   Usual: In this case it is difficult to evaluate the dose because the use of Progesterone for premenstrual syndrome (PMS) is not an FDA-approved use, so there is no established dose. Furthermore, the directions for use lack a frequency of administration. This should be checked and clarified with the prescriber and/or the patient. Progesterone is widely used for this indication, and for this example we will assume that the dose is satisfactory.
2. Check compatibility–stability: As with the Aspirin Suppositories, Progesterone Vaginal Suppositories are an official USP product; the monograph recommends storage in tight, light-resistant containers and in a refrigerator (3). The *USP* formula calls for the addition of 25 mg Silica Gel per suppository to act as a suspending/dispersing agent. This will be needed if the quantity of Progesterone powder needed does not melt/dissolve in the chosen base. The recommended beyond-use date is 90 days after the day on which they were compounded.
3. Procedure Note: Prepare enough material for two extra dosage units.
   a. Select the base for this suppository. The one chosen for this example is Base #4 given in Table 23.2 of Chapter 23. This base is 40% PEG 8000 and 60% PEG 400. Base #5 in that table has been re-

ported to give good results, and manufactured preformulated PEG suppository bases such as Polybase® are readily available.

b.   Calculate the amount of PEG 8000 and PEG 400 needed. Because of the loss that will occur in the compounding procedure, an excess amount of base material must be made. In this case, for PEG base with an approximate density of 1.125 g/mL, the minimum needed would be:

$$2 \ mL/mold \ cavity \times 1.125 \ g/mL \times 8 \ suppositories = 18 \ g$$

Make 30 g of base using the amounts determined below.

PEG 8000: $40\% \times 30 \ g = 12 \ g \ PEG \ 8000$

PEG 8000 is a solid and can be weighed.

PEG 400: $60\% \times 30 \ g = 18 \ g \ PEG \ 400$

PEG 400 is a liquid and is measured volumetrically. s.g. = 1.125 g/mL

$$\frac{1.125 \ g \ PEG \ 400}{1 \ mL \ PEG \ 400} = \frac{18 \ g \ PEG \ 400}{x \ mL \ PEG \ 400}; \ x = 16 \ mL \ PEG \ 400$$

c.   Calculate the amount of active ingredient(s) and excipients needed for the prescription order. Remember to calculate for two extras.

$$8 \times 100 \ mg = 800 \ mg \ progesterone$$

d.   If particle size reduction is needed, weigh an excess amount of drug, triturate, and weigh the amount calculated above.

e.   Before melting the base and combining the ingredients, prepare the suppository mold. Make certain it is clean. Apply a lubricant to the mold if needed. A thin film of vegetable oil spray usually works well.

f.   Put the measured PEGs in a beaker and melt for approximately 1 minute in the microwave oven, or use a warm water bath and heat to approximately 60°C.

g.   Put the weighed drug (800 mg Progesterone) in a small beaker and add approximately one third of the melted PEG base. The Progesterone may melt/dissolve, giving a clear liquid. For drugs that do not melt or dissolve, disperse and suspend the drug throughout the melted base. A suspending agent such as Silica Gel may be used.

h.   Pour the drug-base liquid in the bottoms of eight or fewer mold cavities. Make sure to get complete transfer of all this material to the mold cavities, because this contains the active ingredient.

i.   Q.s. all eight cavities with extra melted PEG base. Overfill the cavities slightly because the base will contract somewhat as it cools.

j.   Allow the suppositories to solidify at room temperature for about 15–20 minutes and then in the refrigerator.

k.   Carefully trim and discard excess material from the top of the mold with a razor blade; this trimmed material is extra melted base used to completely fill the cavities and does not contain any drug.

l.   Remove the suppositories from the mold cavities. We now have eight suppositories that in total contain 800 mg of drug and enough base material for the eight suppositories, but the drug is not uniformly distributed: there may be 150 mg in one suppository and 10 mg or even no drug in another suppository.

m.   Put the eight suppositories in a clean beaker and remelt the material. Stir to obtain a homogeneous mixture.

n.   Now repour the homogeneous mixture. If there were no loss of material in the beaker, you would get exactly eight suppositories. This is never possible and besides, you need to overfill the cavities to compensate for contraction on cooling. Therefore, pour six or seven nicely filled suppository cavities and repeat the congealing and trimming procedure.

o.   If using a disposable mold as a dispensing wrapper, place the suppositories in a dispensing container. If a reusable mold is used, remove the suppositories from the mold cavities. Wrap each suppository in foil or put in individual small plastic bags and place the suppositories in a dispensing container.

➤ *EXAMPLE* Determination of density displacement factors

1. In the example given above, if the suppository mold is calibrated with pure PEG base to obtain a mean weight of PEG base per cavity, and the completed suppositories (containing drug) are now weighed to get a mean weight with drug, a density factor for the drug in this PEG base can be calculated. This is useful so that a double casting method is not needed the next time these are made.

   a. Calibrate the mold for the base by pouring five suppositories with pure base, trimming and removing each suppository from its mold cavity, and weighing each. As with Sample Prescription 31.1, note and record the temperature of the melt so that this fusion temperature can be used each time for this calibration weight, because the density of some bases will vary depending on temperature of the melt. In this example, the temperature of the melt is 60°C, and the average weight per suppository with just PEG base is found to be 2.371 g.

   b. Weigh the six Progesterone suppositories and calculate a mean weight. For this example, the mean weight is 2.356 g. Of this 2.356 g, 0.1 g is Progesterone and the rest, 2.256 g, is PEG base:

   $$2.356 \text{ g Progesterone-PEG} - 0.1 \text{ g Prog} = 2.256 \text{ g PEG}$$

   Note: If progesterone had a density factor of 1.0, 0.1 g of Progesterone would have displaced 0.1 g of PEG and the weight of the Progesterone suppositories would have been the same as that of the suppositories made with just PEG base, 2.371 g.

   c. Calculate the number of grams of PEG base that was displaced by 0.1 g of Progesterone. This is the amount of PEG base in the pure base suppositories minus the amount of PEG base in the Progesterone suppositories:

   $$2.371 \text{ g} - 2.256 \text{ g} = 0.115 \text{ g of PEG base displaced by 0.1 g Progesterone}$$

   d. Calculate the density factor for progesterone in PEG base. This is the number of grams of drug that will displace 1 gram of base.

   $$\frac{0.1 \text{ g Progesterone}}{0.115 \text{ g PEG base}} = \frac{x \text{ g Progesterone}}{1 \text{ g PEG base}}; x = 0.87 \text{ g Progesterone displaces 1 g PEG base}$$

   Note: The above example uses fictitious numbers to illustrate a process for calculating a density factor. The actual experimental density factors for Progesterone are 1.0 with PEG base and 1.25 in Cocoa Butter. These known density factors for Progesterone in two different bases, together with published density factors for drugs in Cocoa Butter (such as those listed in Table 31.1), have been used to estimate density factors for these other drugs in PEG base. For example, the density factor listed for Boric Acid in Cocoa Butter is 1.5. The density factor of Boric Acid in PEG base is estimated as follows:

   $$\frac{1.0 \text{ D.F. Progesterone in PEG base}}{1.25 \text{ D.F. Progesterone in Cocoa Butter}} = \frac{x \text{ D.F. Boric Acid in PEG base}}{1.5 \text{ D.F. Boric Acid in Cocoa Butter}};$$

   $$x = 1.2 \text{ D.F. for Boric Acid in PEG base}$$

SAMPLE PRESCRIPTIONS

➤ **Prescription 31.3**

Contemporary Physicians Group Practice
20 S. Park Street, Triturate, WI 53706
Tel: (608) 555-1333 Fax: (608) 555-1335

℞ # 903

Name *Bonnie Toehouse*	Date *00/00/00*
Address *2530 Talbott Trail*	Age Wt/Ht

℞

     Indomethacin   25 mg
     Fattibase   q. s.

     Dispense 6 suppositories

     Sig: Insert 1 supp pr q 12 hr for arthritis

         B. Butterfield 00/00/00

Refills   3   *Ozzie Wurtz*   M.D.

DEA No. _____

Ingredients Used (for eight suppositories)

Ingredient	Quantity Used	Manufacturer Lot #-Exp Date	Solubility	Dose Comparison		Use in the Prescription
				Given	Usual	
Indomethacin 25 mg Capsules	8 × 25 mg capsule contents	BJF Generics SP3111-mm/yy	Pract. insol. in water; 1 g/50 mL alcohol	25 mg q 12 h	25 mg q 12 h	arthritis
Fattibase®	q.s.	JET Labs SP3112-mm/yy	immisc. w/water and alcohol	—	—	base

Compatibility–Stability/Beyond-Use Date

Stability–Compatibility: Indomethacin Suppositories are official in the USP; Indomethacin in a nonaqueous, inert type of suppository base such as Fattibase® should be very compatible and stable.

Preservative: This is a nonaqueous formulation and no preservative is needed.

Packaging and Storage and Beyond-use date: The *USP* monograph for Indomethacin Suppositories recommends storage in well-closed containers at controlled room temperature (3). Fattibase has a melting point of 96–99°F and the manufacturer of Fattibase® recommends storage in the refrigerator, so Pharmacist Butterfield will recommend that these be stored in the refrigerator. These suppositories are being made with a manufactured dosage form, so Pharmacist Butterfield will use the recommended beyond-use date of 6 months or 25% of the time remaining until the product's expiration date, whichever is earlier (4).

Calculations

Dose/Concentration

Dose of 25 mg two times a day is OK.

Ingredient Amounts

The procedure for this preparation uses the double casting method. Although the quantity of drug per suppository is only 25 mg, this prescription uses the material in Indomethacin capsules, and this contains excipients in addition to the drug, and the powder per unit weighs more than 100 mg. Because the double casting method is used, no precalibration of the mold cavities for the base is needed unless Pharmacist Butterfield would want to calculate a density factory for Indomethacin capsule powder with Fattibase®.

Because a whole number of capsules is needed (25 mg of Indomethacin per dose and Indomethacin available as 25-mg capsules), there are no necessary calculations for amount of active ingredients. Use the contents of eight Indomethacin 25-mg capsules for eight suppositories.

An estimation of total weight of Fattibase® is needed so that a sufficient amount of Fattibase® can be melted. In this case, because material for eight suppositories is being made and a standard mold for rectal suppositories with 2-mL/mold cavity is used, an amount in excess of 14.24 g of Fattibase® should be melted:

Fattibase® has a specific gravity of 0.89

8 supp × 2 mL/supp × 0.89 g/mL = 14.24 g Fattibase® at minimum needed

In the procedure below, 20 g of Fattibase® is melted.

Compounding Procedure

Open a rectal suppository mold and spray the interior very lightly with vegetable oil spray. Reassemble the mold. Empty the contents of eight Indomethacin 25-mg capsules and place the powder in a small beaker. On a class 3 torsion or an electronic balance, weigh approximately 20 g of Fattibase®, put it in a clean beaker or crucible, and melt the Fattibase® on a hot water bath to 50–53°C. Add about one third of the melted Fattibase® to the Indomethacin powder in the beaker and stir to mix. It may be necessary to stir until the mixture is near its congealing point so that the Indomethacin capsule powder remains suspended and maintains a uniform, homogeneous mixture. Note and record the temperature on the melt, 48°C. Pour the mixture into the bottom of eight or fewer mold cavities. If necessary, reheat the mixture and add some extra Fattibase® so that all of the mixture with Indomethacin can be poured into mold cavities. Q.s. the eight cavities with extra Fattibase® at the same temperature as that recorded for the Indomethacin/Fattibase® mixture. Let the suppositories solidify, then finish hardening them in the refrigerator. Remove and trim excess material from the top of the mold with a razor blade. Remove the eight suppositories from the mold and remelt. Stir the mixture to obtain a homogeneous mix. When the melt is at the recorded temperature of 48°C, repour it into six or seven cavities. As before, let the suppositories solidify, then put in a refrigerator for 15–20 minutes to harden. Trim the excess material from the top of the mold with a razor blade and remove the suppositories. Select the six best suppositories. Wrap each suppository in foil, and dispense in a suppository box or other suitable container.

Quality Control

The suppositories are opaque and white, with a smooth surface. Each suppository was weighed and the weight was recorded. The mean weight was 1.756 g, which was close to the estimated weight of 1.78 g for 2-mL suppositories with base material specific gravity of 0.89. The temperature of the melt at pouring was recorded at 48°C.

Labeling

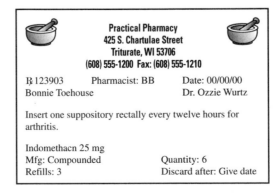

Practical Pharmacy
425 S. Chartulae Street
Triturate, WI 53706
(608) 555-1200 Fax: (608) 555-1210

℞ 123903   Pharmacist: BB   Date: 00/00/00
Bonnie Toehouse   Dr. Ozzie Wurtz

Insert one suppository rectally every twelve hours for arthritis.

Indomethacn 25 mg
Mfg: Compounded   Quantity: 6
Refills: 3   Discard after: Give date

Auxiliary Labels: For Rectal Use; Keep in the Refrigerator;
May cause drowsiness, dizziness

Patient Consultation

Hello, Ms. Toehouse, I'm your pharmacist, Billy Butterfield. Do you have any drug allergies? Are you taking any other medications? What did Dr. Wurtz tell you about this? This suppository is for your arthritis. Unwrap and insert one rectally every 12 hours. For arthritis you should be sure to use these on a regular basis; if you forget to insert one, do so as soon as you remember unless it is close to the time for your next dose; then just skip the missed dose. This drug will reduce inflammation in your joints. When inserting, you may want to hold it in place for a short while so as not to expel the suppository. Have you used suppositories before? I will give you this sheet; it gives some helpful hints on using suppositories (see Fig. 31.1). Common side effects for this medication include drowsiness and dizziness. You may experience some stomach or intestinal upset; if this is bothersome or severe, call Dr. Wurtz. Also discontinue use if you get hives, shortness of breath, tightness in your chest, or any unusual reaction, including headaches and skin rash. (Note: There are a multitude of other possible side effects—see the *USP/DI Vol. I* or other suitable drug information reference for more information.) Don't take any other drugs for your arthritis such as Aspirin, Salicylates, Ibuprofen, or other such drugs. Keep these in the refrigerator and out of the reach of children. Discard any unused suppositories after 6 months (or 25% rule). You may have this refilled three times. Do you have any questions?

➤ **Prescription 31.4**

Contemporary Physicians Group Practice
20 S. Park Street, Triturate, WI 53706
Tel: (608) 555-1333 Fax: (608) 555-1335

R # 906

Name *Joseph Draheim*   Date *00/00/00*

Address *623 San Francisco Circle*   Age *3 y.o.*   Wt/Ht *37 lb, 40"*

R

Promethazine HCl   5 mg
Cocoa Butter   q.s.

Disp. #6 Supp.

Sig: Insert 1 supp pr q 4-6 hr prn nausea and vomiting

B. Schwartz 00/00/00

Refills *NR*   *Hokey* _____   M.D.

DEA No. _____

Ingredients Used (Amounts are for eight suppositories, two extra)

Ingredient	Quantity Used	Manufacturer Lot #-Exp Date	Solubility	Dose Comparison		Use in the Prescription
				Given	Usual	
Promethazine HCl 25 mg tablets	40 mg drug from 336 mg crushed tablet powder	BJF Generics SP3121-mm/yy	fr. sol. in water sol. in alcohol	5 mg q 4–6 hr	4–10 mg q 4–6 hr	antiemetic
Cocoa Butter	7.664 g	JET Labs SP3122-mm/yy	insol. in water sl sol in alcohol	—	—	base, vehicle

Compatibility–Stability/Beyond-Use Date

Stability–Compatibility: Promethazine HCl Suppositories are official in the USP. Promethazine HCl oxidizes in the presence of air and moisture, but in a nonaqueous, inert type of suppository base such as Cocoa Butter it should be quite compatible and stable. Promethazine HCl is subject to light-catalyzed oxidation, so these suppositories should be packaged in tight, light-resistant containers and stored in cool temperatures. Promethazine HCl is very soluble in water, so the release from the fatty base should be satisfactory.

Preservative: This is a nonaqueous formulation and no preservative is needed.

Packaging and Storage and Beyond-use date: The *USP* monograph for Promethazine HCl Suppositories recommends tight, light-resistant containers with storage in a cold place (3). Pharmacist Schwartz will package the suppositories in tight, amber vials and will label that these be stored in the refrigerator. These suppositories are being made with a manufactured dosage form, Promethazine tablets, so Pharmacist Schwartz will use the recommended beyond-use date of 6 months or 25% of the time remaining until the product's expiration date, whichever is earlier (4).

Calculations

Dose/Concentration

The pediatric antiemetic dose of Promethazine HCl in suppositories is given in the *USP DI* as 0.25 to 0.5 mg per kg of body weight or 7.5 to 15 mg per m^2 of BSA every 4 to 6 hours as needed. This patient has a body weight of 37 lbs and a height of 40".

Milligram dose based on dosage in mg/kg:

$$Body\ weight\ in\ kg: \frac{37\ lb}{2.2\ lb/kg} = 16.8\ kg$$

Dose in mg: *0.25 to 0.5 mg/kg* $\times$ *16.8 kg = 4.2 to 8.4 mg*

Milligram dose based on BSA:

Based on Joseph's weight and height, the BSA from the nomogram in Appendix E is 0.68 m^2.

Dose in mg: *7.5 to 15 mg/m^2* $\times$ *0.68 m^2 = 5.1 to 10.2 mg*

The dose of 5 mg, while on the low side, is within the acceptable range. Pharmacist Schwartz may instruct Joseph's mother that if Joseph's nausea and vomiting are not relieved with this dose, she can call him and he will consult with Dr. Hokey about increasing the dose.

Ingredient Amounts (Calculations are for two extras)

These suppositories are being made by the hand-rolling method. They are made to be 1 g each because they are for a 3-year-old child.

Total weight for eight suppositories:

$$1\ g/supp \times 8\ suppositories = 8\ g\ total$$

Weight in mg of Promethazine HCl:

$$5\ mg/supp \times 8\ suppositories = 40\ mg\ Promethazine\ HCl$$

The Promethazine HCl is available as the pure powder, but the pharmacy does not have this in stock and this prescription order is needed immediately. The drug is available in the pharmacy as 25-mg tablets, each weighing 210 mg. For 40 mg of Promethazine HCl, Pharmacist Schwartz will need two tablets (*40 mg $\div$ 25 mg/tablet = 1.6 tablets*).

Amount of crushed tablet powder:

$$\frac{25\ mg\ Promethazine}{210\ mg\ tablet\ powder} = \frac{40\ mg\ Promethazine}{x\ mg\ tablet\ powder}; x = 336\ crushed\ tablet\ powder$$

Weight in g of Cocoa Butter base:

8 g to 0.336 g Promethazine HCl crushed tablet powder = 7.664 g Cocoa Butter

Compounding Procedure

On a class 3 torsion balance or an electronic digital balance, weight two Promethazine HCl 25-mg tablets. Each tablet weighs 210 mg (weights will vary with different manufacturers and lots). Crush the two tablets and weigh 336 mg of crushed tablet powder, containing 40 mg of active ingredient. Weigh 7.664 g of Cocoa Butter. Add a small amount of finely shaved Cocoa Butter to the crushed tablet powder in a glass mortar and triturate well. Add the rest of the finely shaved cocoa butter by geometric dilution and triturate well to form a plastic mass. Remove the mass from the mortar and place it in a piece of clean, white filter paper. Put on plastic disposable gloves. Knead the material to form a plastic mass. Transfer the mass to an ointment slab and, using a clean pill roller or a metal spatula, roll the mass into a cylindrical pipe that is slightly longer than 6 inches. Using a clean razor blade, cut off the irregular ends of the pipe, and then cut the pipe into six equal pieces. Shape with one pointed end and weigh each piece (each should weigh 1 g $\pm$ 5%.) Cut off any excess with a razor blade. Put each in a zippered bag and dispense in an amber vial or powder square with a tight, child-resistant closure.

Labeling

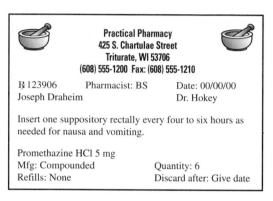

Auxiliary Labels: For Rectal Use; Keep in the Refrigerator;
Make cause drowsiness, dizziness

Patient Consultation

Hello, Mrs. Draheim, I'm Bobby Schwartz, the pharmacist who prepared Joseph's prescription. Does he have any drug allergies? Is he taking any other medications? What did Dr. Hokey tell you about this medicine and how to use it? These are Promethazine HCl suppositories to control his nausea and vomiting. To use these, unwrap one suppository and insert it rectally. Hold it in place for a few moments to allow it to melt. Have you used suppositories before? I will give you an instruction sheet that will give you some helpful hints on administration techniques (see Fig. 31.1). You may give Joseph one suppository every 4 to 6 hours. If he does not seem to be experiencing relief, contact me or Dr. Hokey, as we may have to adjust the dose or try something else. These may make him drowsy, but at this point that may be helpful in allowing him to get some extra rest. Occasionally children on this drug get restless or experience nightmares; if this should happen call me or Dr. Hokey, and if it is bothersome we may try a different drug. Store these in the refrigerator, out of reach of children. Discard any unused suppositories after 6 months (or 25% rule). Dr. Hokey has not ordered any refills on this prescription; I assume that if Joseph does not improve rapidly, Dr. Hokey wants to see him. Do you have any questions?

► **Prescription 31.5**

```
                 Contemporary Physicians Group Practice
                     20 S. Park Street, Triturate, WI  53706
                   Tel: (608) 555-1333  Fax: (608) 555-1335

                                          R # 932

  Name   Rod Robinson                      Date   00/00/00

  Address  312 Campfire Trail              Age    13     Wt/Ht

    R

              Hydromorphone HCl            4 mg
              Fattibase                    q.s.

                   #6 Suppositories
                                          Jean Jones 00/00/00

        Sig:  Insert 1 supp pr q 6-8 hr prn severe pain

  Refills   NR                            Henry Paque              M.D.

  (Schedule II, No red "C")     DEA No.   AP3296577
```

Ingredients Used (Amounts are for 8 suppositories, 2 extra)

Ingredient	Quantity Used	Manufacturer Lot #-Exp Date	Solubility	Dose Comparison Given	Dose Comparison Usual	Use in the Prescription
Hydromorphone HCl	120 mg weighed 24 mg dispensed	JET Labs SP3131-mm/yy	1 g/3 mL water	4 mg rectally q 6–8 hr	3 mg rectally q 4–8 hr	analgesic
Silica Gel	360 mg weighed 96 mg used	JET Labs SP3132-mm/yy	insol in water and alcohol	—	—	diluent, suspending agent, disintegrant
Fattibase®	15.216 g	JET Labs SP3112-mm/yy	immis w/water and alcohol	—	—	base, vehicle

Compatibility–Stability/Beyond-Use Date

Stability–Compatibility: Although not an official USP product, manufactured Hydromorphone HCl suppositories are available in a 3-mg strength. Hydromorphone HCl in a nonaqueous, inert type of suppository base such as Fattibase® should be very compatible and stable.

Preservative: This is a nonaqueous formulation and no preservative is needed.

Packaging and Storage and Beyond-use date: The *USP* monograph for Hydromorphone HCl Tablets recommends storage in tight, light-resistant containers (3), so Pharmacist Jones will dispense these suppositories in a suitable tight, amber vial. Fattibase® has a melting point of 96–99°F, and the manufacturer of Fattibase® recommends storage in the refrigerator, so Pharmacist Jones will recommend that these be stored in the refrigerator. These suppositories are a nonaqueous solid dosage form made with a USP ingredient, so Pharmacist Jones may use a recommended beyond-use date of up to 6 months (4).

Calculations

Dose/Concentration

Dose OK

Ingredient Amounts (Amounts are for eight suppositories, two extra)

This method uses fusion with a calibrated mold.

Determine the mean weight of Fattibase® per mold cavity:

On a warm water bath, slowly heat the Fattibase® to approximately 50–53°C to completely melt the base. Remove the container from the warm water bath and allow the base to cool to 48°C; record this temperature. Pour the pure Fattibase® into five mold cavities. Allow this to solidify; then trim and remove the suppositories. Weigh each suppository on a digital balance (weight recorded below). Calculate the mean weight of Fattibase® per cavity.

Suppository #1	1.911 g
Suppository #2	1.918 g
Suppository #3	1.923 g
Suppository #4	1.903 g
Suppository #5	1.934 g
	9.589 g

Mean weight per suppository: 9.589 g/5 = 1.918 g Fattibase®/suppository

Weight of Hydromorphone HCl in mg: *4 mg/suppository × 8 suppositories = 32 mg*

This amount is below the MWQ, so a dilution and aliquot must be made. Hydromorphone HCl is a controlled substance, so a minimum amount should be weighed, 120 mg. Silica Gel may be used as the diluent so that it can also serve as a suspending and dispersing agent. A convenient amount of Silica Gel to use would be 360 mg.

Total amount of dilution:

120 mg Hydromorphone + 360 mg Silica Gel = 480 mg dilution

Amount of dilution that will contain 32 mg of Hydromorphone HCl:

$$\frac{120 \, mg \, Hydromorphone}{480 \, mg \, dilution} = \frac{32 \, mg \, Hydromorphone}{x \, mg \, dilution}; x = 128 \, mg \, dilution$$

Weight of Fattibase® for eight suppositories:

Note: Because the amount of Hydromorphone HCl–Silica Gel dilution is small in comparison to the weight of the base, any difference in displacement on a gram-for-gram basis will be considered to be negligible.

Multiply the mean weight/cavity by the number of suppositories desired and subtract the weight of the Hydromorphone HCl aliquot. This is the amount of Fattibase® needed for the product.

Total weight for eight suppositories:

8 supp × 1.918 g/supp = 15.344 g for 8 suppositories

Weight of Fattibase® for eight suppositories:

15.344 g − 0.128 g Hydromorphone aliquot = 15.216 g Fattibase® needed

Compounding Procedure

Open a rectal suppository mold and spray the interior very lightly with vegetable oil spray. Reassemble the mold. On a class 3 torsion or an electronic balance, weigh 120 mg of Hydromorphone HCl and 360 mg of Silica Gel. Put the Hydromorphone in a mortar and add the Silica Gel with trituration using geometric dilution. Weigh 128 mg of this mixture and place in a beaker. Weigh 15.216 g of grated Fattibase®. Place the beaker containing the Hydromorphone aliquot on a warm water bath and add the grated Fattibase® to the beaker in portions, melting the Fattibase® with each addition. When all the Fattibase® has been added, stir to mix and continue stirring until the mixture is 50°C and the mixture is uniform. Remove the container of melt from the warm water bath and stir the mixture while allowing the melt to reach 48°C. Pour the melt into seven mold cavities, overfilling slightly. Let the mixture solidify at room temperature, then place in the refrigerator to harden.

When hardened, trim excess material from the top of the mold with a razor blade. Remove the suppositories from the mold cavities. Select the six best suppositories and weigh and record the weight of each as a quality control measure. Wrap each in foil or seal individually in polyethylene bags. Dispense in an amber vial or powder square with a tight, child-resistant closure.

Quality Control

The suppositories are opaque and white, with a smooth surface. Each suppository was weighed and the weight was recorded. The mean weight was 1.779 g, which is close to the estimated weight of 1.78 g for 2-mL suppositories with base material specific gravity of 0.89. The temperature of the melt at pouring was recorded at 48°C.

Labeling

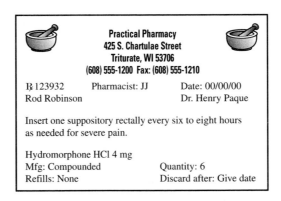

Practical Pharmacy
425 S. Chartulae Street
Triturate, WI 53706
(608) 555-1200 Fax: (608) 555-1210

℞ 123932   Pharmacist: JJ   Date: 00/00/00
Rod Robinson   Dr. Henry Paque

Insert one suppository rectally every six to eight hours
as needed for severe pain.

Hydromorphone HCl 4 mg
Mfg: Compounded   Quantity: 6
Refills: None   Discard after: Give date

Auxiliary Labels: For Rectal Use; Keep in the Refrigerator;
May cause drowsiness, dizziness
Federal Do Not Transfer Label

Patient Consultation

Hello, Mrs. Robinson, I'm your pharmacist, Jean Jones. Does Rod have any drug allergies? What do you know about this medication (or did Dr. Paque tell you anything about it)? Is Rod taking any other medications? This medication is to give him relief from his pain. This drug usually causes drowsiness, so don't be alarmed if he feels this effect. Because he is feeling so ill, this will help him to sleep. Other medications, either prescription or nonprescription, that cause drowsiness will intensify this effect, so be sure to consult me or Dr. Paque before using something like that. Medications like this one sometimes cause stomach upset, even if taken rectally. If this should happen, call Dr. Paque. To administer a dose, unwrap and insert one suppository rectally. This may be repeated every 6 to 8 hours if needed for severe pain. Have you ever given suppositories before? Here is a sheet of helpful instructions (see Fig. 31.1). Don't exceed the prescribed dose; if it is not holding him for 6 hours, call Dr. Paque. You may try supplementing with oral or rectal Acetaminophen. Store these in a refrigerator and out of the reach of children. Discard unused medication after 3 months (give date). There are no refills, but if you need more please contact Dr. Paque. Do you have any questions?

■ Figure 31.1 HOW TO INSERT A RECTAL SUPPOSITORY

1. Wash your hands carefully with soap and warm water.
2. Remove all foil or other wrappings from the suppository to be inserted.
3. Lubricate the tapered (pointed) end of the suppository with a small amount of K-Y® Jelly or other type of lubricating gel, but not petroleum jelly (e.g., Vaseline®). If not available, moisten suppository with a small amount of water.
4. Lie on your side with your lower leg straightened out and upper leg bent forward, toward the stomach. (See drawing A.)
5. Lift upper buttocks to expose rectal area.
6. Gently insert the suppository into your rectum until it passes the sphincter (about 1/2 to 1 inch in infants, and 1 inch in adults). (See drawing B.)
7. Gentle, persistent pressure allows the suppository to remain in place without discomfort.
8. Hold buttocks together for a few seconds and remain lying down for about 15 minutes.
9. Avoid excessive movement or exercise for approximately 1 hour.
10. Wash your hands immediately after inserting the suppository.

NOTE:

*Suppositories should be kept in a tightly closed container and stored in a cool place. (See package for any further storage instructions.)

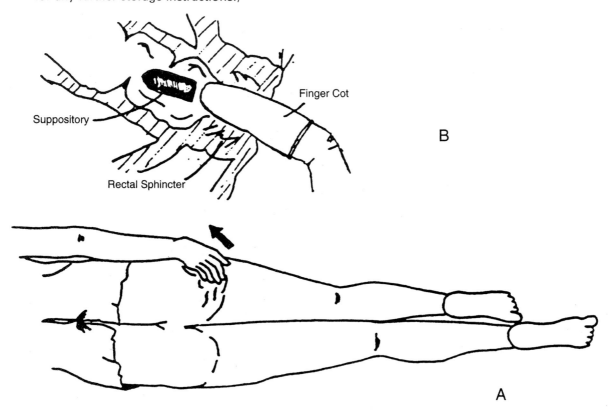

References

1. The 2002 United States Pharmacopeia 25/National Formulary 20. Rockville, MD: The United States Pharmacopeial Convention, Inc., 2001;2222.
2. Plaxco Jr JM. Suppositories. In: King RE, ed. Dispensing of medications, 9th ed. Easton, PA: Mack Publishing Co., 1984;93.
3. The 2002 United States Pharmacopeia 25/National Formulary 20. Rockville, MD: The United States Pharmacopeial Convention, Inc., 2001; Official Monographs.
4. The 2002 United States Pharmacopeia 25/National Formulary 20. Rockville, MD: The United States Pharmacopeial Convention, Inc., 2001;2054.

CHAPTER 32

Parenteral Products

I. INTRODUCTION

A. Parenteral products are those preparations intended for administration by injection through the skin (additional definitions are given later in this chapter).

B. The whole topic of parenteral products, their preparation, manipulation, handling, and use is complex and extremely critical. Because parenteral administration bypasses the natural protective barriers of the skin or alimentary tract, these products have strict requirements not encountered with dosage forms intended for other routes of administration. Unfortunately, over the last 15 to 20 years, there have been a fair number of accidents involving errors in preparing or administering parenteral products. Many of these have been well-publicized cases and have involved everything from dispensing products with microbiological contamination to errors in dosage or giving the wrong drug. In some cases, the accidents illustrated a lack of understanding on the part of the pharmacist or other health care personnel of the recognized standards for handling parenteral products.

C. Although a thorough discussion of the above issues is beyond the scope of this book, this chapter provides an introduction to the topic of parenteral drug products and their administration. A sampling of published standards of practice is given, with directions on how to access the complete documents. Definitions are given to aid the reader in understanding the documents and other parenteral product literature. Sample calculations that are useful for making IV admixtures, injections, and other parenteral preparations and sample medication orders with procedures and labeling are presented at the end of this chapter.

D. A more complete knowledge of current standards and procedures for handling parenteral products is essential for any pharmacist who is either preparing or supervising the preparation, handling, and use of parenteral products; it is the responsibility of such a pharmacist to be knowledgeable about current standards of practice. References are given below with helpful information on parenteral products, devices, equipment, and handling procedures and techniques. The standards of practice are under discussion and revision, so anyone practicing in this area should consult the most up-to-date versions and resources.

   1. American Society of Health-System Pharmacists (ASHP) Technical Assistance Bulletins (TAB)

     The most current Technical Assistance Bulletins from ASHP are available on their Internet site, www.ashp.org.

     a. ASHP Technical Assistance Bulletin on Quality Assurance for Pharmacy-prepared Sterile Products

    b. ASHP Technical Assistance Bulletin on Handling Cytotoxic and Hazardous Drugs

2. National Association of Boards of Pharmacy Model Rules and state laws

    a. NABP Model Rules on Sterile Preparations: NABP Model Rules, which are current in year 2002, are available in the Appendices section of the CD that accompanies this book. Contact NABP or visit their Internet site, www.nabp.org to check for any revisions to their model rules.

    b. State laws: Check the state laws for the state in which you are practicing for current standards and regulations.

3. *USP* Chapters

    a. General Tests Chapter ⟨1⟩ Injections

    b. General Information Chapter ⟨1206⟩ Sterile Drug Products for Home Use is current as of *USP 26–NF 21*, but changes to this chapter have been proposed in the *Pharmacopeial Forum*, including a change in chapter number to ⟨797⟩, which would put this in the section of potentially legally enforceable chapters.

    c. There are various other *USP* chapters of interest for parenteral products, such as ⟨61⟩ Microbial Test Limits, ⟨71⟩ Sterility Tests, ⟨85⟩ Bacterial Endotoxin Test, ⟨151⟩ Pyrogen Test, ⟨1035⟩ Biological Indicators for Sterilization, ⟨1116⟩ Microbiological Attributes of Clean Rooms and Other Controlled Environments, and others.

4. Food and Drug Administration (FDA) documents

    a. "Guideline on Sterile Drug Products Produced by Aseptic Processing" is a formal guidance that was prepared by the FDA Center for Drug Evaluation and Research in June 1987. It is intended for use in the pharmaceutical industry, but a good share of the information in this document is also useful for pharmacists involved in processing sterile preparations. In September 2002 FDA published a revised draft of this guidance. As of the end of 2002, these new guidelines are in the form of a preliminary concept paper, and FDA is receiving comments on it, but a final guidance is expected to be published. These documents and comments on them can be found on FDA's Internet site, www.fda.gov. The site has a search engine that responds with appropriate documents and papers when the name of the document given above is entered.

    b. Other documents may also be useful. One example is ISO 14644–1: Cleanrooms and Associated Controlled Environments, Classification of Air Cleanliness.

5. Reference books (Note: Consult the latest edition of these references)

    a. Buchanan EC, McKinnon BT, Scheckelhoff DJ, Schneider PJ. *Principles of Sterile Product Preparation*. Bethesda, MD: ASHP. This is an excellent book and probably the most complete reference on proper handling of sterile products by pharmacists and health care professionals.

    b. *Remington: The Science and Practice of Pharmacy* has several very useful chapters, including "Sterilization," "Parenteral Preparations," and "Intravenous Admixtures." *Remington* is published by Lippincott Williams & Wilkins, Philadelphia.

    c. Trissel LA, ed. *Handbook on Injectable Drugs*. Bethesda, MD: ASHP. This book gives specific information on individual parenteral products, their content, stability, and compatibility in IV solutions and when combined with other parenteral drug products.

    d. Catania PN, ed. *King Guide to Parenteral Admixtures*. Napa, CA: King Guide Publications, Inc. This is a book with content similar to the *Handbook on Injectable Drugs*, but it comes in a loose-leaf binder and updates are mailed to the subscriber at regular intervals. Information is available through its web site, www.kingguide.com or by phone at 888-546-4484.

    e. Bing CM, ed. *Extended Stability for Parenteral Drugs*. Bethesda, MD: ASHP. As the name implies, this book gives stability information for extended beyond-use dating when this is needed for use at non-institutional sites such as home health care.

    f. Turco S. *Sterile Dosage Forms*. Philadelphia: Lea & Febiger (now Lippincott Williams & Wilkins).

    g. Allen LV Jr. *The Art, Science, and Technology of Pharmaceutical Compounding.* Washington DC: American Pharmaceutical Association. This book has a useful chapter, "Parenteral Preparations," that contains sample standard operating procedures.

  6. Videotapes and Internet sites

    a. ASHP has produced a number of video products on parenteral products.

      (1) Quality Assurance for Pharmacy-Prepared Sterile Products is a general but comprehensive videotape (VHS format) with a useful workbook.

      (2) Safe Handling of Cytotoxic and Hazardous Drugs gives complete coverage of this topic from preparation to product administration, spill cleanup, and management and personnel issues.

      (3) Safe Handling of Sharps shows prevention and handling of needle stick accidents.

      (4) Sterile Product Preparation: A Multimedia Tool was introduced in 2002 to provide a multimedia learning tool that gives practice in simulated experience with sterile product preparation.

    b. Some schools of pharmacy have web sites with video demonstrations for the use of their students in parenteral product laboratories. Often the school will provide access to others if permission is requested. For example, the University of Tennessee College of Pharmacy has a specialty in the area of sterile products and often has continuing education courses and web sites with helpful information.

    c. Some of the companies and private organizations listed in Chapter 12 have videotapes and training courses on preparing and handling sterile products.

II. USES OF PARENTERAL PRODUCTS

A. Parenteral administration offers one alternative when a patient is unable (e.g., unconscious, vomiting) to take medication by mouth.

B. Some drugs must be given parenterally because they are not therapeutically active when taken orally because of inactivation in the gastrointestinal tract or first-pass metabolism by the liver.

C. The parenteral route may be necessary or preferred when drug action is required immediately.

D. In some cases, a drug must be injected because it requires direct delivery to an organ, a lesion, a muscle, or a nerve.

E. Fluids, electrolytes, and/or nutrients may be delivered parenterally for patients who cannot take these orally.

F. Depots of drugs in long-acting drug delivery systems injected into muscle masses may offer superior therapy or convenience.

G. Implantable pumps offer advantages in certain circumstances.

III. DISADVANTAGES OF PARENTERAL THERAPY

A. Manufactured parenteral products are more difficult and costly to produce. Because they must conform to strict requirements for microbiological purity, particulate matter, and pyrogenicity, special manufacturing equipment and facilities are needed.

B. In pharmacies and patient care, special equipment, devices, and techniques are also required for the safe preparation, handling, and administration of parenteral products. Specially trained personnel are needed.

C. Once administered, a parenteral product cannot be removed. Problems with dose or adverse effects may be difficult or impossible to reverse.

D. Any introduction of pathogens into the product during production, preparation, manipulation, or handling or during administration to the patient can have serious and even deadly consequences.

E. Because drug products are being injected directly into tissue, there may be pain or tissue damage associated with the administration.

IV. DEFINITIONS

The following definitions are essential in understanding references, literature, and standards concerning parenteral products. In the area of sterile products, terms often have specific meanings that may not be apparent from the words in the terms. It is important that pharmacists working in this area have a good understanding of these terms.

A. **Parenteral Articles:** "Parenteral articles are preparations intended for injection through the skin or other external boundary tissue, rather than through the alimentary canal, so that the active substances they contain are administered, using gravity or force, directly into a blood vessel, organ, tissue, or lesion. Parenteral articles are prepared scrupulously by methods designed to ensure that they meet Pharmacopeial requirements for sterility, pyrogens, particulate matter, and other contaminants, and, where appropriate, contain inhibitors of the growth of microorganisms. An Injection is a preparation intended for parenteral administration and/or for constituting or diluting a parenteral article prior to administration." (1)—*USP*

B. **Large-volume Intravenous Solution:** Also called large-volume parenterals or LVPs, these are single-dose injections containing more than 100 mL of solution that are intended for intravenous use (1).

C. **Small-volume Injection:** These are injections of 100 mL or less. They may be either single-dose and multidose products (1).

D. **Pyrogen:** A substance that induces a fever in a patient

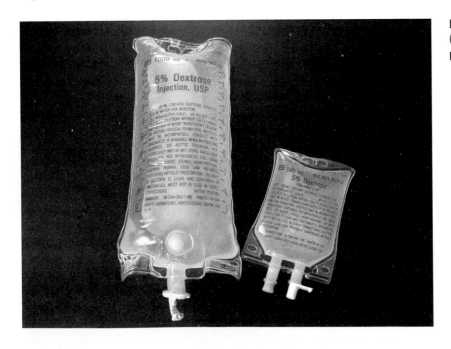

Large-volume parenteral
(LVP) and small-volume
parenteral (minibag).

E. **Endotoxin:** A pyrogenic product present in a bacterial cell wall. These substances are lipopolysaccharides that can be found anywhere live or dead bacteria have been present. As large molecules, they are not destroyed by steam sterilization or bacterial filtration. They can be destroyed on glassware using dry heat sterilization. The most common source of endotoxin material is water that has contained bacterial contamination; the endotoxin can remain after any bacteria are removed or killed. When a solution containing the endotoxin is injected into a patient, it can cause fever and even death.

F. **Sterility:** The absence of viable microorganisms. Because sterility cannot usually be confirmed with certainty, statistical probability is used to describe it.

G. **Sterility Assurance Level (SAL):** This term is used to designate the probability of finding a nonsterile unit (such as a bacterium) following a sterilization step or procedure. Usually it is expressed as a negative power of ten (e.g., 1 in 1 million or 10^{-6}) (2).

H. **Sterilization:** A process or procedure that removes or destroys all viable microorganisms, based on a probability function (2).

I. **Terminal Sterilization:** A procedure carried out at the end of processing, when a product is in its final sealed container, that destroys all viable microorganisms (2). Terminal Sterilization is usually intended to achieve SAL of less than 10^{-6} (4).

J. **Class 100, Class 10,000, and Class 100,000:** The class numbers are used to describe air quality in a designated area. The numbers, such as 100, 10,000, etc., refer to the **number of particles** 0.5 μm or larger per cubic foot of air. A maximum **number of microbes** per cubic foot is also designated for each class, 0.1 or less for Class 100, 0.5 or less for Class 10,000, and 2.5 or less for Class 100,000. There are also other requirements, such as temperature and relative humidity and, when applicable, air exchange and pressure differential, which depend on the class.

K. **Aseptic Processing:** In manufacturing, this term has the following meaning: "Those operations performed between the sterilization of an object or preparation and the final sealing of its package" (2). Because there is no terminal sterilization of the product in its final container, these operations are carried out in "an environment of extremely high quality" (4,5). In practice situations, the term refers to processing operations involving sterile products that are carried out in a laminar airflow workbench or barrier isolator. The *USP* states that such operations be validated using media-fill runs (3).

L. **Laminar Airflow Workbench (LAFW):** Also known as laminar flow hoods, these are workbenches that provide an environment of specially filtered air that sweeps the work area and provides an aseptic work area. Regular room air is drawn through a gross filter (similar to a furnace filter) into an intake opening in the hood; the air then goes through a plenum where the air flow is equalized and is then passed in a unidirectional parallel flow pattern (laminar flow) through a HEPA filter. The air is forced through the HEPA filter and over the work area at a velocity of 90 ft/min, which is sufficient to sweep particulate matter away from the work area. LAFWs are certified to be **Class 100** environments. These workbenches are available either as horizontal or vertical flow hoods.

With **horizontal** flow hoods, the HEPA filter takes up the back, vertical surface of the hood space, and the laminar air blows from the HEPA filter horizontally across the work area and directly at the worker who is standing at the front edge of the hood and working on the workbench surface.

With **vertical** flow hoods, the HEPA filter takes up the top, horizontal surface of the hood space, and the laminar air blows from the HEPA filter downward through the hood space and into intake grills located along the front and back edges of the workbench surface. Vertical flow hoods, sometimes called **biological safety cabinets (BSCs)**, can be used for any aseptic processing, but they are required for working with cytotoxic or other

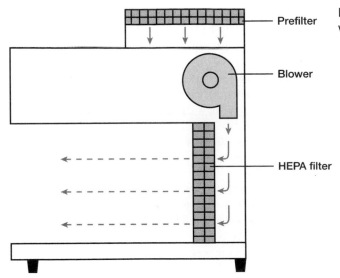

Horizontal laminar airflow workbench (LAFW)

— Prefilter

— Blower

— HEPA filter

Horizontal Flow Hood

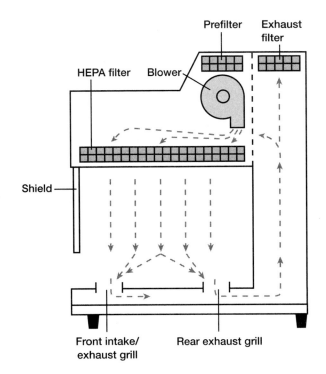

Vertical laminar airflow workbench (LAFW)

Prefilter   Exhaust filter

HEPA filter   Blower

Shield

Front intake/ exhaust grill   Rear exhaust grill

Vertical Flow Hood

hazardous drugs. They have a clear glass or plastic shield that comes part way down the front of the hood space; the clear front shield and the vertical flow pattern with air contained within the hood protect the worker from contamination by drugs being processed within the hood.

M.   **HEPA Filter:** HEPA stands for high-efficiency particulate air. A filter that provides this type of environment is an essential component of both horizontal and vertical laminar airflow workbenches and other aseptic processing areas. For these purposes, the HEPA filters are certified to provide air that is filtered with minimum 0.3-micron particle retaining efficiency of 99.97%.

N. Critical Surfaces: Surfaces that come into contact with sterile product, container, or closures. For example, the needle shaft that is used for transferring a drug solution from a vial to an IV container is a critical surface.

O. Critical Area: This is an area where sterile products, containers, and closures are exposed to the environment. A LAFW is an acceptable critical area.

P. Cleanroom: Also called a **buffer room**, this is a room that is designed and maintained to prevent particulate and microbiological contamination of drug products as they are being prepared or processed. Such a room is assigned and meets air cleanliness classification such as Class 10,000 or Class 100,000. Cleanrooms contain the LAFWs used for aseptic processing of parenteral products. In some cases when parenteral processes present a low risk of contamination, the LAFW may be positioned in what is termed a **controlled area**. While not a separate room, this is a protected area located away from traffic patterns and pharmacy-related nonsterile activities.

Q. Anteroom: This is a room adjacent to the cleanroom; although of high quality, it may have a lesser air cleanliness classification than the cleanroom. For example, if the cleanroom is maintained as a Class 10,000 space, the anteroom may be Class 100,000. Activities in the anteroom include things like washing and gowning and unpacking of cleanroom supply packages. Cardboard boxes and other packaging materials are not brought into cleanrooms because opening and handling them introduces particulates into the environment.

R. Barrier Isolator: Barrier isolators provide a LAFW that is completely enclosed. For the operator, access to the work surface is through glovebox-type portals. Materials and supplies for aseptic processing enter through special air-lock boxes attached to the unit. Models are available that provide either Class 10 or Class 100 environments. Some models provide negative pressure systems for protecting operators from hazardous drugs and chemicals. Because these microenvironments are completely isolated, a cleanroom, anteroom, and special gowning is not required (6).

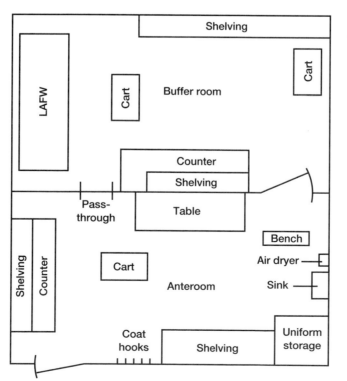

Sample floor plan for a cleanroom and anteroom

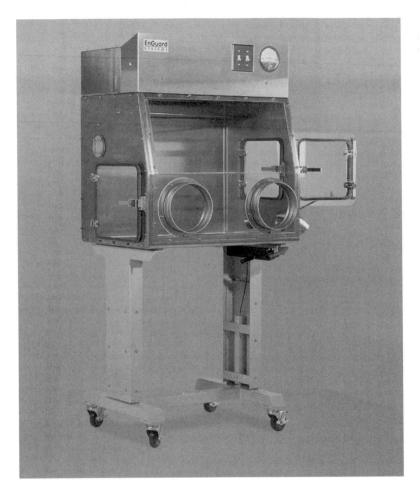

Barrier isolator (photo courtesy of Containment Technologies Group, Inc.)

S.   Risk Levels: This refers to the potential risk to patients caused by the introduction of microbial contamination into a finished sterile product and subsequent opportunity for growth of inadvertently added contaminants. In assigning risk levels, the source and quality of ingredients and environmental and processing factors are considered. ASHP and *USP* each designate three risk levels, Level 1 (called Low Risk in the *USP*) having the least risk potential and Level 3 (called High-Risk Category 2 in the *USP*) having the greatest risk potential. The characteristics of the various risk levels are described in the next section of this chapter.

T.   Validation: In general terms, validation means verifying that a set of procedures gives the intended result under all expected circumstances. With regard to sterile product processing, the *USP* defines it as follows: "The act of validation of a sterilization or aseptic process involves planned testing designed to demonstrate that microorganisms will be effectively destroyed, removed, or prevented from inadvertently being introduced by personnel or by process-related activities" (3).

U.   Media Fill: Both ASHP and *USP* guidelines require media-fill validation of aseptic processing. This is a procedure in which personnel who do aseptic processing prepare a simulated product using culture medium. The simulated product is then incubated to determine if the product was contaminated during the procedure. The media-fill procedure attempts to simulate as closely as possible the exact environmental and process-related conditions and intensity level (e.g., time during the work shift and number of transfers or manipulations required to create a product) of actual practice. The validation procedure should be representative of the greatest risk that might be experienced in an actual practice situation.

V.   **Batch Preparation:** The preparation of multiple units of a sterile product by the same worker during the same time period. For example, if a worker prepares 30 syringes of a given dose of an antibiotic at one time, this is batch preparation. This is in contrast to receiving an individual order for an antibiotic injection for a patient and preparing that one unit for that specific patient.

V.   RISK LEVELS

A.   Both the ASHP Technical Assistance Bulletin (TAB), *Guidelines on Quality Assurance of Pharmacy-Prepared Sterile Products*, and the *USP* General Information Chapter ⟨1206⟩ Sterile Drug Products for Home Use have designated three-tier systems of risk levels to aid pharmacists in making decisions about the use of environmental controls and processing standards when making sterile products.

B.   The risk level system was briefly defined above under the term "Risk Level." The principal features of each risk level for the two systems are given in Table 32.1. Table 32.2 shows a comparison of requirements for the three risk levels in the two systems. The primary focus of each system is described below.

  1.   ASHP's system focuses on the needs and practice environments of institutions such as hospitals. Hospitals and similar institutions in the U.S. vary greatly in size, facilities, scope of practice, and budget. Although patient safety is of paramount importance, the cost/benefit ratio is always a consideration. The TAB tries to take these various factors into consideration.

TABLE 32.1   ASHP and *USP* Risk Levels (published as of December 2002)

ASHP	USP	Examples
RISK LEVEL 1 (RL 1)	**LOW RISK (LR)**	KCl in D5W 250 mL bag
All manufactured sterile starting materials	All manufactured sterile starting materials	
Closed system transfers (Ampules are considered closed systems)	Closed system transfers (Ampules are considered closed systems)	Ampicillin reconstitution for IM injection
Storage–Beyond-use date:		TPN by gravity
Room Temp. ≤ 28 hrs	*Focus: Processing technique*	
Refrigeration ≤ 7 d then use in 24 hr		
Frozen ≤ 30 d then use in 24 hr		
Unpreserved: single patient		
Preserved: may be batch		
Focus: Storage–beyond-use dating and number of patients		
RISK LEVEL 2 (RL 2)	**HIGH RISK I (HR I)**	TPN produced by Automix
Storage-Beyond-use date: Room Temp. > 28 hrs	Numerous manipulations	
	Multiday infusions or pumps	Producing multiple Cefazolin bags
Unpreserved: batch OK		
Automated TPN	Automated TPN	Unpreserved: epidurals
Focus: All multiple patients and extended storage times	*Focus: Multiple manipulations and administration over multiple days*	Portable pump reservoirs
RISK LEVEL 3 (RL 3)	**HIGH RISK II (HR II)**	Cardioplegic Solutions
Non-sterile starting material	Non-sterile starting material	Alum Bladder Irrigations

TABLE 32.2   ASHP and *USP* Guidelines by Risk Level (published as of December 2002)

Guideline	ASHP	USP
RISK LEVELS	RL 1 least potential for risk RL2 RL3 most potential for risk	LR least potential for risk HR I HR II most potential for risk
ANTEROOM	RL 1 not required RL 2 recommended RL 3 required	LR required HR I required HR II required
DESIGNATED AREA FOR PREPARATION THAT CONTAINS THE LAFW	Called Controlled Area RL1 Separate area with limited access RL 2 Separate room, Class 10,000 RL 3 Separate room, Class 10,000 or 100	Called Buffer Room LR Separate room, Class 100,000 HR I Separate room, Class 10,000 HR II Separate room, Class 10,000 or 100
LAFW	Class 100 required for all risk levels	Class 100 required for all risk levels
HOOD RE-CERTIFICATION	Every 6 months	Every 12 months
GARB	RL 1 Clean clothing covers and hair covers required; masks & gloves recommended RL 2 Gowns, gloves, and masks required; shoe covers recommended RL 3 RL 2 plus shoe covers required, all worn only in controlled area	All levels require clean, nonshedding uniforms, including hair covers, shoe covers, and gloves, all worn only in the buffer room. Masks required when using horizontal LAFW's.
PROCESS and PERSONNEL VALIDATION	Annual check-up	LR Personnel validation with media fill runs quarterly HR I & II Personnel quarterly check-up and annual process validation
ENVIRONMENT	RL 1 No requirement RL 2 Positive air pressure 3 written monitoring plan	All levels require positive air pressure & written monitoring plan
QUARANTINE	RL 3 only	HR II only
HANDLING OUTSIDE THE PHARMACY	For all levels pharmacist assures that delivery and end users store products properly	For all levels pharmacist assures that delivery and end users store products properly; patients and caregivers are given complete training in product use

Both guidelines require personnel training, written policies and procedures, quality assurance programs, and documentation

a. For institutional practices, parenteral products can be made and delivered on a frequent basis, and they are handled and administered by trained health care professionals. As a result, short (e.g., 24-hour) beyond-use dates are an option, and there is professional supervision over storage conditions. Short beyond-use dates and storage in a refrigerator means that the opportunity and conditions for growth of any inadvertent microbiological contamination are less. As a result, environmental controls and procedures need not be quite as strict. This can be seen in several requirements for ASHP Risk Level 1 (e.g., allowance for a controlled area instead of a clean room, no requirement for positive room pressure, and no required anteroom). This is helpful because even small hospitals can comply with ASHP Risk Level 1 requirements, and the types of products and the beyond-use dates possible with Risk Level 1 should meet the needs of these institutions.

b. At the other end of the spectrum is Risk Level 3, which includes the risky and more technically difficult product preparation using nonsterile starting materials.

Cardioplegic solutions for open-heart surgery are often made with nonsterile chemicals, but hospitals that engage in this sort of activity are larger institutions with the staff and facilities to comply with the requirements for Risk Level 3 production. Institutions that cannot comply with the requirements for Risk Level 3 should not engage in this type of compounding.

    c. Pharmacists who prepare or supervise the preparation of sterile products in hospitals and similar institutions should be intimately familiar with the standards of this ASHP TAB. As indicated in section I. of this chapter, the most current full text of this document is available on the ASHP web site.

2. As the chapter name implies, *USP* General Information Chapter ⟨1206⟩ Sterile Drug Products for Home Use is focused on parenteral products made for home health care.

    a. As stated in section I., Chapter ⟨1206⟩ is current as of *USP 26–NF 21*. Recently the FDA has encouraged USP to create a chapter on sterile product preparation that is more inclusive than just for home health care. This is part of an effort to bring better quality control to the making of sterile products, and changes to Chapter ⟨1206⟩ have been proposed in the *Pharmacopeial Forum*. As of December 2002, the proposed new document is still in the draft and discovery stage. The changes include an expanded chapter text and a change in number to ⟨797⟩, which would put this chapter in the section of potentially legally enforceable chapters.

    b. In its current form, Chapter ⟨1206⟩ is geared toward home health care. For this reason, the default maximum beyond-use date for stable preparations is 30 days. This is an important issue for home health care because patients are not in-house and some patients may live many miles away; it would be inconvenient and often impossible for them to get a fresh supply of needed products on a daily cycle. Because of this need for longer beyond-use dates, it is essential that the products be prepared in a way to ensure that they are sterile. This is done through very strict environmental and processing controls and quality assurance programs for all three risk levels. These standards are both practical and possible because making products for home health care is an optional practice, and pharmacies that decide to specialize in this type of service realize that they must invest in special facilities and processes to make these products. The development and availability of barrier isolators for use in pharmacies have facilitated providing a physical environment for making sterile products in a more limited space, but **a sterile environment does not ensure sterility; strict aseptic processing and appropriate quality control procedures are essential.**

    c. Because Chapter ⟨1206⟩ is being revised, contact USP for information about the most current version of this document.

VI. PREPARATION OF PARENTERAL PRODUCTS

Although most parenteral products are manufactured by the pharmaceutical industry, many pharmacists, particularly those working in hospitals or home health care practices or those servicing long-term care facilities, routinely handle and manipulate IV admixtures and injections. As indicated previously, these pharmacists require special knowledge and training. Most often this begins in pharmacy school, but there is also on-the-job training plus elective courses, video and multimedia resources, special seminars, and much published literature on this subject. Many of these resources were described in section I. of this chapter. A pharmacist practicing in this specialty area has a special responsibility for knowing and understanding the standards of practice for handling sterile drug products. The outline below gives general procedures in manipulating and compounding parenteral products. These are illustrated in each of the sample medication orders at the end of this chapter. The procedures given here are very basic; anyone compounding sterile products requires advanced instruction using the resources described above. All sample products in this chapter are Risk Level 1; products made in Risk Levels 2 and 3 are beyond the scope of this chapter.

A. Check the dose, including allowable:
   1. Route of administration
   2. Volume of administration
   3. Concentration of solution
   4. Rate of administration

   The section below on parenteral routes of administration gives guidance for some of these factors.

B. Check for stability and compatibility of the product.

C. Perform any additional necessary calculations.

D. Prepare the appropriate labels.

E. Wash and gown.
   1. This should be done in the anteroom if this is available. A "sticky" mat just inside the entrance to the anteroom is helpful in removing loose particles from shoes.
   2. Remove jewelry and wash hands and forearms with germicidal soap.
   3. Don a clean, low-shedding gown, hair covers, and foot covers. Masks may be used but are optional when using a vertical LAFW.

F. Enter the controlled area or cleanroom and put on sterile protective gloves.

G. Wipe down the LAFW using 70% Isopropyl Alcohol and sterile 4 x 4's. Wipe the side surfaces of the inside of the hood first, then the work surface, from back to front. The hood should be turned on at least 30 minutes before using it.

H. Assemble the supplies needed to make the product and take them to the LAFW. Syringes, needles, alcohol wipes, drug products, and IV solutions should be immediately available on clean carts or shelves.

I. Using aseptic technique, prepare the product.
   1. If using a horizontal airflow hood, be sure to work a minimum of 6 inches inside the front edge of the hood.
   2. If using a vertical air flow hood, be sure to work behind the front shield and above the area where the laminar air stream splits to enter the grills at the front and back edges of the work surface for the air to recirculate.
   3. Be careful not to let anything come between a critical surface and the air coming from the HEPA filter. Be aware of placement of supplies and zones of turbulence created by articles in the laminar airflow stream.
   4. Be careful not to touch any critical surfaces such as the shaft or other parts of the needle except its cap, or the syringe tip or any part of the syringe plunger except the disk or lip used to move the plunger.

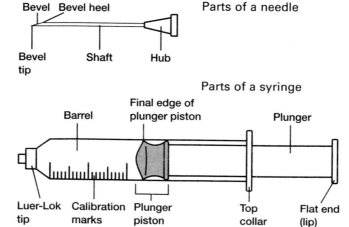

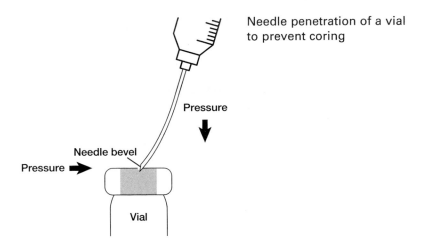

Needle penetration of a vial
to prevent coring

Pressure

Needle bevel

Pressure ➤

Vial

5. Wipe all vials, ampules, and injection ports with alcohol wipes.
   a. Swab the diaphragms of vials from back to front before entering with a needle.
   b. Enter vial diaphragms with the needle bevel up and use slight lateral pressure so the needle tip and heel go in the same hole to prevent coring the diaphragm.
   c. Remember that vials are sealed systems, so it is important to maintain equalized pressure: volume of air or liquid in = volume of liquid or air withdrawn.
   d. When using ampules, eliminate any possible glass shards in the liquid withdrawn by using a filter needle.
   e. When injecting drug solution through the injection port into a large-volume parenteral bag or a minibag, be sure that the needle penetrates both the exterior diaphragm and the inside diaphragm. Also use care to ensure that the needle does not puncture the IV bag.

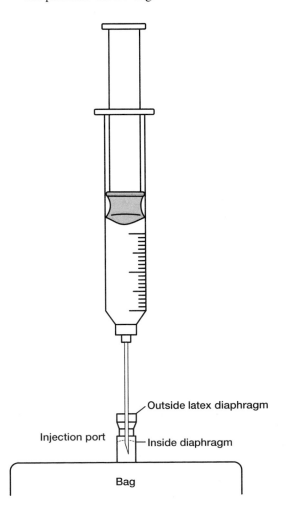

Needle penetration of an IV
injection port

Outside latex diaphragm

Injection port

Inside diaphragm

Bag

J.   Remove the product from the LAFW and immediately apply the appropriate labeling.

K.   Dispose of sharps and other used supplies properly.

VII.   PARENTERAL ROUTES OF ADMINISTRATION

Note: The size of a needle is designated using two numbers, the length in inches of the shaft and the gauge (the diameter of the needle bore).

A.   Intradermal (ID)
  1. Injection area: Located just below the surface of the skin (at the interface between the epidermis and dermis). This route is most often used for skin tests in which systemic absorption is undesirable and could be dangerous (e.g., serious allergic reactions).
  2. Volumes: Limited to small quantities, usually 0.1 mL, but may be as small as 0.02 mL and as large as 0.5 mL.
  3. Syringe sizes: 1-mL syringes, often labeled "tuberculin" because these syringes were used to administer tuberculin skin tests. Unlike other syringes, these are available with and without needles attached. If a syringe is sent to a nursing unit with a needle attached, be certain the needle cover is snapped in place. If it is not sent with a needle, the syringe should be filled with 0.1 mL excess for priming the new needle. The syringe should then be labeled with a statement to this effect: "This syringe contains 0.1 mL excess for priming."
  4. Needle sizes: 25–28 gauge, 3/8- to 5/8-inch length

B.   Subcutaneous (SC, SQ, Sub-Q, Hypo)
  1. Injection area: Subcutaneous fat tissue located beneath the skin between the dermis and muscle. When administering a drug subcutaneously, the skin may be pinched up to avoid giving the drug into the muscle. This route is used for insulin, injectable pain medication, and others where specified.
  2. Volumes: Limited to approximately 1 mL
  3. Syringe sizes: 1 or 3 mL
  4. Needle sizes: Depends on use. Insulin syringes have ultrafine needles of 30 gauge (a 32-gauge needle is planned), 1/2 inch; "hypos" are often 25 gauge, 1/2- to 5/8-inch length. Insulin syringes come with the needle attached. It is left in place for administering the dose after withdrawing the drug from the product vial. For other drugs, the needle used for withdrawing the dose is usually removed; a Luer tip cap is applied; and the nurse or caregiver selects and attaches an appropriate needle at the time of injection. In this case, excess for priming the new needle should be included in the syringe and the syringe labeled to this effect.

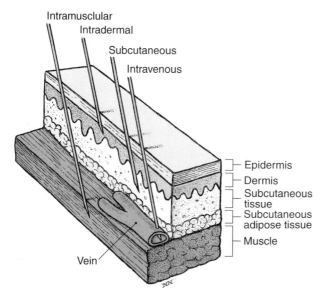

Various parenteral routes of administration (reprinted with permission from Stein SM. Drug administration. In: Boh LE, ed. Pharmacy Practice Manual: A Guide to the Clinical Experience. Philadelphia: Lippincott Williams & Wilkins, 2001)

C. Intramuscular (IM)

1. Injection area: Muscle mass: deltoid (arm), gluteus maximus (buttocks), vastus lateralis (top of leg). Any nonirritating drug can be given by this route.

2. Volumes: The volume administered is limited by the mass of the injected muscle. For adults, up to 2 mL may be given in the deltoid muscle of the upper arm, and up to 5 mL into the gluteal medial muscle of the buttock (these upper limits may be painful). For children, the volumes are more restricted. See Table 32.3 for guidelines. For small children, the vastus lateralis muscle is the recommended muscle because it is the largest muscle mass in children under 3 years of age and it is free of major nerves and vessels. The gluteus maximus is not well developed until a child has walked for at least 1 year. It is also avoided because it has a major large nerve, the sciatic nerve, running through the middle. **For children up to 3 years, the maximum volume is 1 mL.** Keep this in mind when making I.M. injections for children.

3. Syringe sizes: 1–5 mL

4. Needle sizes: 20–22 gauge, 1/2–1 1/2 inches in length

D. Intravenous (IV)

1. Injection areas: Veins. This route is used for fluid, electrolyte, and nutrient replacement; for administration of any drug that needs to get into the circulation immediately; for irritating drugs; and for drugs that require carefully controlled blood levels.

2. Volumes: Obviously, volume is less of a limitation with IV therapy. There are fluid restrictions—about 3 L a day for adults and less for children. Certain disease states further restrict fluid load. The flow rate may also be restricted by the size of the vein chosen for administering the drug.

3. Syringe sizes: 1–60 mL

4. Needle sizes: 20–22 gauge, 1/2–1 1/2 inches in length

5. IV administration is further subdivided into continuous or constant infusion, intermittent, and bolus or IV push. For calculations involving flow rate for continuous or intermittent infusions, see the next section on calculations.

a. Continuous: The drug is added to a large-volume parenteral solution, and the solution is then slowly and continuously dripped into a vein.

(1) Advantages

(a) Allows fluid and drug therapy to be administered simultaneously

(b) Achieves continuous, constant blood levels of the drug

(c) Minimizes vein irritation and trauma, because most drugs are less irritating when in dilute solutions

(d) Continuous infusion is usually less expensive than intermittent or bolus administration because fewer units are needed and less nursing and pharmacy staff time is involved in preparation, processing, and administration.

TABLE 32.3 Guidelines for Maximal Amounts of Solutions to Be Injected into Muscle Tissues (7)

Muscle Group	Birth to 1½ years (cc)	1½ to 3 years (cc)	3 to 6 years (cc)	6 to 15 years (cc)	15 years to adulthood (cc)
Deltoid	Not recommended	Not recommended unless other sites are not available 0.5	0.5	0.5	1
Gluteus maximus	Not recommended	Not recommended unless other sites are not available 1	1.5	1.5–2	2–2.5
Ventrogluteal	Not recommended	Not recommended unless other sites are not available 1	1.5	1.5–2	2–2.5
Vastus lateralis	0.5–1	1	1.5	1.5–2	2–2.5

Howry LB, Bindler RM, and Tso Y: *Pediatric Medications*, Philadelphia, Lippincott, 1981, p. 62.

(2) Disadvantages

    (a) The IV requires greater monitoring because it runs continuously.

    (b) If the IV infiltrates and cannot be continued, part of the dose has not been administered.

    (c) Cannot be used on fluid-restricted patients

    (d) The extended run times cannot be used with certain unstable drugs.

b. Intermittent: The drug is added to an intermediate volume (25–100 mL) and given in an intermediate period of time (15–60 minutes), at **spaced** intervals, such as every 6 hours.

    (1) Advantages

        (a) Requires less monitoring than continuous infusion

        (b) The complete dose is given in a moderate fluid volume and over a moderate period of time; therefore, there is less chance than with bolus administration of toxicity without the disadvantages of continuous administration.

        (c) Many drugs are more stable at moderate concentrations than in the concentrated solutions required by bolus administration.

    (2) Disadvantages

        (a) Fluids and some electrolytes cannot be given this way.

        (b) Drug blood levels are less constant than with continuous administration.

        (c) The method cannot be used for direct administration to an organ or tissue.

        (d) Sometimes impractical for immediate injection in emergency situations

c. IV push or bolus: The drug solution is placed in a syringe and administered in a short period of time (minutes) directly into a vein or IV tubing that goes into a vein. This may be a one-time administration, or it may be repeated at spaced intervals.

    (1) Advantages

        (a) Can be used for immediate injection in emergency situations

        (b) Requires no monitoring of IV fluid administration

        (c) Less expensive than intermittent administration because there is no extra IV tubing or bag

    (2) Disadvantages

        (a) Many drugs are more irritating in these highly concentrated solutions.

        (b) Some drugs are less stable in concentrated solutions.

        (c) Drug toxicity is a greater problem when a total dose is given in a bolus over a short period of time.

        (d) Drug blood levels are less constant than with either continuous or intermittent IV dosing.

        (e) When repeated doses are given, it may require more staff time because at least 2–10 minutes may be needed at the bedside for each dose given.

VIII. CALCULATIONS FOR PARENTERAL PRODUCTS AND ADMINISTRATION

A. For calculations of a general nature, see Chapters 7 through 10 on pharmaceutical calculations. Calculations specific to parenteral products and sample medication orders are given here.

B. Powder Volume

Some parenteral products have limited stability when in solution and are furnished by the product manufacturer as dry powder for reconstitution. At the time the drug is to be administered, a sterile diluent, usually Sterile Water for Injection or Sterile Sodium Chloride for Injection, is added.

The volume that the powder occupies after it is dissolved in solution is called the powder volume. For some drug products, this volume is so small that it is considered negligible no matter what the dilution. For other products it occupies an intermediate volume, in which case the powder volume must be considered when making calculations involving concentrated solutions, but may be ignored with more dilute solutions. For other products the powder volume is substantial and must always be taken into account.

➤ *EXAMPLE*

Although we usually think of powder volume in reference to parenteral products, all powders occupy a volume when dissolved. This is probably most obvious in the oral antibiotic powders for reconstitution. For example, a 100-mL bottle of amoxicillin for oral suspension requires the addition of 60 mL of Purified Water to give 100 mL of a suspension. In this case, the powder volume is 40 mL (100 mL − 60 mL = 40 mL). This information can be very useful. Suppose you wanted to give a dose of 165 mg for a product that has a concentration of 250 mg/5 mL when the product is reconstituted as directed on the bottle or package insert; the volume of the dose would be:

$$\frac{250\,mg}{5\,mL} = \frac{165\,mg}{x\,mL}; x = 3.3\,mL$$

If the pharmacist or prescriber thought that this volume would be difficult for the patient to measure, and that a 1-teaspoonful (5-mL) volume would be more convenient, the product could be reconstituted to give 165 mg/5 mL. This could be done in the following manner:

1. Calculate the total number of mg of amoxicillin in the bottle:

$$\frac{250\,mg}{5\,mL} = \frac{x\,mg}{100\,mL}; x = 5,000\,mg\,/\,bottle$$

2. Calculate the number of mL needed for this amount of drug to give a concentration of 165 mg/5 mL:

$$\frac{165\,mg}{5\,mL} = \frac{5,000\,mg}{x\,mL}; x = 152\,mL\,suspension$$

3. Based on a powder volume of 40 mL, calculate the number of mL of Purified Water that must be added to the bottle to give a final volume of 152 mL:

$$152\,mL - 40\,mL = 112\,mL$$

4. It may be necessary to add the water in two steps, and the partially reconstituted product will probably have to be transferred to a larger bottle to accommodate the total volume of 152 mL.

These same principles may be applied to parenteral powders for reconstitution. The following example illustrates the use of powder volume in a therapeutic situation:

➤ *EXAMPLE*

Rocephin® (ceftriaxone sodium) for Injection is available in 2-g vials for reconstitution. The product package insert states that when 7.2 mL of Sterile Water for Injection is added to this vial, the concentration of the resulting solution is 250 mg/mL. Your medical team wants to give this drug to a 10-month-old, 20-lb child. A drug information reference gives the following dosage information for infants and children: For serious infections (other than meningitis) in children 12 years of age or younger, the recommended dose is 50 to 75 mg/kg/day in divided doses every 12 hours.

1. The medical team is considering giving 75 mg/kg/day IM in two divided doses. The dose in mg of ceftriaxone is first calculated for this child.

$$Weight\ of\ child\ in\ kg : \frac{20\,lb}{2.2\,lb/kg} = 9.09\,kg$$

Based on this weight, the dose for this child is calculated:

mg/day: 9.09 kg × 75 mg/kg/day = 682 mg/day

$$mg/dose : \frac{682\,mg/day}{2\,doses/day} = 341\,mg/dose$$

2. Next, the number of mL of Ceftriaxone for Injection reconstituted as recommended in the product package insert is calculated:

$$\frac{250\,mg}{mL} = \frac{341\,mg}{x\,mL};\ x = 1.36\,mL$$

3. It is decided that this volume is too large to give IM to this child, and it is uncertain if the powder for injection is sufficiently soluble to make a more concentrated IM injection. An IV push administration is being considered. The physician asks if the drug can be made in a concentration of 100 mg/mL. You must now calculate the number of mL of Sterile Water for Injection to add to an unreconstituted 2-g vial to obtain this concentration.

   a. First, calculate the powder volume of the drug in the 2-g vial.
   The volume of injection when reconstituted as directed in the package insert:

   $$\frac{250\,mg}{1\,mL} = \frac{2,000\,mg}{x\,mL};\ x = 8\,mL$$

   Volume of diluent added when reconstituted as directed in the package insert: 7.2 mL

   Powder volume: *8 mL − 7.2 mL = 0.8 mL*

   b. Now calculate the new volume of water to add for reconstitution to give a concentration of 100 mg/mL.
   New volume of injection when reconstituted to give 100 mg/mL:

   $$\frac{100\,mg}{mL} = \frac{2,000\,mg}{x\,mL};\ x = 20\,mL$$

   Powder volume: 0.8 mL
   New volume of diluent to give 100 mg/mL:

   20.0 mL − 0.8 mL = 19.2 mL

   c. As with the previous example, it may be necessary to add the water in two portions, and the partially reconstituted product will probably have to be transferred to a larger bottle or syringe to accommodate the total volume of 20 mL.

C. Calculation of IV Flow Rates
IV administration, either continuous or intermittent, requires that the flow of the IV solution into the patient be regulated at a recommended rate or over a desired or recommended time interval.

   1. One method for controlling rate of flow is to use an IV administration set that has a drip chamber.
   a. An IV administration set is plastic tubing that has a spike adapter on one end that is inserted into a port of the IV bag or bottle, and the other end of the tubing has a needle or similar adapter that accesses the patient's vein. The IV set has a drip chamber of transparent plastic inserted in the tubing immediately below the spike adapter. The orifice from the bottom of the adapter into the drip chamber gives a controlled drop size (e.g., 0.05 mL/drop or 20 drops/mL).
   b. The rate of flow is regulated using a roller clamp on the IV set that controls the number of drops per minute that flow into the drip chamber and through the rest of the tubing and into the patient.

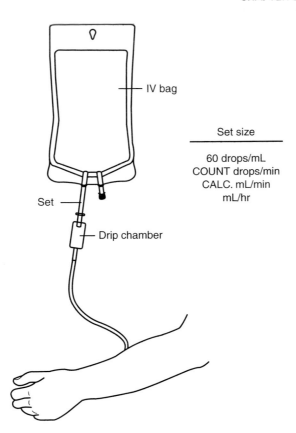

IV administration set with drip chamber

IV bag

Set size

60 drops/mL
COUNT drops/min
CALC. mL/min
mL/hr

Set

Drip chamber

c.   There are two common IV sets: one size gives 20 drops/mL and the other 60 drops/mL; the latter is sometimes called a micro- or a mini-drip set.

d.   The nurse or caregiver counts the number of drops per minute entering the drip chamber and converts this to mL/min using the drops/mL set size. If the rate of flow is either too fast or too slow, this is adjusted using the roller clamp. This process is illustrated with several examples given below and with several of the sample medication orders that follow.

2.   In some circumstances, either precise administration rates or positive pressure is required; in these circumstances infusion devices such as controllers or IV pumps are needed. For infusion devices like this, the desired rate in mL/hr or mL/min is programmed into the device software.

➤ *EXAMPLE*

Given the following order:

KCl 20 mEq in 500 mL D5W. Infuse IV over 8 hours.

The administration set delivers 20 drops/mL.

1. What is the flow rate in mL/hr?

$$500\ mL/8\ hr = 62.5\ mL/hr = 63\ mL/hr$$

2. What is the flow rate in drops/min?

By dimensional analysis:

$$\left(\frac{20\ drops}{mL}\right)\left(\frac{63\ mL}{hr}\right)\left(\frac{hr}{60\ min}\right) = 21\ drops/min$$

➤ **EXAMPLE**

Given the following order:

Ampicillin Na 175 mg in 100 mL 0.9 % NaCl Solution. Infuse IV piggyback over 15 minutes and repeat q 6 hr.

The administration set delivers 20 drops/mL.

1. What is the flow rate in mL/min?

$$100 \ mL/15 \ min = 6.7 \ mL/min$$

2. What is the flow rate in drops/min?

By dimensional analysis:

$$\left(\frac{20 \ drops}{mL}\right)\left(\frac{6.7 \ mL}{min}\right) = 134 \ drops/min$$

By proportion:

$$\frac{20 \ drops}{mL} = \frac{x \ drops}{6.7 \ mL}; x = 134 \ drops$$

Since 6.7 mL will be given in each minute and there are 134 drops in 6.7 mL, the number of drops given in each minute is 134.

➤ **EXAMPLE**

Given the following order:

Nitroglycerin IV 50 mg in 250 mL NSS. Start at 5 mcg/min and titrate dose with respect to response.

The administration set delivers 60 drops/mL.

1. What is the flow rate in mL/hr?

$$\left(\frac{250 \ mL}{50 \ mg \ NTG}\right)\left(\frac{0.005 \ mg \ NTG}{min}\right)\left(\frac{60 \ min}{hr}\right) = 1.5 \ mL/hr$$

2. What is the flow rate in drops/min?

$$\left(\frac{60 \ drops}{mL}\right)\left(\frac{1.5 \ mL}{hr}\right)\left(\frac{hr}{60 \ min}\right) = 1.5 \ drops/min$$

Note: When the administration set delivers 60 drops/mL, the mL/hr = drops/min.

D. Mixing Two or More Drugs in One Syringe
1. Check the doses.
2. Check compatibility.
   a. Check the product package insert, the *Handbook on Injectable Drugs,* or the *King Guide to Parenteral Admixtures* for compatibility information.
   b. Consult prescriber concerning any substantive changes.
3. Special techniques for ensuring proper dose volumes when one or more volumes are small
   a. Examples of common circumstances: Pediatric doses

   Insulin

   Biotech drugs
   b. There are two issues to consider relative to the dose volumes under consideration: 1) amount of dead space in the syringe hub and needle lumen and 2) priming volume.
   c. Dead space in syringe hub and needle lumen
   The volume in the syringe hub varies with the manufacturer and the syringe size. The volume in the needle lumen varies with the manufacturer and the needle

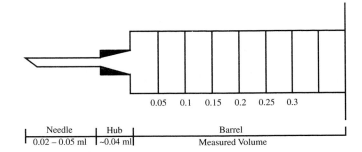

gauge and length. Volumes were checked for various 1-mL syringes and several sizes of needles. The hub and lumen volumes for this sample are given here.

Volume in hub = 0.04 mL

Volume in the lumen of a 1-inch 22-g needle = 0.03 mL

Volume in the lumen of a 1.5-inch 19-g filter needle = 0.05 mL

When you have a small volume for a dose and a serial multiple draw into the same syringe, you will get too much of the first drug (by the volume left in the hub and needle when the first drug is drawn) and not enough of the second drug (by that same volume). Potential errors are shown with the following examples.

(1) Filter needle used and not changed between draws → 0.09 mL

(0.04 mL [hub] + 0.05 mL [needle] = 0.09 mL)

(2) 22-g 1-inch needle used and not changed between draws → 0.07 mL

(0.04 mL [hub] + 0.03 mL [needle] = 0.07 mL)

(3) Any needle used but changed between draws → 0.04 mL

(Just the volume in the syringe hub, since the needle was changed between the draws)

As you can see, for small dose volumes (less than 1.0 mL), dead space can make a significant difference. You can also see that even if you switch needles between draws, you may still get a substantial percent error (from the 0.04-mL dead space in the syringe hub) if one of the dose volumes is very small.

d. Methods of handling dead space with small dose volumes

There are two ways of handling this dead space, depending on the circumstances.

(1) A precise dose is needed.

If a particular dose of each drug is needed, the problem of dead space can be circumvented in the following way.

(a) Draw the proper dose of each drug into separate syringes.

(b) Remove the protective hub cap from the tip of a third syringe, draw back its plunger, and then, using aseptic technique, shoot each drug solution into that third syringe through the hub opening.

By drawing the proper dose volume of each drug into separate syringes, then injecting each into a third syringe, only the correct measured volume of each drug is in the third syringe. The extra dead space volume remains in the original needles and syringes. This is illustrated with Sample Prescription 32.8.

(2) Injections that are given routinely and adjusted based on monitoring parameters

There are some cases for which small volumes are drawn sequentially in the same syringe. A common example is the use of regular and long-acting insulins when given at the same time; administering both injections in one syringe allows the patient to take just one shot. In this case, the use of three syringes would be both complex and expensive for the patient. Because doses are given routinely and are adjusted based on blood glucose levels, as long as the same procedure and sequence of drawing are used, the concern about needle dead space is not germane. It is, however, very important to always use the same sequence and procedure because the dead space still exists and affects the volumes drawn; in this case this is compensated for by adjusting doses by monitoring outcomes. This method is illustrated with Sample Prescription 32.7.

e. Priming volume: In the first example given above, extra volume of each drug solution obviously must be drawn to fill the hub of the third syringe and to prime the new needle that the nurse will apply when administering the drug solution to the patient. This is called "priming volume."

(1) If the drug volumes are **equal,** the priming volume may be split equally, half for each drug. For example, if there are two drugs and the desired priming volume is 0.1 mL, you would use 0.05 mL of each for the priming volume.

(2) If the drug volumes are **unequal,** the priming volume must have the same proportion of each drug solution as is in the dose volume.

For example: Drug A: 0.1 mL dose volume
Drug B: 0.2 mL dose volume
Total dose volume: 0.3 mL

If you desire a priming volume of 0.1 mL, one third of this volume (0.1/0.3 = 1/3) or 0.033 mL must be Drug A and two thirds of this volume (0.2/0.3 = 2/3) or 0.067 mL must be Drug B.

Therefore, to administer 0.1 mL of Drug A and 0.2 mL of Drug B in one syringe, draw 0.13 mL of Drug A in one syringe (0.1 mL for the dose and 0.03 mL for priming volume); draw 0.27 mL of Drug B in a second syringe (0.2 mL for the dose and 0.07 mL for priming volume); shoot these solutions into a third syringe and apply a Luer tip cap. This syringe now contains 0.4 mL (0.13 mL of Drug A + 0.27 mL of Drug B = 0.4 mL). When the nurse gives the 0.3-mL dose, he or she will apply an appropriate needle to the syringe and will fill the syringe hub and the needle. He or she will then depress the syringe plunger to the 0.3-mL mark on the syringe before giving the dose. This is one reason why the volume to be administered should always be indicated on the syringe label.

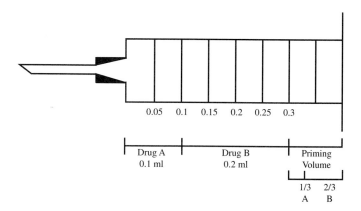

SAMPLE MEDICATION ORDERS

➤ Medication Order 32-1

MEDICAL CENTER HOSPITAL
Triturate, Wisconsin 53706

PATIENT ORDERS

Patient Name: Brett Favrite
History Number: 120579   Room Number: 430
Weight: 175 lbs   Height: 5'11"
Age: 62 y.o.
Attending Physician: R. Farrell

Date	Time	Orders
00/00/00	1700	Give Heparin 5,000 units IV push; then start IV Constant Infusion
		Heparin 15,000 units in 500 mL NSS. Give at a rate of 1,200 units/hr
		Recheck aPPT in AM. *R. Farrell, MD*
		J. Thompson 00/00/00

Materials Needed

1. Drug: Heparin Sodium, 5,000 units/mL, 10-mL vial
2. Primary IV fluid: 0.9% Sodium Chloride Injection, 500-mL bag
3. Syringe(s) used in preparation: 3 mL
4. Needle(s) used in preparation: 22-g 1-inch
5. IV set that delivers 60 drops/mL (mini-drip)

Therapeutic Intent: Anticoagulant

Compatibility–Stability/Beyond-Use Date

Stability–Compatibility: Heparin Sodium is available as an injectable solution that is reported to be stable indefinitely at room temperature. It is also physically compatible and stable in 0.9% Sodium Chloride Injection at the concentration of this constant infusion solution (8).

Packaging and Storage and Beyond-use date: The pharmacy will put a "Store in the refrigerator" label on this unpreserved LVP. The pharmacy will label the bag with its customary 48-hour beyond-use date, which is consistent with the policy of this hospital for IV solutions of this type when labeled for storage in the refrigerator.

Calculations

Dose/Concentration

Recommended dosage in *USP DI*:

Bolus of 35–70 units/kg or 5,000 units by IV injection followed by continuous infusion of 20,000–40,000 units in 1,000 mL of 0.9% Sodium Chloride Injection over 24 hours with usual rate of 1,000 units/hr, but adjusted as determined by results of coagulation tests (9)

Dose ordered:

5,000 units (63 units/kg for this 175-lb [80-kg] man) IV push followed by continuous infusion at 1,200 units/hr and monitored using a PTT coagulation test

Note: Dosing of Heparin varies greatly with the clinical condition and intent of therapy; relatively low doses are used for prophylaxis at the time of surgery and much higher doses with an active thrombolytic or embolic disorder. Many institutions have protocols for Heparin use.

IV flow rate calculations:

mL/hr:
$$\left(\frac{500\ mL}{15,000\ units}\right)\left(\frac{1,200\ units}{hr}\right) = 40\ mL\,/\,hr$$

drops/min:
$$\left(\frac{60\ drops}{mL}\right)\left(\frac{40\ mL}{hr}\right)\left(\frac{hr}{60\ min}\right) = 40\ drops\,/\,min$$

Note: Although IV Heparin flow rates are often regulated using an infusion controller for which the rate is programmed in mL/hr, the above calculation is to give you additional practice in calculating IV flow rate using a drip chamber.

Length of time one bottle will last: $\dfrac{500\ mL}{40\ mL\,/\,hr} = 12.5\ hr$

Ingredient Amounts

Heparin Sodium for IV infusion solution: $\dfrac{5,000\ units}{mL} = \dfrac{1,500\ units}{x\ mL}; x = 3\ mL$

Compounding Procedure

Use aseptic technique in all procedures for preparing this sterile product. Remove jewelry and wash hands and forearms with germicidal soap. Don a clean, low-shedding gown and hair and foot covers; lastly, put on sterile protective gloves. Wipe the surfaces of the LAFW with 70% Isopropyl Alcohol using sterile 4x4's. Assemble all needles and syringes needed, Heparin 5,000 unit/mL-vial, and 500-mL bag of NSS. Wipe all vial diaphragms and IV ports with alcohol wipes. Withdraw 3 mL of Heparin from vial and inject the solution through the injection port into the bag of 0.9% Sodium Chloride Injection. Agitate bag gently to mix. Cover port of LVP bag with seal. Inspect for cloudiness and/or particulate matter. Remove the bag from the hood and place an IV label on the bag.

Quality Control

All volumes are checked and confirmed. The solution is inspected and found to be clear, colorless, and free of any particulates or turbidity.

Labeling

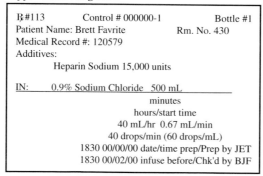

Zipper-closure bag label

R#113   Control # 000000-1   Bottle #1
Patient Name: Brett Favrite   Rm. No. 430
Medical Record #: 120579
Additives:
          Heparin Sodium 15,000 units

IN: 0.9% Sodium Chloride   500 mL
                    minutes
                hours/start time
          40 mL/hr 0.67 mL/min
          40 drops/min (60 drops/mL)
     1830 00/00/00 date/time prep/Prep by JET
     1830 00/02/00 infuse before/Chk'd by BJF

Auxiliary Labels: Keep in the Refrigerator do not freeze, 24-28 hrs if no refrigeration

➤ Medication Order 32-2

MEDICAL CENTER HOSPITAL
Triturate, Wisconsin 53706

PATIENT ORDERS

Patient Name: Bernie Brewer
History Number: 100937 Room Number: 136
Weight: 28 lbs Height: 35"
Age: 3 years–7 months
Attending Physician: Penelope Pixce

Date	Time	Orders
00/00/00	1400	KCl 10 mEq and Calcium Gluconate 1.5 mEq in 250 mL D5W.
		Infuse IV over six hours. *Penelope Pixce, MD*
		J. Thompson 00/00/00

Materials Needed

1. Drugs: KCl, 2 mEq/mL, 20-mL vial
    Calcium Gluconate, 10% 10-mL vial (9.3 mg Ca^{++} or 0.465 mEq Ca^{++}/mL)
2. Primary IV fluid: Dextrose 5% in Water, 250-mL bag
3. Syringe(s) used in preparation: two 5-mL
4. Needle(s) used in preparation: two 22-g 1-inch
5. IV set that delivers 20 drops/mL

Therapeutic Intent: Electrolyte replacement

Compatibility–Stability/Beyond-Use Date

Stability–Compatibility: The pharmacy has both electrolytes available as solutions in multidose vials and the primary IV solution, Dextrose 5% in Water, in a PVC bag.

Potassium Chloride Injection has a neutral pH in the range of 4–8. The solution itself is chemically and physically very stable, and it is physically compatible in D5W with Calcium Gluconate (8). The multidose vials used by this pharmacy contain Methylparaben (0.05%) and Propylparaben (0.005%) as a preservative system, but when diluted in the LVP solution, this would not provide sufficient preservative to protect the preparation from microbial growth. After adding Potassium Chloride Injection to an IV solution, the bag should be inverted several times to ensure adequate mixing.

The product package insert states that Calcium Gluconate 10% Injection is a supersaturated solution of Calcium Gluconate that is maintained in solution through the addition of calcium saccharate tetrahydrate. Because it is a supersaturated solution, it should be inspected prior to use to ensure there is no precipitation. The manufacturer states that crystals may be redissolved by gentle heating in a warm water bath at 60°C. The product used by this pharmacy is a single-use vial that contains no preservative, and the manufacturer states that any unused portion of a vial should be discarded. Calcium Gluconate is compatible when mixed with Potassium Chloride in Dextrose 5% in Water (8).

Packaging and Storage and Beyond-use date: The pharmacy will label this unpreserved LVP "Store in the refrigerator, Do not Freeze." The pharmacy will label the bag with its customary 48-hour beyond-use date, which is consistent with the policy of this hospital for IV solutions of this type.

Calculations

Dose/Concentration

Potassium Chloride

Recommended dosage in *USP DI*:

The usual pediatric dose of KCl for electrolyte replacement or hypokalemia treatment is up to 3 mEq of K^+ per kg of body weight or 40 mEq/m² BSA a day, with the volume of the IV fluid dependent on the body size of the patient (9).

Note that the above dose is an amount per day, and our order is a single infusion over 6 hours. The pharmacist must be sure this single dose does not exceed the maximum and then will have to keep track of the amount given over each day to be sure it does not exceed the maximum given above.

Dose ordered:

Patient weight: *28 lb ÷ 2.2 lb/kg = 12.7 kg*

Patient height: 35 inches

Patient BSA (from nomogram in Appendix E): 0.55 m²

Dose in mEq/kg: *10 mEq/12.7 kg = 0.8 mEq/kg*

Dose in mEq/m² BSA: *10 mEq/0.55 m² = 18.2 mEq/m²*

This dose is OK, well below the maximums recommended. Lab tests for electrolytes will be used to monitor blood levels of both the potassium and calcium, and adjustments will be made as appropriate to the clinical condition of the patient.

Calcium Gluconate

Recommended dosage in *USP DI*:

The usual IV pediatric dose of Calcium Gluconate for hypocalcemia is 200 to 500 mg (19.5 to 48.8 mg of calcium ion). It is administered in a single dose at a rate that does not exceed 47.5 mg of calcium ion per minute. It may be repeated if necessary (9).

Dose ordered:

This order is written in terms of mEq of Calcium Gluconate, so to check the dose, a conversion from mEq to mg of Ca^{++} and/or mg of Calcium Gluconate must be done. The molecular weight of Calcium Gluconate is 430, and there is one calcium ion per molecule. Calcium has an atomic weight of 40.

Dose of 1.5 mEq Ca^{++} in terms of mg of Calcium Gluconate:

$$\left(\frac{430.36\ mg\ Ca\ Gluc.}{mmol\ Ca\ Gluc.}\right)\left(\frac{mmol\ Ca\ Gluc.}{2\ mEq\ Ca^{++}}\right)\left(\frac{1.5\ mEq\ Ca^{++}}{}\right) = 323\ mg\ Ca\ Gluc.$$

Dose of 1.5 mEq Ca^{++} in terms of mg of calcium ion:

$$\left(\frac{40\ mg\ Ca^{++}}{mmol}\right)\left(\frac{mmol}{2\ mEq\ Ca^{++}}\right)\left(\frac{1.5\ mEq\ Ca^{++}}{}\right) = 30\ mg\ Ca^{++}$$

For this drug solution, we also have helpful information in the product package insert. It states that each mL of Calcium Gluconate 10% Injection contains 9.3 mg of calcium (0.465 mEq) as calcium gluconate and calcium saccharate heptahydrate. Therefore, we could use these numbers in making a conversion from mEq calcium to mg of calcium:

$$\frac{0.465\ mEq\ Ca^{++}}{9.3\ mg\ Ca^{++}} = \frac{1.5\ mEq\ Ca^{++}}{x\ mg\ Ca^{++}}; x = 30\ mg\ Ca^{++}$$

This dose is within the recommended range. Since we are giving 30 mg of calcium ion over 6 hours, we do not have to be concerned about the maximum rate of 47.5 mg of calcium ion per minute. Lab tests for electrolytes will be used to monitor blood levels of both the potassium and calcium, and adjustments will be made as appropriate to the clinical condition of the patient.

IV flow rate calculations:

mL/hr: $250\ mL/6\ hr = 41.7 \approx 42\ mL/hr$

drops/min: $\left(\dfrac{20\ drops}{mL}\right)\left(\dfrac{42\ mL}{hr}\right)\left(\dfrac{hr}{60\ min}\right) = 14\ drops/min$

Ingredient Amounts

Potassium Chloride: $\dfrac{2\ mEq\ K^+}{mL} = \dfrac{10\ mEq\ K^+}{x\ mL}; x = 5\ mL$

Calcium Gluconate: $\dfrac{0.465\ mEq\ Ca^{++}}{mL} = \dfrac{1.5\ mEq\ Ca^{++}}{x\ mL}; x = 3.2\ mL$

Compounding Procedure

Use aseptic technique in all procedures for preparing this sterile product. Remove jewelry and wash hands and forearms with germicidal soap. Don a clean, low-shedding gown and hair and foot covers; lastly, put on sterile protective gloves. Wipe the surfaces of the LAFW with 70% Isopropyl Alcohol using sterile 4x4's. Assemble all needles and syringes needed, KCl 2 mEq/mL 20-mL vial, Calcium Gluconate 10% 10-mL vial, Dextrose 5% in Water 250-mL LVP. Wipe all vial diaphragms and IV ports with alcohol wipes. Using appropriate syringes, withdraw 5 mL of KCl from the vial and inject into the port of the 250-mL D5W bag. Agitate the D5W bag by several inversions to mix. Withdraw 3.2 mL of Calcium Gluconate from the vial and inject into the port of the 250-mL D5W bag. Agitate the D5W bag by several inversions to evenly distribute drugs. Cover port of LVP bag with seal. Inspect for cloudiness and/or particulate matter. Remove the bag from the hood and place an IV label on the bag.

Quality Control

All volumes are checked and confirmed. The solution is inspected and found to be clear, colorless, and free of any particulates or turbidity.

Labeling

Zipper-closure bag label

Ŗ 114   Control # 000000-2   Bottle #1
Patient Name: Bernie Brewer   Rm. No. 136
Medical Record #: 100937
Additives:
KCl 10mEq and Calcium Gluconate 1.5 mEq
IN: Dextrose 5% in Water 250 mL
minutes
6 hours/start time
42 mL/hr 0.7 mL/min
14 drops/min (20 drops/mL)
1830 00/00/00 date/time prep/Prep by JET
1830 00/02/00 infuse before/Chk'd by BJF

Auxiliary Labels: Keep in the Refrigerator do not freeze, 24–28 hrs if no refrigeration

➤ **Medication Order 32-3**

MEDICAL CENTER HOSPITAL
Triturate, Wisconsin 53706

<u>PATIENT ORDERS</u>

Patient Name: Ben Capital
History Number: 842926   Room Number: 215-Peds
Weight: 32 lbs   Height: 38"
Age: 3 y.o.
Attending Physician: Patsy Heider, MD

Date	Time	Orders
00-00-00	1600	Na Nitroprusside 50 mg in 250 mL D5W.
		Start at 1.3 mcg/kg/min, then titrate to maintain diastolic
		BP ≤ 100 mm Hg. *Patsy Heider, MD*
		J.Thompson 00/00/00

Materials Needed

1. Drug: Nitroprusside 50 mg/5 mL vial
2. IV fluid: Dextrose 5% in Water, 250 mL
3. Syringes: 3 mL
4. Needles: 22-g, 1 inch
5. Foil or opaque plastic for wrapping IV bag
6. IV set that delivers 60 drops/mL (mini-drip)

Therapeutic Intent: Rapid reduction of blood pressure

Compatibility–Stability/Beyond-Use Date

Stability–Compatibility: Sodium Nitroprusside has been available both as a drug powder for reconstitution and as a solution in a single-use vial. This pharmacy is using a solution product that contains in each 2 mL the equivalent of 50 mg Sodium Nitroprusside Dihydrate in Sterile Water for Injection. The product package insert states that the drug in solution is sensitive to light. The amber single-dose vials are to be stored at controlled room temperature and in the product carton until time of use. The drug solution is not for direct infusion and must be diluted in 250–1,000 mL of Dextrose 5% in Water. Once diluted, the IV bag should be protected from light using a foil or opaque plastic wrap; however, the administration set need not be protected. The freshly diluted solution is stable for 24 hours.

Packaging and Storage and Beyond-use date: The IV bag with freshly prepared drug solution will be wrapped in the brown opaque plastic wrap that accompanies the drug vial. The IV solution will be prepared shortly before it is needed. Because of the slow infusion rate for this medication order, there is sufficient solution in the IV bag to run for approximately 41.7 hours (250 mL ÷ 6 mL/hr = 41.7 hr). However, the expiration time recommended by the manufacturer for the reconstituted and diluted solution is 24 hours, so 24 hours will be the assigned beyond-use date.

Calculations

Dose/Concentration

Recommended dosage in product package insert:

   3 mcg/kg/min and adjusted based on response

   Range: 0.5–10 mcg/kg/min

Dose ordered: 1.3 mcg/kg/min OK, within range

Concentration of drug in IV: 50 mg/250 mL

Weight of patient in kg: *32 lb ÷ 2.2 lb/kg = 14.5 kg*

Based on the drug concentration in IV and the dose in mcg/kg/min, the IV flow rate is:

mL/hr:

$$\left(\frac{250\ mL}{50\ mg\ Na\ Nitroprus.}\right)\left(\frac{0.0013\ mg\ Na\ Nitroprus.}{kg/min}\right)\left(14.5\ kg\right)\left(\frac{60\ min}{hr}\right) = 5.7\ mL/hr$$

drops/min:

$$\left(\frac{60\ drops}{mL}\right)\left(\frac{5.7\ mL}{hr}\right)\left(\frac{hr}{60\ min}\right) = 5.7\ or\ 6\ drops/min$$

Note: Because Nitroprusside is a drug that requires a carefully controlled administration rate, IV flow rates for this type of infusion are usually regulated using an infusion controller for which the rate is programmed in mL/hr. The above calculation is to give you additional practice in calculating flow rates using a drip chamber.

Ingredient Amounts

One vial of 50 mg/2 mL in 250 mL of Dextrose 5% in Water (D5W)

Compounding Procedure

Use aseptic technique in all procedures for preparing this sterile product. Remove jewelry and wash hands and forearms with germicidal soap. Don a clean, low-shedding gown and hair and foot covers; lastly, put on sterile protective gloves. Wipe the surfaces of the LAFW with 70% Isopropyl Alcohol using sterile 4x4's. Assemble all needles and syringes needed, single-dose vial of Na Nitroprusside, 50 mg/2 mL, and 250-mL LVP bag of D5W. Wipe all diaphragms and ports with alcohol wipes. Withdraw 2 mL from the vial of Na Nitroprusside, 50 mg/2 mL. Inject the solution through the injection port into the bag of D5W. Agitate bag gently to mix. Cover port of LVP bag with seal. Inspect the IV bag to be sure the solution is clear with no particulates or haze. Remove the bag from the hood and place a label directly on the IV bag indicating that Na Nitroprusside was added. Wrap the bag with opaque plastic to protect the drug solution from light, and secure the wrap with tape. Attach a patient-specific IV label to the outside of the opaque wrap.

Quality Control

All volumes are checked and confirmed. The solution is inspected and found to be clear, colorless, and free of any particulates or turbidity.

Labeling

Zipper-closure bag label

R#116	Control # 000000-3	Bottle #1
Patient Name: Ben Capital		Rm. No. 215-Peds
Medical Record #: 842926		
Additives:		
	Na Nitroprusside 50 mg	
IN: Dextrose 5% in Water 250 mL		
	minutes	
	hours/start time	
	6 mL/hr micro-drops/min	
	6 drops/min (60 drops/mLset)	
	1700 00/00/00 date/time prep/Prep by JET	
	1700 00/01/00 infuse before/Chk'd by BJF	

Auxiliary Labels: Keep in the Refrigerator do not freeze
(Optional since this is to be used immediately)

➤ **Medication Order 32-4**

MEDICAL CENTER HOSPITAL
Triturate, Wisconsin 53706

<u>PATIENT ORDERS</u>

Patient Name: Rachel Sensible
History Number: 152492   Room Number: 772
Weight: 44 lbs.   Height: 44"
Age: 5 y.o.
Attending Physician: Walter Johnson, MD

Date	Time	Orders
00-00-00	1600	Erythromycin Lactobionate 20 mg/kg/day in equally divided doses
		q 6 hrs. Please dilute each dose in 100 mL minibag and give
		over 1 hour. *Walter Johnson MD*
		J.Thompson 00/0/00

Materials Needed

1. Drug:Erythromycin Lactobionate 1 g/vial
2. IV fluids: 0.9% Sodium Chloride for Injection, 100 mL
3. Syringe: 20-mL and 3-mL
4. Needle: 22-g 1-inch
5. IV set delivers 20 drops/mL

Therapeutic Intent: Antibiotic

Compatibility–Stability/Beyond-Use Date

Stability–Compatibility: Erythromycin Lactobionate is available as a lyophilized powder for reconstitution. The pharmacy is using a 1-g vial. The product package insert states that the 1-g vial should be reconstituted with 20 mL of Sterile Water for Injection; no other reconstitution vehicle should be used, including Bacteriostatic Water for Injection, because precipitation may occur. This solution is stated to be stable for 2 weeks in the refrigerator or 24 hours at room temperature. Because of the irritative properties of the drug, this solution must be diluted before administration. The concentration for continuous infusion is 1 mg/mL, and the concentration for intermittent infusion is 1 to 5 mg/mL, and no less than 100 mL of IV solution should be used. Either 0.9% Sodium Chloride Injection or Lactated Ringer's Injection can be used as is, but if Dextrose 5% in Water or other IV fluid containing Dextrose is used, the pH of the Dextrose solution must be adjusted first with Sodium Bicarbonate Injection 4%. A pH of at least 5.5 is desirable because Erythromycin Lactobionate is unstable in acidic solutions.

Packaging and Storage and Beyond-use date: The reconstituted vial will be stored in the refrigerator and will be given a 48-hour beyond-use date, which is consistent with the policy of this hospital for unpreserved reconstituted sterile solutions. The IV bag will be given an 8-hour beyond-use date as recommended in the product package insert for diluted solutions.

Calculations

Dose/Concentration

Recommended dose given in product package insert: 15–20 mg/kg/day

Dose ordered: 20 mg/kg/day—OK

Weight of patient in kg: *44 lb ÷ 2.2 lb/kg = 20 kg*

Dose per day in mg: $\left(\dfrac{20\ mg\ Erythro.}{kg\,/\,day}\right)\left(\dfrac{20\ kg}{}\right) = 400\ mg\,/\,day$

Each dose in mg: $\left(\dfrac{400\ mg}{day}\right)\left(\dfrac{day}{4\ doses}\right) = 100\ mg\,/\,dose$

Ingredient Amounts

Erythromycin 1-g vial mixed with 20 mL Sterile Water for Injection gives a concentration of 1,000 mg/20 mL = 50 mg/mL

Volume of injection for each 100-mg dose: $\left(\dfrac{mL}{50\ mg\ Erythro.}\right)\left(\dfrac{100\ mg}{dose}\right) = 2\ mL\,/\,dose$

The maximum concentration for intermittent infusion is 1–5 mg/mL. If each 100-mg dose is placed in a 100-mL minibag, the concentration would be 100 mg/100 mL = 1 mg/mL—OK

Flow rate:

Acceptable range given in the product insert: 20–60 minutes ∴ 100 mL given over 1 hr (60 min) is OK.

mL/min: *100 mL/60 min = 1.67 mL/min*

drops/min using a 20 drop/mL set: $\left(\dfrac{20\ drops}{mL}\right)\left(\dfrac{1.67\ mL}{min}\right) = 33\ drops\,/\,min$

Compounding Procedure

Use aseptic technique in all procedures for preparing this sterile product. Remove jewelry and wash hands and forearms with germicidal soap. Don a clean, low-shedding gown and hair and foot covers; lastly, put on sterile protective gloves. Wipe the surfaces of the LAFW with 70% Isopropyl Alcohol using sterile 4x4's. Assemble all needles and syringes needed, 1-g vial of Erythromycin Lactobionate, a vial of Sterile Water for injection, and a 100-mL bag of 0.9% Sodium Chloride Injection. Wipe vial diaphragms and bag ports with alcohol swabs. Use a 20-mL syringe to withdraw 20 mL Sterile Water and inject it into the Erythromycin vial. When the drug is completely dissolved, withdraw 2 mL (100 mg) and add it to the 100-mL bag of Sodium Chloride 0.9%. Agitate and inspect bag. Cover port of LVP bag with seal. Remove the bag from the hood and label the bag appropriately.

Quality Control

All volumes are checked and confirmed. The solution is inspected and found to be clear and free of particulates and turbidity.

Labeling

Zipper-closure bag label

℞#117	Control # 000000-4	Bottle #1
Patient Name: Rachel Sensible	Rm. No. 772	
Medical Record #: 152492		
Additives:		
	Erythromycin Lactobionate 100 mg	
IN:	0.9% Sodium Chloride 10 mL	
	60 minutes	
	1 hours/start time	
	100 mL/hr micro-drops/min	
	33 drops/min (20 drops/mLset)	
	1700 00/00/00 date/time prep/Prep by MB	
	0100 00/01/00 infuse before/Chk'd by BJF	

Auxiliary Labels: Keep in the Refrigerator do not freeze
          (Optional since product insert states this is not suitable for storage)

➤ **Medication Order 32-5**

MEDICAL CENTER HOSPITAL
Triturate, Wisconsin 53706

PATIENT ORDERS

Patient Name: David Drummer
History Number: 202075   Room Number: 783
Weight: 20 lbs   Height: 29"
Age: 1 y.o.
Attending Physician: Franco Kotze, MD

Date	Time	Orders
00-00-00	1600	Penicillin G K 200,000 units IM
		Give 30 min. prior to surgery. *Franco Kotze, MD*
		J. Thompson 00/00/00

Materials Needed

1. Drug: Penicillin G K g 1,000,000 units/vial
2. Reconstitution fluid: Sterile Water for Injection
3. Syringes: 3-mL and 5-mL
4. Needle: 22-g 1-inch

Therapeutic Intent: Antibiotic

Compatibility–Stability/Beyond-Use Date

Stability–Compatibility: Penicillin G Potassium for Injection is available as sterile powder for reconstitution. Although it comes in a variety of vial sizes, our pharmacy has vials that contain1,000,000 units of Pen G K. Acceptable diluents for reconstitution include Sterile Water for Injection, 0.9% Sodium Chloride Injection, and Dextrose Injection (e.g., D5W). The product package insert for the available product states that sterile reconstituted solutions are stable when refrigerated for 1 week, and solutions diluted for IV infusion are stable at room temperature for at least 24 hours. Penicillins are unstable in carbohydrate solutions at alkaline pH, but the sterile powder for injection contains citrate buffers for a desirable pH.

Packaging and Storage and Beyond-use date: The reconstituted vial and the syringe contain drug solution will be stored in the refrigerator and will be given a 48-hour beyond-use date, which is consistent with the policy of this hospital for unpreserved reconstituted sterile solutions.

Calculations

Dose/Concentration

Recommended dosage in *USP DI*:

12,500–25,000 units/kg q 6 hr IM or IV for most indications for infants and children. Certain special indications give other doses (9).

Dose ordered: 200,000 units

Weight of patient in kg: *20 lb ÷ 2.2 lb/kg = 9.1 kg*

Dose for patient in units/kg: *200,000 units/9.1 kg = 21,978 units/kg—OK*

Ingredient Amounts

The reconstitution instructions for the 1,000,000-unit vials with resulting concentrations are:

Diluent Volume:	9.6 mL	Resulting Concentration:	100,000 units/mL
	4.6 mL		200,000 units/mL
	3.6 mL		250,000 units/mL

The manufacturer recommends that for comfort, the concentration for an IM injection not exceed 100,000 units/mL. For this order of 200,000 units, however, this concentration would give a volume of 2 mL, too large a volume for this pediatric patient. (1 mL is the maximum IM volume for children up to the age of 3 years; see Table 32.3). Therefore, we desire to reconstitute this injection with a volume of diluent that will yield a solution that is as dilute as possible without exceeding a 1-mL volume. From the reconstitution information given above, if 4.6 mL of diluent is added, a solution that is 200,000 units/mL results. This is the dilution that should be used, and 1 mL is drawn (+ 0.1 mL to prime the needle).

Compounding Procedure

Use aseptic technique in all procedures for preparing this sterile product. Remove jewelry and wash hands and forearms with germicidal soap. Don a clean, low-shedding gown and hair and foot covers; lastly, put on sterile protective gloves. Wipe the surfaces of the LAFW with 70% Isopropyl Alcohol using sterile 4x4's. Assemble all needles and syringes needed, Penicillin 1,000,000-unit vial, and a vial of Sterile Water for Injection. Wipe all diaphragms with alcohol swabs. From the vial of Sterile Water for Injection, withdraw 4.6 mL with a 5-mL syringe and inject it into the Penicillin vial. Swirl to dissolve completely. Using a fresh 3-mL syringe and needle (this is recommended because with this relatively small dose volume, the Sterile Water, left in the dead space of the original syringe and needle, will dilute the drug solution and result in a subpotent dose), withdraw 1.1 mL of the Penicillin solution (includes 0.1 mL for priming). Remove the needle and put on a Luer tip cap. Remove the syringe from the hood, label the syringe, and place in a labeled zippered bag.

Quality Control

All volumes are checked and confirmed. The final solution is inspected to ensure that it is clear and free of particulates and turbidity.

Labeling

Syringe label

> Penicillin G K 200,000 units/mL   Control # 000000-5
> For IM use
> This syringe contains 0.1 mL excess for priming
> Do not use after 1700 00/02/00

Zipper-closure bag label

> ℞ #118   Control # 000000-5
> David Drummer
> Rm #783   Medical Record #202075
> Penicillin G K 200,000 units/mL   For IM use
> Give 30 minutes prior to surgery
> This syringe contains 0.1 mL excess for priming.
> Do not use after 1700 00/02/00

Auxiliary labels: Keep in the Refrigerator, Do not freeze;
Beyond-use date is 48 hours

➤ **Medication Order 32-6**

MEDICAL CENTER HOSPITAL
Triturate, Wisconsin 53706

PATIENT ORDERS

Patient Name: John Bass
History Number: 120579   Room Number: 508
Weight: 174 lbs   Height: 5'11"
Age: 55 y.o.
Attending Physician: Ima Hack, MD

Date	Time	Orders
00-00-00	1600	Asparaginase 2 units/0.1 mL
		Inject 0.1 mL ID at test site and observe for 1 hour before
		starting treatment. *Ima Hack, MD*
		J. Thompson 0/0/00

Materials Needed

1. Drug: Asparaginase 10,000 IU/vial (Elspar®)
2. Reconstitution fluid: Sterile Water for Injection
3. Syringes: 1-mL, 5-mL, 10-mL
4. Needles: 20-g 1-inch, 25-g 5/8-inch

Therapeutic Intent: Allergy skin test for Asparaginase

Compatibility–Stability/Beyond-Use Date

Stability–Compatibility: May be reconstituted with either Sterile Water for Injection or 0.9% Sodium Chloride Injection. The product contains no preservative.

Storage and Beyond-use date: The reconstituted product should be stored in the refrigerator (2°–8°C). Unused reconstituted product should be discarded after 8 hours or sooner if the solution becomes cloudy (9).

Calculations

Dose/Concentration

Recommended dosage for skin test in *USP DI*: 2 units/0.1 mL as an ID skin test (9)

Note: Because of problems with allergic reactions to this antineoplastic drug, it is recommended that a skin test be used before initiating therapy and also when 1 week or more has intervened between doses of this drug (9).

Dose ordered: Same as above

Ingredient Amounts

An Asparaginase vial contains 10,000 International Units. Reconstitution with 5 mL of Sterile Water gives 10,000 units/5 mL = 2,000 units/mL

Take a minimum measurable quantity of 0.1 mL to give:

$$2000 \text{ units/mL} \times 0.1 \text{ mL} = 200 \text{ units}$$

Put this in an empty sterile vial and add 9.9 mL of Sterile Water for Injection to give a total volume of 10 mL with a concentration of:

$$200 \text{ units/10 mL} = 20 \text{ units/mL} = 2 \text{ units/0.1 mL}$$

Compounding Procedure

Note: Because this is a hazardous drug, this procedure should be done in a biological safety cabinet, not in a horizontal LAFW. Use aseptic technique in all procedures for preparing this sterile product. Remove jewelry and wash hands and forearms with germicidal soap. Don a clean, low-shedding gown and hair and foot covers. For this drug, a cytotoxic compound, double-glove and use a facemask. Wipe down the biological safety cabinet surfaces with 70% Isopropyl Alcohol using sterile 4x4's. Assemble necessary materials. This is a cytotoxic drug: **Do not use the same syringe and/or needle for any of the transfers.** Wipe the diaphragms of vials with alcohol swabs. Reconstitute the 10,000-unit vial of Asparaginase with 5 mL of Sterile Water for Injection. Gently agitate (do not shake) and allow to dissolve. Withdraw 0.1 mL of this solution and transfer to an empty sterile vial. Using a separate needle and syringe, withdraw 9.9 mL of Sterile Water for Injection from a vial and transfer it to the sterile vial containing 0.1 mL of drug solution. Agitate to mix and inspect for clarity. Withdraw 0.1 mL of this solution with a 1-mL tuberculin syringe with an attached 25-g 5/8-inch needle. Cap the needle tightly; because this skin test is dispensed with the administration needle in place, no excess for priming is needed in the syringe. Remove the syringe from the hood and label the syringe. Put the syringe in a zippered bag that is labeled with a patient label and a warning label for chemotherapy drugs.

Quality Control

All volumes are checked and confirmed. The solution is clear and free of turbidity. If gelatinous fibers develop in the solution, it may be filtered without loss of potency using a 5-micron filter (a 0.2-micron filter may not be used).

Labeling

Syringe label

Asparaginase 2 units/0.1 mL   Control # 000000-6 For ID use only. Do not use after 0100 00/01/00

Zipper-closure bag label

R #115   Control # 000000-6 John Bass Rm #508   Medical Record #120579 Asparaginase 2 units/0.1 mL Inject 0.1 mL ID at test site and observe for 1 hour before starting treatment Do not use after 0100 00/01/00

Auxiliary labels: Keep in the Refrigerator, Do not freeze;
Beyond-use date is 8 hours
CATION: CHEMOTHERAPY Handle with Gloves; Dispose of Properly

➤ **Medication Order 32-7**

MEDICAL CENTER HOSPITAL
Triturate, Wisconsin 53706

PATIENT ORDERS

Patient Name: Gudding, Kuba
History Number: 558330   Room Number: 815
Weight: 210 lbs   Height: 6'2"
Age: 64 y.o.
Attending Physician: F. Kohlen, MD

Date	Time	Orders
00-00-00	1300	Insulin injection:
		Mix in one syringe:
		Regular Insulin 30 units and Isophane Insulin 55 units.
		Give subcutaneously Q AM.. *F. Kohlen , MD*
		J. Thompson 00/00/00

Materials Needed

1. Drug: Humulin R Insulin, Humulin N Insulin 100 units/mL, 10-mL vials
2. Syringes: 1-mL insulin syringe

Therapeutic Intent: Antidiabetic agent

Compatibility–Stability/Beyond-Use Date

Stability–Compatibility: When vials of insulin are stored in the refrigerator but protected from freezing, the insulin is stable until the expiration date given on the bottle. Bottles of insulin stored at room temperature and protected from direct sunlight are stable for 1 month (10). These are multidose vials and contain a preservative.

Isophane (NPH) and regular insulin are stable when mixed and are absorbed from the site of injection as if given separately. The mixtures are stable for 1 month at room temperature or for 3 months if refrigerated (10).

When mixing insulin in a single syringe, the Regular insulin is drawn first and then the NPH. One way to remember the order of mixing is to think of a perfect summer day: clear to partly cloudy. Because air must be replaced in each vial equal to the volume removed, this means that mixing insulin in a single syringe requires a special sequence:

Example: Regular insulin needed = x units
                NPH insulin needed = y units

Order of steps:
1. Inject y units of air into NPH vial and take out needle without drawing any insulin into the syringe.
2. Inject x units of air into the Regular insulin vial and withdraw x units of Regular insulin.
3. Insert the needle into the NPH vial, withdraw y units of NPH insulin (total units of insulin in the syringe is now x + y units), and withdraw the needle.

Insulin is routinely drawn sequentially in the same syringe. Because of the small volumes involved and the dead space in the needle and hub of the syringe, it is important to always draw insulin in the same way and use the same brand of syringes. A different dose would also result if the two insulin types were drawn in separate syringes and either given separately or first pooled in a third syringe or vial.

Packaging and Storage and Beyond-use date: If drawn into glass or plastic syringes, mixtures are stable for 7 days at room temperature or 14 days under refrigeration. If drawn into a syringe, the syringe should be stored with the needle pointing upward to prevent the insulin suspension particles from settling into the needle area and plugging the needle. At the time of use, the syringe plunger should be drawn back and the suspension agitated gently to remix the insulins (10). The syringe for this order may be stored at room temperature with a 7-day beyond-use date.

Note: Unlike mixtures of NPH and Regular insulin, mixtures of Lente and Regular insulin should be given immediately after mixing to obtain the desired result (10).

Calculations

Dose/Concentration

Insulin dosage is dependent on the blood glucose testing results of the patient.

Ingredient Amounts

Insulin syringes are marked in units; draw 30 units of Regular Insulin and 55 units of NPH Insulin for a total of 85 units.

Compounding Procedure

Use aseptic technique in all procedures for preparing this sterile product. Remove jewelry and wash hands and forearms with germicidal soap. Don a clean, low-shedding gown and hair and foot covers; lastly, put on sterile protective gloves. Wipe the surfaces of the LAFW with 70% Isopropyl Alcohol using sterile 4x4's. Assemble the materials needed, a U-100 insulin syringe and one 10-mL bottle each of Regular Humulin U-100 Insulin and Humulin N U-100 Insulin. Swab the Insulin Regular and Isophane vial ports with an alcohol swab. Using a 1-mL insulin syringe with attached needle, pull the plunger back to 85 units (0.85 mL). Insert the needle into the Humulin N vial and push in 55 units (0.55 mL) of air so the plunger is now at the 30-unit mark. Withdraw the needle and insert it into the Regular Insulin vial. Push in the remaining volume of air into that vial, and with the vial inverted, draw back the syringe plunger to 30 units (0.3 mL) to withdraw that amount of Regular insulin from the vial. Next, using the same syringe and needle, reenter the Isophane insulin vial and withdraw 55 units (0.55 mL) of insulin from the vial; the plunger should now be at the 85-unit mark. Remove the needle from the vial and recap the needle. Draw back the plunger and rotate to mix. With the needle pointing upward, move the plunger back to the previous marking. Remove all materials from the hood and place a label on the syringe. Place the syringe in a labeled zippered bag.

Quality Control

All volumes are checked and confirmed. The suspension appears cloudy but with no larger crystals or particulates.

Labeling

Syringe label

Humulin R Insulin 30 units and Hymulin N Insulin 55 units/0.85 mL Control #000000-6   For Subcutaneous use Do not use after 1400 00/07/00

Zipper-closure bag label

℞ #120   Control # 000000-6 Kuba Gudding Room 815   Medical Record #558330 Humulin R Insulin 30 units and Humulin N Insulin 55 units/0.85 mL For Subcutaneous Use Give 0.85 mL subcutaneously every morning Do not use after 1400 00/07/00

Auxiliary labels: Store with needle pointing upward
Beyond-use date is 7 days

➤ **Medication Order 32-8**

MEDICAL CENTER HOSPITAL

Triturate, Wisconsin 53706

<u>PATIENT ORDERS</u>

Patient Name: Jason Matthaus
History Number: 526942   Room Number: 783
Weight: 26 lbs   Height: 34"
Age: 2 y.o.
Attending Physician: Franco Kotze, MD

Date	Time	Orders		
00-00-00	1600	Phenobarbital Na	25 mg	Mix in one syringe and
		Glycopyrrolate	~~0.8 mg~~	give 1° prior to surgery
		Promethazine HCl	12 mg	*Franco Kotze, MD*
		Called Dr. Kotze and we agreed to change the above order to give		
		Glycopyrrolate 0.06 mg rather than 0.8 mg. Also will give the		
		Phenobarbital in a separate syringe. *J.Thompson 00/00/00*		

Materials Needed

1. Drugs: Phenobarbital Na 65 mg/mL, 1-mL vial
      Glycopyrrolate 0.2 mg/mL 20-mL vial
      Promethazine HCl 25 mg/mL, 1-mL amp
2. Syringes: 1-mL, 3-mL
3. Needles: 22-g 1-inch needles and a filter needle

Therapeutic Intent: Preoperative sedative with anticholinergic properties

Compatibility–Stability/Beyond-Use Date

Stability–Compatibility: The pharmacy has all three drugs available as injectable solutions, Glycopyrrolate and Phenobarbital Na in vials and Promethazine HCl in an amber ampule.

Glycopyrrolate Injection has a pH of 2–3 and is stable in acid pH but is subject to ester hydrolysis above pH 6. The low pH of its solutions causes precipitation of the neutral weak acid for salts of drugs such as barbiturates (8). The product used by the pharmacy is in a multidose vial and contains a preservative.

Promethazine HCl Injection has a pH in the range of 4-5.5. It is compatible with Glycopyrrolate Injection but incompatible with Phenobarbital Na Injection. Promethazine HCl is photosensitive; its solutions should be protected from light and should be inspected for discoloration and particulates prior to use. It is somewhat subject to sorption, especially if the pH of the solution is increased, but one study showed no loss due to sorption when stored in polypropylene plastic syringes for 24 hours at room temperature when protected from light (8). The product used by the pharmacy is in a single-use ampule and contains no preservative.

Phenobarbital Na Injection has a pH in the range of 8.5-10.5. Its injection formulations use a combination of pH and a cosolvent system containing alcohol and propylene glycol for solubility. The cosolvent systems also provide an antimicrobial preservative system for the injection. Intact vials should be protected from light. Phenobarbital Na Injection is incompatible with both Glycopyrrolate and Promethazine HCl Injections (8).

Packaging and Storage and Beyond-use dating: Because of the incompatibility of Phenobarbital Na with Promethazine HCl and with Glycopyrrolate, the Phenobarbital must be drawn in a separate syringe. Because the Phenobarbital Na Injection is stable and preserved, it can either be given a 7-day beyond-use date and labeled for storage in the refrigerator or a 24-hour dating with storage at room temperature, as is standard practice for this pharmacy with preparations of this type. The Promethazine HCl and Glycopyrrolate will be drawn in a single syringe. *The Handbook of Injectable Drugs* states that this combination is stable for 48 hours at 25°C. Because this is an unpreserved solution, it will be labeled for storage in the refrigerator and with a beyond-use date of 48 hours, as is standard practice for this pharmacy with preparations of this type.

Calculations

Dose/Concentration

Recommended pediatric sedative-hypnotic or preoperative doses from the *USP DI*:

Phenobarbital: IM or IV 1-3 mg/kg body weight

Glycopyrrolate: IM dose of 4.4–8.8 mcg (0.0044–0.0088 mg)/kg body weight

Promethazine HCl: For children 2 years and older, IM dose of 500 mcg (0.5 mg) to 1 mg per kg body weight; or 12.5 to 25 mg: or 1.1 mg/kg when combined with meperidine and an anticholinergic

Dose ordered:

Child's body weight in kg: *26 lb ÷ 2.2 lb/kg = 11.8 kg*

Phenobarbital: *25 mg/11.8 kg = 2.1 mg/kg*—OK, within the recommended range.

Glycopyrrolate: *0.8 mg/11.8 kg = 0.07 mg/kg*—This dose is 10 to 20 times the recommended dose. Therefore, Pharmacist Thompson called Dr. Kotze to have the dose changed to 0.06 mg of Glycopyrrolate, which is: *0.06 mg/11.8 kg* = 0.005 mg/kg, an appropriate dose for this 2-year-old child. Doses like this that are small decimal fractions of a milligram are better written on a microgram basis, 60 mcg as opposed to 0.06 mg, because it is easier to spot decimal point errors.

Promethazine HCl: *12 mg/11.8 kg = 1.0 mg/kg*—OK, within the recommended range

Ingredient Amounts

Na Phenobarbital:

Injectable solution is 65 mg/mL. The volume for the 25-mg dose is:

$$\frac{65\,mg\,Pb}{mL} = \frac{25\,mg\,Pb}{x\,mL}; x = 0.38\,mL + 0.1\,mL\ excess\ for\ priming$$

Glycopyrrolate

Injectable solution is 0.2 mg/mL (or 200 mcg/mL). The volume for the 60-mcg dose is:

$$\frac{200\,mcg\,Glycopy.}{mL} = \frac{60\,mcg\,Glycopy.}{x\,mL}; x = 0.3\,mL + excess\ for\ priming$$

Promethazine HCl:

Injectable solution is 25 mg/mL. The volume for the 12-mg dose is:

$$\frac{25\,mg\,PMZ}{mL} = \frac{12\,mg\,PMZ}{mL}; x = 0.48\,mL + excess\ for\ priming$$

To mix Glycopyrrolate and Promethazine, draw the dose volume of each plus an amount for priming. To get the amount of each solution for priming, find the volume fraction of the drug in the total dose volume and multiply this times the total priming volume of 0.1 mL.

Calculating the priming volume for Glycopyrrolate and Promethazine:

1. Calculate the total volume per dose: *0.3 mL + 0.48 mL = 0.78 mL.*

2. Calculate the volume fraction of Glycopyrrolate: *0.3/0.78 = 0.38.*

3. Calculate the volume fraction of Promethazine: *0.48/0.78 = 0.62.*

4. The priming volume of Glycopyrrolate is its volume fraction times the total priming volume desired: *0.38 × 0.1 mL = 0.038 or 0.04 mL*. The total volume of Glycopyrrolate is the dose volume plus its calculated priming volume: *0.3 mL + 0.04 mL = 0.34 mL*.

5. The priming volume of Promethazine is its volume fraction times the total priming volume desired: *0.62 × 0.1 mL = 0.062 or 0.06 mL*. The total volume of Promethazine is the dose volume plus its calculated priming volume: *0.48 mL + 0.06 mL = 0.54 mL*.

Note: In this case, the final dose volume is close to 1 mL and the individual dose volumes are fairly close to equal, so it would be acceptable to just divide the priming volume equally between the two injections. In cases for which the total dose volume is very small (0.5 mL or less) and/or the individual dose volumes are small but significantly different, this procedure of using the volume fractions to determine the priming volume of each injection should be followed.

Compounding Procedure

Use aseptic technique in all procedures for preparing this sterile product. Remove jewelry and wash hands and forearms with germicidal soap. Don a clean, low-shedding gown and hair and foot covers; lastly, put on sterile protective gloves. Wipe the surfaces of the LAFW with 70% Isopropyl Alcohol using sterile 4x4's. Assemble all materials. Wipe all diaphragms of vials and all ampules with alcohol wipes. With a 1-mL syringe, withdraw 0.48 mL of Phenobarbital Na Injection from its vial. Remove the needle and put on Luer tip cap. In a separate 1-mL syringe, withdraw 0.34 mL of Glycopyrrolate. Replace the needle guard and place the syringe on an alcohol swab. Using a separate syringe and a regular needle, withdraw **an excess** of 0.54 mL Promethazine Injection from its ampule. Switch the needle to a filter needle, fill the new needle with drug solution, and expel the excess volume in the syringe to the 0.54-mL mark. Take a new 3-mL syringe, pull back the plunger to a volume in excess of 0.88 mL. Shoot the 0.34 mL of Glycopyrrolate and the 0.54 mL of Promethazine into this third syringe. Agitate to mix and inspect for solution clarity. Expel any excess air from the syringe. Place Luer cap over the syringe tip. Remove the syringes from the hood and label each syringe, indicating on each syringe label that the syringe contains 0.1 mL excess for priming. Dispense both syringes, properly labeled, into one labeled zip-closure bag.

Quality Control

All volumes are checked and confirmed. The solutions in the syringes are inspected and found to be clear and free of turbidity or particulates.

Labeling

Phenobaribital Na:

Syringe label

> Phenobarbital Na 25 mg/0.38 mL   Control # 000000-8
> For IM use
> This syringe contains 0.1 mL excess for priming
> Do not use after 1700 00/02/00

Zipper-closure bag label

> ℞ #119   Control # 000000-8
> Jason Matthaus
> Room 783   Medical Record #526942
> Phenobarbital Na 25 mg/0.38 mL   For IM Use
> Give 0.38 mL one hour prior to surgery.
> This syringe contains 0.1 mL excess for priming.
> Do not use after 1700 00/02/00

Auxiliary labels: Keep in the refrigerator, Do not freeze (optional since
this is to be used immediately);
Beyond-use date is 48-hours

Glycopyrrolate and Promethazine HCl:

Syringe label

> Glycopyrrolate 60 mcg and Promethazine HCl 12 mg/0.78 mL
> Control #000000-9   For IM use
> This syringe contains 0.1 mL excess for priming
> Do not use after 1700 00/02/00

Zipper-closure bag label

> ℞ #119   Control # 000000-9
> Jason Matthaus
> Room 783   Medical Record #526942
> Glycopyrrolate 60 mcg and Promethazine HCl 12 mg/0.78 mL
> For IM Use.
> Give 0.78 mL IM one hour prior to surgery.
> This syringe contains 0.1 mL excess for priming.
> Do not use after 1700 00/02/00

Auxiliary labels: Keep in the refrigerator, Do not freeze (optional since
this is to be used immediately);
Beyond-use date is 48-hours

➤ **Medication Order 32-9**

MEDICAL CENTER HOSPITAL
Triturate, Wisconsin 53706

PATIENT ORDERS

Patient Name: Hortense Hartman
History Number 849502   Room Number: Outpatient
Weight: 110 lbs   Height: 5'7"
Age: 53 years
Attending Physician: Lance Smitby, MD

Date	Time	Orders
00/01/00	1000	Use standard CMF regimen for breast cancer:
		Day 1, 00/01/00 Cycle 1
		1. Cyclophosphamide 100 mg/m² PO
		Give on days 1 through 14 (00/01/00 through 00/14/00)
		2. Methotrexate 40 mg/m² IV in NS 50 mL. Infuse over 15 minutes.
		Give on days 1 and 8 (00/01/00 and 00/08/00)
		3. Fluorouracil 600 mg/m² IV in NS ~~500 mL~~. Infuse over ~~4 hr~~
		Give on days 1 and 8 (00/01/00 and 00/08/00) *Note change of order*
		Put Fluorouracil in 50 mL NS and infuse over 10 minutes. JET/LS
		4. Ondansetron 24 mg PO and Dexamethasone 20 mg PO 30 minute
		prior to CMF, then Ondansetron 8 mg PO BID and Dexamethasone
		8 mg PO BID × 3 days. May take Ondansetron 8 mg PO q 8 hr
		prn on days 4 thorugh 14. *Lance Smitby, MD*
		J. Thompson 00/01/00

Materials Needed

Cyclophosphamide: 50-mg tablets

Methotrexate:
1. Drug: Methotrexate Injection, 25 mg/mL 10-mL vial
2. Primary Fluid: Sodium Chloride 0.9% in Water for Injection, 50 mL
3. Syringe(s) used in preparation: 3-mL
4. Needle(s) used in preparation: 20-g 1-inch
5. IV set that delivers 20 drops/mL

Fluorouracil:
1. Drug: Fluorouracil Injection 50 mg/mL, 20-mL vial
2. Primary Fluid: Sodium Chloride 0.9% in Water for Injection, 50 mL
3. Syringe(s) used in preparation: 20-mL
4. Needle(s) used in preparation: 20-g 1-inch
5. IV set that delivers 20 drops/mL

Therapeutic Intent: Chemotherapy for breast cancer

Compatibility–Stability/Beyond-Use Date

Cyclophosphamide: Not applicable; these are manufactured tablets for oral use.

Methotrexate Sodium:
Stability–Compatibility: The Methotrexate Na is available as prepared solutions and as a lyophilized powder. The solutions are available both preserved and preservative-free. This pharmacy has 10-mL vials of the preserved solution, which has a concentration of 25 mg/mL. It is compatible with 0.9% Sodium Chloride Solution. The drug is photosensitive; at the concentration used for this order, and when in a PVC bag, it is reported that there is significant loss in 8 to 12 hours unless protected from light (8).
Packaging and Storage and Beyond-use date: Although this drug solution may be stored in the refrigerator, it will be made shortly before use and will be stored at controlled room temperature. Because of its photolability, it will be given a 4-hour beyond-use dating.

Fluorouracil:
Stability–Compatitility: Fluorouracil is available as a prepared solution in a concentration of 50 mg/mL. It is compatible with 0.9% Sodium Chloride Solution. The drug is photosensitive and should be inspected prior to use; the solution is normally colorless to faintly yellow and a slight discoloration does not affect its potency or safety. It should not be used if it is a darker yellow or if there are crystals present. It is stable in PVC bags (8).
Packaging and Storage and Beyond-use date: Although this drug solution may be stored in the refrigerator, and it will be labeled "Store in the refrigerator, Do not Freeze," it will be made shortly before use and will be stored at controlled room temperature until the time of use. If use is delayed, it will be stored in the refrigerator. The pharmacy will label this unpreserved LVP with its customary 48-hour beyond-use date, which is consistent with the policy of this hospital for IV solutions of this type.

Calculations

Dose/Concentration

Pharmacist Thompson consulted the cancer chemotherapy protocol for the CMF (Cyclophosphamide, Methotrexate, and Fluorouracil) regimen in the "Cancer Chemotherapy Update" feature of the journal *Hospital Pharmacy* (11). For the "Classic" or conventional CMF regimen, all the doses, concentrations, and flow rates for this order are within the protocol except the Fluorouracil. This drug is to be administered either IV push over 3 to 5 minutes or by IV infusion over less than 10 minutes. If given by infusion the drug is to be diluted in 50 to 100 mL of 0.9% Sodium Chloride or 5% Dextrose Injection. According to the reference, a short infusion time is essential, and extending it even to 15 minutes will result in a change in the drug's activity. Pharmacist Thompson has consulted with Dr. Smitby, and they have changed the order as indicated on the order sheet. Pharmacist Thompson will calculate the milligram doses for each drug and will transfer the order for the oral Cyclophosphamide tablets to an outpatient prescription order form to be dispensed by the hospital outpatient pharmacy. The IV drugs are given on days 1 and 8 of the 28-day cycle, and Pharmacist Thompson will keep track of the total dose per cycle (80 mg/m^2 for the Methotrexate and 1,200 mg/m^2 for the Fluorouracil).

Doses ordered in mg:

Ms. Hartman's BSA from the nomogram using her weight of 110 lb and height of 5'7" (67"): 1.57 m^2

Cyclophosphamide: *100 mg/m^2 × 1.57 m^2 = 157 mg*

Methotrexate: *40 mg/m^2 × 1.57 m^2 = 63 mg*

Fluorouracil: *600 mg/m^2 × 1.57 m^2 = 942 mg*

IV flow rates:

Methotrexate:

  mL/min: *50 mL/15 min = 3.3 mL/min*

   Drops/minute with a 20 drop/mL set: *20 drops/mL × 3.3 mL/min = 67 drops/min*

Fluorouracil:

   mL/minute: *70 mL/10 min = 7 mL/min* (Note: see below concerning volume)

   Drops/minute with 20 drop/mL set: *20 drops/mL × 7 mL/min = 140 drops/min*

Ingredient Amounts

Methotrexate:

Volume of Injection for 63-mg dose: $\dfrac{25\,mg\,MTX}{1\,mL} = \dfrac{63\,g\,mg\,MTX}{x\,mL}$; $x = 2.5\,mL\,MTX\,Injection$

Fluorouracil:

Volume of Injection for 942-mg dose: $\dfrac{50\,mg\,FU}{1\,mL} = \dfrac{942\,mg\,FU}{x\,mL}$; $x = 18.8\,mL\,FU\,Injection$

Because this volume is significant with respect to the 50 mL of the IV minibag, and because the flow rate of the Fluorouracil should not be extended, a rounded volume of 20 mL is added to the IV volume when calculating the flow rate above.

Cyclophosphamide:

This drug comes in 50-mg tablets. A dose of 150 mg (3 tablets) will be given daily for 14 days. The dose may be given either as a single dose or in divided doses, but it should be given early in the day to minimize exposure of the bladder to a toxic metabolite of the drug. It should be given with 6–8 oz fluid. The prescription order will be written for:

Cyclophosphamide 50 mg tablets **#42**

Sig: Take three tablets each morning with 6 to 8 ounces of liquid for 14 days.

Ms. Hartman will also be given prescription orders for the Ondansetron and Dexamethasone.

Compounding Procedure

Note: Because these are hazardous drugs, these procedures should be done in the biological safety cabinet, not in a horizontal LAFW. Use aseptic technique in all procedures for preparing these sterile products. Remove jewelry and wash hands and forearms with germicidal soap. Don a clean, low-shedding gown and hair and foot covers. For these cytotoxic drugs, double-glove and use a facemask. Wipe down the biological safety cabinet surfaces with 70% Isopropyl Alcohol using sterile 4x4's. Assemble necessary materials. Wipe diaphragms of vials and IV ports with alcohol swabs.

Methotrexate: From a 10-mL vial of Methotrexate 25 mg/mL, withdraw 2.5 mL using a 3-mL syringe and inject it into the port of a 50-mL bag of 0.9% Sodium Chloride Injection. Agitate gently to mix and inspect for solution clarity. Attach a port cover to the additive port. Label the bag with the patient-specific label and a Chemotherapy label and put the bag in a zipper-lock bag.

Fluorouracil: From a 20-mL vial of Fluorouracil 50 mg/mL, withdraw 18.8 mL using a 20-mL syringe and inject it into the port of a 50-mL bag of 0.9% Sodium Chloride Injection. Agitate gently to mix and inspect for solution clarity. Attach a port cover to the additive port. Label the bag with the patient-specific label and a Chemotherapy label and put the bag in a zipper-lock bag.

Quality Control

All volumes are checked and confirmed. The solutions are inspected and found to be clear and free of particulates and turbidity.

Labeling

Zipper-closure bag label

```
℞ #121          Control # 000000-10              Bottle #1
Patient Name: Hortense Hartman      Rm. No. Outpatient
Medical Record #: 849502
Additives:
          Methotrexate 63 mg

IN:     0.9% Sodium Chloride  50 mL
                      15 minutes
                   hours/start time
                  mL/hr  3.3 mL/min
               67 drops/min (20 drops/mL)
           1100 00/01/00 date/time prep/Prep by JET
           1500 00/01/00 infuse before/Chk'd by BJF
```

Auxiliary labels: Keep in the Refrigerator, Do not freeze

Zipper-closure bag label

```
℞ #122          Control # 000000-11              Bottle #1
Patient Name: Hortense Hartman      Rm. No. Outpatient
Medical Record #: 849502
Additives:
          Fluorouracil 942 mg

IN:     0.9% Sodium Chloride  50 mL
                      10 minutes
                   hours/start time
                  mL/hr  7 mL/min
               140 drops/min (20 drops/mL)
           1100 00/01/00 date/time prep/Prep by JET
           1100 00/03/00 infuse before/Chk'd by BJF
```

Auxiliary labels: Keep in the Refrigerator, Do not freeze

References

1. The 2002 United States Pharmacopeia 25/National Formulary 20. Rockville, MD: The United States Pharmacopeial Convention, Inc., 2001;1833.
2. Garkinkle BD, Henley MW. Sterilization. In Gennaro AR, ed. Remington: The science and practice of pharmacy, 20th ed. Philadelphia: Lippincott William & Wilkins, 2000;753.
3. The 2002 United States Pharmacopeia 25/National Formulary 20. Rockville, MD: The United States Pharmacopeial Convention, Inc., 2001;2234–2247.
4. Center for Drug Evaluation and Research. Sterile Drug Products Produced by Aseptic Processing Draft, Preliminary Concept Paper. Rockville, MD: Food and Drug Administration; Sept. 2002, www.fda.gov/cder/dmpq/aseptic-cp.pdf. Accessed December 2002.
5. Center for Drug Evaluation and Research. Sterile Drug Products Produced by Aseptic Processing. Rockville, MD: Food and Drug Administration; June 1987.
6. Moussa M, Rahe H, Lo K. Technology spotlight: barrier isolators. IJPC. 2003;7:42–43.
7. Howry LB, Bindler RM, Tso Y. Pediatric medications. Philadelphia: JB Lippincott, 1981;62.
8. Trissel LA, ed. Handbook of injectable drugs, 12th ed. Bethesda, MD: The American Society of Health-System Pharmacists, 2003.
9. USP DI, Vol. I, 22d ed. Greenwood Village, CO: MICROMEDEX Thomson Healthcare, 2002.
10. Drug facts and comparisons, 2002 ed. St Louis, MO: Facts and Comparisons, 2001;317.
11. Waddell JA, Holder NA, Solimando, DA Jr. Cyclophosphamide, methotrexate, and fluorouracil (CMF) regimen. Hosp Pharm 1999;34: 1268–1277.

CHAPTER 33

Parenteral Nutrition

I. DEFINITIONS

A. As the name implies, **Total Parenteral Nutrition** (TPN), or **Total Nutrition Admixture** (TNA), is IV therapy that provides nutrition to patients who cannot take nourishment by mouth.
  1. The aim of TPN is to replace and maintain by IV infusion essential nutrients when (and **only when**) oral or tube feedings are contraindicated or inadequate. It is used only when necessary because of the risks associated with this therapy and the high cost of this treatment.
  2. Typical situations when TPN is used include:
     a. Severely undernourished patients without oral intake > 1 week
     b. Severe pancreatitis
     c. Severe inflammatory bowel disease (Crohn's disease and ulcerative colitis)
     d. Extensive bowel surgery (i.e., short bowel syndrome)
     e. Small bowel obstruction (SBO)
     f. Pregnancy (in cases of severe nausea and vomiting)
     g. Head-injury patients

B. "All-in-One," "3-in-1," or Total Nutrient Admixtures (TNA) formulations are TPNs that contain IV fat emulsion in the same container with traditional amino acids, dextrose, and electrolytes.

C. Hyperalimentation (HA) is an older term for TPN.

D. PPN stands for Peripheral Parenteral Nutrition. It is described in the Special Topics section later in this chapter.

II. BASIC REQUIREMENTS AND CONSIDERATIONS FOR TPN THERAPY

A. What to give
  1. Basic nutrients and fluid
     a. Dextrose—the major source of calories; each gram of dextrose provides 3.4 kcal.
     b. Amino acids—for the protein synthesis required for tissue growth and repair; each gram of protein provides 4 kcal.

    c. Fat—for required essential fatty acids and as a source of calories; each gram of fat provides 9 kcal.

    d. Basic electrolytes—Na, K, Mg, Ca, phosphate

    e. Vitamins

    f. Trace elements—Cu, Cr, Zn, Mn, Se

  2. Histamine H_2-receptor antagonists—to prevent and treat upper gastrointestinal, stress-related ulceration; these medications are often included in TPN formulations.

B. To avoid exceeding normal daily fluid limitations, the nutrients are usually administered as highly concentrated, hypertonic solutions. To give some perspective, approximate osmolarities (in mOsm/L) of plasma, two large-volume parenteral solutions, and a typical TPN are given here:

Plasma	300
0.9% NaCl	300
D5W	250
TPN (central)	1800

C. Vein damage that would be caused by giving these highly hypertonic TPN solutions is minimized by administering the TPN solution through a large-diameter central vein where blood flow is rapid. This enables the TPN solution to be diluted rapidly as it flows into the body.

  1. The usual position of the central catheter is the superior vena cava. Because this vessel is near vital organs and blood supplies, catheter placement is verified by radiograph.

  2. If a peripheral vein is used for administration of parenteral nutrition, the solution given must be less hypertonic. PPN solutions have osmolarities of approximately 700–900 mOsm/L.

  3. Heparin (3,000 units/day) and hydrocortisone (5 mg/L) are often added to PPN formulations to decrease the risk of thrombophlebitis.

III. NUTRIENTS AND FLUID REQUIREMENTS

The values given in this section are the average 24-hour requirements for an adult. (See also the TPN Example and Table 33.2, TPN Requirement Worksheet, at the end of this chapter.) Reference 1 contains an excellent review of TPN requirements (1). Other good sources of information include the Internet sites of the American Society of Parenteral and Enteral Nutrition (ASPEN) at www.nutritioncare.org and the Baxter Healthcare Corporation at www.nutriforum.com.

A. Body Weight

  1. Actual body weight (ABW) is most commonly used for calculation of fluid and nutritional requirements. When the actual weight of a patient exceeds Ideal Body Weight (IBW) by 30% (i.e., ABW > 130% IBW), an adjusted body weight can be determined for calculation of nutritional requirements. The following equation may be used to calculate adjusted body weight:

Adjusted body weight = (Actual body weight − IBW) 0.25 + IBW

  2. For the equations used to calculate IBW, refer to Chapter 8.

    Note: In the sample calculations for fluid and nutrient requirements given below, a "typical" adult with ABW of 70 kg is used.

B. Fluid Requirements

  1. General: 2,500–3,500 mL for an average adult

                500–2,000 mL for an adult in renal failure (depending on the severity of the disease)

  2. Based on body weight: (two different methods are shown)

    a. **30-35 mL/kg ABW**

      Example: For a 70-kg adult = 30 to 35 mL/kg × 70 kg = 2,100 to 2,450 mL

    b. 1,500 mL/1st 20 kg, then 20 mL/for each kg ABW above the first 20 kg

        Example: For a 70-kg adult = 1,500 mL + (20 mL/kg × 50 kg) = 2,500 mL

C. Protein (Amino Acid) Requirements

    1. General: **0.8 − 2.0 g protein (amino acids)/kg ABW**

        Example: For a 70-kg adult: 0.8 to 2.0 g/kg × 70 kg = 56 to 140 g amino acids.

    2. The amount of amino acids given will depend on the stress level and/or the extent and level of body injury, with 1 g protein/kg given for mild stress and up to 2 g/kg for severe stress.

D. Dextrose

    1. Dextrose is the major source of non-protein kcals, but IV fat is also used.

    2. General requirements

        a. **3–5 mg/kg/min**

            Example: 24-hour dextrose requirement for a 70-kg adult:

$$\left(\frac{3-5\,mg\,Dextrose}{kg\,/\,min}\right)\left(70\,kg\right)\left(\frac{1\,g}{1000\,mg}\right)\left(\frac{1440\,min}{day}\right) = 302 - 504\,g\,Dextrose\,/\,day$$

        Notice that to furnish this amount of dextrose using a 10% Dextrose solution, 3,020 to 5,040 mL per 24 hours would be required, greatly exceeding the normal daily fluid requirements. This is why more concentrated dextrose solutions (20–30% dextrose) are required for TPN therapy; this explains why TPN solutions are so highly hypertonic.

E. IV Fat Emulsion

    1. Available as 10, 20, or 30% emulsions

        a. The 10% product supplies 1 kcal/mL, the 20% product 2 kcal/mL, and the 30% product 3 kcal/mL.

        b. The osmolarity ranges from 200 to 300 mOsmol/L, with glycerin added to make the fat emulsions isotonic.

        c. The 30% product is indicated ONLY for administration as part of a 3-in-1 or TNA.

    2. Uses

        a. Originally, IV fat emulsion was given in one of two ways:

            (1) Administered two or three times/week as a separate IV, not primarily as a calorie source, but to prevent essential fatty acid depletion (EFAD)

            (2) Administered daily

                (a) For patients, such as diabetics, who have difficulty tolerating high dextrose loads, IV fat emulsion was given by constant infusion as a source of calories. It was administered in a separate IV by using a Y-tubing IV administration setup.

                (b) For patients on PPN, IV fat emulsion either was mixed directly with a concentrated TPN solution or the two IVs were run together using Y-tubing. In this case, the fat emulsion served as a calorie source while cutting down on the total osmolarity of the solution.

        b. Now it is recognized that most patients require daily fat, so IV fat emulsion is given on a daily basis to nearly all patients.

        (1) **IV fat should represent 1-4% of the total calories delivered to prevent EFAD.**

        (2) The dextrose, amino acids, electrolytes, and fat emulsion are often incorporated into one container. These are referred to as "All-in-One" or "3-in-1" solutions, or TNAs, and these preparations are infused via a central vein.

            CAUTION: In the spring of 1994, several deaths were reported with patients using these combined solutions. Autopsies showed the presence of precipitated calcium phosphate in the lungs of these patients; apparently the precipitation occurred in the 3-in-1 solutions' and its presence was masked by the fat emulsion. As a result, the FDA has issued guidelines for compounding these solutions (see the *FDA Safety Alert* in Fig. 33.1). An analysis of the factors affecting precipitation of calcium phosphate is given in section IV. C.

(3) When provided on a daily basis, it is recommended that **no more than 30% of the total daily calories be administered as IV fat over a 12- to 24-hour period** to avoid immune dysfunction.

■ **Figure 33.1** FDA Safety Alert

 DEPARTMENT OF HEALTH & HUMAN SERVICES   Public Health Service

Food and Drug Administration
Rockville MD 20857

FDA SAFETY ALERT:
Hazards of Precipitation Associated with Parenteral Nutrition

To: **Hospital Pharmacists**   April 18, 1994
     Hospital Risk Managers
     Hospital Nutritional Support Teams
     Home Health Care Nutrition Support Services
     Hospital Directors of Nursing
     Home Care Pharmacists
     Home Care Nurses
     Physicians

This is to alert you of a concern that precipitate formation in total parenteral nutrition (TPN) admixtures may present a life-threatening hazard to your patients.

The Food and Drug Administration has received a report from one institution of 2 deaths and at least 2 cases of respiratory distress, which developed during peripheral infusion of a three-in-one (amino acids, carbohydrate and lipids) TPN admixture. The admixture contained 10% FreAmine III, dextrose, calcium gluconate, potassium phosphate, other minerals, and a lipid emulsion all of which were combined using an automated compounder. The solution may have contained a precipitate of calcium phosphate. Autopsies revealed diffuse microvascular pulmonary emboli containing calcium phosphate. One literature report cites an adult case of subacute interstitial pneumonitis associated with calcium phosphate precipitates.[1]

TPN solutions are made according to a variety of formulations and compounding protocols. Thus, there are possibilities of calcium phosphate precipitates and many other chemical incompatibilities. Precipitates could develop because of a number of factors such as: the concentration, pH, and phosphate content of the amino acid solutions; the calcium and phosphorous additives; the order of mixing; the mixing process; or the compounder. The presence of a lipid emulsion in the TPN admixture would obscure the presence of any precipitate.

Because of the potential for life threatening events, caution should be taken to ensure that precipitates have not formed in any parenteral nutrition admixtures.

There is a medical need for the use of parenteral nutrition in some patients. Until data can be developed and validated to support specific recommendations for TPN preparation, the FDA suggests the following steps to decrease the risk of additional injuries:

1. The amounts of phosphorous and of calcium added to the admixture are critical. The solubility of the added calcium should be calculated from the volume at <u>the time the calcium is added</u>. It should not be based upon the final volume.

   Some amino acid injections for TPN admixtures contain phosphate ions (as a phosphoric acid buffer). These phosphate ions and <u>the volume at the time the phosphate is added</u> should be considered when calculating the concentration of phosphate additives. Also, when adding calcium and phosphate to an admixture, the phosphate should be added first.

   The line should be flushed between the addition of any potentially incompatible components.

■ **Figure 33.1** *Continued*

2.   A lipid emulsion in a three-in-one admixture obscures the presence of a precipitate. Therefore, if a lipid emulsion is needed, either: (1) use a two-in-one admixture with the lipid infused separately, or (2) if a three-in-one admixture is medically necessary, then add the calcium before the lipid emulsion and according to the recommendations in number 1 above.

     If the amount of calcium or phosphate which must be added is likely to cause a precipitate, some or all of the calcium should be administered separately. Such separate infusions must be properly diluted and slowly infused to avoid serious adverse events related to the calcium.

3.   When using an automated compounding device, the above steps should be considered when programming the device. In addition, automated compounders should be maintained and operated according to the manufacturer's recommendations. Any printout should be checked against the programmed admixture and weight of components.

4.   During the mixing process, pharmacists who mix parenteral nutrition admixtures should periodically agitate the admixture and check for precipitates. Medical or home care personnel who start and monitor these infusions should carefully inspect for the presence of precipitates both before and during the infusion. Patients and caregivers should be trained to visually inspect for signs of precipitation. They also should be advised to stop the infusion and seek medical assistance if precipitates are noted.

5.   A filter should be used when infusing either central or peripheral parenteral nutrition admixtures. At this time, data has not been submitted to document which size filter is most effective in trapping precipitates.

     Standards of practice vary, but the following is suggested: a 1.2 micron air eliminating filter for lipid containing admixtures, and a 0.22 micron air eliminating filter for nonlipid containing admixtures.

6.   Parenteral nutrition admixtures should be administered within the following time frames: if stored at room temperature, the infusion should be started within 24 hours after mixing; if stored at refrigerated temperatures, the infusion should be started within 24 hours of rewarming. Because warming parenteral nutrition admixtures may contribute to the formation of precipitates, once administration begins, care should be taken to avoid excessive warming of the admixture.

     Persons administering home care parenteral nutrition admixtures may need to deviate from these time frames. Pharmacists who initially prepare these admixtures should check a reserve sample for precipitates over the duration and under the conditions of storage.

7.   If symptoms of acute respiratory distress, pulmonary embolus, or interstitial pneumonitis develop, the infusion should be stopped immediately and thoroughly checked for precipitates. Appropriate medical intervention should be instituted. Home care personnel and patients should immediately seek medical assistance.

These recommendations represent the best advice that the FDA can provide at this time. The FDA recognizes there may be alternative safety measures which could be taken to prevent the infusion of precipitates in TPN admixtures. The FDA has requested that industry develop and submit data that will be used to revise relevant labeling (instructions for use) to clarify these issues.

Practitioners who become aware of similar or other drug or device related deaths, serious illnesses and/or serious injuries are asked to notify the FDA. Please submit your reports to MedWatch, Medical Product Reporting Program, by phone at 1-800-FDA-1088 (also call for MedWatch information); by FAX at 1-800-FDA-0178; by modem at 1-800-FDA-7737; or by mail to MedWatch, HF-2, Food and Drug Administration, 5600 Fishers Lane, Rockville, MD 20857.

The Safe Medical Devices Act of 1990 (SMDA) requires hospitals and other facilities to report death, serious illness and injury associated with the use of medical devices. You should follow the procedures established by your facility for such mandatory reporting. Practitioners who become

■ **Figure 33.1** *Continued*

aware of any medical device related adverse event or product problem/malfunction should report to their Medical Device User Facility Reporting person. If it is not reportable under the SMDA, it may be reported directly to MedWatch.

If you have any questions regarding this Safety Alert, please contact Thomas J. McGinnis, RPH, Office of Health Affairs, Food and Drug Administration, 5600 Fishers Lane, Rockville, MD 20857; by phone 1-800-238-7332; or by FAX at 1-800-344-3332.

Sincerely yours,

Murray M. Lumpkin, M.D.
Acting Director
Center for Drug Evaluation
and Research

D. Bruce Burlington, M.D.
Director
Center for Devices and
Radiological Health

3. Disadvantages, cautions, and precautions with IV fat emulsion
   a. A complication similar to an allergic reaction (chills, chest pain, sensation of warmth) occurs rarely (<1%). To check, patients can be started at a slow rate (1 mL/min for 30 minutes) and the product can be discontinued if a reaction occurs. However, this test dose is rarely performed in clinical practice.
   b. It is contraindicated in patients with egg allergies because the emulsion is stabilized with egg phospholipids.
   c. IV preparations containing fat emulsion cannot be filtered with standard 0.22-micron in-line IV filters because these would filter out the fat globules; a 1.2-micron filter is therefore recommended.
   d. There is a limit to the amount of calories that can be supplied by fat; according to the product package insert for IV fat emulsion, the absolute maximum is 60%. All patients need a certain amount of dextrose per day.
   e. It must be used cautiously in patients who have phosphate restrictions (such as patients in renal failure) because it contains approximately 7.5 mM P/500 mL.
   f. It should be used cautiously in patients with a history of hyperlipidemia.
   g. It must be used cautiously in preterm infants because they have immature hepatic function and therefore poor clearance of fat that can accumulate in the lungs. This may be fatal.
   h. Questions exist regarding the immunosuppressant activity of fat emulsion when it is given by bolus infusion (i.e., <6 hours). This does not seem to be a problem when IV fat is given slowly by continuous IV infusion over a 12- to 24-hour period. On the other hand, when IV fat emulsion is administered as a separate infusion in addition to dextrose/amino acids, it should be infused over no longer than 12 hours; this time limit is recommended to prevent the growth of microorganisms that can be inadvertently introduced into the manufacturer's original container during IV administration.
   i. The *USP* monograph for IV Fat Emulsion states that the product should always be examined visually before administration. It should not be used if there is any evidence of creaming, aggregation, coalescence, or any other form of phase separation.

F. Total kcal per day requirement

1. The general requirement for total kcal per day is 25 to 35 kcal/kg ABW.

2. As with the amino acid requirement, the amount of kcal/kg ABW will depend on the patient's stress level, disease state, and level of body injury. This is based on the theory that in certain disease states, more calories are expended.

3. There is some controversy about increasing the level of kcal/kg of ABW based on the level of stress: for example, 25 kcal/kg in mild stress, 30 kcal/kg with moderate stress, and 35 kcal/kg in severe stress. Since dextrose is the major source of calories, you may ask, "Would there be any problem with giving too much dextrose?" Remember from biochemistry:

$$4\ C_6H_{12}O_6\ \text{(excess dextrose)} + O_2 \rightarrow C_{16}H_{32}O_2\ \text{(fat)} + 8\ CO_2 + 8\ H_2O$$

Too much dextrose can result in:

a. Fat deposited in the liver, with the result of liver dysfunction

b. Excess carbon dioxide production with the result of respiratory distress, especially a problem with patients on a ventilator or with chronic obstructive pulmonary disease. If extra calories are needed for a patient with respiratory problems, IV fat should be given directly to avoid excess carbon dioxide production.

c. Generally, these problems develop when dextrose administration exceeds 7 mg/kg/min.

G. Electrolytes, Vitamins, and Trace Elements

1. Sodium: the parenteral recommended daily intake (RDI) is determined by clinical need; the approximate usual range is 1–2 mEq/kg ABW.

a. Sodium is principally an extracellular cation with no established RDI. Its inclusion in the TPN is based upon clinical need.

b. For example, patients with end-stage liver disease, congestive heart failure, or iatrogenic fluid overload may require severe sodium restriction.

c. Conversely, patients with large nasogastric fluid losses, high ileostomy or pancreatic fistula outputs, or significant small bowel losses often require substantial quantities of sodium per day.

2. Potassium: the parenteral RDI is determined by clinical need; the approximate usual range is 1–2 mEq/kg ABW.

a. Potassium is principally an intracellular cation with no established RDI; thus, its inclusion in the TPN is dictated by clinical need.

b. Potassium requirements can be greatly influenced by acid-base status.

   (1) During metabolic acidosis, an excess of hydrogen ions is present in the circulation, and potassium exchanges its intracellular position for hydrogen ions in an attempt to abate the acidemia, thus causing hyperkalemia.

   (2) Conversely, hypokalemia results during metabolic alkalosis.

3. Calcium: parenteral RDI is approximately 10 mEq or 200 mg Ca ion/day.

a. Up to 98% of total body calcium is in bone and can be readily mobilized in times of need under the influence of parathyroid hormone.

b. Certain patients, such as those with severe short bowel syndrome, those requiring massive blood transfusions, etc., may require substantially greater quantities of calcium; such increases given in the TPN admixture should be accomplished gradually.

c. Dosage increases of 5 mEq daily up to a total maximum of 20 mEq/day for acute care are reasonable, and simultaneous monitoring of serum phosphorus is recommended during such times.

4. Magnesium: parenteral RDI is approximately 10 mEq or 120 mg Mg ion/day.

a. Magnesium plasma concentration affects parathyroid hormone secretion, so this ion is closely linked to calcium metabolism.

b. Patients with short bowel syndrome, alcoholics, etc., often require larger doses to achieve magnesium homeostasis; as with calcium, the increased dose can be advanced incrementally by 5 mEq/day up to a total maximum of 40 mEq/day.

5. Phosphorus: parenteral RDI is approximately 30 mmol or 1,000 mg P/day.
   a. The role of phosphorus in physiological processes is diverse; it influences respiration, myocardial function, and platelet, red and white blood cell functions.
   b. In the presence of normal renal function, if phosphate is omitted from TPN formulations, a potentially life-threatening hypophosphatemia can be induced within a week of initiating the TPN therapy.
6. Trace Elements
   a. The normal daily requirements for trace elements are contained in each 3 mL of MTE-5®, which provides 12 mcg of chromium, 1.2 mg of copper, 0.3 mg of manganese, 60 mcg of selenium, and 3 mg of zinc.
   b. In certain conditions, additional selenium (for long-term home TPN) and zinc (for patients with high ileostomy/diarrheal outputs) may be necessary.

IV. SPECIAL TOPICS

A. Peripheral Parenteral Nutrition (PPN)
   1. PPN is given through a peripheral vein, usually in the arm.
   2. Because of the risk of phlebitis, these solutions should have an osmolarity approximately half that of central TPN solutions.
      Approximate osmolarities (in mOsmols/L):

Plasma	300
0.9% NaCl	300
D5W	250
D10W	500
IV fat emulsion	300
TPN	1800
PPN	900

   3. In essence, the electrolyte and IV fat contents of a PPN solution are similar to that for a central TPN, but the amino acid content is cut by approximately half and the dextrose concentration is greatly reduced.
   4. Uses of PPN
      a. PPN may be used to support patients who are able to ingest only a portion of their caloric and protein requirements orally or enterally and when central-vein TPN is not feasible.
      b. PPN is traditionally a short-term therapy (<10 days) because it does not provide total caloric/protein requirements, and these hypertonic solutions are not well tolerated by peripheral veins for extended periods.
      c. PPN is not recommended for patients with severe undernutrition, increased electrolyte needs (especially potassium), fluid restriction, or the need for prolonged IV nutrition support.

B. Special Amino Acid Solutions
   1. Formulas and descriptions of various specialty amino acid solutions can be found in *Drug Facts and Comparisons*. There are special formulations for patients under stress, those with hepatic failure, and those with renal disease.
   2. The use of these specialty products is somewhat controversial. They are usually more expensive than standard formulas, and some practitioners think they offer little significant clinical advantage. Additional information on this subject can be found in the journal article "Value of specialty intravenous amino acid solutions" in the March 15, 1996, issue of the *American Journal of Health-System Pharmacy*.
   3. Amino Acid Solutions for Patients with Hepatic Failure
      a. These solutions contain higher levels of branched-chain amino acids, such as isoleucine, leucine, and valine, and lower levels of aromatic amino acids (tryptophan, phenylalanine) and methionine. An example is HepatAmine®.

    b. This formula modification resulted from an analysis of the plasma content of patients with encephalopathy, a clinical complication found in patients with liver failure. It was noted that in the plasma of these patients, the ratio of aromatic amino acids to branched-chain amino acids is elevated. It was thought that the increased levels of aromatic amino acids may be contributing to the development of liver encephalopathy.

    c. Current recommendations support the use of branched-chain amino acid formulations only in chronic encephalopathy unresponsive to standard amino acid products and pharmacotherapy.

C. Factors Affecting the Precipitation of Calcium Phosphate in TPN Solutions

Calcium and phosphate, two nutritional requirements for TPN solutions, are conditionally compatible. Precipitation depends on numerous factors as described below (see also references 3–15). The chemical equation given here should aid in understanding these factors:

$$HPO_4^{-2} + Ca^{+2} \rightleftarrows H_2PO_4^{-1} + Ca^{+2}$$
$$\downarrow \qquad\qquad\qquad \downarrow$$
$$CaHPO_4\downarrow \qquad\qquad Ca(H_2PO_4)_2$$
$$\text{very insoluble} \qquad \text{relatively soluble}$$

    1. pH of the solution

The pH dependence of the phosphate-calcium precipitation is illustrated in the equation above. Dibasic calcium phosphate ($CaHPO_4$) is very insoluble, whereas monobasic calcium phosphate [$Ca(H_2PO_4)_2$] is relatively soluble. At low pH, the soluble monobasic form ($H_2PO_4^{-1}$) predominates, but as the pH increases, more dibasic phosphate (HPO_4^{-2}) becomes available to bind with calcium and precipitate. Therefore, the lower the pH of the parenteral solution, the more calcium and phosphate that can be solubilized.

    2. Concentration of the calcium

Because it is the free calcium that can form insoluble precipitates, enhanced precipitate formation is expected as the concentration of calcium is increased.

    3. Salt form of the calcium

Although Calcium Gluconate is much more soluble than Calcium Chloride, Calcium Chloride has a much higher percent dissociation. The higher the dissociation, the more free calcium available. The concentration of calcium available for precipitation when added as the Gluconate salt is less than that available when an equimolar amount of calcium is added as the chloride salt. Calcium Gluceptate has no real advantage over the Gluconate salt form.

    4. Concentration of the phosphate

As can be seen in the previous equations, it is the dibasic calcium phosphate salt that is insoluble. The concentration of dibasic phosphate in solution depends on both the total phosphate concentration and the pH of the solution. Potassium Phosphate Injection has a high pH (6.2–6.8) relative to that of Dextrose or Amino Acid solutions. Addition of Potassium Phosphate Injection to a TPN solution not only increases the concentration of the phosphate, but also may increase the pH of the solution, and that favors precipitation.

    5. Concentration of amino acids

Amino acids form soluble complexes with calcium and phosphate, reducing the amount of the free calcium and phosphate available for precipitation. Amino acids also appear to provide an intrinsic buffering system to a TPN solution. Amino Acid formulations have pH's in the range of 4.5–6.5. Those containing higher concentrations of amino acids show less of an increase in pH when phosphate is added and, consequently, an increased tolerance for calcium addition.

    6. Composition of amino acid solutions

Amino acid solutions formulated with electrolytes contain calcium and phosphate, and these must be considered in any projection of compatibility. Some amino acids contain cysteine hydrochloride, which may affect the solubility of calcium and phosphate. Cysteine hydrochloride lowers the pH of the solution, enabling the more soluble monobasic form of phosphate to exist. Therefore, adding cysteine hydrochloride can increase the solubility of calcium and phosphate in a TPN solution.

   7. Concentration of Dextrose in the solution

   Dextrose also forms a soluble complex with calcium and phosphate. It can also act as a weak buffer. The pH of Dextrose solutions is relatively low (4–5) due to the presence of free sugar acids (e.g., gluconic acid) present and formed from the oxidation of the aldehyde moiety on Dextrose during sterilization and storage of Dextrose solutions. Studies have shown that higher concentrations of Dextrose reduce the free calcium and phosphate that can form insoluble precipitates.

   8. Temperature of the solution

   As the temperature is increased, the calcium salts (chloride or gluconate) are dissociated more completely and more calcium ions become available for precipitation. Therefore, an increase in temperature increases the amount or possibility of precipitation. Care must be exercised when transferring these solutions to warmer environments such as neonate nurseries and cribs.

   9. Presence of other additives

   The addition of other drugs to a TPN solution may alter the pH of the solution. Additives may also introduce the possibility of precipitation of other products or incompatibilities with other ions.

   10. Order of mixing

   The FDA recommends that phosphate should be the first electrolyte added to the TNA admixture and calcium should be the last additive.

D.   Vitamins

   1. In April 2001, the FDA amended requirements for marketing of an "effective" adult parenteral multivitamin formulation and recommended changes to the 12-vitamin formulation that has been available for over 20 years.

   2. The new requirements for increased dosages of vitamins B_1, B_6, C, and folic acid as well as addition of vitamin K (creating a 13-vitamin formulation) are based on the recommendations from a 1985 workshop sponsored jointly by the American Medical Association's Division of Personal and Public Health Policy and FDA's Division of Metabolic and Endocrine Drug Products.

   3. Specific modifications of the previous formulation include increasing the provision of ascorbic acid (vitamin C) from 100 mg/day to 200 mg/day, pyridoxine (vitamin B_6) from 4 mg/day to 6 mg/day, thiamine (vitamin B_1) from 3 mg/day to 6 mg/day, folic acid from 400 mcg/day to 600 mcg/day, and addition of phylloquinone (vitamin K) 150 mcg/day.

   4. When using the 12-vitamin formulation, vitamin K can be given individually as a daily dose (0.5-1 mg/d) or a weekly dose (5-10 mg one time per week). Patients who are to receive warfarin for anticoagulation should be monitored more closely when receiving vitamin K to ensure the appropriate level of anticoagulation is maintained.

   5. Multiple vitamins may come in several different forms. They may be packaged as a lyophilized powder intended for reconstitution and dilution in a TPN. They may also be manufactured in two separate vials or in special mix-o-vial units that have two chambers separated by a rubber stopper that can be pushed down when the solutions are to be mixed.

   a.   These special formulations are necessary because of the limited compatibility and stability of several vitamins when combined.

   b.   The multivitamin solutions are mixed together and added to the TPN just before use. Often if the TPN is made at a site that is remote from the care site (e.g., home health care, nursing home), the vitamin unit is sent with the TPN solution and is mixed and added just before the TPN solution is hung.

   c.   The limited stability of the combined multiple vitamins should be considered in assigning a beyond-use date to a TPN solution that contains multiple vitamins.

E. Trace Elements

1. Trace Elements are added to the TPN solution once each day. Trace elements are commercially available as single- or multiple-entity products and in both pediatric and adult formulations.
2. Standard trace element solutions contain Se, Cr, Cu, Mn, and Zn. There are various other trace element solutions that contain Iodine or Molybdenum, alone or in combination, added to the standard trace elements.
3. Patients who have sustained small bowel or large bowel fluid losses should receive supplemental zinc (5-10 mg/d) added separately in addition to the amount in the trace element cocktail (3-5 mg/d).
4. Patients who have hepatic cholestasis should have copper and manganese withheld from the TPN solution because these trace elements are excreted in the bile. Neurological damage from deposition of manganese in the basal ganglia has been reported in PN patients with chronic liver disease or cholestasis.

F. Other Additives: Other components commonly added to TPN solutions include insulin, heparin, hydrocortisone, and histamine H_2-receptor antagonists.

G. Monitoring

1. For an excellent review article on parenteral nutrition monitoring, see "Parenteral Nutrition Monitoring in Hospitalized Patients" (2).
2. Monitoring parameters: See Table 33.1 for a sample TPN monitoring sheet.
    a. Temperature: daily to detect infection or sepsis
    b. Weight: daily to monitor fluid imbalance and maintenance and improvement of clinical condition. Generally, patients should gain only 1–2 pounds per week. Larger weight gains are usually retained fluid or fat from too many calories; a sudden weight gain usually reflects fluid retention.
    c. Nitrogen balance (NB): this monitors nitrogen utilization to determine if the patient's metabolic status is anabolic (buildup) or catabolic (breakdown). It is defined as the difference between the nitrogen intake and nitrogen excretion.

    $$NB = NI - NO$$

    NI is the nitrogen put into the body by TPN and other nutritional sources and NO is the nitrogen excreted by all routes.
    You may see two different, but equivalent, forms of this basic equation in the literature:

    $$NB = NI_{(g/24^\circ)} - (UUN_{(g/24^\circ)} + 4\ g)$$
    or
    $$NB = Protein_{(g/24^\circ)}\ /\ 6.25 - (UUN_{(g/24^\circ)} + 4\ g)$$

    NI is obtained by calculating the number of grams of protein infused in the form of amino acids and multiplying that by 16% (the approximate amount of nitrogen in amino acids). Note that you get the same number by dividing the number of grams of protein or amino acids given by 6.25. The grams of nitrogen can also be determined from the specifications for the particular amino acid solutions being used. This information can be found in the product package insert or the product description in *Drug Facts and Comparisons*.

    UUN stands for Urine Urea Nitrogen, a standard lab test. Urea is the breakdown product of protein.

    4 g is the estimated average loss by other routes, such as through the skin or in feces.

▶ *EXAMPLE*

1. J.S. is a patient receiving a TPN solution that provides 102 g protein per 24 hours. What is his $NI_{(g/24^\circ)}$?

    16% × 102 g Protein = 16.3 g N

    or

    102 g Protein/6.25 = 16.3 g N

TABLE 33.1	TPN Monitoring Sheet

Patient Name: _____ Location: _____ Medical Records #: _____
ABW: _____ IBW: _____ Height: _____ Age: _____
Est. kcal Req./Day _____
Problems & Comments: _____

Frequency		Date	Date	Date	Date	Date	Date	Date	Date	Date
D	WEIGHT (KG)									
D	INPUT (ML/DAY)									
D	OUTPUT (ML/DAY)									
D	TPN INF (ML/DAY)									
D	LIPID INF (ML/DAY)									
D	KCAL (ENTERAL)									
D	TOTAL KCAL									
D	TOTAL PROTEIN (G)									
B	WBC (3.5–10.0)									
W	HCT (40–50)									
	% SEGS									
	% BANDS									
W	PLATELETS (140–380)									
B	PT/PTT (10–13/23–36)									
W	SODIUM (135–144)									
W	POTASSIUM (3.6–4.8)									
W	CHLORIDE (99–108)									
W	CO2 CONTENT (24–33)									
W	GLUCOSE (70–110)									
B	UREA NITROGEN (7–20)									
B	CREATININE (.6–1.3)									
B	CALCIUM (8.8–10.4)									
B	PHOSPHORUS (2.6–4.4)									
B	URIC ACID (4.0–8.0)									
W	CHOLESTEROL (160–310)									
W	TOTAL PROTEIN (6.3–8.0)									
W	ALBUMIN (3.9–5.1)									
W	TOTAL BILI (0–1.4)									
W	GG-TRANSPEP (0–65)									
W	ALKPHOS (35–130)									
W	GO-TRANSAM (0–50)									
W	LDH (90–200)									
W	TRIGLY (<200)									
B	MAGNESIUM (1.7–2.3)									
	Miscellaneous									

Frequency Key: W = weekly   ø No labs drawn   Parameters are the minimum required
                   D = daily   –Values (current rate) may be obtained more often
                   B = biweekly

2. The 24-hour UUN reported by the lab is 9.5 g/24°.
3. Calculate the NB for this patient:

$$NB = 16.3 - (9.5 + 4) = 2.8 \ g$$

What is an acceptable value for NB? Although this depends on the clinical situation, a positive 4–6 g/day in unstressed patients is considered acceptable (2). If the NB is too low or is negative, the TPN formula can be changed to increase the amino acid content.

  d. Plasma proteins: concentrations of serum plasma proteins can be used as a measure of nutritional status because an increase in these reflects protein anabolism.

  (1) Serum albumin is the most commonly determined plasma protein, but its usefulness in monitoring nutritional status is limited because of its long half-life, because the body pool of albumin is large, and because its level in the serum is affected by so many other factors (2).

  (2) Two other plasma proteins, transferrin and prealbumin, have been found to be useful indicators (2).

e. Lab Tests
    (1) Table 33.1 shows a sample TPN monitoring sheet, including the typical frequency of lab tests. The lab tests that are performed and their frequency and normal values vary with the hospital and the clinical condition of the patient. Notice that there are hematologic tests, electrolyte and glucose concentrations, fat-cholesterol monitoring tests, and liver and renal function tests. For more detailed information on lab tests, see the article on monitoring TPN therapy (2).
    (2) Acceptable values for some lab tests may be different for patients on TPN than normal healthy individuals. For example, acceptable blood glucose concentrations are much higher for patients receiving TPN.
    (3) Monitoring of lab values with adjustments of TPN formulas and therapy is becoming a focal point of pharmacist input and participation on the health care team.
f. Clinical Status: how is the patient doing? This is a very important monitoring parameter. A desired clinical outcome of therapy should be determined and all efforts in TPN therapy should be geared toward this end.

➤ *EXAMPLE*

TPN Order

G.D. (Medical Record #200440, Room TLC-480) is a 52-year-old, 176-pound male who is 6'1" tall. He is admitted to the trauma unit after an automobile accident. He is not expected to eat or take tube feedings for >7 days due to multiple injuries to his small bowel. His physician, Dr. Solier, has written the following TPN order:

The prescribed 24-hour TPN is to contain:

Amino Acids	120 g
Dextrose	346 g
Fat	55 g
Sodium Chloride	110 mEq
Potassium Acetate	80 mEq
Sodium Phosphate	30 mmol
Magnesium Sulfate	24 mEq
Calcium Gluconate	10 mEq
Ranitidine	150 mg
Multivitamins	10 mL
Multiple Trace Elements	3 mL

The flow rate for this TPN is 100 mL/hr.

1. Calculate G.D.'s IBW and determine if the TPN requirements should be based on his ABW or an adjusted body weight.
2. Determine if all the nutrients, electrolytes, and fluid volume are within the normal range for G.D. You may ignore the electrolyte contributions in the amino acid solution and in the IV fat emulsion. See the text information in this chapter and Table 33.2, the TPN Requirement Worksheet, for the 24-hour requirements for electrolytes, trace elements, and vitamins. Sample calculations are given below with the results in Table 33.2.
3. This pharmacy will dispense a 24-hour TPN in one IV bag. Calculate the volume in milliliters of each component for each 24-hour bag of this TPN solution. You have the following supplies:

    – Crystalline amino acid solution as Travasol® 10%
    – Dextrose solution as Dextrose 70% in Water
    – IV Fat as IV Fat Emulsion 20%
    – Sterile Water for Injection
    – The concentrations of the various electrolytes and other additives are given in Figure 33.2, the TPN Formula Record.

Sample calculations are given below with the results recorded in Figure 33.2.

TABLE 33.2	TPN Requirement Worksheet

Patient Name: ___GD___   Age: ___52___
Height: ___6'1"___   Weight (ABW): ___176 lbs, 80kg___   IBW: ___80 kg___

Average 24-hour Adult Requirements for TPN Components

Component	Requirement	Amount Ordered	Evaluation
Fluid	30–35 mL/kg	30 mL/kg	OK
Protein (AA)	0.8–2.0 g AA/kg ABW	1.5 g AA/kg ABW	OK
Dextrose	3–5 mg/kg/min	3 mg/kg/min	OK
IV fat	≤ 30% of total kcal	23%	OK
kcal/kg ABW	25–35 kcal/kg ABW	26.9 kcal/kg ABW	OK
Sodium	1–2 mEq/kg ABW	1.9 mEq/kg	OK
Potassium	1–2 mEq/kg ABW	1 mEq/kg	OK
Phosphate	20–40 mmol	30 mmol	OK
Magnesium	8–20 mEq	24 mEq	OK
Calcium	10–15 mEq	10 mEq	OK
Trace Elements	3 mL	3 mL	OK
Vitamins	10 mL unit	10 mL unit	OK

■ **Figure 33.2** Total Parenteral Nutrition Formula Record

Patient Name: *GD*   Location: *TLC-480*   Medical Record # *200440*

Dosing Weight: 80 kg   Administration Date/Time: *00/01/00 @ 1600*

Expiration Date/Time: *00/02/00 @ 1600*   Bag ID #: *001*

Infusion Volume Ordered: *2400 mL*   Infusion Rate: *100 mL/hr*

Base Components	Concentration	Dose Ordered	Volume (mL)
Protein	Travasol 10%	120 g	1200
Dextrose	D70W	346	494
Fat Emulsion	20%	55	275

Additives	Concentration	Dose Ordered	Volume (mL)
Sodium Phosphate	3 mmol P/mL 4 mEq Na/mL	30 mEq	10
Sodium Chloride	4 mEq/mL	110 mEq	27.5
Potassium Acetate	2 mEq/mL	80 mEq	40
Magnesium Sulfate	4 mEq/mL	24 mEq	6
Calcium Gluconate	0.45 mEq/mL	10 mEq	22.2
Adult Multivitamins	-------	10 mL	10
Trace Elements	-------	3 mL	3
Ranitidine	25 mg/mL	150 mg	6

Additives per ion:

Na	150 mEq
K	80 mEq
Mg	24 mEq
Ca	10 mEq
Ac	80 mEq
Cl	110 mEq
P	30 mmol

Sample Calculations for 24-hour Requirements for GD

A. Body Weight
1. Weight in pounds (given): 176 pounds
2. Actual weight in kilograms:

$$\frac{176\ lb}{2.2\ lb/kg} = 80\ kg$$

3. IBW in kilograms: $IBW = 50\ kg + 2.3\ (13") = 79.9\ kg$
G.D.'s current ABW is appropriate for his height; no adjustment is needed.

B. Fluid
1. Volume ordered per day:
100 mL/hr × 24 hr/day = 2,400 mL

2. Fluid requirements: 30–35 mL/kg/day
2,400 mL/80 kg = 30 mL/kg—OK

C. Protein (Amino Acids)
1. Grams of protein ordered per day: 120 g Amino Acids (AA)
2. Protein (AA) requirement: 0.8 to 2.0 g/kg ABW
120 g AA/80 kg ABW = 1.5 g AA/kg ABW—OK
3. Kcal per day from ordered protein:
120 g AA/day × 4 kcal/g AA = 480 kcal/day

D. Dextrose
1. Grams of dextrose ordered per day: 346 g
2. General dextrose requirements: 3–5 mg/kg/min

$$\left(\frac{1000\ mg}{g}\right)\left(\frac{346\ g\ Dextrose}{day}\right)\left(\frac{day}{1440\ min}\right)\left(\frac{}{80\ kg}\right) = 3\ mg/kg/min - OK$$

3. Kcal per day from ordered dextrose:
346 g dextrose/day × 3.4 kcal/g dextrose = 1,176 kcal/day

E. IV Fat
1. Grams of fat ordered per day: 55 g
2. General requirements for IV fat: no more than 30% of total kcal/day
3. Kcal per day from ordered fat:
55 g fat/day × 9 kcal/g fat = 495 kcal/day
4. Total ordered kcal per day:
480 (AA) + 1,176 (dextrose) + 495 (fat) = 2,151 kcal/day
5. % of total kcal as IV fat:
495 kcal/2,151 kcal = 23% of total kcal as IV fat—OK

F. Total kcal/kg ABW per day
1. General requirements for total kcal per day: 25–35 kcal/kg ABW
2. Total ordered kcal/kg ABW per day:
2151 kcal/80 kg ABW = 26.9 kcal/kg/day—OK

G. Electrolytes
1. Phosphorus: the parenteral RDI of ~30 mmol is sufficient for most TPN patients.

30 mmol is ordered —OK

2. Sodium: generally, most patients require 1–2 mEq/kg/day in the TPN.
The Sodium (Na) comes from two sources, the Sodium Chloride (110 mEq) and the Sodium Phosphate (NaP). The Na concentration of the NaP solution is 4 mEq/mL. The volume of NaP to be added to the TPN is based on the desired amount of phosphate,

30 mmol. The volume for this is 10 mL. Therefore, the Na content from the NaP is calculated to be:

4 mEq/mL × 10 mL = 40 mEq Na

The total Na in the 24-hour TPN is calculated to be:

110 mEq (from the NaCl) + 40 mEq (from the NaP) = 150 mEq Na

The amount of Na based on mEq/kg/day is calculated to be:

150 mEq/80 kg ABW = 1.88 mEq/kg—OK

3. **Potassium:** generally most patients require 1-2 mEq/kg/day in the TPN.

    80 mEq is ordered
    80 mEq/80 kg ABW = 1 mEq/kg—OK

4. **Calcium:** the parenteral RDI of ~10 mEq/day is sufficient for most TPN patients. The range is 10-20 mEq/day.

    10 mEq is ordered—OK

5. **Magnesium:** the parenteral RDI of ~10 mEq/day is sufficient for most TPN patients. The range is 8-40 mEq/day.

    24 mEq is ordered —This is within the acceptable range.

Sample Calculations for IV Additives for Each 24-hour Supply of TPN

See Figure 33.2, Total Parenteral Nutrition Formula Record, for concentrations of ingredients.

A. Amino Acids
From Travasol 10%:

$$\frac{10\ g\ AA}{100\ mL\ Travasol} = \frac{120\ g\ AA}{x\ mL\ Travasol}; x = 1200\ mL\ Travasol$$

B. Dextrose
From Dextrose 70% (D 70W):

$$\frac{70\ g\ Dextrose}{100\ mL\ D70W} = \frac{346\ g\ Dextrose}{x\ mL\ D70W}; x = 494\ mL\ D70W$$

C. IV Fat
From IV Fat Emulsion 20%:

$$\frac{20\ g\ Fat}{100\ mL\ IV\ Fat\ Emulsion} = \frac{55\ g\ Fat}{x\ mL\ IV\ Fat\ Emulsion}; x = 275\ mL\ IV\ Fat\ Emulsion$$

D. Sodium Phosphate
From Sodium Phosphate (NaP) 3 mmol P/mL:

$$\frac{3\ mmol\ P}{mL\ NaP} = \frac{30\ mmol\ P}{x\ mL\ NaP}; x = 10\ mL\ NaP$$

E. Potassium Acetate
From Potassium Acetate (KAc) 2 mEq K/mL:

$$\frac{2\ mEq\ K^+}{mL\ KAc} = \frac{80\ mEq\ K^+}{x\ mL\ KAc}; x = 40\ mL\ KAc$$

F. Sodium Chloride
From Sodium Chloride (NaCl) 4 mEq/mL:

$$\frac{4\ mEq\ Na^+}{mL\ NaCl} = \frac{110\ mEq\ Na^+}{mL\ NaCl}\ ; x = 27.5\ mL\ NaCl$$

G. Magnesium Sulfate
From Magnesium Sulfate ($MgSO_4$) 4 mEq/mL:

$$\frac{4\ mEq\ Mg^{+2}}{mL\ MgSO_4} = \frac{24\ mEq\ Mg^{+2}}{x\ mL\ MgSO_4}\ ; x = 6\ mL\ MgSO_4$$

H. Calcium Gluconate
From Calcium Gluconate (CaGluc) 0.45 mEq/mL:

$$\frac{0.45\ mEq\ Ca^{+2}}{mL\ CaGluc} = \frac{10\ mEq\ Ca^{+2}}{x\ mL\ CaGluc}\ ; x = 22.2\ mL\ CaGluc$$

(Note: See Fig. 33.1 for safety alert.)

I. Trace Elements
From MTE-5®: 3 mL

J. Multiple Vitamins
From Infuvite®: 10 mL

K. Ranitidine
From Ranitidine Injection 25 mg/mL:

$$\frac{25\ mg\ Ranitidine}{mL} = \frac{150\ mg\ Ranitidine}{x\ mL}\ ; x = 6\ mL$$

L. Sterile Water for Injection
A total 24-hour fluid volume of 2,400 mL is needed to give the TPN at a rate of 100 mL/hr. Therefore, the volumes of all additives are added and the sum is subtracted from 2,400 mL to determine the amount of Sterile Water for Injection to add for the desired final volume of 2,400 mL.

The volumes of each additive are calculated above and are shown in the last column of Figure 33.2. The sum of these values is 2,093.7 mL ≈ 2,094 mL. Therefore, the volume of Sterile Water for Injection to add is 306 mL:

$$2,400\ mL - 2,094\ mL = 306\ mL$$

References

1. McMahon MM, Farnell MB, Murray JM. Nutritional support of critically ill patients. Mayo Clin Proc 1993;68:911–920.
2. Manzo CB, Dickerson RN. Parenteral nutrition monitoring in hospitalized patients. Hospital Pharmacy 1993;28:561–568.
3. Schuetz DH, King JC. Compatibility and stability of electrolytes, vitamins and antibiotics in combination with 8% amino acids solution. Am J Hosp Pharm 1978;35:33–44.
4. Pinkus TF, Jeffrey LP. Incompatibility of calcium and phosphate in parenteral alimentation solutions. Am J IV Therapy 1976;3:22–24.
5. Henry RS, Jurgens RW, Sturgeon R, et al. Compatibility of calcium chloride and calcium gluconate with sodium phosphate in a mixed TPN solution. Am J Hosp Pharm 1980;37:673–674.
6. Eggert LD, Rusho WJ, MacKay MW, et al. Calcium and phosphorus compatibility in parenteral nutrition solutions for neonates. Am J Hosp Pharm 1982;39:49–53.
7. Fitzgerald KA, MacKay MW. Calcium and phosphate solubility in neonatal parenteral nutrition solutions containing Aminosyn PF. Am J Hosp Pharm 1987;44:1396–1400.

8. Mikrut BA. Calcium and phosphate solubility in neonatal parenteral nutrient solutions containing Aminosyn PF or Trophamine. Am J Hosp Pharm 1987;44:2702–2704.

9. Lenz GT, Mikrut BA. Calcium and phosphate solubility in neonatal parenteral nutrient solutions containing AminosynPF or Trophamine. Am J Hosp Pharm 1988;45:2367–2371.

10. Trissel LA, ed. Calcium and phosphate compatibility in parenteral nutrition, 1st ed. Houston: TriPharma Communications, 2001.

11. Olin BR, Hebel SK, Dombek CE, Kastrup EK, eds. Drug facts and comparisons. St. Louis: JB Lippincott, 1993.

12. McEvoy GK, ed. 93 AHFS Drug Information, Bethesda: American Society of Hospital Pharmacists, 1993.

PART 6

COMPATIBILITY AND STABILITY

CHAPTER 34

Compatibility and Stability of Drug Products and Preparations Dispensed by the Pharmacist

I. DEFINITIONS

A. In *USP* Chapter ⟨1191⟩ Stability Considerations in Dispensing Practice, **stability** is defined as "the extent to which a product retains, within specified limits, and throughout its period of storage and use (i.e., its shelf life), the same properties and characteristics that it possessed at the time of its manufacture" (1).

B. **Physical Properties:** These are the properties of drugs and dosage forms that we can see or test by physical means. Is the drug a solid, a liquid, or a gas? Is it dissolved, suspended, or emulsified, or is it adsorbed to the surface of a container? When a physical change occurs, the same drug or chemical is still present, but its physical state is altered. Pharmaceutical examples of physical changes include a drug precipitating out of solution; a drug adsorbing to the walls of a polyvinyl chloride (PVC) container; and two solid drugs forming a liquid eutectic mixture when triturated together in a mortar.

    1. From a pharmaceutical viewpoint, there are both desirable and undesirable physical changes. When we make a drug solution, we want the physical change of the solid drug dissolving in the chosen solvent. In contrast, when we have an intravenous drug solution, it is unacceptable, and perhaps lethal, for the drug to precipitate out of solution.

    2. Chapter ⟨1191⟩ of the *USP* gives the following criteria for acceptable levels of physical stability: "The original physical properties, including appearance, palatability, uniformity, dissolution, and suspendability, are retained" (1).

C. **Chemical Properties:** The chemical properties of drugs are those manifested by the drug's particular molecular structure. When a chemical change occurs, the original drug molecule is no longer present.

1. Recall from your study of general chemistry some of the types of reactions that occur with inorganic molecules. For example,

   a. Acid-base neutralization reactions such as:
   $$NaOH + HCl \rightarrow Na^+ + Cl^- + H_2O$$

   b. Oxidation–reduction reactions such as:
   $$4\,Fe + 3O_2 \rightarrow 2\,Fe_2O_3 \text{ (rust)}$$

   c. Displacement reactions such as:
   $$NaCl + AgNO_3 \rightarrow Na^+ + NO_3^- + AgCl\downarrow$$

   d. Release of gas such as:
   $$NaHCO_3 + HCl \rightarrow Na^+ + Cl^- + H_2O + CO_2$$

2. Most drugs are complex organic molecules, and chemical changes that occur with them are often more complicated than the simple types shown above; your study of organic and medicinal chemistry has provided you with the detailed knowledge you need to understand and to anticipate many of these changes.

3. Usually we buy drugs of a desired structure, and any change in that structure is undesirable. We then say that degradation or decomposition has occurred. Occasionally, however, we make use of a chemical change to prepare a desired drug preparation, as in making finely divided sulfur and potassium sulfide from solutions of Zinc Sulfate and sulfurated potash when compounding White Lotion:

$$K_2S_3 \bullet K_2S_2O_3 + ZnSO_4 \bullet 7H_2O \rightarrow ZnS + S_2 + K_2SO_4 + K_2S_2O_3 + 7H_2O$$

4. Chapter $\langle 1191 \rangle$ of the *USP* gives the following criteria for acceptable levels of chemical stability: "Each active ingredient retains its chemical integrity and labeled potency, within the specified limits" (1).

TABLE 34.1   References

Books:	Connors KA, Amidon GL and Stella VJ. *Chemical Stability of Pharmaceuticals*, 2nd edition, 1986
	Florey K *Analytical Profiles of Drug Substances*
	King JC *Guide to Parenteral Admixtures*, current edition
	King RE. *Dispensing of Medication*, 1884
	Nahata MC and Hipple TF. *Pediatric Drug Formulations*, current edition
	Trissel LA. *Handbook on Injectable Drugs*, current edition
	Trissel LA. *Trissel's Stability of Compounded Formulations*, current edition
	AHFS Drug Information, current edition
	ASHP Handbook on Extemporaneous Formulations, current edition
	Drug Facts and Comparisons, current edition
	Martindale The complete drug reference (formerly *The Extra Pharmacopoeia*), current edition
	Physicians' Desk Reference, current edition
	Remington: The Science and Practice of Pharmacy, current edition
	The Merck Index, current edition
	United States Dispensatory, no longer in print
	United States Pharmacopeia/National Formulary, current edition
	USP Dispensing Information (USP/DI), Volumes 1 and 3, current edition
Journals:	*American Journal of Health-System Pharmacy**
	Hospital Formulary
	Hospital Pharmacy (Lippincott's)
	International Journal of Pharmaceutical Compounding
	International Journal of Pharmaceutics
	International Pharmaceutical Abstracts
	Journal of Pharmaceutical Science and Technology**
	Journal of Pharmaceutical Sciences
	Journal of Pharmacy Technology
	Journal of Pharmacy and Pharmacology
	Journal of the Parenteral Drug Association
	Pharmaceutical Research

*Former titles include *American Journal of Hospital Pharmacy*, and *Clinical Pharmacy*
**Formerly *Journal of Parenteral Science* and *Technology*
Databases Searches: *International Pharmaceutical Abstracts* and *Medline*
Information on compatibility and stability is also available from drug product manufacturers. The department to contact depends on the organization of the company: Customer Service, Formulation, and R & D (Research and Development) are possibilities. Listings of manufacturers with addresses and telephone numbers are given in the *PDR* and *Facts and Comparisons*, and are also usually available on the Internet site for the company.

D. Microbiological Properties: Drug products should be free of microbiological contamination and should resist any microbial growth.

1. Although certain products, such as parenterals and ophthalmics, are required to be sterile, all drug products should be free of microbiological contamination.

2. For drug products that are labile to the growth of microorganisms introduced during use, preservatives should be added. Preservatives are discussed in Chapter 15.

3. Chapter ⟨1191⟩ of the *USP* gives the following criteria for acceptable levels of microbiological stability: "Sterility or resistance to microbial growth is retained according to the specified requirements. Antimicrobial agents that are present retain effectiveness within the specified limits" (1).

E. References: Table 34.1 gives a list of references that contain helpful information on compatibility and stability of drugs and drug products.

II. RESPONSIBILITY FOR PROVIDING QUALITY DRUG PRODUCTS

A. Providing the public with quality drug products is the joint responsibility of pharmaceutical manufacturers and pharmacists.

B. Standards and guidelines for manufacturing, marketing, handling, and dispensing these products are set by:

1. Federal and state governments through agencies like the FDA and state boards of pharmacy

2. Nonprofit groups and commissions, such as the United States Pharmacopeial Convention, the National Association of Boards of Pharmacy, and the Joint Commission on Accreditation of Healthcare Organizations

3. Professional associations, such as the American Pharmaceutical Association and the American Society of Health-System Pharmacists

C. Responsibility of the Pharmacist

1. In its General Information Chapter ⟨1191⟩ Stability Considerations in Dispensing Practice, the *USP* clearly states that it is the pharmacist's responsibility to ensure that drug products provided to patients meet acceptable criteria of stability. Chapter ⟨1191⟩ is recommended reading for all pharmacy students and pharmacists.

   a. Chapter ⟨1191⟩ outlines those factors that affect product stability. The pharmacist should be conscious of these factors when handling and storing drug products.

   "Each ingredient, whether therapeutically active or pharmaceutically necessary, can affect the stability of drug substances and dosage forms. The primary environmental factors that can reduce stability include exposure to adverse temperatures, light, humidity, oxygen, and carbon dioxide. The major dosage form factors that influence drug stability include particle size (especially in emulsions and suspensions), pH, solvent system composition (i.e., percentage of "free" water and overall polarity), compatibility of anions and cations, solution ionic strength, primary container, specific chemical additives, and molecular binding and diffusion of drugs and excipients" (1).

   b. To help ensure that quality, stable pharmaceutical products are dispensed and used, the *USP* recommends that pharmacists do the following:

   (1) Watch for and comply with expiration dates, rotate stock, and use older products first.

   (2) Store drugs and drug products under recommended environmental conditions.

   (3) Observe products for evidence of instability.

   (4) Properly handle drugs and drug products that require extemporaneous manipulation.

   (5) Package products using recommended containers and closures.

   (6) Educate patients about the proper storage and use of products (1).

2. The pharmacist shares a responsibility with pharmaceutical manufacturers for the stability of manufactured drug products, and pharmacists are encouraged to report any problems with packaging, labeling, or evidence of instability in manufactured drug products to the manufacturer and to the FDA. The report to the FDA can be done easily by going to their web site at www.fda.gov The home page has a selection for product problem reporting. A report may be submitted online or by telephone, or the paper report form can be downloaded and faxed to FDA or sent using a postage-paid addressed form. As of December 2002, the FDA program for reporting drug product problems is called MedWatch, but the agency changes or reorganizes its programs from time to time, so it is best to check their web site for current information.

3. While the *USP* recognizes five types of stability—chemical, physical, microbiological, therapeutic, and toxicological—this chapter concentrates on the first three types because when these are maintained, the other two follow.

4. In the following discussion, the stability and compatibility of both manufactured and extemporaneously prepared drug products are considered, but the major emphasis is on drug preparations made or manipulated by the pharmacist.

III. PHYSICAL CHANGES

A. Liquification of Solid Ingredients

1. Efflorescent Powders: These powders contain water of hydration that may be released when the powders are triturated or when stored in an environment of low relative humidity. The water liberated when the drug or chemical is triturated may cause the powders to become damp or pasty. If water is released to the atmosphere because of low relative humidity, the drug loses its crystallinity and becomes powdery. Furthermore, if water of hydration is given off, a given weight of the resulting powder no longer contains the same amount of drug.
   a. For examples of efflorescent drugs, see Table 34.2.
   b. Strategies for handling these drugs
      (1) Store and dispense these powders in tight containers.
      (2) The anhydrous form of the drug may be substituted for the hydrate, but be sure to make appropriate dose corrections. For example, Sodium Sulfate USP is available as the decahydrate (Glauber's salt) with a molecular weight of 322. The laxative dose of Sodium Sulfate decahydrate is 15 g. If the anhydrous form is substituted (MW = 142), only 6.6 g should be used:

$$\frac{15\,g\,Na_2SO_4 \cdot 10\,H_2O}{322\,g/mol} = \frac{x\,g\,Na_2SO_4\,anhydrous}{142\,g/mol};\quad x = 6.6\,g\,Na_2SO_4\,anhydrous$$

2. Hygroscopic and deliquescent drugs: Hygroscopic drugs or chemicals are solids that absorb moisture from the air. The term "deliquescent" refers to hygroscopic powders that may absorb sufficient moisture to dissolve and form a solution.
   a. For examples of hygroscopic and deliquescent drugs, see Table 34.3.

TABLE 34.2   Efflorescent Powders (2)

Alums	Morphine acetate
Atropine sulfate	Quinine bisulfate
Caffeine	Quinine hydrobromide
Calcium lactate	Quinine hydrochloride
Citric acid	Scopolamine hydrobromide
Cocaine	Sodium acetate
Codeine	Sodium carbonate (decahydrate)
Codeine phosphate	Sodium phosphate
Codeine sulfate	Strychnine sulfate
Ferrous sulfate	Terpin hydrate

King RE: In *Dispensing of Medication*, 9th ed, Mack Publishing Co., Easton, PA, 1984, p. 40.

TABLE 34.3	Hygroscopic and Deliquescent Powders (2)
Ammonium bromide	Pepsin
Ammonium chloride	Phenobarbital sodium
Ammonium iodide	Physostigmine hydrobromide
Calcium bromide	Physostigmine hydrochloride
Calcium chloride	Physostigmine sulfate
Ephedrine sulfate	Pilocarpine alkaloid
Hydrastine hydrochloride	Potassium acetate
Hydrastine sulfate	Potassium citrate
Hyoscyamine hydrobromide	Sodium bromide
Hyoscyamine sulfate	Sodium iodide
Iron and ammonium citrate	Sodium nitrate
Lithium bromide	Zinc chloride

King RE: In *Dispensing of Medication*, 9th ed, Mack Publishing Co., Easton, PA, 1984, p. 40.

b. Strategies for handling these drugs

(1) Store and dispense these drugs in tight containers. This means that powders dispensed as chartulae or divided powders should be sealed in plastic or foil and the packets put in tight containers. This is especially important in humid weather.

(2) For solid compounded formulations, an inert, powdered ingredient that will preferentially absorb water may be added to the formulation. Often there are sufficient other suitable powders in the formulation to fulfill this function. If not, a suitable, inert, water-insoluble (e.g., not lactose) powder may be added. Light magnesium oxide is sometimes used for this purpose and is acceptable, provided the quantity needed is not sufficient to impart a therapeutic laxative effect. When you add extra ingredients, consult with the prescriber. If necessary, make adjustments to maintain the intended dose.

(3) Counsel the patient to store the product or preparation in its original tight container and in a low-humidity environment.

3. Pharmaceutical eutectic mixtures of drugs: A pharmaceutical eutectic mixture is defined as two or more substances that may liquefy when intimately mixed (as with trituration) at room temperature.

a. Under certain conditions, a "damp" powder, a pasty mass, or a liquid may result when two drugs or chemicals, which are solid at room temperature, are triturated together. This interesting phenomenon can easily be explained. It is well known that impurities present in chemicals impart melting points that are lower and less sharp than the melting point of the pure chemical. (Recall from organic chemistry lab that you checked for the purity of a compound by measuring its melting point; a clear, sharp melting point indicated pure compound.) If two or more drugs are triturated together, each may act as an impurity to the other and cause a mutual lowering of the original melting point of each individual compound. If the melting points of the pure compounds are low to begin with, the melting point of the mixture may be below room temperature, and a liquid or paste may result.

b. Whether or not liquification occurs, and the composition of the liquid or paste can both be analyzed using a phase diagram for the specific combination of compounds. For a more thorough discussion of this topic, consult a book of physical pharmacy (3,4). In general, liquification depends on:

(1) Ambient room temperature

(2) Original melting points of the substances

(3) Proportions in which the substances are mixed

(4) Extent and degree of pressure used in trituration

(5) Presence of other ingredients that may sorb any liquid formed

c. For examples of drugs that may form liquid eutectic mixtures, see Table 34.4.

d. There are some cases in which the formation of liquid eutectics is desirable.

(1) The local anesthetic EMLA® Cream owes its success as a topical anesthetic, effective in preventing needle stick pain when drawing blood, to the high con-

TABLE 34.4	Substances That Liquefy When Mixed
Acetaminophen	Lidocaine
Acetanilid	Menthol
Aminopyrine	Phenacetin (Acetophenetidin)
Antipyrine	Phenol
Aspirin	Phenylsalicylate (Salol)
Benzocaine	Prilocaine
Betanaphthol	Resorcinol
Camphor	Salicylic Acid
Chloral hydrate	Thymol

centrations of lidocaine and prilocaine achieved by forming a liquid eutectic mixture of these two components.

(2) There are some solids that have hard crystalline structures that do not reduce to fine powder with direct trituration. An extra compounding step, known as pulverization by intervention (described in Chapter 24, Powders), is needed to make fine particles of this type of ingredient. However, if another ingredient in the formulation forms a liquid eutectic with this crystalline solid, the two can be triturated together and the resulting liquid that is formed can either be adsorbed on an inert solid, as described below, or, if the formulation is a disperse system or a semisolid, the liquid can be directly incorporated in the formulation. This circumvents the need for the pulverization by intervention step. This method is illustrated with Sample Prescription 24.2.

e. Strategies for handling drugs that form liquid eutectic mixtures

(1) Force the liquid eutectic to form, then sorb the liquid onto an inert, high-melting, finely divided solid. This is done by triturating together the eutectic forming drugs to force the formation of the liquid; then an inert powder is added in portions with trituration to sorb the liquid. (As mentioned above, this method is illustrated with Sample Prescription 24.2 and is demonstrated on the CD that accompanies this book.)

(a) If possible, an ingredient already present in the formulation should be used to sorb the liquid.

(b) If no suitable powder is in the formulation, an inert powder may be added. Magnesium carbonate is reported to be the agent of choice, but light or heavy magnesium oxide, calcium phosphate, starch, talc, and lactose may also be suitable (2,3).

(2) An alternative method is to separately triturate each potential eutectic former with an inert powder, such as one of those given above; then the protected powders are mixed together by gentle spatulation.

(3) When you add extra ingredients, consult with the prescriber. If necessary, make adjustments to maintain the intended dose.

B. Polymorphic Reversion

1. There are drugs that can exist in different crystalline structures in the solid state, although they are identical in the liquid or vapor state. Different polymorphic forms of the same substance will exhibit different physical properties, such as melting points and rates of dissolution.

2. Examples include ampicillin, methylprednisolone, hydrocortisone, various sulfa drugs, barbiturates, and many others.

3. Because different polymorphs can give different dissolution rates, the use of different polymorphic forms in a solid dosage form can affect the drug's bioavailability. This is a problem that has long been recognized by the pharmaceutical industry and is one of the reasons behind bioequivalence testing to ensure equivalent therapeutic performance of solid dosage forms made by different manufacturers.

4. The pharmacist should realize that metastable polymorphs are sometimes used in manufacturing solid dosage forms to give more rapid dissolution and improved bioavail-

ability. Manipulation of these products in compounding may result in reversion to the more stable, less soluble, less available polymorph.

5. One common pharmaceutical substance that is notorious because of the problems caused by its polymorphic reversions is Cocoa Butter. Cocoa Butter has several polymorphic forms with melting points of 18°, 24°, 28°–31°, and 34°C. Cocoa Butter is used as a base for making suppositories and must be melted when the suppositories are made by fusion. It can very easily be overheated, and when it is, it solidifies as one of the lower melting polymorphs, which may melt at room temperature, or the suppositories may liquefy when handled by the patient during insertion. To avoid this problem, Cocoa Butter must be melted slowly and carefully, with the temperature not exceeding 34°C.

C. Precipitation from Solution

1. General Principles
   a. As stated at the beginning of this chapter, unintended precipitation of an active ingredient or excipient from solution can be a major hazard with pharmaceutical solutions.

      (1) For oral or topical solutions, if an active ingredient precipitates, the particles will usually settle to the bottom of the bottle so that the initial doses poured from the bottle will be subpotent and the later doses will be superpotent. This can result in either therapeutic failure or toxicity.

      (2) With intravenous solutions, the danger of precipitation can be even greater because insoluble particles can lodge in capillaries and block them, resulting in severe consequences and even death.

   b. Factors that can cause precipitation are discussed below, but it should be realized that pharmaceutical solutions are usually complex, and prediction of precipitation in them is never simple. Numerous reports in journal articles have pointed out that when reading and interpreting compatibility studies involving precipitation, all conditions of the study are relevant and may affect the outcome.

   c. When interpreting compatibility reports it is important to note: 1) the manufacturers of the drugs, 2) their concentrations, 3) the base solution or diluents and their manufacturers, 4) order of mixing, 5) time frames, 6) temperature, and 7) test methods. Changes in any of these factors can alter the results. Two examples:

      (1) The combination of dopamine hydrochloride (DuPont, 12.8 mg/mL) and furosemide (Hoechst-Roussel, 5 mg/mL) had been reported to be compatible when mixed in usual IV solutions. It was later noticed that combining these same drugs in a Y-site administration gave a precipitate. It was subsequently learned that with this particular Y-site administration, one of the drug solutions was from a different manufacturer that used a different buffer, and a different pH resulted (5).

      (2) In a study testing the physical compatibility of a large number of pairs of drug solutions, it was found that while some combinations were always compatible and some combinations were always incompatible, there were some cases for which compatibility depended on the order of mixing the two drug solutions; for some, the length of time after mixing was a factor (initial, 1-hour, and 3-hour testing was done) (6).

2. *Solvent effects:* When a drug is dissolved in a solvent and a second solvent, one in which the drug is poorly soluble, is added, the drug may precipitate.
   a. Typical examples of solvent effects
      Topical: When water or an aqueous solution is added to an alcoholic solution of salicylic acid, precipitation may occur. (The solubility of salicylic acid is 1 g/2.7 mL of alcohol, but only 1 g/460 mL water.)
      Oral: When an aqueous solution or syrup is added to Phenobarbital Elixir, precipitation may occur. (See the tables in Chapter 7 that show the solubility of phenobarbital in various water, alcohol, and glycerin cosolvent systems.)
      Injectables: Digoxin has a water solubility of 0.08 mg/mL. Digoxin Injection is available in a cosolvent system containing 40% Propylene Glycol and 10% Alcohol. If it is diluted with an aqueous injectable solution, precipitation may occur.

TABLE 34.5	Solubility of Diazepam in Varying Dilutions of the Original Formulation Solvent and in Water, D5W, and NS (7)
Solvent	**Solubility (mg/mL)**
100% original	5.2
80% original	1.6
50% original	0.41
20% original	0.11
10% original	0.072
Water	0.053
D5W	0.056
NS	0.045

Unpublished results of Stella VJ and Roberts RD given in *The Handbook of Injectable Drugs*, 4th Ed., p. XVII.

Another drug with similar problems is Diazepam. Diazepam Injection has the following formula:

> 5 mg/mL Diazepam
> 40% Propylene Glycol
> 10% Ethanol
> 5% Benzoic acid/Na Benzoate
> 1.5% Benzyl Alcohol
> q.s. Water   pH = 6.4–6.9

Observe the data in Table 34.5 and note the following results if Diazepam Injection is diluted with an aqueous injection such as Dextrose 5% in Water (D5W). In each case, 1 mL of Diazepam Injection (that is, 5 mg of the drug) is used.

Dilute 50-50:   1 mL Diazepam Injection and 1 mL D5W: 5 mg/2 mL = 2.5 mg/mL, which is >0.41 mg/mL—ppt

Dilute 1:10:   1 mL Diazepam Injection and 9 mL D5W (that is, 10% original): 5 mg/10 mL = 0.5 mg/mL, which is >0.072 mg/mL—ppt

Dilute 1:100:   1 mL Diazepam Injection and 99 mL D5W: 5 mg/100 mL = 0.05 mg/mL, which is approximately equal to 0.056 mg/mL—just at the borderline

b. Usually the problem occurs when water is added to an alcoholic solution of a drug that is poorly soluble in water. The reverse can also be true. For example, Codeine Phosphate is very soluble in water, but it is not very soluble in alcohol. If alcohol is added to an aqueous solution of Codeine Phosphate, the drug may precipitate. This is why cough syrups that contain a large percentage of alcohol to solubilize other water-insoluble ingredients contain Codeine base rather than Codeine Phosphate.

c. Remember that the useful (though approximate) relationship between solubility and solvent volume-fraction is logarithmic, not linear:

$$log\ S_T = vf_{water}log\ S_{water} + vf_{sol}log\ S_{sol}$$

where:
   S_T = total solubility of the drug or chemical
   vf_{water} = volume fraction of water
   S_{water} = solubility of the drug or chemical in water
   vf_{sol} = volume fraction of the other cosolvent
   S_{sol} = solubility of the drug or chemical in the cosolvent

➤ *EXAMPLE*

An Acetaminophen solution is desired with a concentration of 325 mg/5 mL. The pharmacist finds the following solubility information for Acetaminophen in *Remington: The Science and Practice of Pharmacy*: 1 g/70 mL water; 1 g/10 mL alcohol.

1. Express the total desired solubility (S_T) and the solubility in water (S_{water}) and alcohol (S_{alc}) in common terms (e.g., mg/mL):

S_T = 325 mg/5 mL = 65 mg/mL

S_{water} = 1 g/70 mL = 1,000 mg/70 mL = 14.3 mg/mL

S_{alc} = 1 g/10 mL = 1,000 mg/10 mL = 100 mg/mL

2. Recall that the sum of volume fractions = 1

Therefore, $vf_{water} + vf_{alc} = 1$; and $vf_{alc} = 1 - vf_{water}$

3. Substituting in the log solubility equation given above and solving for vf_{water} :

$log\ 65 = (1 - vf_{water})\ log\ 100 + vf_{water}\ log\ 14.3$

$1.813 = (1 - vf_{water})\ (2) + vf_{water}\ (1.155)$

$1.813 = 2 - 2\ vf_{water} + 1.155\ vf_{water}$

$0.845\ vf_{water} = 0.187$

$vf_{water} = 0.187/0.845 = 0.22$, or 22% water and 78% alcohol

Remember that this equation is for pure systems containing the drug and the cosolvent system, and that the result is just a good estimate. In formulation situations we usually have other ingredients present such as sweeteners, flavors, and other active ingredients and excipients. These factors alter the conditions and the results. The use of this equation is illustrated in Sample Prescription 26.5.

    d. Compounding strategies when adding additional solvents to a drug solution

      (1) To maintain a true solution, be sure you are using an appropriate solvent system.

        (a) For solubilities, consult appropriate references, such as *Remington: The Science and Practice of Pharmacy* or *The Merck Index*. If necessary, you may calculate approximate required solvent ratios using the log solubility equation given above.

        (b) If you need to make an aqueous dilution of an injectable drug solution that contains a drug in a cosolvent system, follow the manufacturer's instructions in the product package insert or recommendations in a reference such as *Trissel's Handbook of Injectable Drugs*. For example, the manufacturer of Digoxin Injection recommends that it be diluted with at least a fourfold volume of Sterile Water or the equivalent.

        (c) If information is not available, make a reasonable dilution and observe the solution for a period of time, or dilute the product so that the final concentration of the drug is below its saturation concentration. In all cases, observe the solution and be sure to give sufficient time for redissolution if precipitation occurs.

        (d) Decrease the drug concentration so that the drug is soluble in the solvent system. For systemic medications, remember that if you change the concentration of the active ingredient(s) in the preparation, you must change the volume of the dose administered to give the same quantity of drug.

      (2) For oral or topical products, you may wish to make a suspension. A suspending agent may be required. Remember that a "Shake Well" label is required for disperse systems.

      (3) If you make a substantive change, you should first consult the prescriber.

  3. *pH effects:* Most drugs are weak electrolytes (weak acids or weak bases), and their degree of ionization (i.e., the relative concentration of drug in salt versus free, unionized form) depends on the pH of the solution. When there is a large difference in the solubilities of the two forms, as is usually the case, a problem may occur when you alter the pH of the solution. This can happen when drug solutions with differing pH's are combined or when a drug that generates a different pH is added to the original drug solution.

➤ **EXAMPLE**

1. Chlorpromazine HCl: solubility 1 g/2.5 mL water
   Chlorpromazine base: insoluble in water

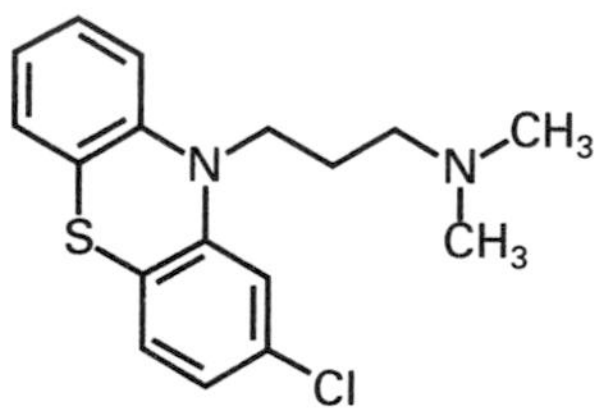

Here you have a drug with high water solubility in its salt form and low water solubility in its free base form (chemical structure shown above). If you were to raise the pH of an aqueous solution of Chlorpromazine HCl, some of the salt form of the drug would be converted to the unionized free form. If the concentration of Chlorpromazine base were to exceed its water solubility, precipitation would occur.

2. Phenobarbital Na: 1 g/mL water
   Phenobarbital (acid): 1 g/1,000 mL water

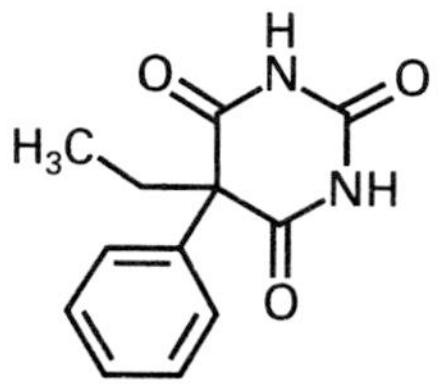

Again, you have a drug with high water solubility in its salt form and low water solubility in its unionized, free form (chemical structure shown above). Here you have the opposite salt type, the salt of a weak acid rather than the salt of a weak base. In this case, if you were to lower the pH of an aqueous solution of sodium phenobarbital, some of the salt form of the drug would be converted to the un-ionized free acid form. If the concentration of phenobarbital acid were to exceed its water solubility, precipitation would occur.

To decide if a possible problem exists, you need to know certain information.

   a. If you do not know, check the solubilities of all the drugs in the solvents involved (that is, the solubilities of both the salt and free forms in the desired solvent or solvent system).

   (1) Even if you have a lot of experience with drugs and their solubilities, this information is not always intuitive; in fact, it can be rather surprising. For example, Codeine and Morphine have chemical structures that are quite similar, yet Codeine base has a water solubility of 1 g/120 mL, whereas the water solubility of Morphine base is 1 g/5,000 mL.

   (2) The solvent system involved is important. In the Chlorpromazine and Phenobarbital examples given previously, there is a good possibility for precipitation if the pH is altered for aqueous solutions. If the solvent system contains sufficient alcohol, precipitation may not occur—even with a change in pH—if the free form is sufficiently soluble in alcohol.

   (3) Sometimes both the salt and the free form are soluble in water and other pharmaceutical solvents such as alcohol. If this is the case, precipitation will not be a problem with a change in pH or solvent system. For example, Ephedrine base and Ephedrine HCl are both soluble in water and in alcohol.

■ Figure 34.1 How to Determine if a Drug is a Neutral Weak Acid or a Neutral Weak Base

MISCONCEPTIONS ABOUT DETERMINING ACID-BASE CHARACTER OF ORGANIC COMPOUNDS

Misconception #1:   If a drug solution has a pH below 7, the drug must be a neutral weak acid, and if the pH of the drug solution is above 7, the drug must be a neutral weak base.

Fact: You cannot tell whether the parent drug is a neutral weak acid or base from the pH of its solutions.

1. It is true that when a pure compound is dissolved in water, if it is a neutral weak acid, the solution will have a pH below 7, and a neutral weak base will give a pH above 7. However, often the neutral species has limited water solubility, so it is usually the salt form that is dissolved, and then the pH of a solution of the salt form varies with the compound.

Examples of some compounds and their salts with pH values of their solutions are given here. Note the variability.

Benzoic Acid, a neutral weak acid, pH of 2.8.
Salt form, Sodium Benzoate, pH of about 8.

Salicyclic Acid, a neutral weak acid, pH of 2.4.
Salt form, Sodium Salicylate, pH of between 5–6.

Phenol, a neutral weak acid, pH of approximately 6.

Chlorpromazine, a neutral weak base with alkaline reaction.
Salt form, Chlorpromazine HCl, pH of about 4.0–5.5.

2. Most manufactured drug solutions, such as injections, have their pH adjusted (e.g., with buffers) to a value for maximum solubility and/or stability of the drug.

Examples:

Cimetidine Injection USP, which is Cimetidine Hydrochloride in Water for Injection, has a pH of 3.8 to 6.0; Cimetidine is a neutral weak base.

Glycopyrrolate Injection USP has a pH between 2.0 and 3.0; Glycopyrrolate is neither an acid nor a base, it is a quaternary ammonium compound.

Pentobarbital Sodium Injection USP has a pH between 9.0 and 10.5; Pentobarbital is a neutral weak acid.

Misconception #2: If a drug has a reported pK_a, it must be a neutral weak acid because pK_b's are reported for neutral weak bases.

Fact: The pK values for both neutral weak acids and neutral weak bases are generally reported as pK_a's. The pK_a value reported for a neutral weak base is actually the pK value for the conjugate acid form of the base. For conjugate acid-base pairs the relationship is:

$$pK_w = pK_a + pK_b$$

Furthermore, one cannot tell from the numerical value of the pK_a whether the compound is a neutral weak acid or a neutral weak base. The following is true:

1. For neutral weak acids, as pK_a decreases, acid strength increases.
2. For neutral weak bases, as the pK_b decreases (and the pK_a of the conjugate acid form increases), base strength increases.

Examples:

Neutral weak acids: Carboxylic acids have pK_a's in the range of 2–6 and are relatively stronger acids than are phenols with pK_a's in the range of 7–11 and thiols with pK_a's in the range of 7–10.

Neutral weak bases: Aliphatic amines have pK_a's in the range of 8–11 (that is, the pK_a of their conjugate acid form) and are relatively stronger bases than are aromatic amines with pK_a's in the range of 4–7.

You cannot tell anything from a numerical value of a pK_a unless you know, using other evidence (such as chemical structure), that the compound in question is a neutral weak acid or is a neutral weak base.

Misconception #3: Since HCl, H_2SO_4, HNO_3, acetic acid, etc., are all acids, therefore, salts that are hydrochlorides, sulfates, nitrates, acetates, etc. must be salts of neutral weak acids.

Fact: The opposite is generally true; compounds that are hydrochlorides, sulfates, nitrates, etc. are usually the salts of neutral weak bases, because salts are formed from the reaction of an acid and a base.

■ **Figure 34.1** *Continued.*

HOW THEN DO YOU TELL IF A COMPOUND IS A NEUTRAL WEAK ACID OR A NEUTRAL WEAK BASE?

1. There are some functional groups that we readily recognize as having essentially neither acidic nor basic properties when in aqueous solution. Examples include, alcohols (R-OH) and polyols (e.g., sugars), ethers (ROR'), esters (RCOOR'), aldehydes (RCHO), ketones (RCOR'), and amides (RCONH$_2$).

2. The are other functional groups that we recognize are acids or have some acidic character. Examples include carboxylic acids (RCOOH), sulfonic acids (RSO$_3$H), phenols (ArOH), thiols (RSH), and imides (RCONHCOR').

3. There are some functional groups that we recognize as bases or have some basic character. Examples include aliphatic amines (R-NH$_2$) and aromatic amines (either ArNH$_2$ or nitrogen as part of an aromatic ring structure).

4. Still, because drug molecules are complex structures, it is often difficult to look at the structure of a drug molecule and decide if it is a weak acid, a weak base, or neither. When this is true, a handy trick is to take note of the name of its salt form and use this information in making a determination.

Recall that in forming a salt, we combine an acid and a base. Now consider the following:

Acid	+	*Base*	=	*Salt*
Mineral Acids		**Neutral Weak Bases**		
HCl		Ranitidine		Ranitidine HCl
HBr		Homatropine		Homatropine HBr
H$_2$SO$_4$		Morphine		Morphine Sulfate
HNO$_3$		Pilocarpine		Pilocarpine Nitrate
H$_3$PO$_4$		Codeine		Codeine Phosphate
Organic Acids				
Malic Acid		Chlorpheniramine		Chlorpheniramine Maleate
Citric Acid		Clomiphene		Clomiphene Citrate
Neutral Weak Acids		Hydroxide Bases		
Phenobarbital		NaOH		Sodium Phenobarbital
Clavulanic Acid		KOH		Potassium Clavulenate
Saccharic Acid		Ca(OH)$_2$		Calcium Saccharate

It can be observed from the above that for the salts of the mineral and organic acids, the parent drug compound is a neutral weak base, and for salts of the hydroxide bases, the parent drug compound is a neutral weak acid. Therefore, when you encounter a drug that has as its salt form a sodium, potassium, calcium, or magnesium salt, the drug itself is most likely a neutral weak acid. Similarly for a salt that is a hydrochloride, sulfate, phosphate, maleate, tartarate, etc., the parent compound is likely a neutral weak base however, there are two notable exceptions in this later case. For this reason, when making a final determination, the chemical structure of the drug must be known.

1. In some cases, for drugs combined with organic acids, the resulting compound may not be a salt, but rather an ester. Examples would be Desoxycortisone Acetate and Clobetasol Proprionate.

2. For some halides, the resulting compound is a quaternary ammonium compound nitrogen covalently bonded to four -R groups with no dissociable proton. Two examples are Benzalkonium Chloride and Demecarium Bromide.

3. Some compounds, such as Sodium Lauryl Sulfate are salts of neutral sting acids and bases; these are not sensitve to pH changes.

In each of these cases, the drugs are neither neutral weak acids nor neutral weak bases, and they are not subject to precipitation of the neutral form by a change in pH.

b. Determine the salt type of the drug: Is the drug the salt of a neutral weak acid or a neutral weak base? In aqueous solutions, precipitation occurs when the salt form is converted to the neutral free form by a change in pH (that is, by raising the pH for the salts of weak bases and by lowering the pH for salts of weak acids). You need to know the salt type of your drug to know if a pH change will be problematic. Because determination of salt type can be difficult, a brief discussion of this with some helpful hints is given in Figure 34.l. For a more thorough discussion of this topic, you may want to read the applicable section in the book *Thermodynamics of Pharmaceutical Systems: An Introduction for Students of Pharmacy* (8).

c. Estimate the resultant pH of the solution. This may be done by checking an appropriate reference or by actual measurement.

(1) If you are adding a pure chemical, check the monograph in *Remington: The Science and Practice of Pharmacy* or *The Merck Index* for the pH of an aqueous solution of that chemical.

(2) If you are adding a manufactured drug solution, the product package insert or a reference like *Trissel's Handbook of Injectable Drugs* often gives helpful information. Drug products often are buffered for stability or solubility purposes, and the pH of their solutions is different than if just pure drug were present in solution.

(3) It is helpful to learn examples of widely used classes of drugs that have distinctly acid or basic pH's. This is especially true for pharmacists who work with IV admixtures. The lists below give some examples of injectable drug solutions that have distinctly acidic or basic pH's:

Drug Solutions That Have Acid pH's
Phenothiazines
Tetracycline HCl
Ascorbic Acid
Glycopyrrolate
Metaraminol Bitartrate
Morphine Sulfate

Drug Solutions that Have Basic pH's
Phenytoin Na
Aminophylline
Sodium Bicarbonate
Sodium Barbiturates

(4) Although you should be careful when adding vehicles and diluents that may affect the pH, be aware that buffer capacity is important. Most drugs and drug solutions have sufficient buffer capacity to overwhelm the pH effects of a neutral, unbuffered liquid vehicle or LVP solution. Relative amounts may be critical. Erythromycin Lactobionate IV is a good example of a product in which solubility is very sensitive both to pH and to concentration when sterile diluent is added for reconstitution.

(5) The pH of the resultant solution under consideration can be checked using either pH paper or a pH meter.

d. Look up the pK_a of the drug under consideration. The Appendices section of the CD that accompanies this book has a long list of pK_a's for drugs and chemicals. Other useful references include books of medicinal chemistry, *Trissel's Stability of Compounded Formulations*, and *The Merck Index*.

e. Calculate the pH of precipitation using the appropriate equation below. Compare this calculated limiting pH with the estimated pH in item **c.** above.

(1) For salts of weak bases use:

$$pK_a = pH - log\left(\frac{S_o}{S_T - S_o}\right)$$

(2) For salts of weak acids use:

$$pK_a = pH - log\left(\frac{S_T - S_o}{S_o}\right)$$

where:

pK_a = the pK_a of the drug (conjugate acid form)
pH = the limit of pH beyond which precipitation will occur at the given value of S_T (i.e., precipitation occurs at pH values lower than this

limit for weak acids, but at pH values above this limit for weak bases)

$S_T =$ the final total concentration of the drug in solution

$S_o =$ the solubility of the un-ionized (neutral) free form of the drug

(3) In using these equations, note that while technically the above concentrations should be expressed in molar units, for the purposes of estimation used in compounding, a weight basis such as mg/mL or w/v% is often used. If more exact estimations are desired, molar quantities should be employed.

(4) Note also that while the pH of precipitation depends on three factors, two of them, the pK_a of the drug and the solubility of the free form (S_o), are properties of the drug and cannot be changed (in a given solvent).

(5) The third factor, the desired final drug concentration (S_T), varies with the situation. It is important to be aware of this when using references such as the *Handbook of Injectable Drugs*. Notice that the C/I (Compatibility/Incompatibility) rating in this reference is given for a particular drug concentration and for a particular vehicle. If these conditions are changed, there may or may not be a problem. Furthermore, in using these ratings, one may think that if a high concentration, such as 500 mg/L, shows compatibility, then surely a lower, more dilute concentration should be OK. This is usually but not always true. Injections usually contain buffers, and sometimes smaller volumes of drug solutions do not have sufficient buffer capacity to maintain the pH at the desired level for solubility when another drug or solution is added.

➤ **EXAMPLE**

In what pH range is it possible to prepare an aqueous solution of chlordiazepoxide having a concentration of 10 mg/5 mL?

1. The solubility of chlordiazepoxide (free base) is 1 g in $>10,000$ mL of water; this is S_o. Chlordiazepoxide HCl is very soluble in water—1 g/10 mL.

2. Chlordiazepoxide has the chemical structure given here:

The salt form of chlordiazepoxide is Chlordiazepoxide Hydrochloride; the drug is a neutral weak base.

3. From literature sources, $pK_a = 4.6$.

4. Express the total desired solubility (S_T) and the limiting solubility of the free base (S_o) in common terms (e.g., in percent):

$S_T = 10$ mg/5 mL $= 200$ mg/100 mL $= 0.2$ g/100 mL $= 0.2\%$

$S_o = 1$ g/10,000 mL $= 0.01$ g/100 mL $= 0.01\%$

5. Using equation (1) above (for neutral weak bases), calculate the pH of precipitatiion:

$$pK_a = pH - log\left(\frac{S_o}{S_T - S_o}\right)$$

$$4.6 = pH - log\left(\frac{0.01}{0.2 - 0.01}\right)$$

$pH = 4.6 + log\ 0.01/0.19 = 4.6 + log\ 0.0526$

$pH = 4.6 - 1.279 = 3.3$

Therefore, the drug is soluble at this desired concentration at any pH **below** 3.3; above this pH, precipitation will occur.

You can confirm that this is a reasonable solution by consulting the monograph for Chlordiazepoxide HCl Injection in the *Handbook of Injectable Drugs*. Here the desired concentration of the drug is higher (5%) and the formulators of the injectable product use both low pH (2.5–3.5) and a cosolvent system of water and propylene glycol to solubilize the drug.

    f. Possible strategies for handling solutions of weak electrolytes

      (1) If possible, control the pH at a desirable level. This may mean keeping incompatible solutions separate.

        (a) For IM injections, draw the drug solutions in separate syringes and give in different sites. This is illustrated with Sample Medication Order 32.8 in Chapter 32.

        (b) For IV injections, give at different times and flush the IV line between additions of the incompatible drug solutions. In some cases, multiple-lumen tubing may be used.

      (2) With oral or topical solutions, a cosolvent may be added if a suitable one is available that will keep the free form of the drug in solution. For example, Phenobarbital Na is soluble in water, but the neutral free acid precipitates in the acid pH of many oral syrups. Alcohol can be added as a cosolvent to keep the free acid in solution. This is illustrated in Example 7.27 in Chapter 7; notice in Table 7.1 that the percentage of alcohol needed to maintain solubility of the Phenobarbital depends on both the concentration of the drug and the pH of the solution. Also, the amount of alcohol needed can often be reduced by the use of a third cosolvent such as glycerin or propylene glycol; this is illustrated for Phenobarbital in Table 7.2.

      (3) For oral or topical solutions, check on the possibility of making a suspension.

      (4) Dilute the final solution so that the concentration of the drug is below the precipitation concentration of the free un-ionized form.

      (5) For injectable drugs that are sensitive to pH changes caused by absorption of CO_2, use short expiration times. Examples include Phenytoin Sodium Injection and Aminophylline Injection.

  4. *Formation of sparingly soluble salts:* When a drug is dissolved in a solvent and another drug is added that forms a sparingly soluble salt with the first drug, precipitation can occur. Precipitation of sparingly soluble salts is actually a chemical rather than a physical change because a new compound is formed, but this subject is included here for completeness in the area of drug precipitations.

    a. Inorganic precipitates

      (1) Remember the general equation for sparingly soluble salts:

$$A_nB_m \rightarrow nA^{+m} + mB^{+n}$$

$$K_{sp} = [A^{+m}]^n [B^{+n}]^m$$

      (2) Some typical pharmacy examples are shown here (shown as associations rather than dissociations):

$$Ag^+ + Cl^- \rightarrow AgCl \downarrow$$

$$Ca(Gluconate)_2 + K_2HPO_4 \rightarrow CaHPO_4 \downarrow + 2K^+ + 2 \text{ gluconate}^{-1}$$

      (3) The example given above with the calcium phosphate can be a serious problem with parenteral nutrition (PN) solutions. In spring 1994, the FDA issued an alert following deaths attributed to the administration of parenteral nutrition solutions containing precipitated calcium phosphate. Note that it is an especially difficult problem to handle because precipitation in these situations depends on so many factors; the *Handbook of Injectable Drugs* lists nine contributing factors, including pH, order of mixing, temperature, calcium salt used, and other ingredients present. A more thorough description of the factors involved is given in Chapter 33, Parenteral Nutrition.

(4) Solubilities for inorganic salts are given in Table 34.6.

b. Precipitation of large cation/large anion compounds

(1) Examples include Heparin Sodium, large antibiotic molecules like Gentamicin Sulfate and Kanamycin Sulfate, quaternary ammonium compounds like Benzalkonium Chloride, Phenylmercuric Nitrate, and many others. For example:

Heparin Na + Gentamicin SO_4 → ppt ↓

(2) Strategies for handling possible precipitation

(a) Check the drug product inserts and available literature. As discussed in the beginning of this section, pay attention to all the details of the test conditions in compatibility reports.

(b) If no information is available, make test solutions first. When combining solutions, carefully monitor for precipitation and observe for a sufficient length of time. Precipitation often is not immediately apparent.

(c) If there will be a change in temperature during storage or use, be sure to test under these conditions also.

(d) If there is any doubt about compatibility, keep the solutions separate. For IM injections, draw the drug solutions in separate syringes and give in different sites. For IV injections, give at different times and flush the IV line between additions of the incompatible drug solutions. In some cases, multiple-lumen tubing may be used. Be especially carefully with Heparin solutions; they are often used as IV flush solutions, and Heparin is incompatible with many other drugs.

c. Drugs with unusual counter ions

(1) Any time you have a drug that is an organic salt with a special or unusual counter ion such as mesylate, lactate, succinate, etc., be cautious when adding a solution of another salt. When a drug manufacturer uses a special salt form, there is a good reason for this, and one reason is that the hydrochloride, sulfate, or other more common salt form of the drug is less soluble. Precipitation is dependent on concentrations and may also vary with other factors such as a pH. Very often such combinations are compatible, but it is wise to be cautious.

(2) One example of this phenomenon involves the drug Dihydroergotamine (DHE) mesylate. There was a published formula for this drug in a nasal solution with Sodium Chloride as the tonicity adjustor, but when the formula was attempted, there was precipitation of the hydrochloride salt of DHE due to the addition of the Sodium Chloride.

TABLE 34.6 Solubilities of Inorganic Salts (9)

Cations	Na	K	NH₄	Mg	Ca	Sr	Ba	Al Mn²⁺	Cr³⁺ Cu²⁺	Fe³⁺ Bi³⁺	Zn²⁺ Hg²⁺	Co²⁺	Ni²⁺ Cd²⁺	Ag	Pb²⁺	Hg⁺
Anions-NO₂	S	S	S	S	S	S	S	S	S	S	S	S	S	S	S	S
-Ac	S	S	S	S	S	S	S	S	S	S	S	S	S	S	S	S
-Cl	S	S	S	S	S	S	S	S	S	S	S	S	I	I	I	I
-SO₄	S	S	S	S	I	I	I	S	S	S	S	S	I	I	I	I
-CO₃	S	S	S	I	I	I	I	I	I	I	I	I	S	I	I	I
-PO₄	S	S	S	I	I	I	I	I	I	I	I	I	I	I	I	I
-S	S	S	S	I	I	I	I	I	I	I	I	I	I	I	I	I
-OH	S	S	S	I	I	I	I	I	I	I	I	I	I	I	I	I

S-soluble. I-insoluble. Soluble in this table includes the USP designations of *very soluble* (1 part of solute in less than 1 part of solvent), *freely soluble* (1 in 1 to 10), *soluble* (1 in 10 to 30), and *sparingly soluble* (1 in 30 to 100). Insoluble includes the USP designations of *slightly soluble* (1 in 100 to 1000), *very slightly soluble* (1 in 1000 to 10,000), and *practically insoluble*, or *insoluble* (1 in more than 10,000).
Reference:
King RE(ed). *Dispensing of Medications*, 9th ed. Easton, PA, Mack Publishing Co., 1984, p 335.

d. Alkaloidal precipitants

(1) Alkaloids include a wide variety of amine drugs of plant origin. Some of our older and more widely used drugs, such as atropine, cocaine, codeine, colchicine, morphine, and ephedrine, are alkaloids. Many are complex molecules that contain other functional groups. Many years ago, when pharmacists had a more limited knowledge of the chemistry of these compounds, they would memorize lists of compounds that would cause alkaloids to precipitate from solution. These included citrate salts, tannins from Wild Cherry Syrup, iodide, and picric acid. Although some of these reactions are simply caused by precipitation of the free, un-ionized base as a result of a change in pH of the solution, other precipitations result from unique reactions.

(2) Possible strategies for handling alkaloidal precipitants vary with the compounds involved. Some pharmaceutical reference books, especially older editions, can be helpful. Often the addition of alcohol prevents precipitation.

5. *Colloids and polymers*

a. Solutions of hydrophilic polymers like Methylcellulose and Acacia depend on hydration through hydrogen-bonding and ion-dipole interactions. These polymers may be dehydrated and precipitated by concentrated electrolyte solutions (especially polyvalent ions) or phenolic compounds. Strategies for handling this type of problem include decreasing the concentration of the electrolyte and/or substituting another polymer gum that is not as easily dehydrated. This subject is discussed in Chapter 18, Viscosity-inducing Agents.

b. For some viscosity-increasing polymers, interactions are required to form the desired gel. For example, Sodium Alginate is gelled with calcium ions, and Carbomer is gelled by the addition of an inorganic (e.g., NaOH) or organic (e.g., Triethanolamine) base. These gels are sensitive to the addition of some other additives or to changes in pH.

c. Amphotericin B forms a colloidal dispersion when reconstituted as directed. Preservative-free Sterile Water for Injection is required. The dispersion may then be diluted with Dextrose 5% in Water. The colloidal dispersion is very sensitive to pH, so the D5W added must have a pH of at least 4.2. Buffers are present in the Amphotericin B formulation to raise the pH of the final solution above 5.0 if the D5W has a pH of at least 4.2; if not, a sterile buffer must be added. The formula for a suitable phosphate buffer is given in the Amphotericin B monograph in the *Handbook of Injectable Drugs*.

d. Erythromycin Lactobionate IV has restrictions similar to those of Amphotericin B. The solubility and stability of the reconstituted Erythromycin Lactobionate IV solution is concentration-dependent; this is why different reconstitution instructions are given for the vial (in which a 5% solution results) and the piggyback (in which 0.5% solution is made).

6. *Effect of temperature*

a. The solubility of most drugs decreases as the temperature of the solution decreases.

(1) Refrigeration is often recommended for solutions of drugs to increase their chemical stability or retard microbial growth, but this may cause problems with precipitation.

(2) Parenteral drugs for which refrigeration is not recommended because of problems with precipitation include Fluorouracil (5-FU), Cisplatin, Cotrimoxazole, Metronidazole, and some brands of Aminophylline.

b. The opposite, though uncommon, can also be true. One example is the precipitation of dibasic calcium phosphate in parenteral nutrition solutions. Calcium phosphate and dibasic calcium phosphate are equilibrium products that result when calcium gluconate and potassium phosphate are added to parenteral nutrition (PN) solutions. Although at room temperature these products may be below the critical concentration for precipitation, if the PN solution is placed in a warm environment such as a neonate crib, the insoluble dibasic calcium phosphate may precipitate from the solution. This unusual phenomenon is due to the fact that the calcium gluconate is more completely dissociated at higher temperatures, and this increases the concentration of calcium ion present in solution and leads to precipitation with the phosphate.

    c. Strategies for preventing precipitation of drug solutions sensitive to temperature changes

        (1) For injectable solutions, check the product package insert or a reference such as the *Handbook on Injectable Drugs.* Warnings concerning temperature effects on precipitation are found in these references. If an extemporaneously prepared sterile product cannot be refrigerated, the beyond-use time may need adjustment.

        (2) For oral or topical solutions, be aware of possible problems when handling solutions at or near the saturation point. If such a solution must be stored or used at a different temperature than that at which it is made, appropriate steps to prevent or handle precipitation may be necessary.

D. Sorption and Leaching

  1. Sorption

    a. Sorption of drugs to containers, closures, IV tubing, bacterial filters, and administration devices can be a problem. Because this reaction cannot be seen, it was not originally recognized. Even now it is not a reaction that can be detected by visual examination.

    b. Adsorption versus absorption: **Adsorption** is solely a surface phenomenon; molecules are concentrating at the interface between phases (liquid-liquid, liquid-solid, gas-solid). In contrast, with **absorption,** the molecules being absorbed are penetrating into the capillary spaces of the absorbing phase (10). Often we do not know whether absorption or adsorption is occurring, so the more general term, sorption, is used. In most instances, it is inconsequential whether absorption or adsorption is occurring.

    c. Drugs may react with either glass or plastic, although generally there are fewer problems with glass.

        (1) With glass the problems can be minimized by coating the glass surface (the process is called silanization) to decrease the number of sites for hydrophilic bonding. Silanization converts the -OH groups on the glass surface to silyl ethers, Si–O–Si.

        (2) With plastics, the most serious problems occur with materials that contain plasticizers. Polyvinyl chloride (PVC) is the plastic that most frequently gives problems. PVC is innately a rigid plastic that is made flexible by the addition of plasticizers such as Di(2-ethylhexyl)phthalate (DEHP) or dioctylphthalate (DOP). Certain drugs partition out of solution and into the liquid plasticizer.

    d. Logically, sorption is dependent on the hydrophilic/lipophilic nature of the drug and the binding site or of the material in the capillary space of the interface.

        (1) A drug's **partition coefficient**, or its relative oil and water solubilities, is sometimes used to predict sorption tendencies.

            (a) Drugs that are poorly water-soluble or lipophilic have a greater tendency to sorb to PVC or dissolve in its plasticizer.

            (b) For example, several of the benzodiazepines, beginning with Diazepam, have been studied quite extensively. Lorazepam, with a water solubility of 0.08 mg/mL, has significant sorption problems both with PVC bags and some other plastics, while another benzodiazepine, Midazolam HCl, which is water-soluble, does not have this difficulty (11-14).

        (2) Sorption and binding are often **pH-dependent**.

            (a) It is easy to see why the amount of binding or partitioning can be pH-dependent in the case of ionizable drugs. Depending on the hydrophilic/lipophilic nature of the binding site or plasticizer, either an ionized or nonionic species will be attracted.

(b) For example, a Chlorpromazine HCl solution with a pH = 5 and stored in PVC bags had only 5% sorption in 1 week at room temperature, but when the pH was adjusted to 7.4, approximately 86% was lost to sorption in the same period. The same behavior has been noted with Midazolam HCl (11,14).

e. Examples of drugs that sorb to glass or plastic surfaces

(1) The first documented cases of sorption involved insulin, nitroglycerin, and diazepam. It is now recognized to be a problem with a wide variety of drugs.

(2) An article published in the *International Journal of Pharmaceutical Compounding* in March 2002 listed the following drugs with significant problems due to sorption to PVC containers and administration sets: Amiodarone, Calcitriol, Diazepam, Isosorbide Dinitrate, Lorazepam, Nicardipine, Nitroglycerin, Propofol, Quinidine Gluconate, Tacrolimus, and Vitamin A. The authors stated that Insulin is not listed because it sorbs to both PVC plastics and to glass and is titrated to the proper dose (15).

(3) Other drugs including Chlorpromazine Hydrochloride, Thiopental Sodium, Bleomycin, and many more also pose problems in this regard. The *Handbook of Injectable Drugs* has a special section in each drug monograph devoted to the drug's sorption potential.

(4) Compatibility problems due to sorption will potentially become increasingly problematic with the development of protein and peptide drugs, many of which may sorb to surfaces.

f. Strategies for handling drugs that sorb to surfaces

(1) Check product package inserts and other references. As stated above, the drug monographs in the *Handbook of Injectable Drugs* each have a section on sorption.

(2) Be suspicious of new drugs from an existing class where sorption problems with other members of that class have been documented.

(3) Special tubing or containers may be used. Consult the product package insert for recommendations. Because these special tubings and containers are expensive, be sure the problem is clinically significant and that it cannot be handled in another way. For example, insulin and nitroglycerin are two drugs with significant sorption problems, but both have their dosages titrated to patient response, so potentially either sorbing or nonsorbing materials could be used (16). There are two situations that require careful consideration:

(a) When using recommended doses for drugs with sorbing problems, be sure to either use the same type of tubing and containers or be prepared to make dosage adjustments. For example, product package inserts for Nitroglycerin Injection state that the usual starting doses that have been reported in clinical studies used PVC administration sets; the use of non-absorbing tubing will result in the need for reduced doses.

(b) Furthermore, be exceedingly careful if it is necessary to switch container or tubing types for a patient stabilized with a drug that has a potential sorption problem.

(4) Because the degree of sorption increases with the length of contact time, the following strategies offer possibilities:

(a) Use short run-times for IVs containing drugs with potential sorption problems.

(b) Add the drug just before the time of administration.

(c) Consider giving the drug by IV push if possible.

(5) The number of binding sites is also a factor, so the use of short administration set tubing can sometimes be helpful. One study with Quinidine Gluconate Injection showed a decrease in sorption from 30% to 3% by using shorter IV tubing (17).

(6) Temperature is another variable that can affect sorption, with sorption increasing with increasing temperature. Temperature can often be controlled to some degree by storing the product in the refrigerator until administration.

2. Leaching

a. In recent years there has been increasing concern about leaching of plasticizers from plastics such as PVC. Of particular concern is DEHP, because it has been classified by the federal Environmental Protection Agency as a probable human carcinogen based on studies done in rodents (18).

b. Drug solutions that contain surfactants or cosolvents are most at risk, because some of these have been found to extract plasticizer from the plastic and contaminate the drug solution.

   (1) For example, the approved labeling for Paclitaxel, which uses a dehydrated alcohol–polyoxyethylated castor oil solvent system, requires use of non-PVC containers and administration sets. The manufacturer of Paclitaxel gives a list of compatible administration sets, tubing, and infusion device components. There is a good discussion of the leaching studies done with this drug in *Trissel's Handbook of Injectable Drugs* (11).

   (2) Other drugs or drug products with potential problems include IV fat emulsion, Vitamin A, cyclosporine, Docetaxel, Propofol, Tacrolimus, and Teniposide, and any others containing surfactants or cosolvents (15,18).

c. Recently the situation with DEHP has been clarified somewhat with a "Dear Colleague" letter sent from the Public Health Service in July 2002. The letter identified the two factors that determine the potential degree of risk to patients exposed to DEHP: 1) patient sensitivity and 2) dose of DEHP received.

   (1) The patients listed at greatest risk are male fetuses and neonatal and peripubertal males. These have been identified because the animal (not human) studies have shown effects on the development of male reproductive systems and the production of normal sperm in young animals. Individuals in this group, as well as pregnant women carrying a male fetus or lactating women nursing a male infant, are considered in the at-risk group.

   (2) The letter also identified procedures that pose the greatest risk of delivering exposure to DEHP from PVC administration materials. They included such things as enteral nutrition, parenteral nutrition with IV fat emulsion in PVC bags, multiple procedures, exchange transfusions, hemodialysis, and several others.

   (3) The letter stated that there is minimal or no risk of DEHP exposure when using PVC bags and tubing with crystalloid fluids (D5W, normal saline, lactated Ringer's injection, etc.).

   (4) The complete document "Safety Assessment of Di(2-ethylhexyl)phthalate (DEHP) Released from PVC Medical Devices" is available on the FDA Center for Devices and Radiological Health (CDRH) web site at www.fda.gov/cdrh/ost/dehp-pvc.pdf, accessed December 2002 (19).

d. Strategies for handling situations where leaching may be a problem

   (1) Containers, administration sets, and device components that do not contain DEHP-plasticized materials can be substituted when there is concern about leaching.

   (2) Examples of such materials include glass, polyolefin, ethylene vinyl acetate (EVA), silicone, polyethylene, and polyurethane (15,19).

   (3) These materials are usually more costly, so the cost:benefit ratio (or risk) should be considered.

IV. CHEMICAL CHANGES

Note: A review of basic chemical kinetics and equations useful in predicting rate of drug degradation is given in Figure 34.2.

A. **Oxidation**

  1. Drug classes susceptible to oxidation include:

  a. Catecholamines (compounds with -OH groups present on adjacent carbon atoms on an aromatic ring; e.g., Epinephrine)

  b. Phenolics (e.g., Phenylephrine, Morphine)

  c. Phenothiazines (e.g., Chlorpromazine, Promethazine)

  d. Olefins (alkenes; i.e., aliphatic compounds w/ double bonds)

  e. Steroids

  f. Tricyclics

  g. Thiols (i.e., sulfhydryl compounds, R-SH; e.g. Captopril)

  h. Miscellaneous (e.g., Amphotericin B, Sodium Nitroprusside, Nitrofurantoin, Tetracycline, Furosemide, Ergotamine, Sulfacetamide, and many others)

■ **Figure 34.2** Review of Chemical Kinetics: Equations for Drug Degradation

1. General Equation

$$Drug[D] + Reactant[R] \rightarrow Product[P]$$

Since the rate of this reaction is dependent on the concentration of two reactants, this is called a 2nd order reaction. The rate equation for this reaction is given by:

$$-\frac{dD}{dt} \propto [D][R] \quad or \quad -\frac{dD}{dt} = K_2[D][R]$$

where K_2 is the 2nd order rate constant

While we try to avoid adding to drug products any reactants that will cause drug degradation, sometimes this is unavoidable. For example, dosage forms, such as solutions, suspensions, and emulsions, require the presence of water, and water is a reactant for hydrolysis reactions; oxygen, a reactant in oxidation reactions, is present in the atmosphere.

2. Apparent 1st order reactions

In aqueous drug products, water is present in large excess so that its concentration is essentially constant. In this case we have kinetics that behave like a 1st order reaction in which, at any given temperature, the rate of reaction is dependent on the concentration of the drug in solution.

The apparent 1st order rate constant is given by:

$$K_1 = K_2[H_2O] \quad where \ [H_2O] \ is \ constant$$

The rate equation for this reaction is then given by:

$$-\frac{dD}{dt} = K_2[D][H_2O] = K_1[D]$$

When we rearrange this equation and integrate over the interval $D_0 \rightarrow D_t$, we get the following equation for apparent 1st order reactions like hydrolysis:

$$In\frac{D}{D_0} = -K_1t \quad or \quad In[D] = In[D_0] - K_1t$$

When we solve this equation for t when D/D_0 is 0.5 (that is, the half-life of the drug product) we get:

$$t_{1/2} = \frac{0.693}{K_1}$$

■ **Figure 34.2** *Continued.*

When we solve this equation for t when D/D_0 is 0.9 (that is, the shelf-life of the drug product) we get:

$$t_{0.9} = \frac{0.105}{K_1}$$

These are important equations, since we can obtain the apparent 1st order rate constant, K_1, from either the half-life or shelf-life of the drug in this product.

3. Apparent Zero order reactions

When the drug is present as a suspension, the concentration of drug in solution, [D], is its solubility. The drug concentration is held essentially constant, because as the drug degrades and therefore is removed from solution, additional drug dissolves from the suspension particles to maintain a saturated solution. Products like this follow apparent zero order kinetics with a rate constant given by:

$$K_0 = K_1[D]$$

where [D] is constant and is equal to the solubility of the drug in solution

The rate equation for an apparent zero order reaction is then given by:

$$-\frac{dD}{dt} = K_0$$

In this case, at a given temperature, the rate is constant and is dependent on the rate constant for the reaction. The drug concentration at any time t is given by:

$$[D] = [D_0] - K_0 t$$

When we solve this equation for t when D/D_0 is 0.5 (that is, the half-life of the drug product) we get:

$$t_{1/2} = \frac{0.5}{K_0}$$

When we solve this equation for t when D/D_0 is 0.9 (that is, the shelf-life of the drug product) we get:

$$t_{0.9} = \frac{0.1[D_0]}{K_0}$$

2. Factors that may affect the rate of oxidation
   a. Presence of oxygen
   b. Light
   c. Heavy metal ions
   d. Temperature
   e. pH
   f. Presence of other drugs or chemicals that can act as oxidizing agents
3. Possible strategies for handling drugs that are subject to oxidation
   a. Protect from oxygen.
      (1) Manufacturers can seal vulnerable drug solutions under nitrogen gas.
      (2) The pharmacist can limit the effect of atmospheric oxygen by using tight containers and by limiting storage time through use of conservative beyond-use dates.

b. Protect from light.

   (1) Use light-resistant containers or syringes.

   (2) Wrap drug containers, IV bags, and syringes with opaque or light-resistant wrappings. Examples of some light-sensitive injectable drug products that may be dispensed in this way include Na Nitroprusside, Chlorpromazine HCl, Amphotericin B, and Doxycycline.

c. Add a metal-chelating agent such as Edetate Disodium (EDTA). This ties up heavy metal ions as chelates, which render the metal ions ineffective as oxidation catalysts (see Chapter 16, Antioxidants). For example, oral liquid preparations of Captopril have been shown to be stabilized using EDTA (20). Sample prescription 28.6 in Chapter 28 illustrates this use. This strategy is not usually used for IV admixtures.

d. Add an antioxidant. Caution should be exercised when doing this because some antioxidants can cause other problems. For example, sodium bisulfite is a useful antioxidant, but it is also a strong nucleophile that initiates other undesirable degradative reactions (see Chapter 16, Antioxidants). This strategy is also not commonly used for IV admixtures.

e. Control storage temperature. Usually the rate of oxidation is more rapid at elevated temperatures and can be retarded by storage of the sensitive product under refrigeration.

f. Control pH. Be careful about mixing drug solutions or adding drugs to a solution when any component is subject to oxidation. Oxidation is most often favored by alkaline pH. For example, when sodium bicarbonate (pH = 7–8.5) is added to the oxidation-sensitive drug norepinephrine, rapid degradation of the norepinephrine results.

g. Keep drugs that are easily oxidized separated from those that are easily reduced. Commercial preparations of parenteral multivitamin preparations illustrate this principle: Folic acid is incompatible with oxidizing agents, reducing agents, and metal ions; cyanocobalamin has limited compatibility with ascorbic acid (about 24 hours), thiamine, and niacinamide. Therefore, injectable multivitamin products are either manufactured as lyophilized powder for injection or are packaged as two separate solutions so the incompatible vitamins can be kept separate until the time of administration.

B. Hydrolysis

1. Drug classes susceptible to hydrolysis include:

   a. Esters, R-CO-O-R (e.g., the local anesthetic "caines" such as procaine and tetracaine, aspirin, belladonna alkaloids, and especially strained ring-systems like the lactones)

   b. Amides, R-CO-NH$_2$, and especially the strained ring-system amides like the lactams (e.g., penicillins)

   c. Imides, R-CO-NH-CO-R′ (e.g., barbiturates)

   d. Thiolesters, R-CO-S-R′

2. Factors that affect the rate of hydrolysis

   a. Presence of water

   b. pH

   c. Presence of general acids and bases (citrate, acetate, phosphate), which are often used as buffers

   d. Concentration of the drug

   e. Temperature

   f. Presence of other components that may catalyze hydrolysis. Dextrose is reported to be a common offender.

3. Strategies for handling drugs subject to hydrolysis

   a. Control exposure to moisture for solid drugs with use of tight containers and desiccants.

b. Control the pH of aqueous formulations. Check the pH of all drug solutions that are to be combined and the usual pH generated by drugs that are to be added. The final pH of a solution can be checked using pH paper.

c. Check appropriate references for possible negative effects of general acids or bases. If this can be a factor in accelerating hydrolysis, avoid adding these compounds as buffers, or limit the amounts used, because this effect is concentration-dependent. Also avoid adding other drug solutions that contain these compounds.

d. Consider drug concentration when this is a factor. Information on this is available in product package inserts and in references such as *The Handbook of Injectable Drugs*. Expiration times may be reduced greatly with concentrated solutions of some drugs subject to hydrolysis. The concentration-dependent rate of hydrolysis of Ampicillin Na is a classic example of this factor.

e. Control storage temperature. The rate of hydrolysis is more rapid at elevated temperatures and can be retarded by storage of the sensitive product under refrigeration. You may need to limit or alter beyond-use dates for drugs subject to hydrolysis, depending on storage conditions.

(1) The Arrhenius equation is a useful tool for estimating the effect of temperature on the rate of hydrolysis.

$$ln\left(\frac{k_2}{k_1}\right) = \frac{E_a(T_2 - T_1)}{R\,T_2\,T_1}$$

where:

k_2 = rate constant for hydrolysis at T_2
k_1 = rate constant for hydrolysis at T_1
E_a = energy of activation for the reaction at the given conditions (concentrations, pH, solvent), in cal-mol^{-1}
R = the gas constant, 1.987 cal/deg-mole
T_1 = temperature in degrees K for rate constant k_1
T_2 = temperature in degrees K for rate constant k_2

(2) Information on half-life and energies of activation for many common drugs can be found in *Chemical Stability of Pharmaceuticals* (21). An analysis of the energies of activation for drugs listed in *Chemical Stability of Pharmaceuticals* was done by the author K.A. Connors. A normal-type distribution curve was found with the lowest E_a at 4,000 cal/mol, the highest at 44,000 cal/mol, and the majority clustered between 17,000 and 26,000 cal/mol.

(3) In a practical sense this is useful information. Consider the following: In pharmacy practice, the situations in which we need to make predictions about changes in stability based on the influence of temperature are often in the area of reconstituted medications, antibiotics, and other drugs of limited stability. Most often it concerns storage under refrigeration versus at room temperature. We can get an approximate quantitative determination of change in shelf life with these changes in storage temperature by solving the Arrhenius equation for the ratio of the rate constants, k_2/k_1, at the two temperatures.

➤ *EXAMPLE*

Set the following parameters in the Arrhenius equation:

T_1 = 278°K (5°C or 41°F, an average refrigerator temperature)

T_2 = 295°K (22°C or 72°F, an average room temperature)

R = 1.987 cal/deg-mol

E_a = 22,000 cal/mol—An average E_a for drugs

$$ln\left(\frac{k_2}{k_1}\right) = \frac{22,000\,(295 - 278)}{1.987\,(295)\,(278)}$$

$$k_2/k_1 = 9.9 \approx 10$$

From this it can be seen that for the "average" drug under "average" conditions, the rate of degradation reactions (such as hydrolysis) is approximately 10 times faster at room temperature than at refrigerator temperatures.

(4) A similar concept has been developed known as Q_{10}.

(a) This is defined as the ratio of the rate constants, k_2/k_1, when the difference in temperature is $10°$.

(b) Values of Q_{10} have been calculated for various energies of activation (E_a) between the normal ambient temperatures of $20°$ to $30°C$ ($68°$ to $86°F$). A list of these values and the development of Q_{10} from the Arrhenius equation is shown in Figure 34.3.

(c) An equation using Q_{10} is also given at the bottom of Figure 34.3 that calculates an estimate of the ratio of the rate constants for any tem-

■ **Figure 34.3** Q_{10} Values and Calculations

Arrhenius Equation: $$In\frac{k_2}{k_1} = \frac{E_a(T_2 - T_1]}{R\,T_2\,T_1}$$ where temperature is in $°K$

Q_{10} is defined as the ratio of k_2/k_1 when the difference in temperature is $10°$:

$$Q_{10} = \frac{k_{(T+10)}}{k_T}$$

Therefore: $$In\,Q_{10} = \frac{E_a(T+10-T)}{R\,(T+10)(T)} = \frac{E_a}{R(T+10)T}\frac{10}{}$$

or $$Q_{10} = e^{\frac{E_a}{R(T+10)T}\frac{10}{}}$$

Using one of these equations you can calculate the Q_{10} values for the $10°$ interval about room temperature ($25°C$) for various E_a Values:

E_a (cal/mol)	Q_{10} (30 to 20°C)
10,000	1.76
12,200	2.0
15,000	2.34
19,400	3.0
20,000	3.11
22,000	3.48
24,500	4.0
25,000	4.12
30,000	5.48

These values can be used with the equation given below to obtain an approximation of the change of rate (k_2/k_1) for various temperature changes.

$$Q_{\Delta T} = Q_{10}^{(\Delta T/10)}$$

For example in going from $278°K$ ($5°C$, refrigerator temperature) to $295°K$ ($22°C$, room temperature), a ΔT of $17°$, for a reaction with E_a of $22,000$ cal/mol, we have

$$Q_{\Delta T} = Q_{10}^{(\Delta T/10)} = 3.48^{17/10} = 3.48^{1.7} = 8.33$$

Note: for more detailed treatment of this subject, see Connors KA, Amidon GL, Stella VJ, *Chemical Stability of Pharmaceuticals, 2nd Ed*, John Wiley & Sons, 1986.

perature change, $Q_{\Delta T}$. Using the same data as was used in the example given above, a k_2/k_1 value of 8.3 is calculated, very close to the 9.9 value calculated using the Arrhenius equation. Either of these methods can be used to get an estimate of the change in rate of a reaction with a change in temperature.

(5) It is extremely important to remember that the energy of activation, E_a, varies with both the drug and the conditions.

    (a) For example, the E_a for the hydrolysis of ampicillin is 16,400 at pH 1.35, 18,300 at pH 4.93, and 22,300 at pH 9.78 (22), which correspond to rate constant ratios (k_2/k_1) of 5.5, 6.8, and 10.2 when going from 5° to 22°C.

    (b) When the true energy of activation for the reaction is known, this should be used.

    (c) Even without known values of energy of activation, it is helpful to have some knowledge of the magnitude of the change of rate of reaction at temperatures of interest; for example, changes in the range of 5 to 15 times for most drugs when going from storage in the refrigerator to room temperature.

C. **Evolution of Gas** (usually CO_2)

    1. Drugs that have problems

        a. Sodium bicarbonate and carbonate buffers are the most common offenders.

        b. Decarboxylation of o- and p-substituted benzoic acids (the antituberculosis drug p-aminosalicylic acid is an example) to give carbon dioxide can also occur.

        c. Note that this effect is actually desired in some preparations, such as effervescent powders and tablets (e.g., Alka Seltzer®).

    2. Strategies for handling this problem

        a. Keep drugs that generate acid pH from sodium bicarbonate and drug products that contain carbonate buffers.

$$NaHCO_3 + H^+ \rightarrow H_2CO_3 \rightarrow H_2O + CO_2 \uparrow$$

        b. For vulnerable solid dosage forms, store and dispense in tight containers.

D. **Displacement**

    1. Cisplatin is the best-known example. It undergoes the following reactions:

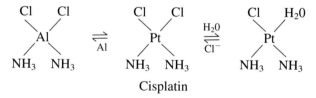

Cisplatin

    2. Strategies in handling Cisplatin and similar drugs

        a. When Cisplatin is diluted (such as in preparing an admixture in an LVP), the solution must have a sodium chloride concentration of at least 0.2% to maintain the chloride ions on the Cisplatin molecule. These ions are essential to the activity of the Cisplatin. Tests have found that 0.45% NaCl or 0.9% NaCl are satisfactory, but not Sterile Water for Injection or D5W. Note that this is a reversible reaction.

        b. Because Aluminum displaces the Platinum when aluminum needles are used, stainless-steel needles must be used for drawing and administering this drug.

E. **Complexation**

    1. Tetracycline is the classic example of a drug that is inactivated by complexation.

        a. This reaction occurs with multivalent ions such as calcium, magnesium, iron, and aluminum.

b. The usual strategy is to keep the drug separate from the offending ions. Tetracyclines should not be mixed with other drug products containing multivalent ions. Furthermore, patients taking tetracyclines (except some synthetic versions) should be counseled to avoid taking the drug with foods or drugs containing multivalent ions, including milk, most breads, iron-containing foods and drugs, and antacids.

2. Aminophylline is an example of a drug that is a complex.

a. In this case, theophylline, the active principle, is complexed in a 2:1 ratio with ethylenediamine. This is done to solubilize the theophylline because this drug has limited water solubility and does not form soluble salts.

b. The complexation is a reversible reaction, and aminophylline may liberate the ethylenediamine. This is especially problematic when the drug is in solution because the theophylline then precipitates out of solution. Injectable solutions of aminophylline contain excess ethylenediamine to ensure that this does not happen, but these solutions should always be inspected for the presence of crystals and should not be used if any are present.

c. The complexation is also pH-dependent.

(1). King's *Dispensing of Medication* reports that Sorenson's phosphate buffer has been used to help maintain the stability of oral solutions of aminophylline (23).

(2) The pH of Aminophylline Injection is maintained with the presence of excess ethylenediamine. The *USP* gives the pH range of injectable solutions of Aminophylline as 8.6–9. The monograph states that excess ethylenediamine may be added, but that no other substance may be added for the purpose of pH adjustment. It also notes that the injection should not be used if crystals are present (24).

3. A third example of a drug that forms complexes is Edetic Acid, also known as ethylenediaminetetraacetic acid or EDTA. Various forms of Edetic Acid are used therapeutically and as stabilizing agents because of the ability of this compound to form complexes with various cations.

a. There are two official injectable products: Edetate Disodium Injection and Edetate Calcium Disodium Injection. The disodium complex is used in emergency situations to treat hypercalcemia because the drug has a complexation site available to complex with and remove the excess calcium in the blood. The calcium disodium complex is used primarily to treat lead poisoning. In this case, the calcium disodium complex is used so that the drug will not remove calcium from the body.

b. EDTA is also used in products subject to oxidation in which metal cations act as catalysts for the oxidation process. EDTA is discussed in more detail in Chapter 16, Antioxidants.

F. Racemization

1. Isomers are compounds that have the same molecular formula (that is, the same number and kind of atoms) but different molecular structures. Enantiomers are isomers that are mirror images of each other. Enantiomers have identical chemical properties except toward optically active reagents and, more importantly in medicine, toward many enzymes, biologic receptors, and membranes. A mixture of equal parts of enantiomers is called a racemate, and the conversion of one enantiomer to a racemate is known as racemization.

2. Examples of drugs that undergo racemization include:

a. Epinephrine: The l-enantiomer has approximately 15–20 times the physiologic activity as the d-enantiomer (25).

b. Some local anesthetics, such as mepivacaine and bupivacaine, undergo racemization (25).

   c. Other well-known drugs are available as both the racemic mixture and as the single enantiomer; examples include amphetamine and dextroamphetamine, albuterol and levalbuterol, and omeprazole and esomeprazole.

  3. Problems exist only when one enantiomer is much more physiologically active than the other **and** when racemization easily takes place. The pharmacist should be aware of this and investigate the literature when handling any drugs that have this potential. In the future, more chiral drugs will be available as pure enantiomers than as racemates.

G. **Epimerization**

  1. Optical isomers that are not superimposable and are not mirror images are called diastereomers. They have different physical properties: different melting points, boiling points, solubilities, and densities. They have the same functional groups and show similar chemical properties but exhibit different rates of reaction. A pair of diastereomers that differ only in the configuration about one carbon atom are called epimers.

  2. One example of a drug that undergoes epimerization is tetracycline. It undergoes reversible epimerization to epitetracycline, a form that has little antibacterial activity. The chemical structures of tetracycline and epitetracycline differ only in the rotation of the -$N(CH_3)_2$ group on the C-4 atom.

  a. Epimerization occurs to an appreciable extent only when tetracycline is in solution. The reaction rate is pH-dependent and is greatest at pH = 3. The rate also depends on temperature and the presence of citrate and phosphate ions. Solutions of Tetracycline Hydrochloride Injection are reported to lose 8–12% of their potency in 24 hours when stored at room temperature (26).

  b. Because epimerization happens only to drug molecules in solution, suspensions of tetracycline are much more stable. Stable oral suspensions can be made by adding a buffer to maintain the pH at a level where the soluble form of tetracycline is minimized. Suspensions of tetracycline at pH 4–7 are reported to be stable for 3 months (26). One recommendation is to use a phosphate buffer with the pH adjusted to approximately 6.

  c. In commercial solutions of tetracycline prescribed for the treatment of acne, the epimerization reaction is controlled by the addition of citric acid for buffering and excess 4-epitetracycline HCl. Because epimerization is a reversible reaction, the excess 4-epitetracycline shifts the equilibrium to prevent the active tetracycline from transforming to the inactive epi form. Extemporaneous topical solutions of tetracycline HCl should probably not be made extemporaneously unless the formulation is known to have ingredients that will control epimerization.

  3. Pilocarpine is another example of a drug that may epimerize with loss of therapeutic activity.

References

1. The 2002 United States Pharmacopeia 25/National Formulary 20. Rockville, MD: The United States Pharmacopeial Convention, Inc., 2001;2231–2234.
2. Ecanow B, Sadik F. Powders. In: King RE, ed. Dispensing of medications, 9th ed. Easton, PA: Mack Publishing Co., 1984;40.
3. Dittert LW, ed. Sprowls' American pharmacy, 7th ed. Philadelphia: JB Lippincott, 1974;333–334.

4. Martin A, Bustamante P. Physical pharmacy, 4th ed. Philadelphia: Lea & Febiger, 1993;41–43.

5. Kohut J III, Trissel LA, Leissing NC. Don't ignore details in drug-compatibility reports. Am J Health-Syst Pharm 1986;53:2339.

6. Oskroba DM, Leissing NC, Trissel LA. An automated process for determining the physical compatibility of drugs. Hosp Pharm 1997;32:1013–1020.

7. Stella VJ, Roberts RD. Unpublished results. In: Trissel LA, ed. Handbook of injectable drugs, 4th ed. Bethesda, MD: The American Society of Hospital Pharmacists, 1986; XVII.

8. Connors KA. Thermodynamics of pharmaceutical systems, An introduction for students of pharmacy. New York: John Wiley & Sons, Inc., 2002;193–202.

9. Booth RE, Dale JK. Compounding and dispensing information. In King RE, ed. Dispensing of medications, 9th ed. Easton, PA: Mack Publishing Co., 1984;335.

10. Martin A, Bustamante P. Physical pharmacy, 4th ed. Philadelphia: Lea & Febiger, 1993:370.

11. Trissel LA, ed. Handbook of injectable drugs, 12th ed. Bethesda, MD: The American Society of Health-System Pharmacists, 2003; Monographs.

12. Trissel LA, Pearson SD. Storage of lorazepam in three injectable solutions in polyvinyl chloride and polyolefin bags. Am J Hosp Pharm 1994;51:368–372.

13. Stiles ML, Allen LV Jr, Prince SJ, Holland JS. Stability of dexamethasone sodium phosphate, diphenhydramine hydrochloride, lorazepam, and metoclopramide hydrochloride in portable infusion-pump reservoirs. Am J Hosp Pharm 1994;51:514–517.

14. Stiles ML, Allen LV Jr, Prince SJ. Stability of deferoxamine mesylate, floxuridine, fluorouracil, hydromorphone hydrochloride, lorazepam, and midazolam hydrochloride in polypropylene infusion-pump syringes. Am J Health-Syst Pharm. 1996;53:1583–1588.

15. Rice SP, Markel JA. A review of parenteral admixtures requiring select containers and administration sets. IJPC 2002;6:120–122.

16. Altavela JL, Haas CE, Nowak DR, Powers J, Gacioch GM. Clinical response to intravenous nitroglycerin infused through polyethylene or polyvinyl chloride tubing. Am J Hosp Pharm 1994;51:490–494.

17. Darbar D, Dell'Orto S, Wilkinson GR, Roden DM. Loss of quinidine gluconate injection in a polyvinyl chloride infusion system. Am J Health-Syst Pharm 1996;53:655–658.

18. Landis NT. Advocacy group targets PVC i.v. equipment. Am J Health-Syst Pharm 1999;56:937–938.

19. Public health notification: PVC devices containing the plasticizer DEHP. Rockville, MD: Public Health Service, Center for Devices and Radiological Health, Food and Drug Administration, July 12, 2002.

20. Lye MYE, Yow KL, et al. Effects of ingredients on stability of captopril in extemporaneously prepared oral liquids. Am J Health-Syst Pharm 1997;54:2483–2487.

21. Connors KA, Amidon GL, Stella VJ. Chemical stability of pharmaceuticals, 2d ed. New York: John Wiley & Sons, 1986; Monographs.

22. Connors KA, Amidon GL, Stella VJ. Chemical stability of pharmaceuticals, 2d ed. New York: John Wiley & Sons, 1986; 202.

23. Booth RE, Dale JK. Compounding and dispensing information. In: King RE, ed. Dispensing of medications, 9th ed. Easton, PA: Mack Publishing Co., 1984;408.

24. The 2002 United States Pharmacopeia 25/National Formulary 20. Rockville, MD: The United States Pharmacopeial Convention, Inc., 2001;118.

25. Alexander KS. Appraisal of product quality. In: King RE, ed. Dispensing of medications, 9th ed. Easton, PA: Mack Publishing Co., 1984;231.

26. Reynolds JEF, ed. Martindale–the extra pharmacopoeia, 30th ed. London: The Pharmaceutical Press, 1993;212–213.

APPENDICES

Abreviations Commonly used in Prescriptions and Medication Orders

Abbrev.	Meaning	Abbrev.	Meaning	Abbrev.	Meaning
a	before	DPT	diphteria, pertussis,	HCT	hematocrit
aa. or ā ā	of each		tetanus	HCTZ	hydrochlorothiazide
ABW	actual body weight	DS	double strength	HEPA	high efficiency particular
a.c.	before meals	d.t.d.	give of such doses		air
ad	up to	DW	distilled water	HR	heart rate
a.d.	right ear	D5NS	dextrose 5% in normal	HRT	hormone replacement
ad lib.	at pleasure, freely		saline (0.9% sodium		therapy
a.m.	morning		chloride)	h.s.	at bedtime
amp.	ampul	D5$\frac{1}{2}$NS or	dextrose 5% in $\frac{1}{2}$	HT	height or hypertension
APAP	Acetaminophen	D5-0.45	normal saline (0.45%	IBW	ideal body weight
aq.	water		NaCl)	ICU	intensive care unit
aq.dist.	distilled water	D5W	dextrose 5% in water	ID	intradermal
a.s.	left ear	DX	diagnosis	IM	intramuscular
ASA	aspirin	EC	enteric coated	INH	isoniozid
ASAP	as soon as possible	ECG or EKG	electrocardiogram	I&O	input and output
ATC	around the clock	EDTA	edetate	inj.	injection
a.u.	each ear	EENT	eyes, ears, nose, throat	IPPD	intermittent positive
b.i.d.	twice a day	EES	erythromycin		pressure breathing
b.i.w.	twice a week		ethylsuccinate	IU or iu	international units
BM	bowel movement	EFAD	essential fatty acid	IV	intravenous
BP	blood pressure		deficiency	IVP	intravenous push or IV
BS	blood sugar	elix.	elixir		pyelogram
BSA	body surface area	e.m.p.	as directed	IVPB	intravenous piggy back
BUN	blood urea nitrogen	EPI	epinephrine	L	liter
BW	body weight	EPO	erythropoietin	LCD	Coal Tar Solution
C	centigrade	ER	emergency room	LR	Lactated Ringer's
c. or c̄	with	et	and		Injection
CA	cancer or cardiac arrest	f. or ft.	make	M.	mix
cap	capsule	F	Fahrenheit	m^2 or M^2	square meter
CBC	complete blood count	FBS	fasting blood sugar	mcg or μg	microgram
cc	cubic centimeter	FFA	free fatty acid	MDI	metered dose inhaler
CCT	crude coal tar	fl or fld	fluid	mEq	milliequivalent
chart or		ft.	make	mg	milligram
chartulate	powder or powder paper	FU or 5-FU	fluorouracil	MI	myocardial infarction
CHF	congestive heart failure	g or Gm	gram	min	minute (s)
CNS	central nervous system	GI	gastro-intestinal	ml or mL	milliliter
comp.	compound	GFR	glomerular filtration rate	MMR	measles, mumps, rubella
COPD	chronic obstructive	gr	grain	MO	mineral oil
	pulmonary disease	gtt, gtts	drop, drops	MOM	milk of magnesia
CPZ	chlorpromazine	GYN	gynecology	mOsm or	
crm	cream	GU	genitourinary	mOsmol	milliosmoles
C&S	culture and sensitivity	H	hypodermic	MR	may repeat
d	day	h or hr	hour	MRX__	may repeat_times
disc or D.C.	discontinue	HA	headache	MS	morphine sulfate or
disp.	dispense	Hb	hemoglobin		multiple sclerosis
div.	divide	HBP	high blood pressure	MVI	multivitamin
DOB	date of birth	HC	hydrocortisone	n	nostril

Abbrev.	Meaning	Abbrev.	Meaning	Abbrev.	Meaning
N&V	nausea and vomiting	pr	rectally	T&C	type and crossmatch
NG	nasogastric	pre-op	before surgery	tab	tablet
NK	none known	p.r.n.	when required or as needed	TAC	Tetracaine, Adrenalin, and Cocaine
no. or No.	number				
noct.	night	PT	physical therapy	tal.	such
non rep. or N.R.	do not repeat or no refills	pulv.	powder	tal. dos.	such doses
		pv	vaginally	tbsp.	tablespoonful
NPO	nothing by mouth	q⁻ or q	every	TCA	tricyclic antidepressant
NS	normal saline	q.d.	every day	TCN	tetracycline
½NS	half-strength normal saline	q.h.	every hour	temp	temperature
		q.i.d.	four times a day	t.i.d.	three times a day
NTG	nitroglycerin	q.o.d.	every other day	t.i.w.	three times a week
NVD	nausea, vomiting & diarrhea	q.s.	a sufficient quantity	TMP/SMX	trimethoprim/ sulfame- thoxizole
		q.s. ad	a sufficient quantity to make		
O.	pint			top	topically
OB-GYN	obstetrics-gynecology	r or R	rectal	TPN	total parenteral nutrition
OC	oral contraceptive	R.L. or R/L	Ringer's Lactate	tr.	tincture
OD	overdose	℞	prescription symbol (recipe or take thou)	tsp.	teaspoonful
o.d.	right eye			U or u	unit(s)
oint.	ointment	s̄ or s	without	UA	urinalysis
o.l.	left eye	sat.	saturated	u.d. or ut dict	as directed
o.s.	left eye	s.i.d.	once a day	ung.	ointment
OR	operating room	Sig.	write on label	URI	upper respiratory infection
OT	occupational therapy	SL	sublingual		
OTC	over-the-counter	SOB	shortness of breath	USP	United States Pharmacopeia
o.u.	each eye	sol.	solution		
o₂	both eyes	s.o.s.	if there is need	UTI	urinary tract infection
oz	ounce (avoirdupois)	SS	saturated solution	UUN	urine urea nitrogen
p or per	by	ss. or s̄s̄	one-half	UV	ultraviolet
Pb	phenobarbital	SSKI	saturated solution of potassium iodide	vol.	volume
p.c.	after meals			VS	vital signs
PCN	penicillin	stat.	immediately	w/	with
p.m.	afternoon; evening	subc, subq, SC or SQ	subcutaneously	w.a. or WA	while awake
p.o.	by mouth			WBC	white blood cell count
post	after	supp.	suppository	wk.	week
post-op	after surgery	susp.	suspension	w/o	without
PPD	purified protein derivative (tuberculin)	SVR	alcohol	X	times
		syr.	syrup	y.o.	year old
PPI	patient package insert	SZ	seizure	ZnO	zinc oxide
PPM	parts per million				

The degree symbol (°) can either indicate degrees of temperature—for example, 98.6°F; or it can mean "hour" or "hours"—for example, "q3°" means every three hours.

APPENDIX B
Common English Titles and Synonyms

English Title	Synonyms	
Acacia	Gum Arabic	
Acetanilid	Antifebrin	
Acetophenetidin	Phenacetin	
Aconite	Monk's Hood	
Agar	Agar-Agar, Vegetable Gelatin	
Alcohol	Spiritus Vini Rectificatus, S.V.R.	95% Ethanol
Aluminum Acetate Solution	Burow's Solution	
Aminoacetic Acid	Glycine	
Aminopyrine	Amidopyrine	
Ammonia Liniment	Hartshorn Liniment	
Ammonium Acetate Solution	Spirit of Mindererus	
Ammonium Carbonate	Baker's Salt	
Ammonium Chloride	Ammonium Muriate, Sal ammoniac	
Antimony Potassium Tartrate	Tartar Emetic	
Antipyrine	Phenazone	
Areca	Betel Nut	
Aromatic Elixir	Simple Elixir	
Arsenic Trioxide	Arsenous Acid, White Arsenic	
Ascorbic Acid	Vitamin C, Cevitamic Acid	
Aspidium	Male Fern	
Belladonna Leaf	Deadly Nightshade Leaf	
Belladonna Tincture	Belladonna Leaf Tincture	
Bentonite	Mineral Soap, Soap Clay	
Benzaldehyde	Artificial Almond Oil	
Benzoic Acid	Flowers of Benjamin	
Benzoic and Salicylic Acid Ointment	Whitfield's Ointment	
Bismuth Magma	Milk of Bismuth	
Bismuth Subcarbonate	Basic Bismuth Carbonate	
Bismuth Subnitrate	Basic Bismuth Nitrate	
Bismuth Subgallate	Dermatol	
Calamine	Prepared Calamine	
Precipitated Calcium Carbonate	Precipitated Chalk	
Calcium Hydroxide	Slaked Lime	
Calcium Hydroxide Solution	Lime Water	
Camphor	Gum Camphor	
Camphor and Soap Liniment	Soap Liniment	
Capsicum	Cayenne Pepper	
Carboxymethylcellulose Sodium	CMC	
Cascara Sagrada	Rhamus Purshiana	
Castor Oil	Oleum Ricini	
Prepared Chalk	Drop Chalk	
Chlorobutanol	Chloretone	
Chondrus	Irish Moss	
Cinnamon Oil	Oil of Cassia	
Citric Acid Syrup	Syrup of Lemon	
Coal Tar	Crude Coal Tar, CCT	
Coal Tar Topical Solution	Liquor Carbonis Detergens, LCD	
Cocaine Hydrochloride	Cocaine Muriate	
Cod Liver Oil	Oleum Jecoris Aselli	
Codeine	Methylmorphine	
Colocynth	Bitter Apple	
Copaiba Mixture	Lafayette Mixture	
Purified Cotton	Absorbent Cotton	
Creosote	Beechwood Creosote	
Cupric Sulfate	Blue Vitriol	
Dextrose	d-Glucose	
Diethylstilbestrol	Stilbestrol	
Digitalis	Foxglove	
Diagnostic Diphtheria Toxin	Schick Test Toxin	

English Title	Synonyms
Ergonovine Maleate	Ergotrate Maleate
Eriodictyon	Yerba Santa
Estrone	Theelin
Ethyl Aminobenzoate	Benzocaine, Anesthesin
Ethyl Nitrite Spirit	Sweet Spirit of Nitre
Eucalyptol	Cineol
Eugenol	Oil of Clove
Ferric Chloride Tincture	Tincture of Iron
Ferric Subsulfate Solution	Monsel's Solution
Ferrous Carbonate Pills	Blaud's Pills
Ferrous Sulfate	Green Vitriol
Glycerin	Glycerol
Glycyrrhiza	Licorice Root
Green Soap	Soft Soap
Hamamelis Water	Witch Hazel
Hydrastis	Golden Seal
Hydrochloric Acid	Muriatic Acid
Hyoscyamus	Henbane
Strong Iodine Solution	Lugol's Solution
Iodine Tincture	Mild Tincture of Iodine
Ipecac and Opium Powder	Dover's Powder
Iron and Ammonium Acetate Solution	Basham's Solution
Iron, Quinine and Strychnine Elixir	Elixir I.Q. and S.
Lactose	Milk Sugar
Lanatoside C	Digilanid C
Lanolin	Woolfat
Lead Acetate	Sugar of Lead
Lead Subacetate Solution	Goulard's Extract
Lemon Tincture	Lemon Peel Tincture
Lime	Calcium Oxide, Quicklime
Lime Liniment	Carron Oil
Sulfurated Lime Solution	Vleminckx' Solution
Linseed	Flaxseed
Lobelia	Indian Tobacco
Magnesia Magma	Milk of Magnesia
Magnesium Citrate Solution	Citrate of Magnesia
Magnesium Sulfate	Epsom Salt
Menadione	Synthetic Vitamin K
Menthol	Peppermint Camphor
Red Mercuric Oxide	Red Precipitate
Yellow Mercuric Oxide	Yellow Precipitate
Mild Mercurous Chloride	Calomel, Protochloride of Mercury
Compound Mild Mercurous Chloride Pills	Compound Cathartic Pills
Mercury Bichloride	Corrosive Sublimate, Mercuric Chloride
Mercury	Quicksilver
Mild Mercurial Ointment	Blue Ointment
Ammoniated Mercury	White Precipitate
Methyl Salicylate	Wintergreen Oil, Gaultheria Oil
Methylrosaniline Chloride	Gentian Violet, Crystal Violet
Mineral Oil	Heavy Liquid Petrolatum, Parrafin Oil
Myristica	Nutmeg
Nicotinic Acid	Niacin
Nitric Acid	Aqua Fortis, Spirit of Nitre
Nitrohydrochloric Acid	Aqua Regia
Nitrous Oxide	Laughing Gas
Olive Oil	Sweet Oil
Opium Tincture	Laudanum, Deodorized Opium Tincture
Compound Opium and Glycyrrhiza Mixture	Brown Mixture
Paregoric	Camphorated Opium Tincture
Peppermint Spirit	Essence of Peppermint
Compound Pepsin Elixir	Compound Digestive Mixture
	Elixir Lactated Pepsin
Pepsin and Renin Elixir	Essense of Pepsin
Phenol	Carbolic Acid
Phenyl Salicylate	Salol

English Title	Synonyms
Physostigmine Salicylate	Eserine Salicylate
Plantago Seed	Psyllium Seed
Polyethylene Glycol	Carbowax®
Polysorbate	Tween®
Sulfurated Potash	Liver of Sulfur
Potassium Arsenite Solution	Fowler's Solution
Potassium Bitartrate	Cream of Tartar
Potassium Chlorate Gargle with Iron	Golden Gargle
Potassium Nitrate	Saltpeter
Potassium Sodium Tartrate	Rochelle Salt
Resorcinol	Resorcin
Riboflavin	Vitamin B_2
Ringer's Solution	Isotonic Solution of 3 Chlorides
Rose Oil	Attar of Roses
Rosin	Colophony
Saccharin	Gluside
Sanguinaria	Bloodroot
Scopolamine Hydrobromide	Hyoscine Hydrobromide
Purified Siliceous Earth	Purified Kieselguhr, Diatomaceous Earth
Toughened Silver Nitrate	Lunar Caustic
Medicinal Soft Soap	Green Soap
Soft Soap Liniment	Tincture of Green Soap
Sodium Bicarbonate	Baking Soda
Compound Tablets of Sodium Bicarbonate	Soda Mint Tablets
Sodium Bicarbonate and Calcium Carbonate Powder	Sippy Powder No. 1
Sodium Bicarbonate and Magnesium Oxide Powder	Sippy Powder No. 2
Sodium Biphosphate	Monosodium Phosphate, Monobasic Sodium Phosphate
Sodium Borate	Borax
Compound Sodium Borate Solution	Dobell's Solution
Sodium Carbonate	Sal Soda, Soda Ash, Washing Soda
Sodium Phosphate	Disodium Hydrogen Phosphate, Dibasic Sodium Phosphate
Sodium Saccharin	Soluble Saccharin
Sodium Sulfate	Glauber's Salt
Sodium Thiosulfate	Sodium Hyposulfite, "hypo"
Sublimed Sulfur	Flowers of Sulfur
Sulfuric Acid	Oil of Vitriol
Syrup	Simple Syrup
Taraxacum	Dandelion Root
Theobroma Oil	Cocoa Butter
Thiamine HCl	Vitamin B_1
Tragacanth	Gum Tragacanth
Trinitrophenol	Picric Acid
Whiskey	Spiritus Frumenti
White Lotion	Lotion Alba
White Petrolatum	Petrolatum Alba
White Wax	Bleached Beeswax
Yellow Wax	Beeswax
Wool Fat	Anhydrous Lanolin
Hydrous Wool Fat	Hydrous Lanolin
Yellow Lotion	Yellow Wash
Zinc Gelatin	Zinc Gelatin Boot
Zinc Oxide	Flowers of Zinc
Zinc Oxide Paste	Lassar's Plain Zinc Paste
Zinc Oxide Paste with Salicylic Acid	Lassar's Paste
Zinc Sulfate	White Vitriol

APPENDIX C
WEIGHTS AND MEASURES

METRIC MEASURES

In 1960, a conference was held to create a single system of weights and measures for the entire world. The International System of Units, *SI units,* were adopted. The meter (symbolized *m*) is the fundamental unit of both the International System of Units and the Metric System. The basic units of both volume and weight are derived from the meter. The basic unit for volume is the liter (*L*); it is the volume of 1,000 cubic centimeters (often written cc). The basic unit for weight is the gram (*g*); it is the weight of 1 cm^3 of water at 4° C. Other metric units of length, volume, or weight are achieved by applying prefixes to the appropriate basic unit. The prefix specifies a power of ten which is multiplied times the basic unit. For example, the prefix *milli* is associated with a 10^{-3} multiple, so that a *millimeter* is 10^{-3} meters, a *milligram* is 10^{-3} grams, and a *milliliter* is 10^{-3} liters.. Prefixes for SI units, together with their associated powers of ten, and their symbols are given here. Below are the metric units of length, volume, and weight most commonly used in pharmacy and medicine.

Power of Ten	Prefix	Symbol
10^{18}	exa	E
10^{15}	peta	P
10^{12}	tera	T
10^{9}	giga	G
10^{6}	mega	M
10^{3}	kilo	k
10^{2}	hecto	h
10	deka	da
1	No prefix (basic unit)	
10^{-1}	deci	d
10^{-2}	centi	c
10^{-3}	milli	m
10^{-6}	micro	μ
10^{-9}	nano	n
10^{-12}	pico	p
10^{-15}	femto	f
10^{-18}	atto	a

METRIC MEASURES OF LENGTH

100 centimeter (cm) = 1 meter (m)
10 millimeters (mm) = 1 centimeter (cm)
1,000 micrometers (μm) = 1 millimeter (mm)

METRIC MEASURES OF VOLUME

1,000 milliliters (mL) = 1 liter (L)
1,000 microliters (μL) = 1 milliliter (mL)

METRIC MEASURES OF WEIGHT

1,000 gram (g) = 1 kilogram (kg)
1,000 milligrams (mg) = 1 gram (g)
1,000 micrograms (μg or mcg) = 1 milligram (mg)

THE COMMON SYSTEMS

Two other systems of measurement, while not official, are used in the United States. The avoirdupois system is the common system of weights—pounds and ounces—used in commerce and daily life. The apothecary system of volume—pints, quarts, gallons—is the common system for commerce and household measurement. The apothecary system of weights is used only in pharmacy and medicine. While these are no longer official systems of measurement and their use is strongly discouraged, there are practitioners (and older compounding formulas) that use these systems. As a result, pharmacists should know about them; ignorance of these systems could lead to serious errors in interpretation or measurement

APOTHECARY MEASURE OF VOLUME

60 minims (ɱ) = 1 fluidrachm or fluidram (flȝ or ȝ*)
8 fluidrachms = 1 fluidounce (fl ℥ or ℥ or oz)
16 fluidounces = 1 pint (pt or O)
2 pints (32 fluidounces) = 1 quart
4 quarts (8 pints) = 1 gallon (gal or C)

APOTHECARY MEASURE OF WEIGHT

20 grains = 1 scruple (☆)
3 scruples (60 grains) = 1 drachm or dram (ȝ)
8 drachms (480 grains) = 1 ounce (℥)
12 ounces (5760 grains) = 1 pound (℔)

AVOIRDUPOIS MEASURE OF WEIGHT

437.5 grains (gr) = 1 ounce (oz)
16 ounces (7,000 grains) = 1 pound (lb)

HOUSEHOLD MEASURES OF VOLUME

3 teaspoonfuls (t or tsp or ȝ*) = 1 tablespoonful (T or tbsp.)
2 tablespoonfuls = 1 fluidounce (fl ℥ or ℥ or oz)
8 fluidounces (8 oz) = 1 cup (Cu)
2 cups (16 oz) = 1 pint (pt or O)
2 pints (32 oz) = 1 quart (qt)
4 quarts (128 oz) = 1 gallon (gal or C)

HOUSEHOLD MEASURES OF WEIGHT

16 ounces (oz) = 1 pound (lb)

HOUSEHOLD MEASURES OF LENGTH

12 inches (in or ″) = 1 foot (ft or ′)
3 feet = 1 yard (yd)

CONVERSION EQUIVALENTS OF VOLUME

1 teaspoonful (t or tsp or ȝ*) = 5 milliliters (mL)
1 tablespoonful (T or tbsp.) = 15 milliliters (mL)
1 mL = 16.23 ɱ
1 ɱ = 0.06 mL
1 fluidrachm (fl ȝ*) = 3.69 milliliters   {4 mL}
1 fluidounce (oz. or fl ℥) = 29.57 milliliters   {30 mL}
1 pint (16 oz) = 473 milliliters   {480 mL}
1 quart (32 oz) = 946 milliliters
1 gallon (128 oz) = 3785 milliliters

CONVERSION EQUIVALENTS OF WEIGHT

1 gram (g) = 15.432 grains (gr)
1 kilogram (kg) = 2.20 pounds (Avoir.)
1 grain = 64.8 mg   {65 or 60 mg}
1 ounce (oz) (Avoir.) = 28.35 grams   {30 g}
1 ounce (℥) (Apoth.) = 31.1 grams
1 pound (Avoir.) = 454 grams
1 pound (Apoth.) = 373 grams
1 pound (Avoir.) = 7000 grains
1 pound (℔) (Apoth.) = 5760 grains
1 grain Apothecary = 1 grain Avoirdupois

CONVERSION EQUIVALENTS OF LENGTH

1 m = 39.37 in
1 in = 2.54 cm

* Use of the ʒ symbol as an abbreviation for teaspoon: Although a fluid dram (ʒ) contains 3.69 mL, it is common practice for practitioners to use the dram symbol (ʒ) **in the Sig** or Directions for Use portion of a prescription document as an abbreviation for teaspoonful. In Chapter ⟨1221⟩ Teaspoon of the *USP* it states, "For household purposes, an American Standard Teaspoon has been established by the American National Standards Institute as containing 4.93 ± 0.24 mL (1)." Therefore, the ʒ symbol, when used in the Sig portion of the prescription order, means 5 mL.

The use of such symbols, with dual meanings, should be discouraged. Even more hazardous is the use in the Sig of the apothecary ounce symbol (℥) as an abbreviation for 30 mL or two tablespoonfuls, and the use of the apothecary symbol for one-half ounce (℥ ss) as an abbreviation for 15 mL or one tablespoonful. In this case, pharmacists have mistakenly interpreted the ℥ symbol as an abbreviation for one tablespoonful, giving a dose that is one-half of that which was intended.

USE OF SIGNIFICANT FIGURES

In the table above, the values given in brackets { } are approximations that are often used in pharmacy practice and compounding. This is permissible in most cases. For example, if a prescription order calls for one ounce of ointment, the pharmacist may compound and dispense 30 grams rather than 28.35 grams (avoirdupois ounce) or 31.1 grams (apothecary ounce). However, if a **compounding formula** is written in either the apothecary or avoirdupois system, it is recommended that the formula be converted to the metric system, and in this circumstance, conversion factors with **three significant figures** are required. For a detailed discussion of significant figures, consult a book on pharmacy calculations or analysis. A few basic definitions and examples are given here.

Absolute number: A number taken at its face value, that is a counting number.

Denominate number: A number that specifies a quantity in terms of a unit of measurement, such as 3 in 3 grams.

Significant figures: The figures of a number that begin with the first figure to the left that is not a zero and end with the last figure to the right that is not a zero or is a zero that is known or considered to be exact. Significant figures express the value of a denominate number as accurately as possible or as needed for an intended purpose.

Examples of conversion equivalents with **three significant figures** from the table above are given here:
1. 1 g = 15.4 gr
2. 1 kg = 2.20 lb (the more accurate value is 2.205 lb, so the zero in this case is significant)
3. 1 gr = 64.8 mg (the more accurate value is 64.799 mg)
4. 1 oz = 28.3 g (the more accurate value is 28.3495 g)

While not required, if conversion equivalents with more than three significant figures are known, these obviously may be used, and with the use of calculators, the math is easily accomplished. More accurate conversion factors are given in the miscellaneous tables section of *The Merck Index* and other similar references.

When performing mathematical operations with a denominate number, there are standard rules for determining the number of significant figures to report in the final answer. This is especially important in reporting scientific data. In compounding, the number of significant figures recorded is often limited by the measuring equipment used. For example, if you were to measure the volume for 8 doses of 0.34 mL each, the volume would be 2.72 mL (8 × 0.34 mL = 2.72 mL), but it would be ridiculous to report that you measured 2.72 mL in a 10 mL graduate because this device does not measure to that degree of accuracy. It would be equally inappropriate to report that you weighed 324.9 mg of powder on a Class 3 Torsion balance because this instrument does not have that level of accuracy. Good judgement with the use of significant figures should be used in recording, reporting, and labeling of drug preparations.

---

1. The 2003 United States Pharmacopeia 26/National Formulary 21. Rockville, MD: The United States Pharmacopeial Convention, Inc., 2002:2439.

APPENDIX D
Approximate Solubilities—Descriptive Terms

Descriptive Term	Parts of Solvent Required for 1 Part of Solute
Very soluble	Less than 1
Freely soluble	From 1 to 10
Soluble	From 10 to 30
Sparingly soluble	From 30 to 100
Slightly soluble	From 100 to 1000
Very slightly soluble	From 1000 to 10,000
Practically insoluble or insoluble	Greater than or equal to 10,000

Source: The 2003 United States Pharmacopeia 26/National Formulary 21, Rockville, MD: The United States Pharmacopeial Convention, Inc. 2002:8.

APPENDIX E

Nomograms for Determination of Body Surface Area from Height and Weight

For Children

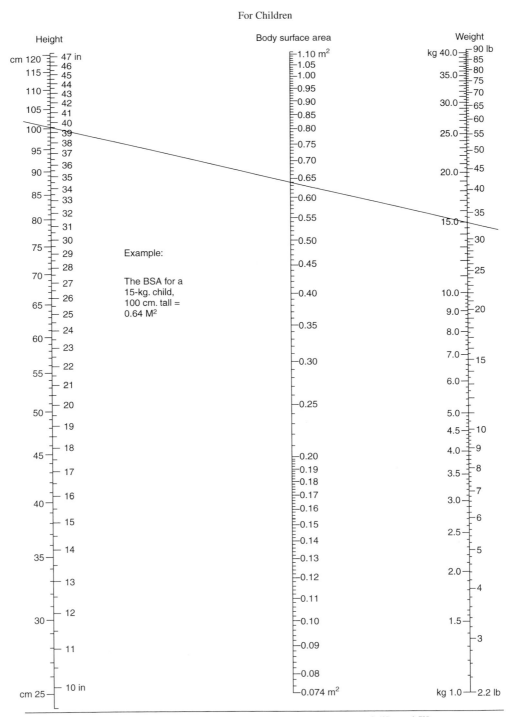

Example:

The BSA for a
15-kg. child,
100 cm. tall =
0.64 M²

From the formula of Du Bots and Du Bots, *Arch. intern. Med.*, 17, 863 (1916): $S = W^{0.425} \times H^{0.725} \times 71.84$, or
$\log S = \log W \times 0.425 + \log H \times 0.725 + 1.8564$ (S = body surface in cm², W = weight in kg, H = height in cm).

For Adults

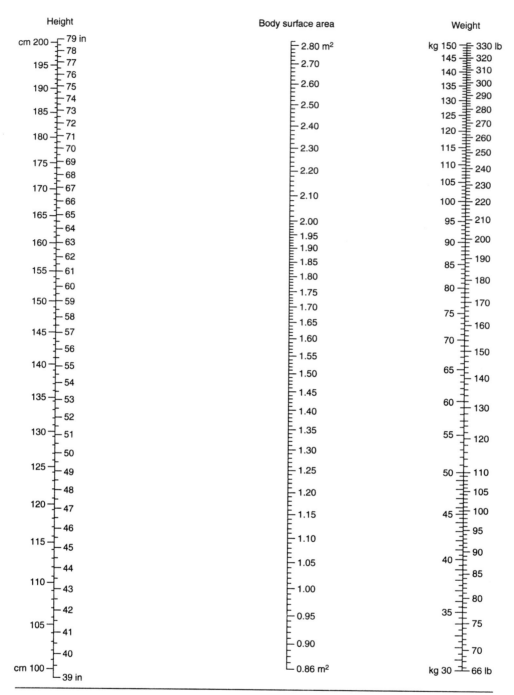

Height	Body surface area	Weight
cm 200 — 79 in	2.80 m²	kg 150 — 330 lb

From the formula of Du Bots and Du Bots, *Arch. intern. Med.,* 17, 863 (1916): $S = W^{.425} \times H^{.725} \times 71.84$, or log S = log $W \times 0.425$ + log $H \times 0.725$ + 1.8564 (S = body surface in cm², W = weight in kg, H = height in cm).

E.2

APPENDIX F

Normal Weight and Height Measurements for Children
Weight in pounds and *kilograms;* Height in inches and *centimeters*
(P = percentile)

Age		BOYS			GIRLS		
		P_{05}	P_{50}	P_{95}	P_{05}	P_{50}	P_{95}
At Birth[1]	Weight	5.7	7.5	8.8	5.8	7.1	9.0
		2.60	*3.40*	*4.01*	*2.64*	*3.20*	*4.06*
	Length	18.5	19.9	20.9	18.5	19.5	20.9
		47.0	*50.5*	*53.0*	*47.0*	*49.5*	*53.0*
1 Month[1]	Weight	7.5	8.9	10.4	7.4	8.5	9.9
		3.42	*4.04*	*4.73*	*3.36*	*3.86*	*4.50*
	Length	20.5	21.5	22.4	20.0	20.9	22.3
		52.0	*54.5*	*57.0*	*50.7*	*53.2*	*56.7*
2 Months[1]	Weight	9.4	11.0	12.5	9.0	10.5	12.1
		4.27	*4.98*	*5.69*	*4.07*	*4.75*	*5.50*
	Length	21.9	22.8	23.8	21.2	22.2	23.4
		55.5	*58.0*	*60.4*	*53.9*	*56.5*	*59.5*
3 Months[1]	Weight	11.4	13.2	15.2	10.6	12.2	14.2
		5.18	*6.00*	*6.90*	*4.80*	*5.53*	*6.46*
	Length	23.0	24.0	25.0	22.6	23.4	24.8
		58.3	*61.0*	*63.6*	*57.4*	*59.5*	*63.0*
4 Months[1]	Weight	12.8	15.1	17.1	11.5	13.8	16.4
		5.82	*6.84*	*7.77*	*5.22*	*6.24*	*7.43*
	Length	23.7	25.4	26.4	23.4	24.4	25.4
		60.1	*64.5*	*67.0*	*59.5*	*62.0*	*64.6*
5 Months[1]	Weight	13.6	16.2	18.3	13.2	15.4	17.3
		6.19	*7.37*	*8.29*	*6.00*	*7.00*	*7.86*
	Length	24.6	26.2	27.2	24.4	25.2	26.4
		62.5	*66.5*	*69.0*	*62.0*	*64.0*	*67.0*
6 Months[1]	Weight	14.9	17.9	19.8	14.0	16.5	19.0
		6.74	*8.12*	*8.98*	*6.34*	*7.48*	*8.62*
	Length	25.2	27.0	28.2	25.0	26.2	27.4
		64.1	*68.5*	*71.6*	*63.5*	*66.5*	*69.6*
7 Months[1]	Weight	15.9	18.4	20.2	14.8	17.4	20.1
		7.19	*8.36*	*9.15*	*6.72*	*7.87*	*9.13*
	Length	25.7	27.6	28.8	25.6	26.8	28.0
		65.2	*70.0*	*73.2*	*65.1*	*68.0*	*71.0*
8 Months[1]	Weight	16.8	19.8	21.8	15.7	18.2	21.5
		7.63	*8.97*	*9.88*	*7.10*	*8.24*	*9.74*
	Length	26.3	28.1	29.3	26.2	27.4	28.7
		66.9	*71.5*	*74.5*	*66.5*	*69.5*	*73.0*
9 Months[1]	Weight	17.6	20.7	22.9	16.1	18.9	21.8
		8.00	*9.37*	*10.40*	*7.30*	*8.58*	*9.88*
	Length	27.1	28.7	29.8	26.7	28.0	29.1
		68.8	*73.0*	*75.8*	*67.9*	*71.0*	*74.0*
10 Months[1]	Weight	17.6	20.7	23.5	16.8	19.3	22.2
		8.00	*9.40*	*10.66*	*7.60*	*8.74*	*10.07*
	Length	27.5	28.9	30.4	27.0	28.3	29.4
		69.9	*73.5*	*77.1*	*68.5*	*72.0*	*74.7*

Age		BOYS			GIRLS		
		P05	P50	P95	P05	P50	P95
11 Months[1]	Weight	18.7	22.0	23.9	17.1	20.2	24.0
		8.50	*10.00*	*10.86*	*7.77*	*9.14*	*10.90*
	Length	28.1	29.7	30.6	27.8	28.9	30.2
		71.3	*75.5*	*77.8*	*70.5*	*73.5*	*76.6*
12 Months[1]	Weight	18.7	22.2	25.0	18.1	21.0	25.0
		8.50	*10.09*	*11.36*	*8.22*	*9.51*	*11.33*
	Length	28.1	30.1	31.3	28.0	29.4	30.5
		71.4	*76.5*	*79.5*	*71.0*	*74.7*	*77.5*
15 Months[1]	Weight	20.8	24.0	28.5	19.7	22.4	25.6
		9.45	*10.90*	*12.93*	*8.92*	*10.15*	*11.61*
	Length	29.6	31.5	32.5	29.5	30.7	31.9
		75.2	*80.0*	*82.5*	*75.0*	*78.0*	*81.0*
18 Months[1]	Weight	22.3	24.9	29.3	21.1	24.1	28.7
		10.12	*11.31*	*13.29*	*9.56*	*10.95*	*13.00*
	Length	30.9	32.7	34.1	30.7	32.1	33.9
		78.4	*83.0*	*86.5*	*78.0*	*81.5*	*86.0*
2 Years[1]	Weight	24.1	27.6	31.8	22.1	26.7	31.0
		10.91	*12.53*	*14.43*	*10.03*	*12.10*	*14.05*
	Length	33.1	34.4	37.1	32.7	34.6	36.0
		84.0	*87.5*	*94.3*	*83.0*	*88.0*	*91.4*

1. Heimendinger J., Helv. paediat. Acta, **19**, 406 (1964). From measurements made in the period 1957–1962 in northwest Switzerland on 341 boys and 326 girls mostly of German-Swiss descent.

Normal Weight and Height Measurements for Children
Weight in pounds and *kilograms;* Height in inches and *centimeters*
(P = percentile)

Age			BOYS			GIRLS		
		P_{05}	P_{50}	P_{95}	P_{05}	P_{50}	P_{95}
$2^1/_2$ years[2]	Weight	20.5	29.8	39.0	21.4	28.9	36.4
		9.3	*13.5*	*17.7*	*9.7*	*13.1*	*16.5*
	Height	33.1	36.4	39.6	32.6	35.8	39.0
		84.1	*92.4*	*100.7*	*82.9*	*91.0*	*99.1*
3 years[2]	Weight	23.1	32.2	41.2	22.7	31.5	40.3
		10.5	*14.6*	*18.7*	*10.3*	*14.3*	*18.3*
	Height	34.7	37.9	41.1	34.1	37.5	40.8
		88.2	*96.3*	*104.4*	*86.7*	*95.2*	*103.7*
$3^1/_2$ years[2]	Weight	25.8	34.6	43.4	24.0	33.7	43.4
		11.7	*15.7*	*19.7*	*10.9*	*15.3*	*19.7*
	Height	36.1	39.4	42.6	35.5	38.9	42.3
		91.7	*100.0*	*108.3*	*90.1*	*98.8*	*107.5*
4 years[2]	Weight	27.8	36.8	45.9	25.8	35.9	46.1
		12.6	*16.7*	*20.8*	*11.7*	*16.3*	*20.9*
	Height	37.4	40.7	44.1	36.8	40.3	43.8
		95.0	*103.5*	*112.0*	*93.4*	*102.3*	*111.2*
$4^1/_2$ years[2]	Weight	30.0	39.2	48.5	27.6	38.1	48.7
		13.6	*17.8*	*22.0*	*12.5*	*17.3*	*22.1*
	Height	38.6	42.1	45.6	38.1	41.7	45.2
		98.0	*106.9*	*115.8*	*96.9*	*105.8*	*114.7*
5 years[2]	Weight	32.2	41.7	51.1	29.8	40.3	50.9
		14.6	*18.9*	*23.2*	*13.5*	*18.3*	*23.1*
	Height	39.8	43.4	47.0	39.6	43.0	46.4
		101.1	*110.2*	*119.3*	*100.5*	*109.2*	*117.9*
$5^1/_2$ years[2]	Weight	34.2	44.1	54.0	31.7	42.8	53.8
		15.5	*20.0*	*24.5*	*14.4*	*19.4*	*24.4*
	Height	40.9	44.6	48.4	40.8	44.3	47.8
		103.9	*113.4*	*122.9*	*103.7*	*112.6*	*121.5*
6 years[2]	Weight	36.2	46.3	56.4	32.8	45.4	58.0
		16.4	*21.0*	*25.6*	*14.9*	*20.6*	*26.3*
	Height	42.0	45.9	49.7	41.7	45.6	49.5
		106.8	*116.5*	*126.2*	*106.0*	*115.9*	*125.8*
$6^1/_2$ years[2]	Weight	37.7	48.7	59.7	32.8	48.1	63.3
		17.1	*22.1*	*27.1*	*14.9*	*21.8*	*28.7*
	Height	43.1	47.0	50.9	42.6	46.9	51.2
		109.6	*119.5*	*129.4*	*108.3*	*119.2*	*130.1*
7 years[2]	Weight	39.7	51.1	62.6	34.8	51.8	68.8
		18.0	*23.2*	*28.4*	*15.8*	*23.5*	*31.2*
	Height	44.2	48.2	52.2	43.9	48.2	52.5
		112.3	*122.4*	*132.5*	*111.5*	*122.4*	*133.3*
$7^1/_2$ years[2]	Weight	40.3	53.6	66.8	36.8	55.6	74.3
		18.3	*24.3*	*30.3*	*16.7*	*25.2*	*33.7*
	Height	45.3	49.3	53.3	45.2	49.4	53.5
		115.1	*125.2*	*135.3*	*114.9*	*125.4*	*135.9*

F.3

Age		BOYS			GIRLS		
		P05	P50	P95	P05	P50	P95
8 years[2]	Weight	40.6	55.8	71.0	38.8	58.9	78.9
		18.4	*25.3*	*32.2*	*17.6*	*26.7*	*35.8*
	Height	46.3	50.4	54.4	46.6	50.5	54.4
		117.7	*128.0*	*138.3*	*118.3*	*128.2*	*137.1*
8½ years[2]	Weight	39.0	58.2	77.4	40.3	61.3	82.2
		17.7	*26.4*	*35.1*	*18.3*	*27.8*	*37.3*
	Height	47.5	51.5	55.4	47.5	51.5	55.5
		120.6	*130.7*	*140.8*	*120.7*	*130.8*	*140.9*
9 years[2]	Weight	41.2	60.6	80.0	42.5	63.5	84.4
		18.7	*27.5*	*36.3*	*19.3*	*28.8*	*38.3*
	Height	48.5	52.5	56.5	48.4	52.4	56.5
		123.2	*133.3*	*143.4*	*122.9*	*133.2*	*143.5*
9½ years[2]	Weight	41.9	63.1	84.2	45.2	66.1	87.1
		19.0	*28.6*	*38.2*	*20.5*	*30.0*	*39.5*
	Height	49.3	53.5	57.6	49.1	53.3	57.5
		125.3	*135.8*	*146.3*	*124.7*	*135.4*	*146.1*
10 years[2]	Weight	43.9	67.2	90.6	46.7	69.4	92.2
		19.9	*30.5*	*41.1*	*21.2*	*31.5*	*41.8*
	Height	50.2	54.4	58.7	49.8	54.1	58.5
		127.4	*138.3*	*149.2*	*126.4*	*137.5*	*148.6*
10½ years[2]	Weight	45.4	72.1	98.8	47.0	72.8	98.5
		20.6	*32.7*	*44.8*	*21.3*	*33.0*	*44.7*
	Height	50.8	55.4	59.9	50.2	54.9	59.7
		129.1	*140.6*	*152.1*	*127.4*	*139.5*	*151.6*
11 years[2]	Weight	50.5	77.2	103.8	48.3	76.7	105.2
		22.9	*35.0*	*47.1*	*21.9*	*34.8*	*47.7*
	Height	51.5	56.2	60.9	50.7	55.8	60.9
		130.8	*142.7*	*154.6*	*128.9*	*141.8*	*154.7*
11½ years[2]	Weight	53.6	82.2	110.9	50.5	81.1	111.8
		24.3	*37.3*	*50.3*	*22.9*	*36.8*	*50.7*
	Height	52.0	57.0	62.0	51.5	57.0	62.6
		132.0	*144.7*	*157.4*	*130.7*	*144.8*	*158.9*
12 years[2]	Weight	56.9	87.1	117.3	53.6	86.0	118.4
		25.8	*39.5*	*53.2*	*24.3*	*39.0*	*53.7*
	Height	52.6	57.9	63.2	52.6	58.5	64.4
		133.5	*147.0*	*160.5*	*133.5*	*148.5*	*163.5*
12½ years[2]	Weight	59.3	92.2	125.0	56.9	91.3	125.7
		26.9	*41.8*	*56.7*	*25.8*	*41.4*	*57.0*
	Height	53.3	59.1	64.8	53.7	59.6	65.6
		135.3	*150.0*	*164.7*	*136.3*	*151.5*	*166.7*
13 years[2]	Weight	63.7	97.2	130.7	61.5	97.7	133.8
		28.9	*44.1*	*59.3*	*27.9*	*44.3*	*60.7*
	Height	54.3	60.4	66.5	55.0	60.7	66.3
		138.0	*153.4*	*168.8*	*139.8*	*154.1*	*168.4*
13½ years[2]	Weight	67.9	102.1	136.2	66.8	104.3	141.8
		30.8	*46.3*	*61.8*	*30.3*	*47.3*	*64.3*
	Height	55.6	61.8	68.0	56.5	61.5	66.5
		141.2	*157.0*	*172.8*	*143.6*	*156.3*	*169.0*
14 years[2]	Weight	72.5	107.1	141.8	74.3	110.5	146.6
		32.9	*48.6*	*64.3*	*33.7*	*50.1*	*66.5*
	Height	57.0	63.2	69.4	57.8	62.3	66.7
		144.8	*160.6*	*176.4*	*146.9*	*158.2*	*169.5*

Age			BOYS		GIRLS		
		P_{05}	P_{50}	P_{95}	P_{05}	P_{50}	P_{95}
$14^1/_2$ years[2]	Weight	75.6	112.2	148.8	81.3	114.2	147.0
		34.3	*50.9*	*67.5*	*36.9*	*51.8*	*66.7*
	Height	58.3	64.5	70.6	58.9	62.9	66.9
		148.2	*163.8*	*179.4*	*149.7*	*159.8*	*169.9*
15 years[2]	Weight	81.1	117.1	153.0	87.1	117.3	147.5
		36.8	*53.1*	*69.4*	*39.5*	*53.2*	*66.9*
	Height	59.8	65.7	71.5	59.4	63.4	67.4
		151.9	*166.8*	*181.7*	*151.0*	*161.1*	*171.2*
$15^1/_2$ years[2]	Weight	86.9	122.1	157.4	90.4	119.7	149.0
		39.4	*55.4*	*71.4*	*41.0*	*54.3*	*67.6*
	Height	61.3	66.7	72.1	59.3	63.8	68.3
		155.8	*169.5*	*183.2*	*150.6*	*162.1*	*173.6*
16 years[2]	Weight	92.4	127.2	162.0	92.2	121.5	150.8
		41.9	*57.7*	*73.5*	*41.8*	*55.1*	*68.4*
	Height	62.5	67.6	72.7	59.5	64.1	68.7
		158.8	*171.7*	*184.6*	*151.2*	*162.9*	*174.6*
$16^1/_2$ years[2]	Weight	99.9	132.1	164.2	93.5	123.2	153.0
		45.3	*59.9*	*74.5*	*43.4*	*55.9*	*19.4*
	Height	63.5	68.3	73.0	59.7	64.4	69.1
		161.3	*173.4*	*185.5*	*151.6*	*163.5*	*175.4*
17 years[2]	Weight	104.9	134.0	163.1	94.8	124.6	154.3
		47.6	*60.8*	*74.0*	*43.0*	*56.5*	*70.0*
	Height	64.0	68.6	73.2	59.7	64.5	69.3
		162.6	*174.3*	*186.0*	*151.7*	*163.8*	*175.9*

2. Heimendinger J., Helv. patediat. Acta, 19, suppl. 13 (1964). From measurements made in the period 1956–1957 on 2150 boys and 2150 girls in Basel, Switzerland.

National Center for Health Statistics Growth Charts

Birth to 36 months: Boys
Length-for-age and Weight-for-age percentiles

NAME _____

RECORD # _____

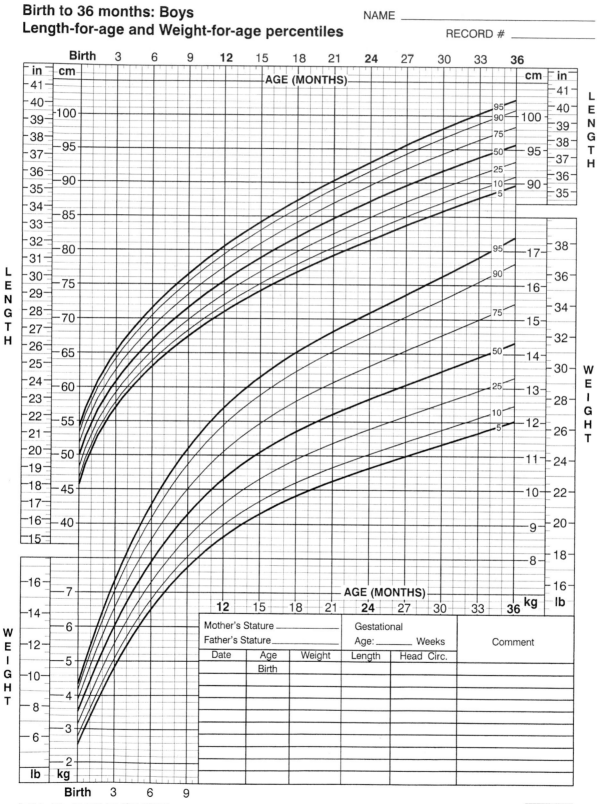

Published May 30, 2000 (modified 4/20/01).
SOURCE: Developed by the National Center for Health Statistics in collaboration with
the National Center for Chronic Disease Prevention and Health Promotion (2000).
http://www.cdc.gov/growthcharts

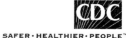

SAFER · HEALTHIER · PEOPLE™

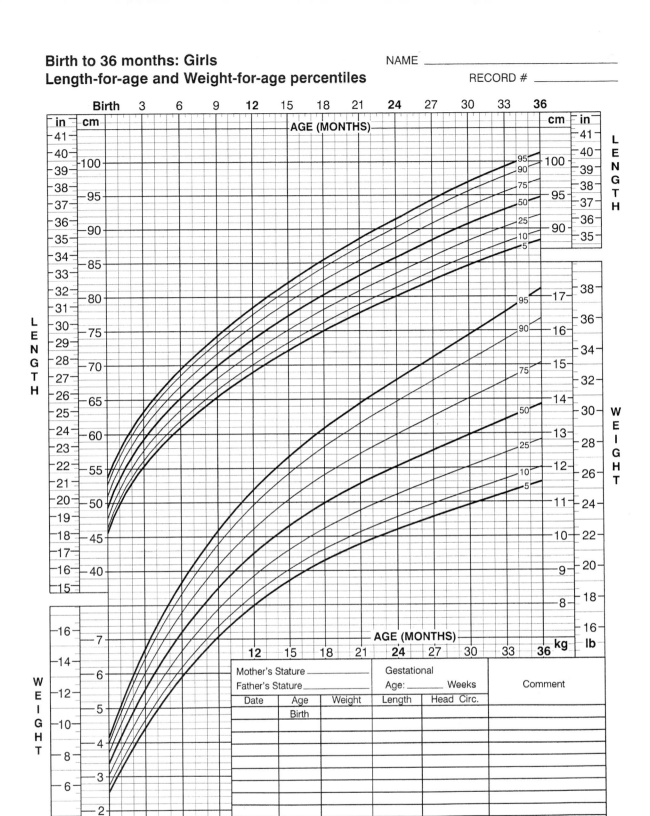

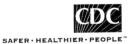

Published May 30, 2000 (modified 4/20/01).
SOURCE: Developed by the National Center for Health Statistics in collaboration with
the National Center for Chronic Disease Prevention and Health Promotion (2000).
http://www.cdc.gov/growthcharts

G.2

2 to 20 years: Boys
Stature-for-age and Weight-for-age percentiles

NAME _____

RECORD # _____

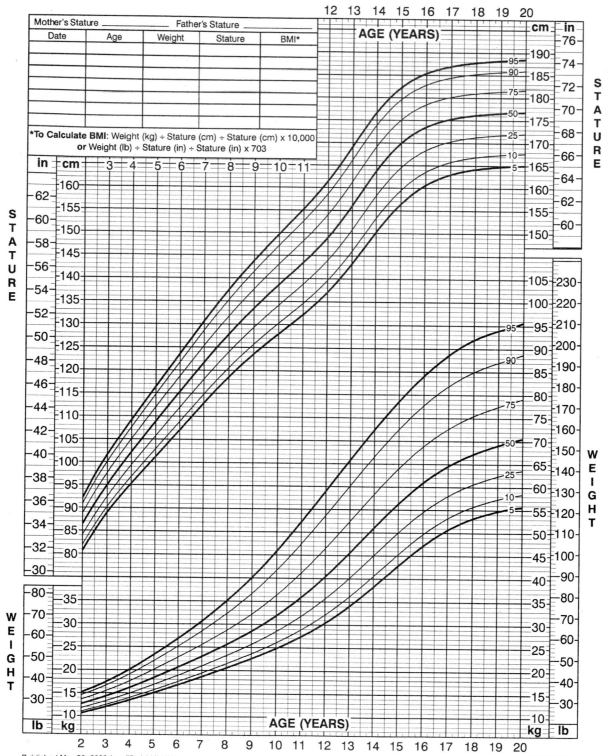

*To Calculate BMI: Weight (kg) ÷ Stature (cm) ÷ Stature (cm) x 10,000
or Weight (lb) ÷ Stature (in) ÷ Stature (in) x 703

Mother's Stature _____ Father's Stature _____

Date	Age	Weight	Stature	BMI*

Published May 30, 2000 (modified 11/21/00).
SOURCE: Developed by the National Center for Health Statistics in collaboration with
the National Center for Chronic Disease Prevention and Health Promotion (2000).
http://www.cdc.gov/growthcharts

CDC

SAFER · HEALTHIER · PEOPLE™

2 to 20 years: Girls
Stature-for-age and Weight-for-age percentiles

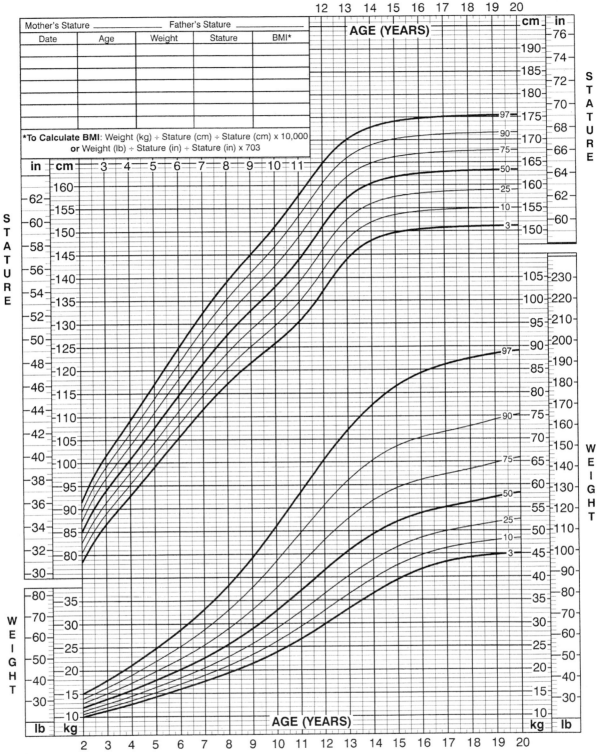

Mother's Stature _____ Father's Stature _____

Date	Age	Weight	Stature	BMI*

*To Calculate BMI: Weight (kg) ÷ Stature (cm) ÷ Stature (cm) x 10,000
or Weight (lb) ÷ Stature (in) ÷ Stature (in) x 703

AGE (YEARS)

STATURE

WEIGHT

Revised and corrected November 21, 2000.
SOURCE: Developed by the National Center for Health Statistics in collaboration with
the National Center for Chronic Disease Prevention and Health Promotion (2000).
http://www.cdc.gov/growthcharts

G.4

ISOTONICITY VALUES

CHEMICAL	MW	$E^{1\%}_{NaCl}$	V^{1g}	$\Delta\,T_f^{1\%}$	% Iso-osmotic Concentration
Acetylcysteine	163.20	0.20	22.2	0.11	4.58%
Alcohol USP (95%)	46.07	0.65	72.2	0.37	1.39%
Alcohol, dehydrate	46.07	0.70	77.8	0.40	1.28%
Alum, potassium	474.39	0.18	20.0	0.10	6.35%
Amantadine hydrochloride	187.71	0.31	34.4	0.18	2.95%
Aminoacetic acid (Glycine)	75.07	0.41	45.6	0.23	2.20%
Aminocaproic acid	131.18	0.26	28.9	0.14	3.52%
p-Aminohippuric acid	194.19	0.13	14.4	0.07	
Aminophylline Dihydrate	456.46	0.17	19.0	0.10	
p-Aminosalicylate sodium	153.14	0.29	32.2	0.16	3.27%
Amitriptyline hydrochloride	313.87	0.18	20.0	0.10	
Ammonium chloride	53.50	1.08	120.0	0.64	
Ammonium phosphate, dibasic	132.06	0.55	61.1	0.31	1.76%
Amobarbital sodium	248.26	0.25	27.8	0.14	3.6%
Amphetamine sulfate	368.50	0.22	24.3	0.12	4.23%
Ampicillin sodium	371.39	0.16	17.8	0.09	5.78%
Anileridine hydrochloride	425.40	0.19	21.1	0.10	5.13%
Antazoline phosphate	363.36	0.20	22.2	0.11	
Antimony potassium tartrate	333.93	0.18	20.0	0.10	
Antipyrine	188.23	0.17	19.0	0.09	6.81%
Antistine hydrochloride	301.81	0.18	20.0	0.11	
Apomorphine hydrochloride	312.79	0.14	15.7	0.08	
L-Arginine hydrochloride	210.66	0.30	33.3	0.17	3.43%
Ascorbic acid	176.12	0.18	20.0	0.11	5.94%
Atropine sulfate	694.85	0.13	14.3	0.07	8.85%
Bacitracin	NA	0.05	5.6	0.02	
Barbital sodium	206.18	0.30	33.3	0.17	3.12%
Benoxinate hydrochloride	344.88	0.18	20.0	0.10	
Benzalkonium chloride	360(ave)	0.16	17.8	0.09	
Benzethonium chloride	448.09	0.05	5.6	0.02	
Benztropine mesylate	403.54	0.21	23.3	0.11	
Benzyl alcohol	108.14	0.17	18.9	0.09	
Betazole hydrochloride	184.07	0.51	56.7	0.29	1.91%
Bethanechol chloride	196.68	0.39	43.3	0.22	3.05%
Boric acid	61.84	0.50	55.7	0.29	1.9%
Bretylium tosylate	414.36	0.14	15.6	0.08	
Bromodiphenhydramine hydrochloride	370.72	0.17	18.9	0.10	
Brompheniramine maleate	435.32	0.09	10.0	0.05	
Bupivacaine hydrochloride	342.90	0.17	18.9	0.09	5.38%
Butabarbital sodium	234.23	0.27	30.0	0.15	3.33%
Butacaine sulfate	710.95	0.20	22.3	0.12	
Caffeine	194.19	0.08	9.0	0.05	
Caffeine and sodium benzoate	NA	0.25	29.0	0.28	
Calcium chloride, anhydrous	110.99	0.70	77.8	0.40	1.29%
Calcium chloride · $2H_2O$	147.02	0.51	56.7	0.29	1.70%
Calcium gluconate · H_2O	448.39	0.16	17.7	0.09	
Calcium lactate · $5H_2O$	308.30	0.23	25.7	0.14	4.5%
Calcium levulinate · $2H_2O$	306.32	0.27	30.0	0.15	
Calcium pantothenate	476.54	0.19	21.1	0.10	5.6%
Camphor	152.23	0.20	22.3	0.12	
Capreomycin sulfate	NA	0.04	4.4	0.02	
Carbachol	182.65	0.36	40.0	0.20	2.82%
Carbenicillin disodium	422.36	0.20	22.2	0.11	4.40%
Cefamandole nafate	512.50	0.14	15.6	0.07	
Cefazolin sodium	476.49	0.13	14.4	0.07	
Ceforanide	519.56	0.12	13.3	0.06	

CHEMICAL	MW	$E^{1\%}_{NaCl}$	V^{1g}	$\Delta T_f^{1\%}$	% Iso-osmotic Concentration
Cefotaxime sodium	477.45	0.15	16.7	0.08	
Cefoxitin sodium	449.44	0.16	17.8	0.09	
Ceftazidime · 5H$_2$O	636.65	0.09	10.0	0.04	
Ceftizoxime sodium	405.39	0.15	16.7	0.08	
Ceftriaxone sodium	661.60	0.13	14.4	0.07	
Cefuroxime sodium	446.37	0.13	14.4	0.07	
Cephalothin sodium	418.42	0.17	18.9	0.09	6.80%
Cephapirin sodium	445.45	0.13	14.4	0.07	7.80%
Chloramphenicol	323.14	0.10	11.0	0.06	
Chloramphenicol sodium succinate	445.19	0.14	15.6	0.07	6.38%
Chlordiazepoxide hydrochloride	336.22	0.22	24.4	0.12	5.50%
Chlorobutanol, hydrated	177.47	0.24	26.7	0.14	
Chloroprocaine hydrochloride	307.22	0.20	22.2	0.10	
Chloroquine phosphate	515.87	0.14	15.6	0.08	7.15%
Chlorpheniramine maleate	390.87	0.17	18.9	0.08	
Chlorpromazine hydrochloride	355.33	0.10	11.1	0.05	
Chlortetracycline hydrochloride	515.35	0.10	11.1	0.06	
Citric acid	192.13	0.18	20.0	0.09	5.52%
Clindamycine phosphate	504.97	0.08	8.9	0.04	10.73%
Cocaine hydrochloride	339.82	0.16	17.7	0.09	6.33%
Codeine phosphate	406.38	0.14	15.6	0.07	7.29%
Colistimethate sodium	1749.82	0.15	16.7	0.08	6.73%
Cromolyn sodium	512.34	0.14	15.6	0.08	
Cupric sulfate · 5H$_2$O	249.69	0.18	20.0	0.09	6.85%
Cupric sulfate, anhydrous	159.61	0.27	30.0	0.15	4.09%
Cyclizine hydrochloride	302.85	0.20	22.2	0.12	
Cyclopentolate hydrochloride	327.85	0.20	22.2	0.11	5.30%
Cyclophosphamide	279.10	0.10	11.1	0.06	
Cytarabine	243.22	0.11	12.2	0.06	8.92%
Deferoxamine mesylate	656.79	0.09	10.0	0.04	
Demecarium bromide	716.61	0.12	13.3	0.06	
Dexamethasone sodium phosphate	516.42	0.17	18.9	0.09	6.75%
Dexchlorpheniramine maleate	390.87	0.15	16.7	0.08	
Dexpanthenol	205.25	0.18	20.0	0.10	5.60%
Dextroamphetamine sulfate	368.50	0.23	25.6	0.13	4.16%
Dextrose, anhydrous	180.16	0.18	20.0	0.10	5.05%
Dextrose, monohydrate	198.17	0.16	17.7	0.09	5.51%
Diatrizoate sodium	635.90	0.09	10.0	0.04	10.55%
Dibucaine hydrochloride	379.92	0.13	14.3	0.08	
Dicloxacillin sodium monohydrate	510.32	0.10	11.1	0.06	
Dicyclomine hydrochloride	345.96	0.18	20.0	0.10	
Diethanolamine	105.14	0.31	34.4	0.17	2.90%
Diethylcarbamazine citrate	391.42	0.14	15.6	0.08	6.29%
Dihydrostreptomycin sulfate	1461.43	0.06	6.7	0.03	21.4%
Dimethyl sulfoxide	78.13	0.42	46.7	0.24	2.16%
Diphenhydramine hydrochloride	291.81	0.27	22.0	0.15	
Dipivefrin hydrochloride	387.90	0.17	18.9	0.09	
Dobutamine hydrochloride	337.84	0.18	20.0	0.10	
Dopamine hydrochloride	189.64	0.30	33.3	0.17	3.11%
Doxapram hydrochloride monohydrate	432.98	0.12	13.3	0.07	
Doxycycline hyclate	1025.89	0.12	13.3	0.07	
Dyclonine hydrochloride	325.88	0.24	26.7	0.13	
Dyphylline	254.24	0.10	11.1	0.05	
Echothiopate iodide	383.23	0.16	17.8	0.09	
Edetate disodium	372.24	0.23	25.6	0.13	4.44%
Edetate calcium disodium	374.28	0.21	23.3	0.12	4.50%
Edrophonium chloride	201.70	0.31	34.4	0.17	3.36%
Emetine hydrochloride	553.56	0.10	11.0	0.06	
Ephedrine hydrochloride	201.69	0.30	33.3	0.18	3.2%
Ephedrine sulfate	428.54	0.23	25.7	0.13	4.54%
Epinephrine bitartrate	333.29	0.18	20.0	0.09	5.7%
Epinephrine hydrochloride	219.66	0.29	32.3	0.16	3.47%
Ergonovine maleate	441.49	0.16	17.8	0.08	
Erythromycin lactobionate	1092.25	0.07	7.8	0.04	
Ethylenediamine	60.10	0.44	48.9	0.25	
Ethylhydrocupreine hydrochloride	376.92	0.17	19.0	0.09	

CHEMICAL	MW	$E^{1\%}_{NaCl}$	V^{1g}	$\Delta T_f^{1\%}$	% Iso-osmotic Concentration
Ethylmorphine hydrochloride	385.88	0.16	17.7	0.08	6.18%
Eucatropine hydrochloride	327.84	0.18	20.0	0.11	
Ferrous gluconate	482.18	0.15	16.7	0.08	
Fluorescein sodium	376	0.31	34.3	0.18	3.34%
Fluorouracil	130.08	0.13	14.4	0.07	
Fluphenazine dihydrochloride	622.63	0.14	15.6	0.08	
D-Fructose	180.16	0.18	20.0	0.10	5.05%
Gallamine triethiodide	891.54	0.08	8.9	0.04	
Gentamycin sulfate	NA	0.05	5.6	0.03	
L-Glutamic acid	147.13	0.25	27.8	0.14	
Glycerin	92.09	0.35	37.7	0.20	
Glycine (also Aminocetic acid)	75.07	0.41	45.6	0.23	2.19%
Glycopyrrolate	398.34	0.15	16.7	0.08	7.22%
Heparin sodium	NA	0.07	7.8	0.04	12.2%
Histamine phosphate	307.14	0.25	27.8	0.14	4.1%
Homatropine hydrobromide	356.26	0.17	19.0	0.09	5.67%
Homatropine methylbromide	370.29	0.19	21.1	0.10	
Hydralazine hydrochloride	196.64	0.37	41.1	0.21	
Hydromorphone hydrochloride	321.81	0.22	24.4	0.12	6.39%
Hydroxyamphetamine hydrobromide	232.12	0.26	28.9	0.15	3.71%
8-Hydroxyquinoline sulfate	388.40	0.21	23.3	0.11	9.75%
Hydroxyzine hydrochloride	447.84	0.25	27.8	0.13	6.32%
Hyoscyamine hydrobromide	370.29	0.19	21.1	0.10	
Hyoscyamine sulfate	712.86	0.15	16.7	0.08	
Imipramine hydrochloride	316.88	0.20	22.2	0.11	
Indigotindisulfonate sodium (Indigo carmine)	466.36	0.30	33.3	0.17	
Iopamidol	777.09	0.03	3.3	0.01	
Isoetharine hydrochloride	275.77	0.23	25.6	0.13	4.27%
Isometheptene mucate	492.65	0.18	20.0	0.09	4.95%
Isoniazid	137.14	0.25	27.8	0.14	4.35%
Isopropyl alcohol	60.10	0.53	58.9	0.30	1.71%
Isoproterenol sulfate	556.63	0.14	15.6	0.07	6.65%
Kanamycin sulfate	582.59	0.07	7.8	0.04	
Ketamine hydrochloride	274.19	0.21	23.3	0.12	4.29%
Labetalol hydrochloride	364.87	0.19	21.1	0.10	
Lactic acid	90.08	0.41	45.6	0.23	2.3%
Lactose monohydrate	360.31	0.07	7.7	0.04	9.75%
Levobunolol hydrochloride	327.85	0.12	13.3	0.07	
Levorphanol tartrate	443.50	0.12	13.3	0.06	
Lidocaine hydrochloride	288.82	0.22	24.4	0.12	4.42%
Lincomycin hydrochloride	443.01	0.16	17.8	0.09	6.60%
Lithium carbonate	73.89	1.06	117.8	0.6	0.92%
Mafenide hydrochloride	222.72	0.27	30.0	0.15	3.55%
Magnesium chloride · 6 H$_2$O	203.30	0.45	50.0	0.26	2.02%
Magnesium sulfate · 7H$_2$O	246.47	0.17	19.0	0.09	6.3%
Magnesium sulfate, anhydrous	120.37	0.32	35.6	0.18	3.18%
Mannitol	182.17	0.17	18.9	0.09	5.07%
Menadiol sodium diphosphate	530.18	0.25	27.8	0.14	
Menthol	156.26	0.20	22.3	0.12	
Meperidine hydrochloride	283.79	0.22	24.3	0.12	4.8%
Mepivacaine hydrochloride	282.82	0.21	23.3	0.11	4.6%
Mercury bichloride	271.50	0.13	14.3	0.07	
Mesoridazine besylate	544.75	0.07	7.8	0.04	
Metaraminol bitartrate	317.30	0.20	22.2	0.11	5.17%
Methacholine chloride	195.69	0.32	35.7	0.18	3.21%
Methadone hydrochloride	345.92	0.18	20.0	0.10	8.59%
Methamphetamine hydrochloride	185.69	0.37	41.0	0.20	2.75%
Methanamine	140.19	0.23	25.6	0.12	3.68%
Methicillin sodium	420.42	0.18	20.0	0.09	6.00%
Methionine	149.21	0.28	31.1	0.16	
Methocarbamol	241.25	0.10	11.1	0.06	

H.3

CHEMICAL	MW	E$^{1\%}_{NaCl}$	V^{1g}	Δ T$_f$$^{1\%}$	% Iso-osmotic Concentration
Methotrimeprazine hydrochloride	364.94	0.10	11.1	0.06	
Methyldopa ethyl ester hydrochloride	275.73	0.21	23.3	0.12	4.28%
Methylergonovine maleate	455.52	0.10	11.1	0.05	
Methylphenidate hydrochloride	269.77	0.22	24.4	0.12	4.07%
Methylprednisolone sodium succinate	496.54	0.09	10.0	0.05	
Metoclopramide hydrochloride	354.27	0.15	16.7	0.08	
Metycaine hydrochloride	292.82	0.20	22.3	0.12	
Mezlocillin sodium	561.57	0.11	12.2	0.06	
Mild silver protein	—	0.17	20.0	0.09	
Minocycline hydrochloride	493.95	0.10	11.1	0.05	
Monoethanolamine	61.08	0.53	58.9	0.30	1.70%
Morphine hydrochloride	375.84	0.15	16.7	0.08	
Morphine sulfate	758.82	0.14	15.6	0.07	
Nafcillin sodium	436.47	0.14	15.6	0.07	
Naloxone hydrochloride	363.84	0.14	15.6	0.08	8.07%
Naphazoline hydrochloride	246.73	0.27	25.7	0.15	3.99%
Neomycin sulfate	NA	0.12	12.3	0.06	
Neostigmine bromide	303.20	0.22	20.0	0.12	
Neostigmine methyl sulfate	334.39	0.20	22.2	0.10	5.22%
Netilmicin sulfate	1441.56	0.07	7.8	0.04	
Nicotinamide	122.13	0.26	29.0	0.14	4.49%
Nicotinic acid	123.11	0.25	27.8	0.14	
Novobiocin sodium	634.62	0.08	8.9	0.04	
Orphenadrine citrate	461.50	0.13	14.4	0.07	
Oxacillin sodium	441.44	0.17	18.9	0.09	6.64%
Oxycodone hydrochloride	351.82	0.14	15.6	0.08	7.4%
Oxymetazoline hydrochloride	296.84	0.22	24.4	0.12	4.92%
Oxymorphone hydrochloride	337.81	0.16	17.8	0.08	
Oxytetracycline hydrochloride	496.91	0.14	15.6	0.08	
Papaverine hydrochloride	375.86	0.10	11.1	0.06	
Paraldehyde	132.16	0.25	27.8	0.14	3.65%
Pentazocine lactate	375.51	0.15	16.7	0.08	
Pentobarbital sodium	248.26	0.25	27.8	0.14	
Penicillin G sodium	356.38	0.18	20.0	0.11	
Penicillin G Procaine	588.71	0.10	11.0	0.06	
Penicillin G potassium	372.47	0.18	20.0	0.11	
Phenacaine hydrochloride	352.85	0.20	17.7	0.10	
Pheniramine maleate	356.42	0.16	17.8	0.09	
Phenobarbital sodium	254.22	0.24	26.7	0.13	
Phenol	94.11	0.35	39.0	0.19	2.8%
Phentolamine mesylate	377.47	0.17	18.9	0.09	8.23%
Phenylephrine hydrochloride	203.67	0.32	32.3	0.18	3.0%
Phenylethyl alcohol	122.17	0.25	27.8	0.14	
Phenylpropanolamine hydrochloride	187.67	0.38	42.2	0.21	2.6%
Physostigmine salicylate	413.46	0.16	17.7	0.09	
Physostigmine sulfate	648.45	0.13	14.3	0.07	7.74%
Pilocarpine hydrochloride	244.72	0.24	26.7	0.13	4.08%
Pilocarpine nitrate	271.27	0.23	25.7	0.13	
Piperacillin sodium	539.54	0.11	12.2	0.06	
Piperocaine hydrochloride	297.82	0.21	23.3	0.12	
Polyethylene glycol 300	NA	0.12	13.3	0.06	6.73%
Polyethylene glycol 400	NA	0.08	8.9	0.04	8.50%
Polyethylene glycol 1500	NA	0.06	6.7	0.03	10.00%
Polyethylene glycol 1540	NA	0.02	2.2	0.01	
Polyethylene glycol 4000	NA	0.02	2.2	0.00	
Polymyxin B sulfate	NA	0.09	10.0	0.04	
Polysorbate 80	NA	0.02	2.2	0.01	
Polyvinly alcohol (99% hydrolyzed)	NA	0.02	2.2	0.00	
Potassium acetate	98.15	0.59	65.5	0.34	1.53%
Potassium chloride	74.55	0.76	84.3	0.43	1.19%
Potassium iodide	166.02	0.34	37.7	0.20	2.59%
Potassium nitrate	85.11	0.56	62.2	0.32	1.62%
Potassium permanganate	158.04	0.39	43.3	0.22	
Potassium phosphate, dibasic anhydrous	174.18	0.46	51.1	0.26	2.11%
Potassium phosphate, monobasic	136.09	0.44	48.9	0.25	2.18%

CHEMICAL	MW	$E^{1\%}_{NaCl}$	V^{1g}	$\Delta T_f^{1\%}$	% Iso-osmotic Concentration
Potassium sorbate	150.22	0.41	45.6	0.23	2.23%
Potassium sulfate	174.27	0.44	48.9	0.25	2.11%
Potassium thiocyanate	97.18	0.59	65.5	0.34	1.52%
Povidone	NA	0.01	1.11	0.00	
Pralidoxime chloride	172.62	0.32	35.6	0.18	2.87%
Pramoxine hydrochloride	329.87	0.18	20.0	0.10	
Prilocaine hydrochloride	256.78	0.22	24.4	0.12	4.18%
Procainamide hydrochloride	271.79	0.22	24.4	0.12	
Procaine hydrochloride	272.77	0.21	23.3	0.12	5.05%
Prochlorperazine edisylate	564.15	0.06	6.7	0.03	
Promazine hydrochloride	320.89	0.13	14.4	0.07	
Promethazine hydrochloride	320.89	0.18	20.0	0.11	
Propantheline bromide	448.40	0.11	12.2	0.06	
Proparacaine hydrochloride	330.85	0.15	16.7	0.08	7.46%
Propoxycaine hydrochloride	330.86	0.19	21.1	0.11	
Propranolol hydrochloride	295.80	0.20	22.2	0.12	
Propylene glycol	76.10	0.43	47.8	0.25	2.10%
Pyridostigmine bromide	261.12	0.22	24.4	0.12	4.13%
Pyridoxine hydrochloride	205.64	0.36	40.0	0.20	
Pyrilamine maleate	401.47	0.18	20.0	0.10	
Quinidine gluconate	520.58	0.12	13.3	0.06	
Quinidine sulfate	782.96	0.10	11.1	0.06	
Quinine bisulfate	422.50	0.09	10.0	0.05	
Quinine hydrochloride	396.91	0.14	15.7	0.07	
Ranitidine hydrochloride	350.87	0.18	20.0	0.10	
Resorcinol	110.11	0.28	31.1	0.16	3.3%
Riboflavin phosphate (sodium)	514.36	0.08	8.9	0.04	
Ritodrine hydrochloride	323.81	0.20	22.2	0.11	
Scopolamine hydrobromide	438.32	0.12	13.3	0.06	7.85%
Secobarbital sodium	260.27	0.24	26.7	0.13	3.9%
Silver nitrate	169.89	0.33	36.7	0.19	2.74%
Sodium acetate	136.08	0.46	51.1	0.26	2.03%
Sodium acetate, anhydrous	82.03	0.77	85.5	0.44	1.18%
Sodium ascorbate	198.11	0.32	35.6	0.18	2.99%
Sodium benzoate	144.11	0.40	44.3	0.23	2.25%
Sodium bicarbonate	84.00	0.65	72.3	0.38	1.39%
Sodium bisulfite	104.06	0.61	67.7	0.35	1.5%
Sodium borate · 10H$_2$O	381.37	0.42	46.7	0.24	2.6%
Sodium carbonate, anhydrous	105.99	0.70	77.8	0.40	1.32%
Sodium carbonate, monohydrated	124.00	0.60	66.7	0.34	1.56%
Sodium carboxymethyl cellulose	NA	0.03	3.3	0.01	
Sodium chloride	58.45	1.00	111.0	0.58	0.9%
Sodium citrate	294.10	0.31	34.4	0.17	3.02%
Sodium iodide	149.89	0.39	43.3	0.22	2.37%
Sodium lactate	112.06	0.55	61.1	0.31	1.72%
Sodium lauryl sulfate	288.38	0.08	8.9	0.04	
Sodium metabisulfite	190.10	0.67	74.4	0.38	1.38%
Sodium nitrate	84.99	0.68	75.7	0.39	1.36%
Sodium nitrite	69.00	0.84	93.3	0.48	1.08%
Sodium phosphate, dibasic anhydrous	141.98	0.53	59.0	0.30	1.75%
Sodium phosphate, dibasic · 2H$_2$O	178.05	0.42	46.7	0.24	2.23%
Sodium phosphate, dibasic · 7H$_2$O	268.08	0.29	32.3	0.16	3.33%
Sodium phosphate, dibasic · 12H$_2$O	358.21	0.22	24.3	0.12	4.45%
Sodium phosphate, monobasic anhydrous	119.98	0.46	51.1	0.26	2.1%
Sodium phosphate, monobasic (NaH$_2$PO$_4$ · H$_2$O)	138.00	0.43	44.3	0.24	2.21%
Sodium phosphate, monobasic dihydrate	156.01	0.36	40.0	0.20	2.77%
Sodium propionate	96.07	0.61	67.7	0.35	1.47%
Sodium salicylate	160.11	0.36	40.0	0.20	2.53%
Sodium succinate	162.05	0.32	35.6	0.18	2.90%
Sodium sulfate · 10H$_2$O	322.19	0.26	28.9	0.14	3.95%
Sodium sulfate, anhydrous	142.04	0.54	60.0	0.30	1.78%
Sodium sulfite, exsiccated	126.04	0.65	72.3	0.37	
Sodium tartrate · 2H$_2$O	230.08	0.33	36.7	0.19	2.72%
Sodium thiosulfate · 5H$_2$O	248.18	0.31	34.4	0.18	2.98%
Spectinomycin hydrochloride	495.35	0.16	17.8	0.09	5.66%

H.5

CHEMICAL	MW	$E^{1\%}_{NaCl}$	V^{1g}	$\Delta T_f^{1\%}$	% Iso-osmotic Concentration
Streptomycin sulfate	1457.40	0.07	7.7	0.03	
Strong silver protein	NA	0.08	9.0	0.04	
Succinylcholine chloride · 2H$_2$O	397.34	0.20	22.2	0.11	4.48%
Sucrose	342.30	0.08	9.0	0.04	9.25%
Sulbactam sodium	255.22	0.24	26.7	0.14	3.75%
Sulfacetamide sodium	254.24	0.23	25.7	0.14	
Sulfadiazine sodium	272.26	0.24	26.7	0.13	4.24%
Sulfamerazine sodium	286.29	0.23	25.7	0.13	4.53%
Sulfamethazine sodium	300.31	0.21	23.3	0.12	
Sulfanilamide	172.21	0.22	24.3	0.13	
Sulfapyridine sodium	271.27	0.23	25.6	0.13	4.55%
Sulfathiazole sodium	304.33	0.22	24.3	0.12	4.82%
Tannic acid	NA	0.03	3.3	0.01	
Tartaric acid	150.09	0.25	27.8	0.14	3.9%
Terbutaline sulfate	548.65	0.14	15.6	0.08	6.75
Tetracaine hydrochloride	300.82	0.18	20.0	0.11	
Tetracycline hydrochloride	480.91	0.14	15.7	0.07	
Tetrahydrozoline hydrochloride	236.75	0.28	31.1	0.16	
Theophylline · H$_2$O	198.18	0.10	11.1	0.05	
Theophylline sodium glycinate	NA	0.31	34.4	0.18	2.94%
Thiamine hydrochloride	337.27	0.25	27.8	0.13	4.24%
Thiethylperazine maleate	631.77	0.09	10.0	0.05	
Thiopental sodium	264.32	0.27	30.0	0.15	3.5%
Thioridazine hydrochloride	407.04	0.05	5.6	0.02	
Thiotepa	189.22	0.16	17.8	0.09	5.67%
Ticarcillin disodium	428.40	0.20	22.2	0.11	4.62%
Timolol maleate	432.49	0.13	14.4	0.07	
Tobramycin	467.52	0.07	7.8	0.03	
Tolazoline hydrochloride	196.68	0.34	37.8	0.19	3.05%
Trifluoperazine dihydrochloride	480.43	0.18	20.0	0.10	
Triflupromazine hydrochloride	388.89	0.09	10.0	0.05	
Trimeprazine tartrate	747.00	0.06	6.7	0.03	
Trimethobenzamide hydrochloride	424.93	0.10	11.1	0.06	
Tripelennamine hydrochloride	291.83	0.30	24.3	0.17	
Tromethamine	121.14	0.26	28.9	0.15	3.41%
Tropicamide	284.36	0.09	10.0	0.05	
Tubocurarine chloride · 5H$_2$O	785.77	0.13	14.4	0.07	
Urea	60.06	0.52	57.8	0.30	1.73%
Vancomycin hydrochloride	1485.71	0.05	5.6	0.02	
Verapamil hydrochloride	491.06	0.13	14.4	0.07	
Warfarin sodium	330.31	0.17	18.9	0.09	6.10%
Xylometazoline hydrochloride	280.84	0.21	23.3	0.12	4.68%
Zinc chloride	136.30	0.61	67.8	0.35	
Zinc phenolsulfonate	555.84	0.18	20.0	0.11	
Zinc sulfate · 7H$_2$O	287.56	0.15	16.7	0.08	7.65%
Zinc sulfate, dried	161.46	0.23	25.6	0.13	4.52%

MW is the molecular weight of the drug.

$E^{1\%}_{NaCl}$ is the sodium chloride equivalent of the drug at 1% concentration (Values may vary slightly with concentration).

V^{1g} is the volume in mL of isotonic solution that can be prepared by adding water to 1.0 g of the drug.

$\Delta T_f^{1\%}$ is the freezing point depression of a 1% solution of the drug.

The values in this table have been obtained from the data of:
1. Hammarlund ER, Pedersen-Bjergaard K. J. Am. Pharm. Assoc., Pract. Ed. 1958; 19:39.
2. Hammarlund ER, Pedersen-Bjergaard K. J. Am. Pharm. Assoc., Sci. Ed. 1958; 47:107–114.
3. Hammarlund ER, Pedersen-Bjergaard K. J. Pharm. Sci. 1961; 50:24–30.
4. Hammarlund ER, Deming JD, Pedersen-Bjergaard K. J. Pharm. Sci. 1965; 54:160–162.
5. Hammarlund ER, Van Pevenage GL. J. Pharm. Sci. 1966; 55:1448–1451.
6. Fassett WE, Fuller TS, Hammarlund ER. J. Pharm. Sci. 1969; 58:1540–1542.
7. Sapp C, Lord M, Hammarlund ER. J. Pharm. Sci. 1975; 64:1884–1886.
8. Hammarlund ER. J. Pharm. Sci. 1981; 70:1161–1163.
9. Hammarlund ER. J. Pharm. Sci. 1989; 78:519–520.
10. The Merck Index, 11th Ed., Merck, Rahway, NJ, 1989, pp. MISC 79 to MISC 103, and other sources.

APPENDIX I
CODE OF ETHICS FOR PHARMACISTS*

PREAMBLE

Pharmacists are health professionals who assist individuals in making the best use of medications. This Code, prepared and supported by pharmacists, is intended to state publicly the principles that form the fundamental basis of the roles and responsibilities of pharmacists. These principles, based on moral obligations and virtues, are established to guide pharmacists in relationships with patients, health professionals, and society.

I.   A pharmacist respects the covenantal relationship between the patient and pharmacist.

Considering the patient-pharmacist relationship as a covenant means that a pharmacist has moral obligations in response to the gift of trust received from society. In return for this gift, a pharmacist promises to help individuals achieve optimum benefit from their medications, to be committed to their welfare, and to maintain their trust.

II.   A pharmacist promotes the good of every patient in a caring, compassionate, and confidential manner.

A pharmacist places concern for the well-being of the patient at the center of professional practice. In doing so, a pharmacist considers needs stated by the patient as well as those defined by health science. A pharmacist is dedicated to protecting the dignity of the patient. With a caring attitude and a compassionate spirit, a pharmacist focuses on serving the patient in a private and confidential manner.

III. A pharmacist respects the autonomy and dignity of each patient.

A pharmacist promotes the right of self-determination and recognizes individual self-worth by encouraging patients to participate in decisions about their health. A pharmacist communicates with patients in terms that are understandable. In all cases, a pharmacist respects personal and cultural differences among patients.

IV.   A pharmacist acts with honesty and integrity in professional relationships.

A pharmacist has a duty to tell the truth and to act with conviction of conscience. A pharmacist avoids discriminatory practices, behavior or work conditions that impair professional judgment, and actions that compromise dedication to the best interests of patients.

V.   A pharmacist maintains professional competence.

A pharmacist has a duty to maintain knowledge and abilities as new medications, devices, and technologies become available and as health information advances.

VI.   A pharmacist respects the values and abilities of colleagues and other health professionals.

When appropriate, a pharmacist asks for the consultation of colleagues or other health professionals or refers the patient. A pharmacist acknowledges that colleagues and other health professionals may differ in the beliefs and values they apply to the care of the patient.

VII. A pharmacist serves individual, community, and societal needs.

The primary obligation of a pharmacist is to individual patients. However, the obligations of a pharmacist may at times extend beyond the individual to the community and society. In these situations, the pharmacist recognizes the responsibilities that accompany these obligations and acts accordingly.

VIII. A pharmacist seeks justice in the distribution of health resources.

When health resources are allocated, a pharmacist is fair and equitable, balancing the needs of patients and society.

---

* Adopted by the membership of the American Pharmaceutical Association October 27, 1994.

INDEX

Page numbers in *italics* denote figures; those followed by a "t" denote tables.